NOVEL
APPROACHES
TO CANCER
CHEMOTHERAPY

This is a volume in
CELL BIOLOGY
A series of monographs

Editors: D. E. Buetow, I. L. Cameron, G. M. Padilla, and A. M. Zimmerman

A complete list of the books in this series appears at the end of the volume.

NOVEL APPROACHES TO CANCER CHEMOTHERAPY

Edited by

Prasad S. Sunkara

Merrell Dow Research Institute
Cincinnati, Ohio

1984

ACADEMIC PRESS, INC.

(Harcourt Brace Jovanovich, Publishers)

Orlando   San Diego   New York   London
Toronto   Montreal   Sydney   Tokyo

ACADEMIC PRESS, INC.
Orlando, Florida 32887

United Kingdom Edition published by
ACADEMIC PRESS, INC. (LONDON) LTD.
24/28 Oval Road, London NW1 7DX

Library of Congress Cataloging in Publication Data
Main entry under title:

Novel approaches to cancer chemotherapy.

    Includes index.
    1. Cancer--Chemotherapy. I. Sunkara, Prasad S.
[DNLM: 1. Antineoplastic Agents--therapeutic use.
2. Neoplasms--drug therapy. QZ 267 N937]
RC271.C5N68 1984   616.99'4061   84-9292
ISBN 0-12-676980-X (alk. paper)

PRINTED IN THE UNITED STATES OF AMERICA

84 85 86 87   9 8 7 6 5 4 3 2 1

Contents

Contributors   xi

Preface   xiii

1 Interferon and Cancer: Current use and Novel Approaches

W. ROBERT FLEISCHMANN, JR., GARY R. KLIMPEL, STEPHEN K. TYRING,
WILLIAM R. VOSS, AND SAMUEL BARON

I.	Introduction	1
II.	Interferon Clinical Trials	5
III.	Combination Therapies	6
IV.	A Murine B_{16} Melanoma Model for Assessment of Therapy of Lymph Node Metastases	10
V.	Potential for Direct Cytolysis of Tumor Cells by Interferon	12
VI.	Activation of NK Cells	14
VII.	Interferon and Hematopoiesis	15
VIII.	Conclusions	16
	References	16

2 Monoclonal Antibodies in the Diagnosis and Treatment of Cancer

FRANCES M. DAVIS AND POTU N. RAO

I.	Introduction	24
II.	Methodology	27
III.	Diagnostic Uses of Monoclonal Antibodies	39
IV.	Therapeutic Uses of Monoclonal Antibodies	53
V.	Conclusions	66
	References	67

3 Inhibitors of Polyamine Biosynthesis as Antitumor and Antimetastatic Agents

PRASAD S. SUNKARA AND NELLIKUNJA J. PRAKASH

I.	Introduction	94
II.	Polyamine Biosynthesis	94
III.	Polyamine Catabolism	96
IV.	Polyamines in Growth and Development	97
V.	Polyamines and Differentiation	98
VI.	Polyamines and Cell Cycle	100
VII.	Polyamine Biosynthesis in Normal and Transformed Cells	100
VIII.	Inhibitors of Polyamine Biosynthesis	103
IX.	Activity of DFMO against Experimental Tumors	109
X.	DFMO and Clinical Cancer	116
XI.	Summary	117
	References	117

4 Prostaglandin, Thromboxane, and Leukotriene Biosynthesis: Target for Antitumor and Antimetastatic Agents

KENNETH V. HONN AND LAWRENCE J. MARNETT

I.	Introduction: Arachidonic Acid Metabolism	128

II.   Modulators of Arachidonate Metabolism as
      Chemopreventative Agents: Inhibition of
      Tumor Initiation   133
III. Inhibition of Tumor Promotion   135
IV.   Overview of the Metastatic Cascade   138
V.   Prostacyclin, Thromboxanes, and Tumor
      Cell Metastasis   141
VI.   Conclusion   152
      References   153

5   Liposomes as a Drug Delivery System in Cancer Therapy

GEORGE POSTE, RICHARD KIRSCH, AND PETER BUGELSKI

I.   Introduction   166
II.   Liposomes   168
III.   Therapy of Experimental Animal Tumors
       Using Liposomes Containing Antineoplastic Drugs   172
IV.   Liposome Targeting   181
V.   Tumor Cell Heterogeneity and Cancer Therapy   198
VI.   Ligand-Directed Targeting of Liposomes
       within the Vascular Compartment   202
VII.   Passive Targeting of Liposome-Encapsulated Drugs
       to Mononuclear Phagocytes and Augmentation
       of Host Resistance to Tumors and
       Microorganisms   203
VIII. Physicochemical Targeting of Liposomes in
       Cancer Chemotherapy   208
IX.   Liposomes and Drug Delivery to Lymph Nodes   210
X.   Liposome Toxicity and Adverse Complications
       of Liposome Uptake by Mononuclear Phagocytes   212
XI.   Clinical Trials and Commercial Development
       of Liposomes as Drug Carriers   215
XII.   Conclusions   219
       References   221

6 Macrophage Activation by Lymphokines: Usefulness as Antimetastatic Agents

EUGENIE S. KLEINERMAN AND ISAIAH J. FIDLER

I.	Introduction	232
II.	Interaction of Macrophages with Heterogeneous Neoplasms	233
III.	Manipulations of Macrophages for Treatment of Metastases	235
IV.	Activation of Tumoricidal Properties of Human Monocytes *in Vitro* by Liposome-Encapsulated Human Lymphokines	237
V.	Selective Destruction of Tumor Cells by Human Monocytes Activated with Liposome-Encapsulated MAF	241
VI.	Conclusions	243
	References	244

7 Tuftsin: A Naturally Occurring Immunomodulating Antitumor Tetratpeptide

KENJI NISHIOKA

I.	Introduction	251
II.	Biology and Chemistry of Tuftsin	252
III.	Antitumor Activity of Tuftsin	258
IV.	Antimicrobial Activity of Tuftsin	262
V.	Concluding Remarks	263
	References	264

8 5α-Reductase: A Target Enzyme for Prostatic Cancer

VLADIMIR PETROW AND GEORGE M. PADILLA

I.	Introduction	270
II.	Historical Background	271

	III.	The Androgen Receptor and the Mechanism of Action of Androgens within the Prostatic Cell	276
	IV.	5α-Reductase, Dihydrotestosterone, and the Human Prostate	277
	V.	Dihydrotestosterone and Prostatic Cancer	280
	VI.	Steroid Biochemistry of the Normal Prostatic Cell	282
	VII.	Hormone Sensitivity of the Neoplastic Prostatic Cell	286
	VIII.	A New Approach to Palliative Treatment of Prostate Cancer	288
	IX.	5α-Reductase as a Target Enzyme for Prostatic Cancer	289
	X.	5α-Reductase Inhibitors Active *in Vivo*	291
	XI.	Summary	297
		Addendum	298
		References	298

9 Aromatase: A Target Enzyme in Breast Cancer

J. O'NEAL JOHNSTON AND BRIAN W. METCALF

	I.	Introduction	307
	II.	Aromatase System	309
	III.	Biological Evaluations	317
	IV.	Summary	324
		References	324

10 Cell Membranes: Targets for Selective Antitumor Chemotherapy

SUSAN J. FRIEDMAN AND PHILIP SKEHAN

	I.	Is Cancer a Disease of Abnormal Growth or of Cell Recognition?	329
	II.	Membrane Targets and Strategies for Selective Antitumor Therapy	333
	III.	Summary	345
		References	346

11 Intervention of Sodium Flux as a Target for Cancer Chemotherapy

IVAN L. CAMERON

I.	Introduction	355
II.	Ionic Differences between Normal and Tumor Cells	356
III.	Common Ionic Events Associated with the Stimulation of Quiescent Cells to Divide	360
IV.	Properties and Mode of Action of Amiloride	362
V.	Effect of Amiloride on Inhibition of Normal and Tumor Cell Proliferation	363
VI.	Search for Other Blockers of Electrolyte Flux as Potential Inhibitors of Cell Proliferation	364
	References	372

Index	375

Contributors

Numbers in parentheses indicate the pages on which the authors' contributions begin.

Samuel Baron (1), Department of Microbiology, The University of Texas Medical Branch at Galveston, Galveston, Texas 77550

Peter Buglelski (165), Smith Kline & French Laboratories, Philadelphia, Pennsylvania 19101

Ivan L. Cameron (355), Department of Cellular and Structural Biology, The University of Texas Health Science Center at San Antonio, San Antonio, Texas 78284

Frances M. Davis (23), Department of Chemotherapy Research, M. D. Anderson Hospital and Tumor Institute, The University of Texas System Cancer Center, Houston, Texas 77030

Isaiah J. Fidler[1] (231), Cancer Metastasis and Treatment Laboratory, Litton Biomedics, Inc.—Basic Research Program, Frederick Cancer Research Facility, National Cancer Institute, Frederick, Maryland 21701

W. Robert Fleischmann, Jr. (1), Department of Microbiology, The University of Texas Medical Branch at Galveston, Galveston, Texas 77550

Susan J. Friedman (329), Department of Pharmacology, and Oncology Research Group, Faculty of Medicine, University of Calgary, Calgary, Alberta T2N 4N1, Canada

Kenneth V. Honn (127), Department of Radiology and Department of Radiation Oncology, Wayne State University, Detroit, Michigan 48202

J. O'Neal Johnston (307), Merrell Dow Research Institute, Cincinnati, Ohio 45215

Richard Kirsch (165), Smith Kline & French Laboratories, Philadelphia, Pennsylvania 19101

[1]Present address: Department of Cell Biology, M.D. Anderson Hospital and Tumor Institute, The University of Texas System Cancer Center, Houston, Texas 77030.

Eugenie S. Kleinerman[2] (231), Laboratory of Molecular Immunoregulation, Biological Response Modifiers Program, Frederick Cancer Research Facility, National Cancer Institute, Frederick, Maryland 21701

Gary R. Klimpel (1), Department of Microbiology, The University of Texas Medical Branch at Galveston, Galveston, Texas 77550

Lawrence J. Marnett (127), Department of Chemistry, Wayne State University, Detroit, Michigan 48202

Brian W. Metcalf[3] (307), Merrell Dow Research Institute, Cincinnati, Ohio 45215

Kenji Nishioka (251), Department of General Surgery/Surgical Research Laboratory and Department of Biochemistry, M. D. Anderson Hospital and Tumor Institute, The University of Texas System Cancer Center, Houston, Texas 77030

George M. Padilla (269), Department of Physiology, Duke University Medical Center, Durham, North Carolina 27710

Vladimir Petrow (269), Department of Pharmacology, Duke University Medical Center, Durham, North Carolina 27710

George Poste (165), Smith Kline & French Laboratories, Philadelphia, Pennsylvania, and Department of Pathology and Laboratory Medicine, University of Pennsylvania School of Medicine, Philadelphia, Pennsylvania

Nellikunja J. Prakash (93), Merrell Dow Research Institute, Cincinnati, Ohio 45215

Potu N. Rao (23), Department of Chemotherapy Research, M.D. Anderson Hospital and Tumor Institute, The University of Texas System Cancer Center, Houston, Texas 77030

Philip Skehan (329), Department of Pharmacology, and Oncology Research Group, Faculty of Medicine, University of Calgary, Calgary, Alberta T2N 4N1, Canada

Prasad S. Sunkara (93), Department of Chemotherapeutics, Merrell Dow Research Institute, Cincinnati, Ohio 45215

Stephen K. Tyring (1), Department of Microbiology, The University of Texas Medical Branch at Galveston, Galveston, Texas 77550

William R. Voss (1), Department of Microbiology, The University of Texas Medical Branch at Galveston, Galveston, Texas 77550

[2]Present address: Department of Cell Biology, M.D. Anderson Hospital and Tumor Institute, the University of Texas System Cancer Center, Houston, Texas 77030.

[3]Present address: Smith Kline & French Laboratories, Philadelphia, Pennsylvania 19101.

Preface

The major aim of this book is to collate in one source new and emerging theories in tumor biology and to discuss their potential usefulness in developing new therapeutic approaches to cancer therapy. It is clear that a selective therapeutic attack on cancer cells is possible only when the basic differences between cancer and normal cells are well understood. In recent years a number of biological and biochemical differences have been discovered. This monograph illustrates how interaction among researchers in different areas of biology, immunology, and biochemistry can help develop selective therapeutic agents against cancer.

Each chapter stresses a unique property of a cancer cell and describes in detail how a novel therapeutic approach can be developed. Chapters 1, 2, 5, 6, and 7 deal with new emerging areas of cancer therapy such as the use of interferon, monoclonal antibodies, liposomes, lymphokines, and immunomodulators (tuftsin), respectively. The other six chapters deal with some of the newly identified biochemical and enzyme targets in cancer cells such as polyamines (Chapter 3), prostaglandin, thromboxane, and leukotrienes (Chapter 4), 5α-reductase (Chapter 8), aromatase (Chapter 9), cell membrane glycoproteins (Chapter 10), and sodium flux (Chapter 11). These chapters dealing with the biochemical approaches include recent developments which should provide the reader with new and rational approaches to cancer therapy.

I hope this book will stimulate biologists, biochemists, immunologists, and molecular biologists to interact with one another to exploit the unique properties of cancer cells in order to develop new approaches to cancer therapy.

I am extremely grateful to Anne C. Hagan for her assistance in editing the volume. My special thanks go to the contributing authors for their enthusiasm and willingness to write about their work.

Prasad S. Sunkara

NOVEL APPROACHES TO CANCER CHEMOTHERAPY

Edited by

Prasad S. Sunkara

Merrell Dow Research Institute
Cincinnati, Ohio

1984

ACADEMIC PRESS, INC.

(Harcourt Brace Jovanovich, Publishers)

Orlando   San Diego   New York   London
Toronto   Montreal   Sydney   Tokyo

ACADEMIC PRESS, INC.
Orlando, Florida 32887

United Kingdom Edition published by
ACADEMIC PRESS, INC. (LONDON) LTD.
24/28 Oval Road, London NW1 7DX

Library of Congress Cataloging in Publication Data
Main entry under title:

Novel approaches to cancer chemotherapy.

    Includes index.
    1. Cancer--Chemotherapy. I. Sunkara, Prasad S.
[DNLM: 1. Antineoplastic Agents--therapeutic use.
2. Neoplasms--drug therapy. QZ 267 N937]
RC271.C5N68 1984   616.99'4061   84-9292
ISBN 0-12-676980-X (alk. paper)

PRINTED IN THE UNITED STATES OF AMERICA

84 85 86 87   9 8 7 6 5 4 3 2 1

NOVEL APPROACHES TO CANCER CHEMOTHERAPY

1

Interferon and Cancer: Current Use and Novel Approaches

W. ROBERT FLEISCHMANN, JR., GARY R.
KLIMPEL, STEPHEN K. TYRING, WILLIAM R.
VOSS, AND SAMUEL BARON

Department of Microbiology
The University of Texas Medical Branch at Galveston
Galveston, Texas

I.	Introduction	1
II.	Interferon Clinical Trials	5
III.	Combination Therapies	6
IV.	A Murine B_{16} Melanoma Model for Assessment of Therapy of Lymph Node Metastases	10
V.	Potential for Direct Cytolysis of Tumor Cells by Interferon	12
VI.	Activation of NK Cells	14
VII.	Interferon and Hematopoiesis	15
VIII.	Conclusions	16
	References	16

I. INTRODUCTION

Interferons (IFN's) have been attracting considerable attention for their anti-tumor properties. However, they are named and classified on the basis of their antiviral properties. They are defined as proteins that exert "virus nonspecific, antiviral activity at least in homologous cells through cellular metabolic processes involving synthesis of both RNA and protein" (Stewart *et al.*, 1980). Three antigenically distinct types of interferon are recognized (Baron *et al.*,

1

Novel Approaches to Cancer Chemotherapy
Copyright © 1984 by Academic Press, Inc.
All rights of reproduction in any form reserved.
ISBN 0-12-676980-X

1982). IFN-α is produced by B cells, null cells, and macrophages upon exposure to B-cell mitogens, viruses, foreign cells, or tumor cells. IFN-β is produced by fibroblasts upon exposure to viruses or foreign nucleic acids. IFN-γ is produced by T cells and perhaps by null cells stimulated with T-cell mitogens, specific antigens, or interleukin 2 (IL 2).

All three interferon types exhibit antitumor and immunoregulatory properties in addition to their antiviral properties. They do, however, differ in their relative activities. For example, IFN-γ induces the antiviral state more slowly than either IFN-α or IFN-β (Dianzani *et al.*, 1978). Also, IFN-γ has been shown in laboratory studies to have more potent immunosuppressive (Sonnenfeld *et al.*, 1977) and antitumor activities than either IFN-α or INF-β (Salvin *et al.*, 1975; Crane *et al.*, 1978; Blalock *et al.*, 1980; Fleischmann, 1982) (see later). This high potency of IFN-γ antitumor activity observed in model systems raises the prospect that the use of IFN-γ in the clinic may greatly increase the effectiveness of interferon therapy.

A considerable amount of study has been directed toward understanding the mechanisms by which the interferon system functions. Figure 1 depicts a working model for the induction and antiviral action of interferon. In this model, interferon is induced by an event occurring during viral replication. The cellular

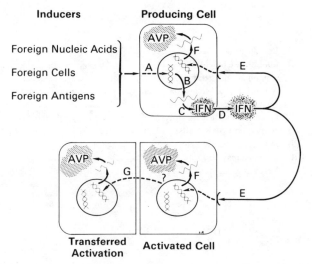

Fig. 1. Cellular events of the induction, production, and action of interferon (IFN). Inducers of IFN react with cells to derepress the IFN gene(s) (A). This leads to the production of mRNA for IFN (B). The mRNA is translated into the IFN protein (C) that is secreted into the extracellular fluid (D), where it reacts with the membrane receptors of cells (E). The IFN-stimulated cells derepress genes (F) for effector proteins (AVP) that establish antiviral resistance and other cell changes. The activated cells also stimulate contacted cells (G) by a still unknown mechanism to produce AVP. (Reproduced with permission from Baron *et al.*, *Texas Reports on Biology and Medicine* **41**, 1–12, 1982.)

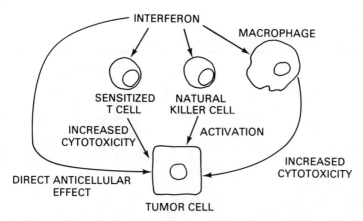

Fig. 2. Antitumor activity of interferon. Interferon has both direct and indirect effects on tumor cells. Interferon has direct anticellular effects by blocking tumor cell growth and, in some cases, causing direct cytolysis of the tumor cells. Interferon's indirect effects are mediated by cytotoxic effector cells such as macrophages, natural killer (NK) cells, and sensitized T cells.

genome is derepressed to produce a specific mRNA, which is then translated to produce interferon. The interferon is released into the surrounding fluid by the producing cell, where it can now interact with specific receptors on the surface of responding cells to initiate a series of events, involving synthesis of both mRNAs and proteins, which lead to the establishment of the antiviral state. The figure also details another interesting feature of interferon action. The interferon responding cell may transfer a signal to a neighboring cell, which causes the neighboring cell to develop an antiviral state without directly interacting with interferon.

The antitumor action of interferon is more complex than the antiviral action. The model just given may serve as a general model for the direct anticellular action of interferon, even to the transfer of antitumor activity from a responding cell to a neighboring cell (Lloyd *et al.*, 1983). However, in addition to its direct effect on the tumor cell, interferon acts on tumor cells indirectly through its activation of the host's cell-mediated immunity system (Fig. 2). Thus, interferon activates and enhances the antitumor activity of natural killer (NK) cells (Trinchieri *et al.*, 1978; Gidlund *et al.*, 1978; Svet-Moldavsky and Chernyakhovskaya, 1967; Djeu *et al.*, 1979) and macrophages (Chapes and Tompkins, 1979; Stanwick *et al.*, 1980; Schultz, 1980). Unfortunately, interferon also protects tumor cells from the cytolytic action of these cells (Trinchieri *et al.*, 1981). It is the sum of these positive and negative, direct and indirect interferon actions that constitutes the antitumor activity of interferon. An understanding of these interactions should enable us to maximize the antitumor activity of interferon and to exploit its potential fully.

TABLE I

Cellular Changes Associated with Interferon Treatment

Change	Reference
Decreased cap methylation	Sen *et al.*, 1977; Sharma and Goswami, 1981
2'5'-Oligoadenylate synthetase production	Baglioni *et al.*, 1982; Ball and West, 1982; Dougherty *et al.*, 1982; Revel *et al.*, 1982; Silverman *et al.*, 1982
Endonuclease (RNase L) activation	Baglioni *et al.*, 1982; Ball and West, 1982; Dougherty *et al.*, 1982; Revel *et al.*, 1982; Silverman *et al.*, 1982
Protein kinase activation	Ohtsuki, 1982; Samuel, 1982
Phosphodiesterase activation	Schmidt *et al.*, 1979
Glycosyltransferase inactivation	Maheshwari *et al.*, 1981
Membrane lipid changes	Pottathil *et al.*, 1980; Chandrabose *et al.*, 1982
Selective decrease in tRNA iso-accepting species	Zilbertstein *et al.*, 1976

A number of cellular changes following interferon treatment have been identi-fied (Table I). However, the precise roles that these changes play in mediating the varied activities of interferon are unknown. Two enzymatic activities have been identified that are induced by interferon (reviewed in Ball and West, 1982; Baglioni *et al.*, 1982; Dougherty *et al.*, 1982; Ohtsuki, 1982; Revel *et al.*, 1982; Samuel, 1982; Silverman *et al.*, 1982). These enzymes have been suggested to be responsible for the antiviral and the direct anticellular activities of interferon. The first is a protein kinase that catalyzes the phosphorylations of the α subunit of protein synthesis initiation factor eIF-2 and of the ribosome-associated protein P1. The second is a $2',5'$-oligoadenylate synthetase that synthesizes the unique oligonucleotide $2',5'$-oligo(A), which in turn activates an endoribonuclease that cleaves viral and cellular RNAs. Unfortunately, there seems to be no simple correlation between the induction, by interferon, of these enzymatic activities and the establishment of either the antiviral or growth-inhibitory effects of inter-feron (Wood and Hovanessian, 1979; Verhaegen *et al.*, 1980; Hovanessian *et al.*, 1981; Vandenbussche *et al.*, 1981). In certain cells, kinase activity seems to be required for both of these interferon effects, while in other cells they occur in the absence of detectable kinase activity. Further, high constitutive levels of synthetase activity can be found in cells in the absence of the antiviral state, and both enzymes can be induced with no inhibition of growth observed. Additional mechanisms must be at play and, indeed, several additional but uncharacterized interferon-induced proteins are detectable in the interferon-treated cells (Gupta *et al.*, 1979; Rubin and Gupta, 1980; Weil *et al.*, 1983). An understanding of the mechanisms by which interferon exerts its antiviral, immunoregulatory, and anticellular activities must await the characterization of these proteins.

II. INTERFERON CLINICAL TRIALS

Interferon has been employed in a number of clinical trials examining both the antiviral and the antitumor potentials of interferon therapy. Table II summarizes a number of clinical trials that have demonstrated the antitumor potential of interferon. While few complete remissions have been induced, positive effects of interferon have been observed, especially for juvenile laryngeal papillomatosis, nodular lymphocytic leukemia, breast cancer, and multiple myeloma.

Certainly these results are encouraging and support the need for further study of interferon therapy, but they do not as yet indicate that interferon is a cure for cancer. For example, IFN-α appears to be highly efficacious against juvenile laryngeal papillomatosis. However, it should be noted that this effect represents tumor management and not cure, since recurrence of the tumor occurs in all cases upon cessation of interferon therapy. Also, in one study with this tumor (Goepfert *et al.*, 1982), an initially potent antitumor effect of the interferon was seen in 10 of 12 patients, but it was sustained during the 7-month course of interferon therapy in only four of the 12 patients. Similar results have been observed for other types of responding tumors. While more controlled trials are needed, this raises the possibility that tumors may become refractory to the interferon treatment. Thus, long-term interferon management of tumors may not be as

TABLE II

Tumors Sensitive to IFN Therapy

Tumor	Reference
Juvenile laryngeal papilloma	Gobel *et al.*, 1981; Haglund *et al.*, 1981; Goepfert *et al.*, 1982
Nasopharyngeal carcinoma	Treuner *et al.*, 1980
Multiple bladder papilloma	Scorticatti *et al.*, 1982
Multiple myeloma	Mellstedt *et al.*, 1979; Gutterman *et al.*, 1980
Malignant lymphoma	Merigan *et al.*, 1978; Gutterman *et al.*, 1980
Acute leukemia	Hill *et al.*, 1979
Mammary carcinoma	Borden *et al.*, 1980; Gutterman *et al.*, 1980
Ovarian carcinoma	Einhorn *et al.*, 1982
Kaposi's sarcoma	Krown *et al.*, 1983
Prostate cancer	Gutterman and Quesada, 1982
Colon cancer	Gutterman and Quesada, 1982
Renal cell carcinoma	Gutterman and Quesada, 1982

efficacious as these clinical trials might suggest. Further investigations, including more follow-up studies on the clinical trial patients who responded to interferon therapy, are needed to address this concern.

While the early clinical trials suggest that interferon therapy may be of limited effectiveness, these trials have employed only IFN-α and IFN-β. Laboratory studies suggest that IFN-γ may be more potent against certain tumors than either IFN-α or IFN-β (Salvin *et al.*, 1975; Crane *et al.*, 1978; Blalock *et al.*, 1980; Fleischmann, 1982). Thus, it is interesting to speculate that HuIFN-γ may be a far more potent agent against selected tumors than is either HuIFN-α or HuINF-β, and that forthcoming clinical studies may show it to be highly efficacious.

Another consideration involves the possible development of an interferon-refractory state during IFN-α therapy. Laboratory studies have shown that tumors refractory to one interferon type may retain their sensitivity to another interferon type. For example, murine L1210R cells, which are resistant to the antiviral and anticellular activity of IFNα/β, retain their sensitivity to IFN-γ (Ankel *et al.*, 1980). It may be possible to bring this observation to the clinic. One type of interferon could be used to obtain an initial antitumor response. A second type could be used sequentially to suppress the tumor further and perhaps cure the patient. This procedure could also be employed to drive a tumor that becomes refractory to the first interferon back into remission.

There are two major concerns that should be addressed before IFN-γ can be evaluated in clinical trials. One, an inhibitor of interferon action is produced concurrently with IFN-γ in both mouse and human systems (Fleischmann *et al.*, 1979b and unpublished observations). *In vitro* studies suggest that this inhibitor blocks the antitumor action of the interferon and greatly reduces its effectiveness. This inhibitor should be quantitated and, if possible, removed from IFN-γ preparations before they are used in clinical trials. Failure to take into account the inhibitor could make it difficult to evaluate accurately the antitumor effectiveness of IFN-γ. Second, *in vitro* studies suggest that IFN-γ is a more potent suppressor of bone marrow function than IFN-α/β in the mouse system (Klimpel *et al.*, 1982). Since bone marrow suppression is one of the major side effects of interferon therapy in humans, it may be necessary to follow bone marrow function carefully during phase I trials in order not to endanger the patient. Despite these concerns, IFN-γ has the potential to be an effective antitumor agent.

III. COMBINATION THERAPIES

There are a number of novel approaches by which interferon might be used to enhance the effectiveness of antitumor therapies. The first involves the use of combinations of IFN-γ and either IFN-α or IFN-β to achieve a synergistic enhancement or potentiation of the antitumor activity of the interferons. Potentiation was first described *in vitro* in the mouse system as an enhancement of the antiviral state (Fleischmann *et al.*, 1979a). Potentiation has since been shown to occur both *in vivo* and *in vitro* in the mouse, to be functionally identical in the human and in the mouse by *in vitro* studies, and to affect the antitumor and immunoregulatory properties of interferon (Fleischmann *et al.*, 1979a, 1980; Brysk *et al.*, 1981; Klimpel *et al.*, 1982; Fleischmann, 1982; Weigent *et al.*, 1983; Fleischmann *et al.*, 1984b). Mixtures of IFN-γ and either IFN-α or IFN-β potentiate; mixtures of IFN-α and IFN-β give only additive effects (Fleischmann *et al.*, 1984b). Figure 3 illustrates potentiation of the *in vivo* antitumor activity of interferon. DBA/2 mice were inoculated subcutaneously with 10^5 P-388 leukemia cells and treated with mock IFN, IFN-γ alone, IFN-α/β alone, or the combination of IFN-γ plus IFN-α/β (Fleischmann *et al.*, 1980). The tumors developed as a solid mass, and tumor size was monitored. Treatment with

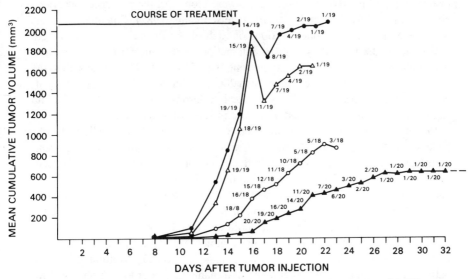

Fig. 3. Effect of combined immune and virus-induced interferons on the rate of P-388 tumor development in DBA/2 mice. Each mouse was inoculated sc with 10^5 P-388 tumor cells, and they were then divided into four groups of 18 to 20 mice each. Mice were inoculated 3 hr before tumor injection and daily for 15 days thereafter at the approximate site of tumor injection with mock interferon (●), immune interferon (△, 25 U/day), virus-induced interferon (○, 25,000 U/day), or a combination of immune (25 U/day) and virus-induced (25,000 U/day) interferons (▲). Volume of the primary tumor was determined for each mouse on the indicated days after tumor cell injection. Data were plotted as the linear increase in mean cumulative tumor volume. Mean cumulative tumor volumes were determined within each group by averaging the tumor size of all surviving mice with the final tumor size of all mice that had died. Fractions indicate number of survivors/total number of mice at the indicated times after tumor injection for each treatment group. (Reproduced with permission from Fleischmann *et al.*, JNCI, *Journal of the National Cancer Institute* **65**, 963–966, 1980.)

IFN-α/β alone significantly delayed tumor growth. A low level of IFN-γ was chosen, which by itself did not affect tumor growth. When the IFN-γ was combined with IFN-α/β, the antitumor activity of the interferons was markedly enhanced as seen by the significant delay in tumor growth with the combination as compared to either interferon alone. Survival times were also followed and showed a similar pattern. IFN-α/β provided a significant increase in time of survival. The dose of IFN-γ employed provided no increase in survival time. The combination of interferons provided an enhanced survival time when compared to that observed with either of the interferons employed alone.

These *in vivo* studies demonstrated the practical application of combination interferon therapy, but they did not address the mechanism of action of potentiation nor did they provide any quantitation of the potentiation effect. Therefore, the system was subdivided for *in vitro* study. The effect of combination interferon treatment on the direct anticellular activity of interferon was examined (Table III). Mouse B_{16} melanoma cells were cloned in the presence of various concentrations of IFN-γ and IFN-α/β (Fleischmann, 1982). Potentiation levels were dependent on the concentrations of each of the interferons and thus were indicative of the mutual synergistic interaction of the interferons. The highest potentiation observed in this experiment was 214-fold. This means that the observed interferon effect was more than 200 times greater than expected considering the arithmetic sum of the separate interferons. Moreover, there was no suggestion that this represented a maximum level of potentiation.

Recent studies employing paired sets of nonmalignant and malignant cells have shown that interferon treatment, particularly combination interferon treatment, has a much greater antiproliferative effect on the malignant cells (Fleischmann *et al.*, 1984a). Thus, combination interferon treatment appeared to differentiate sharply between nonmalignant and malignant cells, suggesting that low levels of interferon employed in combination might have a higher therapeutic index than high levels of either interferon employed separately.

The effect of combination interferon treatment on the activation of cytotoxic effector cells was also examined (Weigent *et al.*, 1983). Natural killer cell activation was found to be potentiated in a manner parallel to that observed for the direct anticellular effect. Thus, combination interferon therapy potentiates both direct and indirect antitumor activities of interferon.

The second novel approach involves the use of the combination of interferon and chemotherapy. Many chemotherapeutic agents have their most potent effect when cells are just entering or in the S phase. Interferons have been shown to block progression of the cell through the G_1 phase (Sokawa *et al.*, 1977; Creasey *et al.*, 1980; Leandersson and Lundgren, 1980). It is enticing to consider that sequential treatment with interferon and an appropriate chemotherapeutic agent like BCNU [1,3-bis(2-chloroethyl)-1-nitrosourea; carmustine] (Barranco and Humphrey, 1971) might prove to be highly synergistic. The following sequence of events might be postulated to occur. Administration of interferon by iv drip

TABLE III

Concentration Dependence of Potentiation of Anticellular Effects of Interferon[a]

Parameter	IFN-γ Concentration		IFN-α/β Concentration		
Control replication units (%)	100	95	88	76	59
Observed IFN titer (U/ml)[b]	0	0.1	0.2	0.3	0.7
Control replication units (%)	99	75	48	36	30
Observed IFN titer (U/ml)	<0.1	0.4	1.1	1.7	2.5
Expected IFN titer (U/ml)	—	0.1	0.2	0.3	0.7
Fold potentiation	—	4.0	5.5	5.7	3.6
Control replication units (%)	78	40	30	25	16
Observed IFN titer (U/ml)	0.3	1.4	2.5	3.3	7.5
Expected IFN titer (U/ml)	—	0.4	0.5	0.6	1.0
Fold potentiation	—	3.5	5.0	5.5	7.5
Control replication units (%)	52	21	19	12	3.7
Observed IFN titer (U/ml)	0.9	4.5	5.4	12	107
Expected IFN titer (U/ml)	—	1.0	1.1	1.2	1.6
Fold potentiation	—	4.5	4.9	10	67
Control replication units (%)	28	15	13	4.5	1.2
Observed IFN titer (U/ml)	2.7	8.2	11	74	729
Expected IFN titer (U/ml)	—	2.8	2.9	3.0	3.4
Fold potentiation	—	2.9	3.8	25	214

[a]Reproduced with permission from W. R. Fleischmann, Jr. (1982) *Cancer Research* **42**, 869–875.
[b]Anticellular units of interferon.

freezes the dividing cells in the G_1 phase. Upon cessation of interferon treatment, interferon is rapidly cleared from the body fluids, and the cells are released in synchrony from their interferon block. Administration of the chemotherapeutic agent kills the dividing cells as they enter their most sensitive phase. Repeated, periodic administration of interferon and the chemotherapeutic agent kills those growing tumor cells that were not synchronized by the previous treatment and those previously resting tumor cells that are newly activated to enter the cell cycle. Indeed, mouse studies with a transplantable leukemia have shown that interferon can be an effective adjuvant to chemotherapy (Chirigos and Pearson, 1973). As a further consideration, the use of interferon in combination therapy may allow the replacement of more toxic agents in the chemotherapeutic cocktail.

The third novel approach involves the pretreatment of patients with interferon prior to surgery. By its very nature, surgery is a traumatic invasive procedure. The period of recovery from surgery may be a time of risk for the patient if this trauma mimics the trauma induced by burns (even small burns) (Kay, 1957; Ninnemann *et al.*, 1978; Baker *et al.*, 1979; Meakins *et al.*, 1979; Suzuki and

Pollard, 1982). The individual may suffer a period of immunosuppression during which small metastases existing prior to surgery may begin to grow unchecked. Pretreatment of the patient could serve to have a direct antitumor effect on metastases (particularly those in the lymph nodes) to kill them before surgery. It might also affect the primary tumor to limit the potential for generation of metastatic cells by the surgery. Further, it might activate the patient's cell-mediated immune system to kill metastatic cells and offset the immunosuppressive effects of surgery. Administration of interferon immediately after surgery might also beneficially boost the activity of the patient's cytotoxic effector cells.

These proposed uses of interferon in combination therapy are highly speculative. No supporting evidence is yet available for the use of interferon in combination with surgery. Perhaps future studies will be able to document its utility. Mouse studies do suggest that the use of interferon in combination with chemotherapeutic agents may have utility for humans and thus potential for the clinic (Chirigos and Pearson, 1973). Further, considerable evidence from laboratory studies does suggest that the use of combination interferon therapy (potentiation) dramatically increases the antitumor activities of the interferons. Thus, it may have considerable potential for the clinic. If it is effective *in vivo* in humans and if the side effects are not too severe, combination interferon therapy might raise the antitumor activity to a level that would be highly efficacious.

IV. A MURINE B$_{16}$ MELANOMA MODEL FOR ASSESSMENT OF THERAPY OF LYMPH NODE METASTASES

Successful surgical treatment of cancer often is limited because of residual lymph node metatases remaining after removal of the primary tumor. In order to determine the parameters of metastatic spread of tumor cells and to evaluate methods by which those metastases can be treated, it is first necessary to develop model systems in animals. To establish such a model system, the time of metastatic spread of B$_{16}$ melanoma from the calf and from the footpad to the popliteal lymph nodes was determined (W. R. Voss, W. R. Fleischmann, Jr., S. J. Stanley, and S. Baron, unpublished observations). Metastatic spread from the primary site of tumor inoculation (5×10^5 cells) to regional lymph nodes and beyond was measured by mortality, gross and histological examination, and culture of tumor cells from lymph nodes. When the tumor was inoculated subcutaneously in the calf and amputated at the knee (below the popliteal lymph nodes) within 1 hr, 80% of the mice died with a mean death day of 32.8 (Fig. 4). This finding indicated that the tumor spreads from its local site very early after implantation. To determine whether this spread was to the popliteal area, the

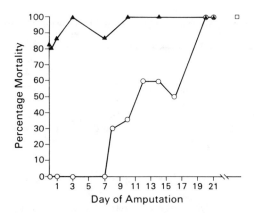

Fig. 4. Kinetics of B_{16} melanoma spread from calf. Percentage mortality of C57BL/6 mice inoculated subcutaneously in calf with B_{16} melanoma (5×10^5 cells) and with amputation at various days below (▲) and above (○) popliteal lymph nodes. □, Unamputated controls.

experiment was repeated but with amputation just above the popliteal area, also as shown in Fig. 4. Metastatic spread beyond the popliteal nodes occurred only after day 7 in the majority of mice inoculated in the calf and amputated above the popliteal lymph nodes. That melanoma cells were actually in the popliteal node was confirmed by culture of the tumor cells from the node. Thus, to establish a model with only popliteal metastases, the primary calf tumor could be removed between days 0 and 7 by amputation below the knee.

Because the metastatic tumor was localized to the lymph node, it was next possible to evaluate the effectiveness of treatment with high concentrations of chemotherapeutic agents delivered to the localized tumor site. B_{16} melanoma cells inoculated into the calf area were treated locally (into tumor inoculation site) or systematically (intraperitoneally) with interferon, the interferon inducer poly(I):poly(C), or the chemotherapeutic agent BCNU (carmustine) daily on days 1–10. Removing the primary tumor surgically and injecting antitumor agents into the amputation stump allowed the agents to pass through the lymphatic system and achieve high concentration at the sites of metastatic implantation in the regional lymph nodes. Protection against both local tumors and popliteal metastases was consistently greater with local rather than systemic therapy either when the primary tumor was or was not removed prior to therapy (Table IV). These findings identify the conditions for a metastatic model of regional lymph nodes metastases and also demonstrate that local chemotherapy is more effective than systemic therapy. This model is a new tool with which to identify local therapies that may eradicate lymph node metastases so that the most effective treatments identified in animals may be tested clinically in humans.

TABLE IV

Comparison of Local versus Systemic Therapy of B_{16} Melanoma in C57BL/6 Mice (No Amputations)[a]

Treatment (days 1–10)	Intraperitoneal		Tumor	
	Mean day of death	Mortality (%)	Mean day of death	Mortality (%)
BCNU 167 μg	36.1	100	>120[b]	0
IFN α/β 10,000 U	25.8	100	31.6	100
Poly(I):poly(C) 50 μg	25.7	100	37.2	100
Placebo	25.4	100	25.7	100

[a]Inoculation of groups of 10 mice on day 0 with 5×10^5 B_{16} melanoma cells injected subcutaneously into calf.

[b]All mice surviving with no detectable tumor.

V. POTENTIAL FOR DIRECT CYTOLYSIS OF TUMOR CELLS BY INTERFERON

The complete eradication of a tumor mass and its attendant metastases is difficult to achieve. If complete eradication of tumors by interferon is accomplished, it is more likely to result from the direct and indirect cytolytic effects of interferon than from the cytostatic effects of interferon. Recent studies have evaluated the potential of IFN-γ to cause the direct cytolysis of tumor cells. MuIFN-γ and HuIFN-γ preparations have recently been shown to have a direct cytolytic activity against a number of tumor and normal cells (Tyring *et al.*, 1982). The cytolytic activity of MuIFN-γ was investigated on 11 murine tumor cell lines. A 20-fold difference was found between the most sensitive cell type, P-388 lymphoma, versus the most resistant type, C127v leukemia. A number of normal mouse cells were also found to have low to intermediate sensitivity to the cytolytic action of IFN-γ. Direct cytolysis did not occur using MuIFN-α or MuIFN-β with any of the 11 cell lines tested. Another report has shown that cytotoxic activity does occur with these interferons for one cell type (Ito and Buffet, 1981). As seen in Fig. 5, treatment with high concentrations of MuIFN-γ (i.e., 2900 U/ml) results in complete lysis of P-388 lymphoma cells within 24 hr, while treatment with lower concentrations (i.e., 700 U/ml) results in a reversible inhibition of cell growth.

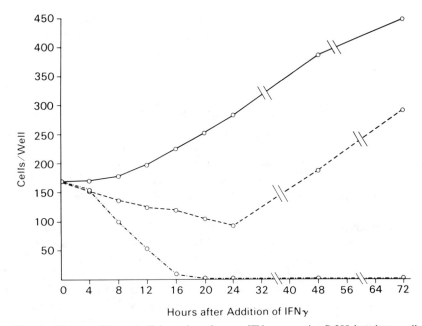

Fig. 5. Kinetics of the anticellular action of mouse IFN-γ on murine P-388 lymphoma cells. Cells treated with 700 U/ml of IFN-γ (dashed line) were significantly different from controls (solid line) at hours 12 through 72 ($p < .05$; Student's t test). Cells treated with 2900 U/ml of IFN-γ (dotted and dashed line) were significantly different from controls at hours 8 and 12 ($p < .05$) and at hours 16 through 72 ($p < .01$). (Reproduced with permission from Tyring et al., *International Journal of Cancer* **30**, 59–64, 1982.)

These findings indicate that direct cytolysis is yet another of the distinctive activities of IFN-γ. The findings also offer the potential for application of direct cytolysis to the therapy of tumors. Since IFN-γ-induced cytolysis does not distinguish between tumor and normal cells, effective therapy would require selective delivery of the IFN-γ to the tumor cells. One obvious selective delivery could be intratumor injection of IFN-γ when the tumor is localized and accessible. Possible examples include skin tumors and brain tumors during surgery.

More speculatively, selective delivery might be developed by cloning and injecting T lymphocytes with specific affinity for tumor cells. After attachment to the tumor cell, the T cell would produce IFN-γ. An advantage of such a delivery mechanism is that IFN secreted into intercellular spaces achieves the high concentrations (Dianzani et al., 1977) needed for cytolysis. Thus, the adjacent tumor cell would be exposed to cytolytic concentrations of IFN-γ, but the more distant normal cell would be exposed only to lower concentrations of diffusing IFN-γ.

A direct test of efficacy soon may be possible when high concentrations of IFN-γ are produced commercially and injected directly into tumors.

VI. ACTIVATION OF NK CELLS

Attention has recently begun to focus on the possible employment of natural killer (NK) cells in cancer therapy. NK cells are large, granular lymphocytes that have the ability to recognize and lyse, without prior sensitization, various tumor cell lines, as well as virus-infected normal cells. NK cells are believed to play an important role not only in immunosurveillance against cancer but also in resistance to viral infections (Herberman *et al.*, 1975; Herberman and Holden, 1978).

It is now clear that human NK cells represent a heterogeneous population of cells (Herberman, 1980; Herberman and Ortaldo, 1981). Early studies defined human NK cells as nonadherent cells lacking characteristics of mature B cells, T cells, or macrophages (Pross and Baines, 1977; West *et al.*, 1977). Studies of cell surface markers on human NK cells using monoclonal antibodies have indicated that NK cells that lyse K562 targets have markers associated with cells of the T lineage (OKT11A and OKT10) (Zarling and Kung, 1980; Zarling *et al.*, 1981) as well as antigens associated with cells of the macrophage lineage (OKM1) (Kay and Horwitz, 1980; Zarling *et al.*, 1981). Another antigen, Leu 7, is also expressed on human NK cells (Abo and Balch, 1981).

NK cells (Leu 7 $^+$ cells) have been shown to be unresponsive to mitogens and alloantigens (Abo and Balch, 1982). However, NK activity can be augmented by pretreatment of NK cells with IFN (Djeu *et al.*, 1979), interleukin 2 (IL 2) (Henney *et al.*, 1981), or mixtures of IFN and IL 2 (Kuribayashi *et al.*, 1981). IL 2 has been shown to induce IFN-γ production by NK cells (Handa *et al.*, 1983). IL 2 has also been shown to be a growth factor for NK cells (Timonen *et al.*, 1982). This has allowed for continuous cell lines to be developed that have NK cell killing activity and for cloned NK cell lines to be established (Dennert, 1980; Nabel *et al.*, 1981).

A study using a cloned mouse NK cell line has shown that when these cells were adoptively transferred to mice, the development of B_{16} tumor colonies in the lungs of such mice were inhibited by 50 to 80% (Warner and Dennert, 1983). Even more impressive was the finding that adoptively transferred cloned NK cells could almost totally inhibit the development of radiation-induced thymic leukemia (Hanna and Fidler, 1980). This, as well as other studies (Talmadge *et al.*, 1980; Hanna and Burton, 1981), clearly indicates that NK cells and/or cloned NK cells can be valuable tools for controlling the growth and metastasis of certain tumor cells.

The fact that IFN can enhance NK cell activity, activate macrophages, and enhance antibody-dependent cellular cytotoxicity (ADCC, which can be mediated by NK cells, macrophages, and/or granulocytes) is appealing for clinical trials using IFN. Unfortunately, tumor cells are not all equivalent in their susceptibility to NK cell or macrophage killing (Herberman *et al.*, 1975; Heberman, 1980). More importantly, some tumor cells pretreated with IFN become resistant to NK cell killing (Trinchieri and Santoli, 1978). This protection has been shown in the human system to be dose dependent, to be reversible when IFN is removed, and to require de novo RNA and protein synthesis.

All of the important considerations just mentioned could be used to design approaches to antitumor therapy where IFN and NK cells are used in combination. In one such approach, peripheral blood NK cells would be purified from early diagnosed cancer patients. These cells would be grown *in vitro* in the presence of IFN and IL 2 until sufficient numbers were obtained. Tumor cells obtained from biopsy would then be assessed for NK-cell susceptibility and for growth inhibition and/or lysis by IFN treatment. Tumor cells treated with IFN would also be assessed for their susceptibility to NK cells. Thus, patients with tumors that did not become resistant to NK-cell attack would be given IFN therapy *in vivo* plus NK cells that were grown and activated by *in vitro* culture with IL 2 and IFN. Patients with tumor cells that become resistant to NK-cell attack and/or resistant to IFN anticellular effects would be given only NK cells followed by chemotherapeutic agents. An alternative approach might be to give NK cells to patients immediately following surgery. These NK cells might help prevent metastasis of the tumor and/or kill tumor cells that have migrated to other areas of the body. Another approach that has been explored involves the immobilization of interferon in a perfusion chamber, where it can activate NK cells *in vivo* over a period of several weeks (Langvad *et al.*, 1980).

In theory, the foregoing approaches appear reasonable, since NK cells are believed to play an important role in immunosurveillance against cancer. However, NK cells have also been shown to suppress both T- and B-lymphocyte responses *in vitro* (Tilden *et al.*, 1983). This, along with other observations, has led to the belief that NK cells may also play an important role in immunoregulation (Hansson *et al.*, 1981, 1982). Thus, the approach just outlined may also have important limitations.

VII. INTERFERON AND HEMATOPOIESIS

Granulocytopenia has been a major problem associated with patients receiving human leukocyte IFN for antineoplastic therapeutic trials (Greenberg *et al.*, 1976; Gutterman *et al.*, 1980). Many studies have shown that IFN (α and/or β) inhibits murine and human erythroid and granuloid progenitor cells (McNeill and Gresser, 1983; Gallien-Lartigue *et al.*, 1980; Dandoy *et al.*, 1981; Verma *et al.*,

1981). Proliferation of murine pluripotent hematopoietic stem cells has also been inhibited by IFN α/β (Gidali *et al.*, 1981). Studies on the effect of different types of IFN on macrophage and granulocyte colony formation (CFU-C) *in vitro* using mouse bone marrow cells, have shown that IFN-γ is much more potent (50- to 100-fold) than IFN-α/β at inhibiting CFU-C formation, and that IFN-α/β and IFN-γ synergize in suppressing CFU-C formation (Klimpel *et al.*, 1982). Interestingly, inhibition mediated by all of these IFN's (IFN-α/β, and/or IFN-γ) was dependent on the amount of colony-stimulating factor (CSF) present in the culture system. These findings may be important for future clinical trials using IFN and where bone marrow function might be suppressed. Thus, a novel approach to overcome IFN-mediated suppression of bone marrow function might be to give the patient CSF. This might serve two roles. It could offset the suppressive effects of IFN and could allow normal or increased levels of lymphoid and/or myeloid cells to be produced in the patient. These cells, which contain different effector cells, could in turn be acted upon by IFN to develop higher antitumor cell activity.

VIII. CONCLUSIONS

Interferons have shown some promise as antitumor agents in humans; however, their full potential may not yet have been achieved. IFN-γ is just becoming available for clinical use. IFN-γ employed alone and in combination with IFN-α may dramatically increase interferon's activity. Interferon treatment combined with chemotherapy and interferon treatment combined with surgery may also give enhanced antitumor activity. Further, metastatic cells may be successfully attacked by interferon administration via the lymph system draining the site of the primary tumor. Also, direct cytolysis of tumor cells in the primary tumor may be obtainable by intratumor administration of interferon. Additionally, cytotoxic effector cells, such as NK cells, may be activated *in vitro* or *in vivo* by interferon treatment to give an enhanced level of killing of tumor cells in the primary tumor in metastases. Finally, it may be possible to employ colony-stimulating factor in combination with interferon to antagonize specifically the bone marrow-suppressive effects of interferon and to stimulate the production of increased levels of cytotoxic effector cells. Thus, a variety of novel approaches to interferon therapy may be of value for the management of human tumors.

REFERENCES

Abo, T., and Balch, C. M. (1981). A differentiation antigen of human NK and K cells identified by a monoclonal antibody (HNK-1). *J. Immunol.* **127**, 1024–1029.

Abo, T., and Balch, C. M. (1982). Characterization of HNK-1+ (Leu-7) human lymphocytes. II. Distinguishing phenotypic and functional properties of natural killer cells from activated NK-like cells. *J. Immunol.* **129,** 1758–1761.

Ankel, H., Krishnamurti, C., Besancon, F., Stefanos, S., and Falcoff, E. (1980). Mouse fibroblast (type I) and immune (type II) interferons: Pronounced differences in affinity for gangliosides and in antiviral and antigrowth effects on mouse leukemia L-1210R cells. *Proc. Natl. Acad. Sci. U.S.A.* **77,** 2528–2532.

Baglioni, C., Nilsen, T. W., Maroney, P. A., and de Farra, F. (1982). Molecular mechanisms of action of interferon. *Tex. Rep. Biol. Med.* **41,** 471–478.

Baker, C. C., Miller, C. L., and Trunkey, D. D. (1979). Predicting fatal sepsis in burn patients. *J. Trauma* **19,** 641–648.

Ball, L. A., and West, D. K. (1982). 2'5'-Oligoadenylate synthetase in interferon-treated chick cells. *Tex. Rep. Biol. Med.* **41,** 487–492.

Baron, S., Dianzani, F., and Stanton, G. J. (1982). General considerations of the interferon system. *Tex. Rep. Biol. Med.* **41,** 1–12.

Barranco, S. C., and Humphrey, R. M. (1971). The effects of 1,3-bis(2-chloroethyl)-1-nitrosourea on survival and cell progression in Chinese hamster cells. *Cancer Res.* **31,** 191–195.

Blalock, J. E., Georgiades, J. A., Langford, M. P., and Johnson, H. M. (1980). Purified human immune interferon has more potent anticellular activity than fibroblast or leukocyte interferon. *Cell. Immunol.* **49,** 390–394.

Borden, E., Dao, T., Holland, J., Gutterman, J. U., and Merigan, T. C. (1980). Interferon in recurrent breast carcinoma: Preliminary report of the American Cancer Society Clinical Trials Programs. *Proc. Am. Assoc. Cancer Res.* **21,** 187.

Brysk, M. M., Tschen, E. H., Hudson, R. D., Smith, E. B., Fleischmann, W. R., Jr., and Black, H. S. (1981). The activity of interferon on ultraviolet light-induced squamous cell carcinomas. *J. Am. Acad. Dermatol.* **5,** 61–63.

Chandrabose, K. A., Cuatrecasas, P., and Pottathil, R. (1982). Interferon mediated changes in lipid metabolism. *Tex. Rep. Biol. Med.* **41,** 499–505.

Chapes, S. K., and Tompkins, W. F. (1979). Cytotoxic macrophages induced in hamsters by vaccinia virus: Selective cytotoxicity for virus-infected targets by macrophages collected late after immunization. *J. Immunol.* **123,** 303–310.

Chirigos, M. A., and Pearson, J. W. (1973). Cure of murine leukemia with drug and interferon. *JNCI, J. Natl. Cancer Inst.* **51,** 1367–1368.

Crane, J. L., Jr., Glasgow, L. A., Kern, E. R., and Youngner, J. S. (1978). Inhibition of murine osteogenic sarcomas by treatment with type I or type II interferon. *JNCI, J. Natl. Cancer Inst.* **61,** 871–874.

Creasey, A. A., Bartholomew, J. C., and Merigan, T. C. (1980). Role of G_0–G_1 arrest in the inhibition of tumor cell growth by interferon. *Proc. Natl. Acad. Sci. U.S.A.* **77,** 1471–1475.

Dandoy, F., DeMaeyer, E., and DeMaeyer-Guignard, J. (1981). Antiproliferative action of interferon on murine bone marrow-derived macrophages is influenced by the genotype of the marrow-donor. *J. Interferon Res.* **1,** 263–270.

Dennert, G. (1980). Cloned lines of natural killer cells. *Nature (London)* **287,** 47–49.

Dianzani, F., Viano, I., Santiano, M., Zucca, M., and Baron, S. (1977). Effect of cell density on development of the antiviral state in interferon-producing cells: A possible model of *in vivo* conditions. *Proc. Soc. Exp. Biol. Med.* **155,** 445–448.

Dianzani, F., Salter, L., Fleischmann, W. R., Jr., and Zucca, M. (1978). Immune interferon activates cells more slowly than does virus-induced interferons. *Proc. Soc. Exp. Biol. Med.* **159,** 94–97.

Djeu, J. Y., Heinbaugh, J. A., Holden, H. T., and Herberman, R. B. (1979). Augmentation of mouse NK cell activity by interferon and interferon inducers. *J. Immunol.* **122,** 175–181.

Dougherty, J. P., Samanta, H., Floyd-Smith, G., Broeze, R., Jayeram, B. M., and Lengyl, P. (1982). Enzymology of interferon action. The $(2'-5')(A)_n$ synthetase–RNAse L pathway. *Tex. Rep. Biol. Med.* **41**, 443–451.

Einhorn, N., Cantell, K., Einhorn, S., and Strander, H. (1982). Human leukocyte interferon therapy for advanced ovarian carcinoma. *Cancer Clin. Trials* **5**, 167–172.

Fleischmann, W. R., Jr. (1982). Potentiation of the direct anticellular activity of mouse interferons: Mutual synergism and interferon concentration dependence. *Cancer Res.* **42**, 869–875.

Fleischmann, W. R., Jr., Georgiades, J. A., Osborne, L. C., and Johnson, H. M. (1979a). Potentiation of interferon activity by mixed preparations of fibroblast and immune interferon. *Infect. Immun.* **26**, 248–253.

Fleischmann, W. R., Jr., Georgiades, J. A., Osborne, L. C., Dianzani, F., and Johnson, H. M. (1979b). Induction of an inhibitor of interferon action in a mouse lymphokine preparation. *Infect. Immn.* **26**, 949–955.

Fleischmann, W. R., Jr., Kleyn, K. M., and Baron, S. (1980). Potentiation of antitumor effect of virus-induced interferon by mouse immune interferon preparations. *JNCI, J. Natl. Cancer Inst.* **65**, 963–966.

Fleischmann, W. R., Jr., Newton, R. C., Fleischmann, C. M., Colburn, N. H., and Brysk, M. M. (1984a). Discrimination between nonmalignant and malignant cells by combinations of IFN-γ plus IFN-α/β. *J. Biol. Response Modifiers* **3**, 397–405.

Fleischmann, W. R., Jr., Schwarz, L. A., and Fleischmann, C. M. (1984b). Requirement for IFN gamma in potentiation of interferon's antiviral and anticellular activities: Identity of mouse and human systems. *J. Interferon Res.* **4**, 265–274.

Gallien-Lartigue, O., Carrez, D., DeMaeyer, E., and DeMaeyer-Guignard, J. (1980). Strain dependence of the antiproliferative action of interferon on murine erythroid precursors. *Science* **209**, 292–293.

Gidali, J., Feher, I., and Talas, M. (1981). Proliferation inhibition of murine pluripotent haemopoietic stem cells by interferon or poly I:C. *Cell Tissue Kinet.* **14**, 1–7.

Gidlund, M., Orn, A., Wigzell, H., Senik, A., and Gresser, I. (1978). Enhanced NK cell activity in mice injected with interferon and interferon inducers *Nature (London)* **273**, 759–761.

Gobel, U., Arnold, W., Wahn, V., Treuner, J., Jungens, H., and Cantell, K. (1981). Comparison of human fibroblast and leukocyte interferon in the treatment of severe laryngeal papillomatosis in children. *Eur. J. Pediatr.* **137**, 175–176.

Goepfert, H., Gutterman, J. U., Dichtel, W. J., Sessions, R. B., Cangir, A., and Sulek, M. (1982). Leukocyte interferon in patients with juvenile laryngeal papillomatosis. *Ann. Otol. Rhinol. Laryngol.* **9**, 431–436.

Greenberg, H. B., Pollard, R. B., Lutwick, L. I., Gregory, P. B., Robinson, W. S., and Merigan, T. C. (1976). Effect of human leukocyte interferon on hepatitis B virus infection in patients with chronic active hepatitis. *N. Engl. J. Med.* **295**, 517–522.

Gupta, S. L., Rubin, B. Y., and Holmes, S. L. (1979). Interferon action: Induction of specific proteins in mouse and human cells by homologous interferons. *Proc. Natl. Acad. Sci. U.S.A.* **76**, 4817–4821.

Gutterman, J., and Quesada, J. (1982). Clinical investigation of partially pure and recombinant DNA derived leukocyte interferon in human cancer. *Tex. Rep. Biol. Med.* **41**, 626–633.

Gutterman, J. U., Blumenschein, G. R., Alexanian, R., Yap, H. Y., Buzdar, A. V., Cavanillas, F., Hortobagyi, G. N., Distefano, A., Hersh, E. M., Rasmussen, S. L., Harmon, M., Kramer, M., and Pestka, S. (1980). Leukocyte interferon-induced tumor regression in human metastatic breast cancer, multiple myeloma, and malignant lymphoma. *Ann. Intern. Med.* **93**, 399–406.

Haglund, S., Lundquist, P. G., Cantell, K., and Strander, H. (1981). Interferon therapy in juvenile laryngeal papillomatosis. *Arch. Otolaryngol.* **107**, 327–332.

Handa, K., Suzuki, R., Matsui, H., Shimizu, Y., and Kumagai, K. (1983). Natural killer (NK) cells as a responder to interleukin 2 (IL 2). II. IL 2-induced interferon γ production. *J. Immunol.* **130**, 988–992.

Hanna, N., and Burton, R. C. (1981). Definitive evidence that natural killer (NK) cells inhibit experimental tumor metastasis *in vivo*. *J. Immunol.* **127**, 1754–1758.

Hanna, N., and Fidler, I. J. (1980). Role of natural killer cells in the destruction of circulating tumor emboli. *JNCI, J. Natl. Cancer Inst.* **65**, 801–809.

Hansson, M., Kiessling, R., and Andersson, B. (1981). Human fetal thymus and bone marrow contain target cells for natural killer cells. *Eur. J. Immunol.* **11**, 8–12.

Hansson, M., Beran, M., Andersson, B. and Kiessling, R. (1982). Inhibition of *in vitro* granulopoiesis by autologous allogeneic human NK cells. *J. Immunol.* **129**, 126–132.

Henney, C. S., Kuribayashi, K., Kern, D., and Gillis, S. (1981). Interleukin-2 augments natural killer cell activity. *Nature (London)* **291**, 335–338.

Herberman, R. B., ed. (1980). "Natural Cell-Mediated Immunity against Tumors." Academic Press, New York.

Herberman, R. B., and Holden, H. T. (1978). Natural cell-mediated immunity. *Adv. Cancer Res.* **27**, 305–377.

Herberman, R. B., and Ortaldo, J. R. (1981). Natural killer cells: Their role in defense against disease. *Science* **214**, 24–30.

Herberman, R. B., Nunn, M. E., Holden, H. T., and Lavrin, D. H. (1975). Natural cytotoxic reactivity of mouse lymphoid cells against syngeneic and allogeneic tumors. II. Characterization of effector cells. *Int. J. Cancer* **16**, 230–240.

Hill, N. O., Loeb, E., Pardue, A. S., Dorn, G. L., Khan, A., and Hill, J. M. (1979). Response of acute leukemia to leukocyte interferon. *J. Clin. Hematol. Oncol.* **9**, 137–149.

Hovanessian, A. G., Meurs, E., and Montagnier, L. (1981). Lack of systematic correlation between the interferon mediated antiviral state and the levels of 2-5A synthetase and protein kinase in three different types of murine cells. *J. Interferon Res.* **1**, 179–190.

Ito, M., and Buffet, R. F. (1981). Cytocidal effect of purified fibroblast interferon on tumor cells *in vitro*. *JNCI, J. Natl. Cancer Inst.* **66**, 819–825.

Kay, G. D. (1957). Prolonged survival of a skin homograft in a patient with very extensive burns. *Ann. N. Y. Acad. Sci.* **64**, 767–774.

Kay, H. D., and Horwitz, D. A. (1980). Evidence by reactivity with hybridoma antibodies for a probable myeloid origin of peripheral blood cells active in natural cytotoxicity and antibody-dependent cell-mediated cytotoxicity. *J. Clin. Invest.* **66**, 847–851.

Klimpel, G. R., Fleischmann, W. R., Jr., and Klimpel, K. D. (1982). Gamma interferon (IFNγ) and IFNα/β suppress murine myeloid colony formation (CFU-C): Magnitude of suppression is dependent upon level of colony-stimulating factor (CSF). *J. Immunol.* **129**, 76–80.

Krown, S. E., Real, F. X., Cunningham-Rundles, S., Myskowski, P. L., Koziner, B., Fein, S., Mittelman, A., Oettgen, H. F., and Safai, B. (1983). Preliminary observations on the effect of recombinant leukocyte A interferon in homosexual men with Kaposi's sarcoma. *N. Engl. J. Med.* **308**, 1071–1076.

Kuribayashi, K., Gillis, S., Kern, D. E., and Henney, C. S. (1981). Murine NK cell cultures: Effects of interleukin-2 and interferon on cell growth and cytotoxic reactivity. *J. Immunol.* **126**, 2321–2327.

Langvad, E., Hyden, H., Peterson, J. K., Jordal, R., and Olsen, G. (1980). Extracorporeal interferon therapy in malignant melanoma. *Arzneim.-Forsch.* **30**, 1245–1246.

Leandersson, T., and Lundgren, E. (1980). Antiproliferative effect of interferon on a Burkitt's lymphoma cell line. *Exp. Cell Res.* **130**, 421–426.

Lloyd, R. E., Blalock, J. E., and Stanton, G. J. (1983). Cell-to-cell transfer of interferon-induced antiproliferative activity. *Science* **221**, 953–955.

McNeill, T. A., and Gresser, I. (1973). Inhibition of haemopoietic colony growth by interferon preparations from different sources. *Nature (London), New Biol.* **244**, 173–174.

Maheshwari, R. K., Vijay, I. K., Olden, K., and Friedman, R. M. (1981). Assay of glycosyltrans-ferase activities in microsomal preparation from cells treated with interferon. *In* "Methods in Enzymology" (S. Pestka, ed.), Vol. 79B, pp. 302–306. Academic Press, New York.

Meakins, J. L., Christou, N. V., Shizgal, H. M., and MacLean, L. D. (1979). Therapeutic ap-proaches to anergy in surgical patients: Surgery and levamisole. *Ann. Surg.* **190,** 286–296.

Mellstedt, H., Ahre, A., Bjorkolm, M., Holm, G., Johansson, B., and Strander, H. (1979). Inter-feron therapy in myelomatosis. *Lancet* **I,** 245–247.

Merigan, T. C., Sikora, K., Breeden, J. H., Levy, R., and Rosenberg, S. A. (1978). Preliminary observations on the effect of human leukocyte interferon in non-Hodgkin's lymphoma. *N. Engl. J. Med.* **299,** 1449–1453.

Nabel, G., Bucalo, L. R., Allard, J., Wigzell, H., and Cantor, H. (1981). Multiple activities of a cloned cell line mediating natural killer cell function. *J. Exp. Med.* **153,** 1582–1591.

Ninnemann, J. L., Fisher, J. C., and Frank, H. A. (1978). Prolonged survival of human skin allografts following thermal injury. *Transplantation* **25,** 69–72.

Ohtsuki, K. (1982). A biological role of interferon-induced protein kinases. *Tex. Rep. Biol. Med.* **41,** 493–498.

Pottathil, R., Chandrabose, K. A., Cuatrecassas, P., and Lang, D. J. (1980). Establishment of the interferon-mediated antiviral state: Role of fatty acid cyclooxygenase. *Proc. Nat. Acad. Sci. U.S.A.* **77,** 5437–5440.

Pross, H. F., and Baines, M. G. (1977). Spontaneous human lymphocyte-mediated cytotoxicity against tumor target cells. *Cancer Immunol. Immunother.* **3,** 75–85.

Revel, M., Kimchi, A., Friedman, M., Wolf, D., Merlin, G., Panet, A., Rapaport, S., and Lapidot, Y. (1982). Cell-regulatory function of interferon induced enzymes: Antimitogenic effect of (2'-5') oligo-A, growth related variations in (2'-5') oligo-A synthetase, and isolation of its mRNA. *Tex. Rep. Biol. Med.* **41,** 452–462.

Rubin, B. Y., and Gupta, L. S. (1980). Interferon-induced proteins in human fibroblasts and development of the antiviral state. *J. Virol.* **34,** 446–454.

Salvin, S. B., Youngner, J. S., Nishio, J., and Neta, R. (1975). Tumor suppression by a lymphokine released into the circulation of mice with delayed hypersensitivity. *JNCI, J. Natl. Cancer Inst.* **55,** 1233–1236.

Samuel, C. E. (1982). Molecular mechanisms of interferon action: Interferon-mediated phosphoryla-tion of ribosome-associated protein P_1 and protein synthesis initiation factor eIF-2. *Tex. Rep. Biol. Med.* **41,** 463–470.

Schmidt, A., Chernajovsky, Y., Shulman, L., Federman, P., Berissi, H., and Revel, M. (1979). An interferon-induced phosphodiesterase degrading (2'5') oligoadenylate and the C-C-A terminus of tRNA. *Proc. Natl. Acad. Sci. U.S.A.* **76,** 4788–4792.

Schultz, R. M. (1980). Macrophage activation by interferons. *Lymphokine Rep.* **1,** 63–97.

Scorticatti, C. H., De De La Pena, N. C., Bellora, O. G., Mariotto, R. A., Casabe, A. R., and Comolli, R. (1982). Systemic IFN-alpha treatment of multiple bladder papilloma grade I or II patients: Pilot study. *J. Interferon Res.* **2,** 339–343.

Sen, G. C., Shaila, S., Le Bleu, B., Brown, G. E., Desrosiers, R. C., and Lengyl, P. (1977). Impairment of reovirus mRNA methylation in extracts of interferon-treated Ehrlich ascites tumor cells: Further characteristics of the phenomenon. *J. Virol.* **21,** 69–83.

Sharma, O. K., and Goswami, B. B. (1981). Inhibition of vaccinia mRNA methylation by 2',5'-linked oligo (adenylic acid) triphosphate. *Proc. Natl. Acad. Sci. U.S.A.* **78,** 2221–2224.

Silverman, R. H., Cayley, P. J., Wrenschner, D. H., Knight, M., Gilbert, C. S., Brown, R. E., and Kerr, I. M. (1982). 2-5A (pppA2'p5'A2'p5'A) in interferon-treated encephalomyocarditis virus-infected mouse L-cells. *Tex. Rep. Biol. Med.* **41,** 479–486.

Sokawa, Y., Watenabe, Y., Watenabe, Y., and Kawade, Y. (1977). Interferon suppresses the transition of quiescent 3T3 cells to a growing state. *Nature (London)* **268,** 236–238.

Sonnenfeld, G., Mandel, A. D., and Merigan, T. C. (1977). The immunosuppressive effect of type II mouse interferon preparations on antibody production. *Cell. Immunol.* **34**, 193–206.

Stanwick, T. L., Campbell, D. E., and Nahmias, A. J. (1980). Spontaneous cytotoxicity mediated by human monocyte–macrophages against human fibroblasts infected with herpes simplex virus—Augmentation by interferon. *Cell. Immunol.* **53**, 413–416.

Stewart, W. E., II, Blalock, J. E., Burke, D. C., Chany, C., Dunnick, J. K., Falcoff, E., Friedman, R. M., Galasso, G. J., Joklik, W. K., Vilcek, J. T., Youngner, J. S., and Zoon, K. C. (1980). Interferon nomenclature. *Nature (London)* **286**, 110.

Suzuki, F., and Pollard, R. B. (1982). Alterations of interferon production in a mouse model of thermal injury. *J. Immunol.* **129**, 1806–1810.

Svet-Moldavsky, G. J., and Chernyakhovskaya, I. J. (1967). Interferon and the interaction of allogeneic normal and immune lymphocytes with L cells. *Nature (London)* **215**, 1299–1300.

Talmadge, J. E., Meyers, K. M., Prieur, D. J., and Starkey, J. R. (1980). Role of NK cells in tumor growth and metastasis in *beige* mice. *Nature (London)* **284**, 622–624.

Tilden, A., Abo, T., and Balch, C. M. (1983). Suppressor cell function of human granular lymphocytes identified by the HNK-1 (LEU-7) monoclonal antibody. *J. Immunol.* **130**, 1171–1175.

Timonen, T., Ortaldo, J. R., Stadler, B. M., Bonnard, G. D., Sharrow, S. O., and Herberman, R. B. (1982). Cultures of purified human natural killer cells: Growth in the presence of interleukin 2. *Cell. Immunol.* **72**, 178–185.

Treuner, J., Niethammer, D., Dannecker, G., Hagmann, R., Neef, V., and Hofschneider, P. H. (1980). Successful treatment of nasopharyngeal carcinoma with interferon. *Lancet* **I**, 817–818.

Trinchieri, G., and Santoli, D. (1978). Antiviral activity induced by culturing lymphocytes with tumor-derived or virus-transformed cells: Enhancement of human natural killer cell activity by interferon and antagonistic inhibition of susceptibility of target cells to lysis. *J. Exp. Med.* **147**, 1314–1333.

Trinchieri, G., Santoli, D., Dee, R. R., and Knowles, B. B. (1978). Antiviral activity induced by culturing lymphocytes with tumor derived or virus-transformed cells. Identification of the antiviral activity as interferon and characterization of the human effector lymphocyte subpopulation. *J. Exp. Med.* **147**, 1299–1313.

Trinchieri, G., Granato, D., and Perussia, B. (1981). Interferon-induced resistance of fibroblasts to cytolysis mediated by natural killer cells: Specificity and mechanism. *J. Immunol.* **126**, 335–340.

Tyring, S., Klimpel, G. R., Fleischmann, W. R., Jr., and Baron, S. (1982). Direct cytolysis by partially-purified preparations of immune interferon. *Int. J. Cancer* **30**, 59–64.

Vandenbussche, P., Divizia, M., Verhaegen-Lewalle, M., Fuse, A., Kuwata, T., De Clercq, E., and Content, J. (1981). Enzymatic activities induced by interferon in human fibroblast cell lines differing in their sensitivity to the anticellular activity of interferon. *Virology* **111**, 11–22.

Verhaegen, M., Divizia, M., Vandenbussche, P., Kuwata, T., and Content, J. C. (1980). Abnormal behavior of interferon-induced enzymatic activities in an interferon-resistant cell line. *Proc. Natl. Acad. Sci. U.S.A.* **77**, 4479–4483.

Verma, P. S., Spitzer, G., Zander, A. R., Gutterman, J. U., McCredie, K. B., Dicke, K. A., and Johnston, D. A. (1981). Human leukocyte interferon preparation-mediated block of granulopoietic differentiation *in vitro*. *Exp. Hematol. (Copenhagen)* **9**, 63-76.

Warner, J. F., and Dennert, G. (1983). Effects of a cloned cell line with NK activity on bone marrow transplants, tumour development and metastasis *in vivo*. *Nature (London)* **300**, 31–34.

Weigent, D. A., Langford, M. P., Fleischmann, W. R., Jr., and Stanton, G. J. (1983). Potentiation of lymphocyte natural killing by mixtures of alpha or beta interferon with recombinant gamma interferon. *Infect. Immun.* **40**, 35–38.

Weil, J., Epstein, C. J., Epstein, L. B., Sedmak, J. J., Sabran, J. L., and Grossberg, S. E. (1983). A unique set of polypeptides is induced by γ interferon in addition to those induced in common with α and β interferons. *Nature (London)* **301,** 437–439.

West, W. H., Cannon, G. B., Kay, H. D., Bonnard, G. D., and Herberman, R. B. (1977). Natural cytotoxic reactivity of human lymphocytes against a myeloid cell line: Characterization of effector cells. *J. Immunol.* **118,** 355–361.

Wood, J. N., and Hovanessian, A. G. (1979). Interferon enhances 2′-5′ A synthetase in embryonal carcinoma cells. *Nature (London)* **282,** 74–76.

Zarling, J. M., and Kung, P. L. (1980). Monoclonal antibodies which distinguish between human NK cells and cytotoxic T lymphocytes. *Nature (London)* **288,** 394–396.

Zarling, J. M., Clouse, K. A., Biddison, W. E., and Kung, P. C. (1981). Phenotypes of human natural killer cell populations detected with monoclonal antibodies. *J. Immunol.* **127,** 2575–2580.

Zilberstein, A., Dudock, B., Berissi, H., and Revel, M. (1976). Control of messenger RNA translation by minor species of leucyl-tRNA in extracts from interferon-treated L cells. *J. Mol. Biol.* **108,** 43–54.

2

Monoclonal Antibodies in the Diagnosis and Treatment of Cancer

FRANCES M. DAVIS AND POTU N. RAO

Department of Chemotherapy Research
M. D. Anderson Hospital and Tumor Institute
The University of Texas System Cancer Center
Houston, Texas

I.	Introduction	24
	A. Definition of Monoclonal Antibodies	24
	B. Advantages of Monoclonal Antibodies Compared to Conventional Antisera	25
II.	Methodology	27
	A. Mouse Monoclonal Antibodies	28
	B. Human Monoclonal Antibodies	36
	C. Antibodies with Dual Specificities	38
III.	Diagnostic Uses of Monoclonal Antibodies	39
	A. Serological Markers	39
	B. Immunohistology	40
	C. Radiolocalization of Tumors (Tumor Imaging)	51
IV.	Therapeutic Uses of Monoclonal Antibodies	53
	A. *Ex Vivo* Treatment of Bone Marrow for Transplantation	54
	B. Serotherapy	57
	C. Targeting of Drugs, Toxins, and Radionuclides	62
	D. Immunological Manipulation	63
	E. Factors Influencing Therapeutic Efficiency	64
	F. Viruses in MAb Preparations Used for Therapy	66
V.	Conclusions	66
	References	67

Novel Approaches to Cancer Chemotherapy

I. INTRODUCTION

In 1975, Kohler and Milstein described a method for the immortalization of a single antibody-producing cell in such a way that it and its progeny continued to secrete the same antibody. The significance of this discovery, like the one by Watson and Crick (1953), was immediately and widely recognized. It has been seminal in the development of new methods of cancer diagnosis and treatment, as well as in studies on the process of carcinogenesis and on the biology of normal and neoplastic cells and tissues. Today there are reproducible methods for the production of monoclonal antibodies (MAb), and they are being improved continually. The antibodies produced are already in use for cancer diagnosis and treatment and can be expected to be used increasingly in the future.

The purpose of this chapter is to describe what monoclonal antibodies are and how they are produced, with particular emphasis on aspects related to the diagnosis and therapy of cancer, and to review the preliminary preclinical and clinical studies in which MAb have been used. Excellent reviews can be found on methods for production and screening of MAb (Goding, 1980; Staines and Lew, 1980; Yelton and Scharff, 1981; Foster, 1982; Galfre and Milstein, 1981; Reading, 1982; Zola and Brooks, 1982; Damjanov and Knowles, 1983; Kozbor and Roder, 1983), and on diagnostic and therapeutic uses of MAb (McMichael and Bastin, 1980; Diamond et al., 1981; Edwards, 1981; Diamond and Scharff, 1982; McMichael and Fabre, 1982; Mitchell and Oettgen, 1982; Neville et al., 1982; Ritz and Schlossman, 1982; Sikora, 1982; Thurlow and McKenzie, 1983; Levy and Miller, 1983b; Olsson, 1983). In the rapidly developing field of MAb, another review may serve the purpose of including the latest advances and developments. This chapter will emphasize the use of MAb to tumor-specific or tumor-associated antigens, but will also describe how MAb that are not strictly specific for tumor cells can be used for accurate diagnosis and staging, as well as for therapy.

A. Definition of Monoclonal Antibodies

The antibodies produced by a clone of cells derived from a single cell are called monoclonal antibodies. Such a clone secretes only one antibody, and all the antibody molecules secreted by the cells are identical in amino acid sequence and antigen-binding properties. Different antibody-producing cells secrete antibodies of different amino acid sequences that bind to different antigenic sites, or epitopes. When an animal mounts an immune response to an antigen, many such clones of cells are activated to secrete antibodies to various epitopes on the antigen, and these antibodies are polyclonal in origin. The antibodies in the serum are a mixture of different antibodies to the same antigen and to unrelated antigens to which the animal has had an immune response. Under ordinary circumstances, individual antibody-producing cells cannot be isolated and propagated as individual clones of cells secreting monoclonal antibodies, and so these antibodies cannot be studied or used as purified proteins.

One exception is myeloma or plasmacytoma cell lines, which are derived from animals with tumors of antibody-producing cells and can be grown in tissue culture. Although studies of the myeloma proteins secreted by the tumors into the serum of patients or by clones of tumor cells into tissue culture medium have been instrumental in deciphering the structure and assembly of immunoglobulins, there are few cases in which the antigen has been identified. The seminal publications of Kohler and Milstein (1975, 1976) described a means of immortalizing single cells producing antibodies of preselected specificity. Their method involves the fusion of antibody-producing cells from immunized mice with cultured mouse myeloma cells to yield cell hybrids, or hybridomas, that can propagate indefinitely and continue to secrete the same antibody. Mouse hybridoma clones secreting MAb of interest in tissue culture can then be grown as solid or ascites tumors in mice to increase antibody yield.

B. Advantages of Monoclonal Antibodies Compared to Conventional Antisera

A comparison of some of the properties of conventional antisera and monoclonal antibody preparations is presented in Table I. Conventional antisera are obtained by bleeding immunized animals and allowing the blood to clot, leaving fluid, noncellular serum. In practice, an immunoglobulin fraction obtained by salt fractionation and ion exchange chromatography (Zola and Brooks, 1982) is usually utilized. Monoclonal antibodies are pure, homogeneous, totally reproducible reagents, available forever in unlimited supply. Thus, the same antibodies can be used by laboratories throughout the world. Indeed, the commercial marketing of MAb is a growth industry (Anonymous, 1979).

One of the most important advantages of monoclonal antibodies is the potential for identification and purification of antigens that may not have been previously recognized. They can be produced from animals immunized with very complex mixtures of antigens. This is possible because each MAb reacts with a single antigenic determinant, not with multiple determinants on multiple components of the immunizing material, as do conventional antisera. For example, MAb produced after immunization of animals with whole cells or cell membrane preparations from melanoma (Chee et al., 1982), sarcoma (Brown, 1983), and gastrointestinal cancer (Steplewski et al., 1981; Magnani et al., 1982) have been used to recognize and characterize biochemically several tumor-associated antigens that had not been identified previously. MAb specific for a single 110-kilodalton protein associated with the Golgi apparatus were obtained after immunization of a mouse with whole-gerbil fibroma cells that had been extracted with

TABLE I

Comparison of Properties of Monoclonal Antibodies and Conventional Antisera

		Monoclonal antibodies	
Property	Conventional antisera	Tissue culture supernatant	Ascites fluid
Concentration of immunoglobulin	10 mg/ml	0.1–200 μg/ml[a]	0.6–10 mg/ml
Concentration of immunoglobulin of desired specificity	0.1–1.0 mg/ml	0.1–200 μg/ml	0.1–10 mg/ml
Reproducibility	Batch-to-batch variability in epitopes recognized, binding kinetics, etc.	Absolute	
Cross-reactivity	Partial, due to common antigenic determinants on different antigens	Binding to single determinant; no cross-reactivity unless same determinant is present and then cross-reactivity complete	
Supply	Limited to each animal and each bleed	Unlimited	
Immunoglobulin properties	Typical spectrum of all; average behavior varies	Only one antibody class and subclass, with individual properties selected by screening method.	

[a]In serum-free or immunoglobulin-free medium. Otherwise, 1 mg/ml in medium containing 10% serum.

Triton X-100 (Lin and Queally, 1982). In fact, the exquisite specificity of MAb has been used by Hansen and Beavo (1982) to identify conformationally distinct forms of cyclic nucleotide phosphodiesterase. We have produced MAb to mitosis-specific antigens that bind only when the antigens are phosphorylated (Davis *et al.*, 1983b).

Perhaps the most obvious disadvantage of MAb is that they may vary in their reactivity depending on the type of immunological assay used. Thus, it is not uncommon to find that MAb that are reactive in one assay, such as immunofluorescence, may not be reactive in another assay, such as a dot blot binding assay (Hawkes *et al.*, 1982; Naiem *et al.*, 1982), or after some other treatment protocol or fixation method (Silver and Elgin, 1979; Foster *et al.*, 1982b; Frankel *et al.*, 1982; Hancock *et al.*, 1982; Naritoku and Taylor, 1982). The reactivity of an antibody in any system depends on the particular properties of the individual MAb–epitope pair, since there is only one antibody of the same class, subclass, and amino acid sequence that recognizes only that single epitope. For example, most monoclonal IgG's will not precipitate most antigens, because the extensive cross-linking needed to form large, insoluble complexes cannot occur. A monoclonal IgM may activate the complement pathway very well, but cannot bind to staphylococcal protein A for purification. An individual epitope recognized by MAb in alcohol-fixed frozen sections of biopsy specimens may be masked, altered, or denatured in formaldehyde-fixed, paraffin-embedded sections. This problem becomes even more complex when attempts are made to use MAb as therapeutic agents. An antibody that efficiently detects and binds to tumor cells *in vitro* under one set of conditions may not do so under another set of conditions (Kammer, 1983) or *in vivo* (Thierfelder *et al.*, 1983; Haskell *et al.*, 1983), or may be efficiently bound but may not have any biological effect (Thorpe and Ross, 1982; Trowbridge and Domingo, 1981).

Since only one antigenic determinant is recognized by each MAb, cross-reactivity with other antigens is usually absent. However, in some cases unexpected cross-reactivities have been observed. For example, Dulbecco *et al.* (1981) reported that an MAb to a lymphocyte cell surface antigen, Thy-1, cross-reacted with intermediate filaments in the cells. Such cross-reactivity is thought to be due to the presence of usual or unusual amino acid sequences that form identical or similar epitopes on unrelated proteins (Brown, 1982; Nigg *et al.*, 1982).

II. METHODOLOGY

The purpose of this section is to describe the general techniques used to produce MAb and to consider some of the variables that have been investigated that may be of importance in cancer diagnosis and therapy.

The most common methodology used for obtaining monoclonal antibodies is derived directly from that originally described by Kohler and Milstein (1975). It involves fusion of the spleen cells from a preimmunized mouse with cells of a cultured mouse myeloma cell line. The myeloma cells used lack the enzyme hypoxanthine phosphoribosyltransferase (HPRT), so that hybrids are selectable in medium containing hypoxanthine, aminopterin, and thymidine (HAT) (Littlefield, 1964). Hybrid clones are screened for antibody binding to the cells used as immunogen. Hybridoma clones secreting antibodies to the immunogen are subcloned, and milligram quantities of MAb are produced from ascites fluid in mice. There are many variables in this procedure, including choice of immunogen, method of immunization, type of myeloma cells to be used as the immortal parent, hybrid selection, fusogen, method of screening for antibody-secreting clones, method of subcloning, and method of mass production of antibodies. Monoclonal antibodies from many species, including human (Levy and Dilley, 1978), rabbit (Yarmush *et al.*, 1980), rat (Garcia-Perez and Smith, 1983), hamster (Sanchez-Madrid *et al.*, 1983), and cow (Srikumaran *et al.*, 1983), have been produced by fusion of lymphocytes from immune donors with mouse myeloma cells, although selection of interspecific hybridoma clones secreting antibodies of preselected specificity occurs at very low frequency. Rat myeloma cell lines that can be used to produce rat monoclonal antibodies have been described (Galfre *et al.*, 1979; Bazin, 1982; Smedley *et al.*, 1983). Human MAb may have some advantages over mouse MAb in the diagnosis and treatment of cancer, and the recent availability of suitable human myeloma cell lines (reviewed by Olsson and Kaplan, 1983), as well as the ability to immortalize human antibody-secreting lymphocytes with Epstein–Barr virus (EBV) (reviewed by Kozbor and Roder, 1983), promises the production and widespread use of human MAb. Finally, antibodies with dual specificities that can react with two epitopes on cells, or that could be used to carry drugs (Raso, 1982; Ghetie and Moraru, 1983) also show potential in cancer diagnosis and therapy.

A. Mouse Monoclonal Antibodies

1. Immunization

a. Immunization in Vivo. Most of the MAb that are available today are the products of fusion of cells from animals immunized *in vivo* with complex mixtures of antigens. The antigens have been poorly defined and immunization parameters poorly understood. The enormous potential of MAb methodology is indicated by the fact that so many interesting and useful MAb have been produced by immunization with whole cells, cell homogenates, or complex mixtures of antigens. These MAb are used to define the antigens present on different cell types or to detect differences in antigens on tumor and normal cells.

Immunization of animals with whole cells is commonly accomplished by the intraperitoneal injection of $1–2 \times 10^7$ live or fixed cells. One or more booster injections are given at 1- to 6-week intervals. Spleens from the animals are excised, and the dissociated cells are fused 3–5 days following the final booster immunization. Kohler and Milstein (1975) used an initial intraperitoneal injection of 0.2 ml packed sheep red blood cells followed 1 mo later by an intraperitoneal booster and fusion of spleen cells 4 days later.

More complex protocols have been reported. Each group usually tries a variety of immunization protocols and reports one or more that have worked for them. For example, Minna *et al.* (1981) used six weekly injections of 2×10^7 live cells: the first dose was given subcutaneously in complete Freund's adjuvant, the next four intraperitoneally, and the final booster intravenously. Spleen cells were fused 3 days later. Since MAb reacting with soluble antigens or antigens on the surface of living cells may not necessarily react with the same determinants after the tissues are fixed and embedded (Naiem *et al.*, 1982), Williams *et al.* (1982) immunized with human primitive endoderm cells fixed with formol-saline, since their purpose was to obtain antibodies that could be used to detect antigens histochemically in fixed sections of germ cell neoplasms.

Immunization with such complex mixtures of antigens depends on the large antibody repertoire of the animal immunized. Inbred mice can make an estimated $1-5 \times 10^7$ different antibodies (Klinman and Press, 1975; Lerner, 1982), with perhaps $1-8 \times 10^3$ different antibodies to the same determinant (Kreth and Williamson, 1973; Kohler, 1976). However, some animals may not mount an important immune response to some antigens. When mice were immunized with preimplantation mouse embryos, Shevinsky et al. (1982) were unable to obtain mouse MAb to SSEA-3, a stage-specific cell surface mouse embryonic glycoprotein antigen that is also found on the surface of human teratocarcinoma cells. MAb to SSEA-3 could be obtained by immunizing rats with preimplantation mouse embryos or mice with human embryonal carcinoma cells.

In complex mixtures of antigens, such as whole-tumor cells, there are usually a few immunodominant components to which much of the response will be directed; therefore, many of the MAb selected will also be against the immunodominant epitopes (Milstein and Lennox, 1980). Thus, mice immunized with human cells yield many hybridomas producing MAb to human major histocompatibility antigens (Dippold et al., 1980; Thompson et al., 1982a). Some attempts have been made to block the major immunogens immunologically to allow detection of minor or less immunogenic components (Foster, 1982). For example, Kennett and Gilbert (1979) precoated human neuroblastoma cells used for immunization with anti-human antibodies to attempt to reduce the response to "human" antigens.

Monoclonal antibodies to some well-characterized, biochemically defined, tumor-associated antigens have been produced in an attempt to obtain antibodies to antigenic determinants with greater specificity for tumor cells. Thus, antibodies to purified human α-fetoprotein (AFP) (Uotila et al., 1980), carcinoembryonic antigen (CEA) (Accolla et al., 1980; Hedin et al., 1982a), and placental alkaline phosphatase (Pl-ALP) (Slaughter et al., 1981) have been reported. Immunizations required 50–100 μg of purified antigen. Although the four MAb to α-fetoprotein do not distinguish between different α-fetoproteins, and therefore could be reacting either with the same epitope or with epitopes common to all α-fetoproteins (Uotila et al., 1980), eight MAb to carcinoembryonic antigen recognized six different epitopes (Hedin et al., 1982a), and six MAb to placental alkaline phosphatase recognized six epitopes and could be used to distinguish between different isozymes (Slaughter et al., 1981). MAb to cell surface, tumor-associated antigens can also react with different epitopes on the same molecule (Webb et al., 1983).

Immunization with synthetic peptides (Lerner, 1982; Schmitz et al., 1982) has been used to produce polyclonal and monoclonal antibodies with preselected submolecular binding specificities, and the majority of these antibodies also bind to the native molecule. This capability may be important, because studies on oncogenes and oncogene products as markers and causes of cancer (reviewed by Bishop, 1982) have demonstrated that the oncogene product in a human bladder carcinoma cell line differs from the normal cellular counterpart by a single amino acid (Tabin *et al.*, 1982; Taparowsky *et al.*, 1982).

b. Immunization **in Vitro.**   Immunization of cells *in vitro*, by incubation of dissociated spleen cells with antigen in culture, in the presence of growth factors produced by thymocytes (reviewed by Reading, 1982), was first reported by Hengartner *et al.* (1978). Immunization *in vitro* is especially valuable when the quantities of antigen are limited, when antigenicity is weak, or when suppression or tolerance *in vivo* is responsible for the failure of immunization to "self" antigens. Thus, Luben *et al.* (1982) were able to obtain MAb by immunizing with picomoles of antigen. Another advantage is that immunization can normally be accomplished in 5 days. Although 80% of the MAb obtained from such experiments are IgM, more IgG antibodies can be obtained after prolonged immunization (Pardue *et al.*, 1983).

c. Increasing the Frequency of Antigen-Specific Hybridomas.   Even with hyperimmunization, only a small proportion of the cells in the spleen are "activated" or actually secreting immunoglobulin (Damjanov and Knowles, 1983). Yet, Kohler and Milstein (1975) found that 50% of their hybrids were making new immunoglobulins, and 20% of these were making antibodies specific for the immunizing cells. It is fortunate that "activated" cells fuse much more readily than resting spleen cells (Goding, 1980), although the specific characteristic that causes increased fusion is unknown. Nevertheless, in most fusions only 10–20% of the hybrids are making antibodies to the immunizing cells, and only a small percentage of these may be specific for the cell type used. Schnegg *et al.* (1981) screened 345 hybridoma clones after fusion of spleen cells from a mouse immunized with human glioma cells. Of these, 36 (10%) reacted with glioma cells as well as nonglioma cells, and only 3 (0.9%) were relatively glioma specific. Minna *et al.* (1981) screened 3041 hybridoma clones after immunization with small cell lung carcinoma cells and only 1.4% of them were lung cancer specific.

Because of the low frequency of hybridoma clones secreting immunoglobulins specific for the immunizing cells, various methods to increase their frequency by enriching for antibody precursor or antibody-producing lymphocytes before fusion have been developed (reviewed by Siraganian *et al.*, 1983). Bankert *et al.* (1980) coated the parental myeloma cells with antigen to promote binding to and fusion with antigen-reactive spleen cells. The number of positive clones obtained per 10^6 spleen cells fused was increased 50-fold by the adoptive transfer of cells from an immunized mouse into a sublethally irradiated, syngeneic host, which was then given a booster immunization (Fox *et al.*, 1981, 1982). Alternatively, cells from immunized animals have been cultured with antigen *in vitro* before fusion (Fox *et al.*, 1982) in an attempt to increase the number and/or fusion frequency of spleen cells producing the desired antibody. Feder *et al.* (1983) devised a method using bromodeoxyuridine and Hoechst 33258, followed by irradiation with ultraviolet light, to eliminate nonspecifically stimulated spleen cells before *in vitro* immunization with antigen in serum-free medium to increase the frequency of antigen-specific hybridomas.

2. Fusion Partners and Fusion Agents

A variety of mouse myeloma cell lines have been used as fusion partners, and some of those most commonly used are listed in Table II. The choice of the myeloma parent is based on several properties of the cells, including how well and how quickly the cells and their hybrids grow, ability to fuse, high levels and stability of antibody secretion by the hybrids, and the availability of a selection system so that hybrid cells will grow under conditions that parental cells will not.

Myeloma lines that do not produce and secrete antibodies themselves have been developed, so that the antibodies secreted by hybridomas are strictly monoclonal. The first four mouse cell lines listed in the table have been used successfully in many laboratories and depend on the HAT (hypoxanthine–aminopterin–thymidine) selection system devised by Littlefield (1964). Parental cells lacking either hypoxanthine phosphoribosyltransferase (HPRT) or thymidine kinase (TK) must depend on the de novo synthesis of nucleotide precursors for nucleic acid synthesis, and this de novo pathway can be blocked by aminopterin.

TABLE II

Myeloma Cell Lines for Hybridoma Production

Species	Cell line	Ig Secreted	Selectable marker	References
Mouse	P3- x63-Ag 8.653	—	HPRT$^-$	Kearney *et al.*, 1979
(BALB/c)	SP2/0-Ag 14	—	HPRT$^-$	Shulman *et al.*, 1978
	FO	—	HPRT$^-$	Fazekas de St. Groth and Scheidegger, 1980
	S 194/5XXO.BU.5	—	TK$^-$	Trowbridge, 1978
	FOX-NY	—	APRT$^-$, HPRT$^-$	Taggart and Samloff, 1983
Rat	IR 983F	—	HPRT$^-$	Bazin, 1982
	Y3-Ag 1.2.3	κ	HPRT$^-$	Galfre *et al.*, 1979
Human	SKO-007	ε, κ	HPRT$^-$	Olsson and Kaplan, 1980
	GM-1500 6TG-2	γ^2, κ	HPRT$^-$	Croce *et al.*, 1980
	KR-4	γ, κ	HPRT$^-$, oua^R	Kozbor *et al.*, 1982
	LICR-LON-HMy2	γ^1, κ	HPRT$^-$	Edwards *et al.*, 1982

One of the major problems with hybridomas is that antibody secretion is frequently unstable, since the karyotype of the hybrid clones is unstable and the chromosomes with the antibody genes may be segregated. Thus, frequent cloning and subcloning for antibody producers may be required. Taggart and Samloff (1983) have recently described a novel system using adenine phosphoribosyltransferase [AMP:pyrophosphate phosphoribosyltransferase (EC 2.4.2.7); APRT] selection as described by Liskay and Patterson (1978) to circumvent this problem. The beauty of the Taggart and Samloff (1983) system is in the translocation of the gene for APRT to the chromosome bearing the active immunoglobulin heavy-chain genes in their strain of mice. Since loss of the chromosome bearing the antibody gene is accompanied by loss of the ability of the hybrids to grow in selective media, the hybridoma cultures are stable for antibody production. In addition, this method eliminates the loss of large numbers of hybridomas segregating the chromosomes bearing the HPRT and TK genes, which have nothing to do with antibody production per se.

Fusion between adjacent cells in a population occurs spontaneously at low frequency, but the fusion frequency can be increased by viruses, such as Sendai virus, and chemical agents that affect the membranes, such as lysolecithin and polyethylene glycol (PEG). Kohler and Milstein (1975) initially used Sendai virus, which has been reported to yield primarily IgM-secreting hybridomas (Fazekas de St. Groth and Scheidegger, 1980), possibly because IgG-secreting lymphocytes do not have sufficient Sendai virus receptors to be fused efficiently. PEG is the agent most commonly used (Galfre et al., 1977, Gefter et al., 1977; Kennett, 1979), although the fusion frequency depends on the molecular weight of PEG, the concentration, duration, and temperature of exposure, the presence of other substances such as dimethyl sulfoxide, and even the manufacturer and lot number of the PEG (Fazekas de St. Groth and Scheidegger, 1980).

The addition of feeder layers of cells has been reported to reduce the variability in and possibly increase the recovery of hybrid clones (Fazekas de St. Groth and Scheidegger, 1980). However, if all conditions for hybridoma growth are ideal, there is no need for feeder layers of cells; besides, the hybrid clones may become dependent on the feeder layer (Minna et al., 1981). Spleen cells from nonimmunized animals (Zola and Brooks, 1982), thymocytes (Oi and Herzenberg, 1980), peritoneal macrophages (Fazekas de St. Groth and Scheidegger, 1980), and irradiated human fibroblasts (Brodsky et al., 1979) have been used as feeder layers. Hormones (Kennett et al., 1978) and conditioned media (Astaldi et al., 1980) are sometimes added to promote clonal growth.

3. Screening of Clones

The fusion mixture is usually plated into 100 to 1000 wells in multiwell plates (24 wells or 96 wells/plate). The goal in plating is to have no more than one clonogenic hybrid cell per well. Colonies with about 10^3 cells are visible within 2 to 3 weeks. Most investigators screen for secreted antibody in the supernatant rather than antibody-producing cells, which may have immunoglobulin bound to the membrane (Parks *et al.*, 1979), because the relationship between surface Ig and antibody secretion is not understood. Screening the culture supernatant in the wells for hybridomas secreting the desired antibodies is a very critical step. One problem is that antibodies may be produced not only by hybrid cells but also by surviving spleen cells not involved in fusion. The most important consideration, however, is colony growth. If the sample is taken too early, the antibody concentration in the supernatant may be too low; overgrown colonies may result in colony death. Usually there is 1 week or less during which the colony size is optimum for testing as well as for colony survival. Therefore, the screening method used should be rapid and adaptable to handle large numbers of samples.

Various screening methods have been developed to provide the necessary speed and convenience. Most tests used for screening are indirect but depend primarily on the binding of antibody to antigen, rather than on secondary interactions, such as complement fixation. Most screening methods are designed so that the second antibody reacts with all desired classes of mouse immunglobulin, as in the case of indirect immunofluorescence or radiolabeled anti-immunoglobulin tests. The primary consideration in the choice of a screening method is that the screen should be appropriate to the intended use of the antibody. For antibodies intended to be used in the diagnosis and treatment of cancer, three types of screening assays are commonly used. To screen for antibodies to previously unidentified antigens, whole-cell binding assays (Williams *et al.*, 1977; Schneider and Eisenbarth, 1979; Stoker *et al.*, 1978; Stocker and Heuser, 1979) and immunohistology (Naiem *et al.*, 1982) have been used. To screen for antibodies to antigens that have been characterized and purified, radioimmunoassays or enzyme-linked immunoassays (Saunders, 1979; Tsu and Herzenberg, 1980) have been used. Some investigators (Rotblat *et al.*, 1983) have recommended the use of two screening assays to avoid missing some reactive clones. Other types of screening assays that have been used include enzyme inhibition (Glode *et al.*, 1981; Thorgeirrson *et al.*, 1983), indirect immunoprecipitation using a staphylococcal protein A immunoadsorbent (Kessler, 1975), immunoblot methods in combination with electrophoresis (Towbin *et al.*, 1979; Pearson and Anderson, 1983; Tsang *et al.*, 1983), the adherence of antigen-coated red blood cells (Kohler and Milstein, 1975; Sharon *et al.*, 1979), and complement-dependent cytotoxicity (Ved Brat *et al.*, 1980; Wiels *et al.*, 1981).

a. Whole-Cell Binding Assays. Since the aim of many studies is to develop monoclonal antibodies that can detect antigens on the surface of tumor cells not found on corresponding normal cells, the most commonly used assays are whole-cell binding assays using either live or glutaraldehyde-fixed cells either in suspension or attached to plastic. Cells from various sources are screened in replica, and the specificity of binding is assessed using positive and negative controls.

The cells are incubated with test MAb, washed, and incubated with a second antibody to mouse immunoglobulins, which is either radioactively labeled with ^{125}I or linked to an enzyme such as β-galactosidase, alkaline phosphatase, glucose oxidase, or horseradish peroxidase. After unbound second antibody is washed away, bound radioactivity is determined by counting or autoradiography, or the cells are incubated in the presence of enzyme substrates that yield colored reaction products. The method yields quantitative data on the extent of binding of the test MAb to the various cell types. Glutaraldehyde-fixed cells can be post-fixed in alcohol or acetone so that intracellular as well as cell surface antigens can be detected. For example, whole-cell binding assays have been used to produce monoclonal antibodies reactive with myeloid leukemia cells (Dicke et al., 1982; Johnson and Shin, 1983), small cell lung carcinoma cells (Minna et al., 1981), breast carcinoma cells (Colcher et al., 1981), and colorectal carcinoma cells (Herlyn et al., 1979). Glassy et al. (1983) have recently described a more sensitive, more versatile, and faster enzyme immunofiltration assay in whch whole cells or solubilized antigens are immobilized on glass fiber filters. This method utilizes a filtration manifold as an incubation filtration device. Other whole-cell binding assays use screening on a fluorescence-activated cell sorter (Parks et al., 1979) or microscopic immunofluorescence (Boucheix et al., 1983), both of which allow analysis at the single-cell level.

b. Immunohistology. Indirect immunohistology is the screening method of choice for MAb to antigens exhibiting a recognizable subcellular localization, particularly if their solubilization characteristics are unknown or if the primary purpose is to select antibodies that can be used for immunohistochemistry. Cyto-centrifuge slides, cryostat sections, or formaldehyde-fixed, paraffin-embedded sections are fixed with acetone or methanol, then incubated with test MAb, followed by washing and addition of an indicator antibody that has been conjugated to a fluorochrome or to an enzyme (such as peroxidase or alkaline phosphatase) that yields an insoluble reaction product. Naiem et al. (1982) have emphasized that immunohistological screening on cryostat tissue sections has particular value in identifying antibodies to tissue structures that are difficult to solubilize, such as basement membranes, in providing information on specificity of binding to surfaces of different target cell types present in the section, and can provide a rigorous test that the hybridoma subclones are making the desired antibody. Epstein and Clevenger (1984) have used this method to obtain monoclonal antibodies to nuclear antigens, and we have used indirect immunofluorescence to identify MAb for nucleoli (Davis et al., 1983a) and for intracellular mitosis-specific proteins (Davis et al., 1983b).

c. Binding to Solubilized Antigens. If the antigens have been characterized, are known to be soluble, and can be purified, the most sensitive screening method is a radiolabeled or enzyme-linked immunosorbent assay in which the antigens are immobilized on microtiter plates (Hedin *et al.*, 1982a), immunoassay cuvets (Chee *et al.*, 1982), or nitrocellulose paper (Hawkes *et al.*, 1982). Once the antigens are immobilized, the assay is completed as for the whole-cell binding assay. This assay has been used to screen for antibodies to carcinoembryonic antigen (Kupchik *et al.*, 1981; Hedin *et al.*, 1982a), α-fetoprotein (Uotila *et al.*, 1980), placental alkaline phosphatase (Slaughter *et al.*, 1981), and cytochrome *P*-450 (Park *et al.*, 1982). The assay can also be used to screen for MAb to unpurified and unidentified soluble antigens, as used by Clarke *et al.* (1982) to screen for MAb to marker antigens for prostatic acinar cells in culture. In contrast, Locker and Motta (1983) have immobilized hybridoma supernatant immunoglobulins on diazobenzyloxymethyl paper; they used ^{125}I-labeled antigen.

4. Subcloning and Mass Production of Antibodies

As soon as a hybridoma culture is found to be positive for a desired antibody, the hybridoma should be subcloned immediately. Antibody-producing hybridoma clones may be overgrown in a culture by cells of another clone in wells containing two or more colonies or by nonproducing variants. Nonproducing variants may arise by loss of the chromosomes carrying genes for immunoglobulin or for drug selection as described earlier (Section II,A,2).

Three essentially different methods have been used for subcloning. Limiting dilution is the most commonly used method: hybridoma cells are plated at a dilution so that there is only one viable cell per well, usually in the presence of unstimulated or irradiated spleen or peritoneal exudate cells (Reading, 1982) or monocytes (Brodin *et al.*, 1983). Subcloning has also been successfully accomplished by plating cells in semisolid agar (Goding, 1980) and by selection of individual antibody-producing cells using the fluorescence-activated cell sorter (Parks *et al.*, 1979).

Large quantities of MAb may be prepared either in tissue culture or by growing the hybridoma as a tumor in mice. Production in cell culture yields antibodies that are strictly monoclonal, particularly if serum-free media are used (Murakami *et al.*, 1982; Cleveland *et al.*, 1983). Underwood *et al.* (1983) have used serum-containing medium depleted of staphylococcal protein A-binding proteins to produce MAb with protein A affinity. Large-scale production in tissue culture has been accomplished by Nilsson *et al.* (1983), who used hybridoma cells trapped in agar microbeads. Fazekas de St. Groth (1983) described the automated production of monoclonal antibodies in serum-free medium in a cytostat. Antibody yields of 0.64 to 43.25 mg immunoglobulin/day were obtained from 500-ml cultures of cells at about 10^6 cells/ml.

Large quantities of antibody may also be obtained by injecting the malignant hybridoma clones into syngeneic mice (Zola and Brooks, 1982). Subcutaneous injections give rise to solid tumors, and antibody is released into the serum. Intraperitoneal injections give rise to ascites tumors yielding fluids rich in antibodies. Tumors generally take 7–14 days to grow, even if the animal has been immunosuppressed or pristane primed. Antibody yields usually range from 1 to 10 mg/ml in the presence of many other mouse serum proteins, including normal mouse immunoglobulins. Nevertheless, the hybridoma-produced MAb is the major constituent. Witte and Ber (1983) have used intrasplenic inoculation of as few as 10^4 hybridoma cells in unprimed mice to obtain efficient hybridoma ascites production.

For many purposes, culture fluid or ascites fluid may be used without antibody purification. However, for labeling with radioactive or fluorescent tags, or for injection into humans, purification of antibody by standard methods (Zola and Brooks, 1982) is required.

B. Human Monoclonal Antibodies

Human MAb have been produced by the immortalization of lymphocytes from peripheral blood (Croce et al., 1980; Eisenbarth et al., 1982), lymph nodes draining tumors (Sikora and Wright, 1981; Glassy et al., 1983), lymphocytes infiltrating tumors (Sikora et al., 1982), and other lymphoid tissues such as tonsils (Chiorazzi et al., 1982) and spleen (Olsson and Kaplan, 1980). Technical aspects have been reviewed (Cambon-de-Mouzon and Olsson, 1983; Olsson et al., 1983; Olsson and Kaplan, 1983). Primary immunization of human lymphocytes in vitro has not yet yielded human hybridomas (Kozbor and Roder, 1983), but nonspecific mitogenic stimulation of lymphocytes from immune donors (Shoenfeld et al., 1982) and secondary in vitro immunization of cells from previously immunized donors (Osband et al., 1982; Kozbor and Roder, 1983) have been successful. Two methods for human lymphocyte immortalization are available: fusion to human myeloma cells in culture, and EBV-induced transformation.

1. Advantages of Human MAb Compared to Mouse MAb

There are two main advantages in using human MAb for the diagnosis and treatment of cancer. Human antibodies are clearly preferable for serotherapy to prevent sensitization with xenoantisera. Although the magnitude of the immune responses to mouse MAb in patients treated with it compares favorably with responses observed with conventional serotherapy (Nadler et al., 1980c), many of the patients to whom mouse MAb have been administered for diagnosis or therapy have developed some anti-mouse immunoglobulin (Farrands et al., 1982; Sears et al., 1982c) that has apparently contributed to less marked uptake of diagnostic antibodies in the tumors (Larson *et al.*, 1983) and to the failure of therapy in some cases (Dillman *et al.*, 1982a,b). Human antibodies are therefore also preferable for radioimmunodetection of tumor if repeated scans are anticipated.

It may also be expected that the human response to polymorphic surface determinants may be to a wider range of antigens than the immunodominant determinants recognized by the mouse. Tumor-specific or tumor-associated antigens may be much easier to identify using human MAb. Patients certainly respond to their own tumors, but the efficacy of the immune response may be variable.

Other advantages in using human MAb include the possibility of using autoantibodies to select anti-idiotype antibodies to suppress autologous or transplantation antigens, and obtaining basic knowledge about the spectrum of the human antibody repertoire.

Although there is no readily available system for growth of human hybridomas as ascites fluids, the use of a cytostat as described by Fazekas de St. Groth (1983) could be used to produce large quantities of human MAb. Alternatively, nude mice or immunosuppressed mice could be used.

2. Cell Lines Available for Human Hybridomas

Olsson and Kaplan (1980) first reported a human–human hybridoma producing human MAb. A number of human cell lines have been used as fusion partners for the production of human hybridomas (reviewed by Kozbor and Roder, 1983). All of the human lines presently available secrete some immunoglobulin, and none of these is clearly superior in terms of fusion frequency, cloning efficiency, and rate, efficiency, or class of immunoglobulin produced. Four available cell lines are listed in Table II. The KR-4 cell line of Kozbor *et al.* (1982) has been selected from the HPRT⁻ GM 1500 6TG-2 cell line used by Croce *et al.* (1980) and is doubly marked with ouabain resistance. This cell line will probably become widely used as the combination of EBV transformation and fusion with a human myeloma parental cell line becomes more widespread (see later). Cote *et al.* (1983) compared the LICR-LON-HMy2 cell line with the SKO-007 cell line and found that although there was a four-fold difference in the frequency of hybridoma clones, the numbers of immunoglobulin secretors and classes were comparable.

3. Transformation of Human Lymphocytes with Epstein–Barr Virus

Miller and Lipman (1973) reported that EBV-containing culture supernatants from marmoset cells were able to transform normal human peripheral blood lymphocytes. This methodology was put to use to obtain human monoclonal antibodies (Luzzati *et al.*, 1977; Steinitz *et al.*, 1977). Two strategies are in use. One strategy depends on the selection or enrichment of antigen-binding lymphocytes, which are then transformed by EBV (Steinitz *et al.*, 1977, 1979, 1980; Crawford *et al.*, 1983a). This method can be used to select for various classes of antibody produced (Steinitz and Klein, 1980). This method also selects for the amount of surface immunoglobulin of B cells before fusion. However, it is not yet known what the relationship is between the amount of surface immunoglobulin and the amount of secretory immunoglobulin. Therefore, Rosen *et al.* (1983) advocate the transformation of all the B cells and subsequent cloning and testing of supernatants for antibody.

Until recently, transformation of lymphocytes with EBV was not widely used to produce human MAb, because antibody production is relatively unstable and the quantity is frequently low (Kozbor and Roder, 1983). Kozbor *et al.* (1982) have used a combination of EBV immortalization followed by fusion with a human myeloma cell line to increase the stability and the amount of antibody production. To do this they devised a method to select against the immortal EBV-transformed cells in the fusion mixture by developing the doubly marked KR-4 cell line, which is resistant to ouabain. Since ouabain resistance is a dominant trait, only the hybrids survive in a fusion mixture in the presence of aminopterin (kills the KR-4 cells) and ouabain (kills the EBV-transformed lymphocytes). The hybridomas produced four- to eightfold more antibody than the EBV-transformed parental cells and have remained stable.

C. Antibodies with Dual Specificities

Multivalent antibodies with dual specificities may become very important in cancer therapy, particularly in using antibodies to deliver drugs or toxins (Raso, 1982), or in cases where two antibodies may be able to bind with higher affinity or exert more of an effect than either alone (Jonker *et al.*, 1983a; Ehrlich *et al.*, 1982). There are two ways of preparing antibodies with dual specificities. IgG molecules with two different binding sites can be prepared by disulfide reduction and reannealing of a mixture of the antibodies (Ghetie and Moraru, 1983). An alternative method would be the fusion of two antibody-producing hybridomas to produce a "quadroma" (Reading, 1983). Selection of the hybrids from such a fusion would of course require selectable markers in the two parental cell lines. For example, hybridomas of the KR-4 cell line could be selected that are ouabain resistant but have segregated the HPRT$^+$ gene contributed by the lymphocyte parent, since none of the drug-resistant genes are linked to antibody production. Such cells could then be fused with any other human hybridoma line.

III. DIAGNOSTIC USES OF MONOCLONAL ANTIBODIES

Conventional antisera are currently used in three areas for diagnosis of cancer: (1) serological assays for tumor-associated antigens, such as carcinoembryonic antigen (CEA), α-fetoprotein (AFP), acidic isoferritins, and for assays of circulating antigen-specific immune complexes, (2) immunohistopathology for tumor-associated antigens as well as for determining the cell type of the tumor itself, and (3) tumor localization, using total-body scintigraphy. MAb can be expected to replace conventional antisera in all of these applications. At the very least, the constant supply of antibodies of identical structure, behavior, and binding characteristics offers an advantage over conventional antisera, provided that the MAb chosen have high affinity and high specificity. MAb to CEA or placental alkaline phosphatase have compared favorably with conventional antisera in the clinic (Mach *et al.*, 1981; Naritoku and Taylor, 1982; Wahl *et al.*, 1983). Moreover, the exquisite specificity of MAb for single epitopes may identify individual antigenic determinants on the tumor-associated antigens that are more specific for tumor tissues. The greatest potential of MAb, however, is in uncovering new antigens: tumor-specific or tumor-associated antigens, and antigens on normal cells that can be used to determine the tissue or cell type in which tumor originated.

A. Serological Markers

Serological detection of tumor-specific or tumor-associated antigens is useful for early diagnosis of disease by screening risk groups, as well as in diagnosis, prognosis, and disease monitoring. For example, antibodies to AFP have been used to screen patients with cirrhosis of the liver for hepatoma (Lehmann and Wegener, 1979), since AFP is a characteristic marker for hepatoma. The concentration of CEA in the serum correlates with tumor mass and is a useful marker for monitoring at least a subset of patients with colorectal carcinoma to detect early recurrence (NIH consensus statement: Goldenberg *et al.*, 1981). Although AFP and CEA are not tumor specific, they are tumor associated, and clinically useful, both in assessing the extent of disease and in determining tumor type. MAb to AFP (Uotila *et al.*, 1980) and CEA (Accolla *et al.*, 1980; Kupchik *et al.*, 1981; Hedin *et al.*, 1982a) that have very-high-affinity binding have been produced. Moreover, the MAb to CEA bind to at least six different epitopes, suggesting the possibility that the clinical usefulness of CEA might be improved by increasing the disease-related specificity (Hedin *et al.*, 1983).

Another serological marker for colorectal, gastric, and pancreatic carcinoma has been described by Koprowski *et al.* (1981). The antigen is a glycolipid (Falk *et al.*, 1983) present in the sera of the cancer patients and, like CEA, can be used for longitudinal evaluation of patients (Herlyn *et al.*, 1982; Sears *et al.*, 1982a). Steplewski *et al.* (1981) have also reported that four glycolipid antigens characteristic of colon carcinoma and five glycoprotein antigens of melanoma are shed into tissue culture medium. These results suggest that a number of tumor-associated antigens that have been detected at the surface of tumor cells may be released into the serum, where they could be used as markers. However, antigens that are also present on normal cells may appear in the circulation only when there are tumors of those cell types. For example, circulating human mammary epithelial antigens have been detected in patients with breast cancer (Ceriani *et al.*, 1982).

B. Immunohistology

Tumor pathology is the cornerstone of diagnosis, classification, and subsequent therapy, and MAb will be of enormous value in this area. As described earlier (Section II, A,3,a), most of the assays used to detect MAb are whole-cell binding assays, and most of the MAb so far described react with previously unrecognized and undefined antigens. Some of these MAb are to tumor-associated antigens and can be used to distinguish tumor cells from normal cells of the same cell type (Koprowski *et al.*, 1979, 1981). Some of these MAb are antibodies to normal cell antigens that are also present in or on tumor cells. These antigens can be used to distinguish different tissue or lineage origins for tumors that are morphologically similar (Pizzolo *et al.*, 1980) and to describe the differentiation status of the tumor (Greaves, 1981). They can also be used to detect metastatic tumor cells in distant sites, such as cells with breast epithelial markers in lymph nodes or bone marrow (Foster *et al.*, 1982a,b). The variability in individual epitope expression by tumors (Albino *et al.*, 1981; Wikstrand *et al.*, 1983) and the availability of multiple MAb with characteristic binding to different tumor or tissue types will lead increasingly to the use of panels of MAb for diagnostic immunohistology (Jonak *et al.*, 1982; Kemshead *et al.*, 1983a).

The effect of the fixation method on the reactivity of antibodies is usually much more pronounced for MAb than for conventional antisera, so that some MAb that bind to alcohol-fixed cryostat sections do not bind to formaldehyde-fixed, paraffin-embedded sections (Foster *et al.*, 1982b; Frankel *et al.*, 1982; Hancock *et al.*, 1982; Naritoku and Taylor, 1982). Unless the MAb used for immunohistology are screened on cells that are also pretreated in the same way, there is no way of knowing whether an individual antibody will react. In any case, it is certain that MAb of interest for immunohistology will be produced with other goals in mind as well, such as treatment. Therefore, the optimum conditions for use of each MAb will need to be determined before use. Nevertheless, some potentially interesting antibodies do not work at all in immunohistology (Papsidero *et al.*, 1983).

1. Tumor-Associated Antigens

No antibody yet produced has been proven to be completely tumor specific, able to distinguish dysplastic lesions from *in situ* carcinoma, and able to react with all kinds of tumor cells (Old, 1981). A pancarcinoma antigen detected by a MAb has been described (Ashall *et al.*, 1982; McGee *et al.*, 1982; Woods *et al.*, 1982), but results from several laboratories (Burnett *et al.*, 1983; Krausz *et al.*, 1983; Pallesen *et al.*, 1983; Simpson *et al.*, 1983) show that it is not as specific for malignant neoplasms as originally thought. Colcher *et al.* (1981) have also described some MAb that react with a broad spectrum of carcinomas. A human malignancy-associated nucleolar antigen has been detected in a wide variety of tumor cell types and not in normal cells (Davis *et al.*, 1979, 1983a; Busch *et al.*, 1979), but MAb to this antigen have not yet been reported, and the rabbit antisera so far utilized for detection of this antigen have been subject to batch-to-batch variability. They also could not be made as widely available as MAb can be.

Many MAb have been described that react with cells of a specific tumor type, with little or no reactivity to corresponding normal cells (reviewed by Mitchell and Oettgen, 1982). Some of the tumor-associated antigens of this type are included in Table III. For example, Sikora and Wright (1981) produced human MAb from patients with lung cancer that reacted with membranes from lung cancer cells but not with membranes from normal lung tissue of the same patient. While many of the antigens recognized have not yet been characterized biochemically, those that have been characterized have been either high molecular weight proteins, often with sugar moieties containing the antigenic sites, or nonproteinaceous gangliosides or glycolipids. For example, Soule *et al.* (1983) prepared MAb to breast carcinoma cell lines that react with a phosphorylated glycoprotein of 126 kilodaltons that was not detectable in normal mammary epithelium or control cell lines. Magnani *et al.* (1982) described a marker for gastrointestinal cancer that reacted with adenocarcinomas of the colon (12 of 12), stomach (4 of 5), and pancreas (4 of 7), but not with esophageal carcinomas (0 of 5), normal colon and gastric mucosae, pancreas, liver, kidney, or bone marrow. The antigen was identified as an oligosaccharide. In addition, antibodies raised to tumors of one tissue type are frequently but unpredictably detectable on cells of other tumor types (Chee *et al.*, 1982; Magnani *et al.*, 1982; Ball *et al.*, 1983). Some MAb seem to be able to distinguish benign from malignant lesions (Chee *et al.*, 1982; Teramoto *et al.*, 1982). For example, in one study using human MAb to breast carcinoma antigens, a moderate to strong reaction was elicited with primary (54 of 67) and metastatic (20 of 20) lesions, but not with benign lesions (3 of 20) (Teramoto *et al.*, 1982). It may be that the benign lesions that

TABLE III

Tumor-Associated Antigens of Human Cells Detected Using Monoclonal Antibody Probes

Tumor type	Antigen identity[a]	Source of MAb	In serum	In tumors		In normal cells	References
				Same type	Other types		
Pancarcinoma	gp350, gp390 (Ca1)	Mouse	N.D.[b]	+	+	−	Ashall et al., 1982; McGee et al., 1982; Woods et al., 1982
	N.D.	Mouse	N.D.	+	+	+	Ved Brat et al., 1980
	N.D.	Mouse	N.D.	+	+	−	Colcher et al., 1981
Breast	gp80−>400	Mouse (2)[c]	N.D.	+	−	+	Burchell et al., 1983
	gpp126	Mouse	N.D.	+	+	−	Soule et al., 1983
	p220−400	Mouse	N.D.	+	+	−	Nuti et al., 1982
	N.D.	Mouse (11)	N.D.	+	±	−	Colcher et al., 1981
	N.D.	Mouse	N.D.	+	+	+	Papsidero et al., 1983
	N.D.	Mouse	N.D.	+	−	−	Papsidero et al., 1983
	N.D.	Mouse (5)	N.D.	+	N.D.	−	Schlom et al., 1982
	N.D.	Human	N.D.	+	+	−	Schlom et al., 1980, 1982; Wunderlich et al., 1981; Teramoto et al., 1982
Gastrointestinal Colorectal	p25 + p27	Mouse	+	+	−	−	Thompson et al., 1983
	gp200−370 (CEA)	Mouse	+	+	+	+	Accolla et al., 1980; Lockhart et al., 1980; Kupchik et al., 1981; Hedin et al., 1982a; Haskell et al., 1983

	Lacto-N-fuco-pentaose III	Rat	N.D.	+	—	—	Smedley et al., 1983
	Monosialo-ganglioside	Mouse	+	+	—	—	Brockhaus et al., 1982
		Mouse	N.D.	+	—	—	Koprowski et al., 1979, 1981; Magnani et al., 1981, 1982; Atkinson et al., 1982; Herlyn et al., 1982; Sears et al., 1982a; Lindholm et al., 1983
	Glycolipid	Mouse (3)	N.D.	+	—	+	Koprowski et al., 1979; Falk et al., 1983
	N.D.	Mouse (2)	N.D.	+	—	+	Herlyn et al., 1979; Atkinson et al., 1982; Burtin and Nardelli, 1983
	N.D.	Mouse	N.D.	—	—	—	Thompson et al., 1983
	N.D.	Mouse	N.D.	—	+	+	Thompson et al., 1983
	N.D.	Mouse	N.D.	+	+	—	Embleton et al., 1981; Farrands et al., 1982
Liver	gp65–70 (AFP)	Mouse	+	+	+	+	Tsung et al., 1980; Uotila et al., 1980
Pancreas	N.D.	Mouse	N.D.	+	+	—	Metzgar et al., 1982
Genitourinary							
Cervical	N.D.	Human	N.D.	+	+	—	Glassy et al., 1983
Choriocarcinoma	hCG	Mouse	+	+	—	+	Light et al., 1983
Germ cell	gp200	Mouse	N.D.	+	—	—	Williams et al., 1982
	Carbohydrate (SSEA-3)	Rat	N.D.	+	—	—	Shevinsky et al., 1982; Damjanov et al., 1982
	N.D.	Mouse	N.D.	+	—	+	Edwards et al., 1980

(continued)

43

TABLE III (*Continued*)

Tumor type	Antigen identity[a]	Source of MAb	In serum	In tumors Same type	In tumors Other types	In normal cells	References
Ovary	PI-ALP	Mouse	+	+	+	+	Johnson et al., 1981; Slaughter et al., 1981; McLaughlin et al., 1982, 1983
Prostate	N.D.	Mouse	N.D.	+	–	–	Bast et al., 1981
	p54	Mouse	N.D.	+	+	+	Ware et al., 1982; Webb et al., 1983
	PAP	Mouse	+	+	–	+	Choe et al., 1982; Lee et al., 1982; Lin et al., 1983
	N.D.	Human	N.D.	+	+	–	Glassy et al., 1983
Yolk sac	Carbohydrate (SSEA-1)	Mouse	N.D.	+	–	+	Solter and Knowles, 1978; Gooi et al., 1983
Leukemia							
Leukemia	p24	Mouse	N.D.	+	+	+	Kersey et al., 1981
	gp100	Rat	N.D.	+	–	+	Lebacq and Bazin, 1983
	N.D.	Mouse	N.D.	+	–	+	Ball et al., 1983
	N.D.	Mouse (8)	N.D.	+	–	–	Funderud et al., 1983
cALL	p65-J5	Mouse	N.D.	+	–	+	Ritz et al., 1980a; Liszka et al., 1981
T-ALL	p28	Mouse	N.D.	+	–	+	Levy et al., 1979
	p45	Mouse	N.D.	+	–	+	McMichael et al., 1979; Bradstock et al., 1980

Type	Marker	Species				References
	p65	Mouse	N.D.	+	+	Royston et al., 1980
AMML	N.D.	Mouse	N.D.	+	−	Deng et al., 1982; Seon et al., 1983
Myeloid	N.D.	Mouse	N.D.	+	−	Uchanska-Ziegler et al., 1981
	p44	Mouse	N.D.	−	−	Aota et al., 1983
	N.D.	Mouse	N.D.	+	N.D.	Johnson and Shin, 1983
Lymphoma	p20 + p75	Mouse	+	+	−	Nadler et al., 1980a
	Protein	Mouse	N.D.	+	+	Forster et al., 1982
Burkitt	Glycolipid	Rat	N.D.	+	−	Wiels et al., 1981
Lung	p11.5 + p25.5	Mouse	N.D.	+	−	Brenner et al., 1982
	p31	Mouse (2)	N.D.	+	+	Mulshine et al., 1983
	p119 + p149	Mouse	N.D.	+	+	Mazauric et al., 1982
	p126	Mouse	N.D.	+	+	Mazauric et al., 1982
	Lacto-N-fucopentaose III	Mouse	N.D.	+	+	Cuttitta et al., 1981; Minna et al., 1981; Huang et al., 1983a
	N.D.	Rat	N.D.	−	+	Minna et al., 1981
	N.D.	Mouse	N.D.	+	−	Brenner et al., 1982
	N.D.	Mouse (6)	N.D.	+	+	Brown and Moore, 1982
	N.D.	Mouse	N.D.	−	−	Brown and Moore, 1982
	N.D.	Human (9)	N.D.	+	N.D.	Sikora and Wright, 1981; Sikora et al., 1983
Neuroectodermal	OFA-1	Human	+	+	−	Irie et al., 1982
		Human	+	+	+	Irie et al., 1982
Astrocytoma	p145	Mouse	N.D.	+	+	Cairncross et al., 1982
	p265	Mouse	N.D.	+	+	Cairncross et al., 1982
	N.D.	Mouse (2)	N.D.	+	+	Cairncross et al., 1982
Glioma	N.D.	Mouse (2)	N.D.	+	−	Schnegg et al., 1981
	N.D.	Human (3)	N.D.	+	−	Sikora et al., 1982
	N.D.	Human (4)	N.D.	+	+	Sikora et al., 1982, 1983; Phillips et al., 1983

(continued)

TABLE III (*Continued*)

Tumor type	Antigen identity[a]	Source of MAb	In serum	In tumors Same type	In tumors Other types	In normal cells	References
Melanoma	p28	Mouse	N.D.	+	−	−	Steplewski et al., 1982
	p50–70	Mouse	N.D.	+	+	+	Dippold et al., 1980
	p60	Mouse	N.D.	+	+	−	Mitchell et al., 1982; Steplewski et al., 1982
	gp94	Mouse	N.D.	+	+	−	Imai et al., 1980
	gp95	Mouse	N.D.	+	+	+	Dippold et al., 1980
	p97	Mouse	N.D.	+	+	−	Brown et al., 1980; Woodbury et al., 1980; Larson et al., 1983
	p100	Mouse	N.D.	+	+	−	Bumol et al., 1982; Chee et al., 1982; Morgan and McIntyre, 1983
	p116 + p29 + p26 + p95	Mouse	N.D.	+	−	−	Koprowski et al., 1978; Steplewski et al., 1979; Mitchell et al., 1980, 1981; Thompson et al., 1982b
	gp150	Mouse	N.D.	+	+	+	Dippold et al., 1980
	p196	Mouse	N.D.	+	+	−	Steplewski et al., 1982
	gp250	Mouse	+	+	−	−	Reisfeld et al., 1980; Morgan et al., 1981; Morgan and McIntyre, 1983

Type	Antigen	Species					Reference
	p260 + p240 + p220	Mouse	N.D.	+	−	−	Koprowski et al., 1978; Mitchell et al., 1980
	Ganglioside–glycolipid	Mouse	N.D.	+	−	−	Dippold et al., 1980; Yeh et al., 1982
	HMW-MAA	Mouse (4)	+	+	−	−	Giacomini et al., 1983; Wilson et al., 1983
	Nevocellular	Mouse	N.D.	+	−	+	Sorg et al., 1983
	Nevocellular	Mouse	N.D.	+	+	−	Sorg et al., 1983
	Neural	Mouse	N.D.	+	+	+	Sorg et al., 1983
	Endothelial	Mouse	N.D.	+	+	+	Sorg et al., 1983
	Epidermal	Mouse	N.D.	+	+	+	Sorg et al., 1983
	N.D.	Mouse	N.D.	−	−	−	Yeh et al., 1979
	N.D.	Mouse (3)	N.D.	+	+	+	Carrel et al., 1980
Neuroblastoma	N.D.	Mouse	N.D.	+	−	−	Medrano et al., 1983
	N.D.	Mouse	N.D.	+	−	+	Kennett and Gilbert, 1979
Wilms' tumor	N.D.	Human	N.D.	+	+	−	Glassy et al., 1983
Sarcoma							
Histiocytoma	p102	Mouse	N.D.	+	+	−	Brown, 1983
Leiomyosarcoma	N.D.	Mouse	N.D.	+	−	−	Deng et al., 1981
Osteogenic	N.D.	Mouse	N.D.	+	+	+	Embleton et al., 1981; Farrands et al., 1982
	N.D.	Mouse (3)	N.D.	+	−	−	Hosoi et al., 1982

[a] Abbreviations used: p, protein; gp, glycoprotein; gpp, phosphoglycoprotein; CEA, carcinoembryonic antigen; AFP, α-fetoprotein; hCG, human chorionic gonadotrophin; J5, antibody to cALL antigen; Pl-ALP, placental alkaline phosphatase; SSEA, stage-specific embryonic antigen; PAP, prostatic acid phosphatase; OFA, oncofetal antigen; HM-MAA, high molecular weight melanoma-associated antigen. Numbers represent (molecular weight of polypeptides) $\times 10^3$.

[b] N.D., not determined or not reported.

[c] Numbers in parentheses represent number of different clones isolated.

reacted were "preneoplastic," and detection of carcinoma *in situ* and even preneoplastic lesions may indeed be possible with MAb (Damjanov *et al.*, 1982).

Many of the MAb are diagnostically useful, and some have already been used therapeutically, although many of the MAb to tumor-associated antigens are of low affinity (Glassy *et al.*, 1983). In addition, as with CEA, there may be a low level of staining with normal cells. The J5 antibody to the common acute lymphocytic leukemia antigen (cALL), which has been used therapeutically, typically reacts with 3 to 5% of normal cells (Ritz *et al.*, 1980a). In other cases it is clear that a tumor-associated antigen can be a normal antigen that is modified. Nowinski *et al.* (1980) and Cooper (1982) have described a system in which a terminal sialic acid residue in normal cells is not added in neoplastic cells, exposing an immunodominant saccharide moiety. Brown (1983) has described a 102-kilodalton sarcoma-associated antigen found only in tumors or membranes of first-trimester fetuses but not in normal adult tissues. However, the antibodies detect a small amount of a normal liver protein of 107 kilodaltons.

2. Lineage Markers

MAb reacting with tissue-specific or lineage markers are also of evident diagnostic utility. Many such antibodies to various tissues have been described, including embryonic and germ cells (Williams *et al.*, 1982; Paiva *et al.*, 1983), brain and nerve tissue (Jonak *et al.*, 1982; Carter *et al.*, 1983; Trojanowski and Lee, 1983), breast (Foster *et al.*, 1982a,b; Menard *et al.*, 1983), prostate (Clarke *et al.*, 1982; Lillehoj *et al.*, 1982), pancreas (Eisenbarth *et al.*, 1982; Parsa *et al.*, 1982), thyroid (Bellet *et al.*, 1983), kidney and urinary tract (Chapman *et al.*, 1983; Garcia-Perez and Smith, 1983; Hancock and Atkins, 1983), and melanocytes (Dippold *et al.*, 1980). There are large panels of MAb to various blood cell types, such as lymphocytes (Trucco *et al.*, 1978; Kung *et al.*, 1979; Lampson and Levy, 1979; McMichael *et al.*, 1979; Brooks *et al.*, 1980; Stashenko *et al.*, 1980; Abramson *et al.*, 1981; Forster *et al.*, 1981; Nadler *et al.*, 1980a, 1981a,b; Anderson *et al.*, 1983; Chan *et al.*, 1983; Kasai *et al.*, 1983; Rumpold *et al.*, 1983; Tilden *et al.*, 1983; Zola *et al.*, 1983), monocytes and macrophages (Breard *et al.*, 1980; Mannoni *et al.*, 1982; Bettelheim *et al.*, 1982; Nunez *et al.*, 1982; Clement *et al.*, 1983; Dimitriu-Bona *et al.*, 1983; Flotte *et al.*, 1983; Gooi *et al.*, 1983; Huang *et al.*, 1983a; Russell *et al.*, 1983; Skubitz *et al.*, 1983; Talle *et al.*, 1983), platelets and megakaryocytes (McEver *et al.*, 1980; Vainchenker *et al.*, 1982; McGregor *et al.*, 1983), and endothelial cells (Auerbach *et al.*, 1982), as well as MAb to erythrocyte antigens (Brockhaus *et al.*, 1981; Crawford, *et al.*, 1983b; Finan *et al.*, 1983; Hansson *et al.*, 1983; Young *et al.*, 1983) and globin (Stamatoyannopoulos *et al.*, 1983). The MAb to human lymphocytes have been grouped into phenotypic clusters (Beverley, 1983; Funderud *et al.*, 1983; McKenzie and Zola, 1983). MAb to antigens of the major histocompatibility locus are also being developed (Nadler *et al.*, 1981c; Daar and Fabre, 1983).

As with the tumor-associated antigens, many of these antigens have been identified as carbohydrates or glycolipids like the blood group antigens that are found on many cell types (Gooi *et al.*, 1983; Hakomori, 1983; Huang *et al.*, 1983b; Menard *et al.*, 1983), or are yet to be characterized biochemically.

MAb to antigens shared on normal and tumor cells are being used in various ways for cancer diagnosis. One of the most obvious uses is identifying the phenotype or differentiation state of the abnormal cells. For example, studies have been done to identify the nature of the cells in Hodgkin's disease (Aisenberg and Wilkes, 1982), or to describe the phenotype of hairy cells (Janckila *et al.*, 1983; Worman *et al.*, 1983). Lymphocyte markers on cells of chronic (Perri *et al.*, 1983) and acute lymphocytic leukemia (Greaves, 1981; Foon *et al.*, 1982; Knowles and Halper, 1982; Martin *et al.*, 1982; Venuta *et al.*, 1983; Warnke and Link, 1983), and malignant lymphoma (Aisenberg and Wilkes, 1981; Habeshaw *et al.*, 1983) have been used to phenotype the cells in an effort to correlate differentiation markers and treatment efficacy (Reinherz *et al.*, 1980; Bernard *et al.*, 1981; van der Reijden *et al.*, 1983). Other studies have demonstrated unusual constellations of markers on leukemia cells (Bettelheim *et al.*, 1982; Armitage *et al.*, 1983; Foa *et al.*, 1983). Naiem *et al.* (1983) used MAb to dendritic reticulum cells to distinguish cases of follicular lymphoma of germinal center cell origin from B-cell lymphomas of nongerminal center cell origin. Although the dendritic reticulum cells are not lymphoma cells, their presence or absence in the lesion determined by using the MAb was diagnostic for lymphoma of germinal center cell origin.

MAb to lymphocyte subsets are also being used to evaluate the effect of disease and therapy on the immunological competence of cancer patients (Bernengo *et al.*, 1983; Mills and Cawley, 1983). Robbins and Fudenberg (1983) commented on this work, emphasizing the surprising level of complexity of the regulatory interactions among T-cell subsets that has been revealed using MAb.

Another common diagnostic application of MAb to normal cell antigens is their use in differentiating anaplastic carcinomas from high-grade lymphomas (Pizzolo *et al.*, 1980). Battifora and Trowbridge (1983) demonstrated the utility of such an approach using a single MAb to a leukocyte common antigen found on hematopoietic cells: lymphomas were positive for the antigen (40 of 40), whereas nonlymphomatous tissue samples were negative (110 of 110).

Similarly, MAb specific for individual types of cells can be used to demonstrate the presence of malignant tumor cells in the blood or bone marrow (Dearnaley *et al.*, 1981). For example, Jonak *et al.* (1982) used MAb to detect neuroblastoma cells in the bone marrow. MAb to epithelial cells have been used to distinguish carcinoma cells from reactive mesothelial cells in serous effusions

(Epenetos *et al.*, 1982a). The early detection of metastatic cells may be important for starting systemic therapy early.

MAb to blood group and major histocompatibility antigens may be useful in the evaluation of the degree of malignancy. Several studies have reported a correlation between the increasing degree of malignancy and the progressive loss or increasing expression of these antigens on colorectal cancer cells. Brockhaus *et al.* (1981) and Finan *et al.* (1983) noticed that the expression of the Le[b] and other blood group antigens in gastrointestinal carcinomas was decreased as the degree of malignancy increased. Similar studies have been reported using MAb to HLA and Ia antigens of the major histocompatibility locus, where antigen expression in malignant and some premalignant lesions was increased (Ruiter *et al.*, 1982; Thompson *et al.*, 1982a). Daar and Fabre (1983) demonstrated the anomalous patchy expression of HLA-DR on some colorectal cancer cells, although HLA-DR is absent from normal colorectal epithelium. They suggested that the presence of HLA-DR might augment the immunogenicity of tumor-specific antigens. However, HLA-ABC were absent from tumors of very poor prognosis. Daar and Fabre (1983) suggested that the absence of HLA-ABC from these tumors might contribute to the poor prognosis because of the MHC restriction phenomenon that requires the simultaneous presence of both HLA-ABC self and target antigens; the absence of HLA-ABC might render the cancer cells no longer susceptible to cytotoxic T-cell action.

MAb to major histocompatibility antigens may also prove to be useful in identifying persons at risk for some types of cancer. For example, Winchester *et al.* (1983) have shown an association of susceptibility to hairy cell leukemia, chronic lymphocytic leukemia, and Hodgkin's lymphoma with some Ia determinants, suggesting that human major histocompatibility locus gene products can influence susceptibility to some kinds of cancer, a relationship similar to the defined association between the major histocompatibility haplotype and leukemogenesis in the mouse.

3. Panels of Monoclonal Antibodies

As more MAb are produced and characterized, panels of MAb will be used increasingly for diagnosis. One of the reasons for the use of panels of MAb is the presence of different markers on different subsets of cells. It is clear that the diagnosis of various classes of acute lymphoblastic leukemia depends on the use of a number of monoclonal antibodies, since each type or differentiation stage of lymphocyte has been shown to carry a characteristic combination of MAb-defined markers (Greaves, 1981; Foon *et al.*, 1982; van der Reijden *et al.*, 1983). Another reason for the use of panels of MAb is the heterogeneity of expression of antigens on tumor cells. Albino *et al.* (1981) established six melanoma cell lines from the same patient, and showed that only one of them bound antibodies to a tumor-specific antigen. Wikstrand *et al.* (1983) have demonstrated the persistence of low-antigenic clones in a glioma cell line. The occasional and anomalous cross-reactivity of MAb is another reason for the use of panels of MAb in diagnosis. It is also possible that the malignant cells might be shown to have a unique combination of markers, that could only be demonstrated with panels of antibodies. Thus, Jonak *et al.* (1982) used a combination of monoclonal antibodies to detect neuroblastoma cells in the bone marrow. Kemshead *et al.* (1983a) used a panel of eight MAb to neuroblastoma antigens and five MAb to leukemia-lymphoma antigens to differentiate between leukemia and infiltrating neuroblastoma in the bone marrow of two patients. Conventional histopathological investigations had failed to give a clear answer. One case was defined as leukemia on the basis of reactivity of two of five anti-leukemia MAb and zero of eight antineuroblastoma MAb. The other was defined as neuroblastoma, with reactivity of seven of eight antineuroblastoma MAb, but zero of five antileukemia MAb. Gatter and Mason (1982) used a panel of seven MAb to six antigens, including intracellular intermediate-filament antigens, and indirect immunofluorescence to arrive at the unequivocal diagnosis of high-grade lymphoma or nonlymphoma in five very difficult cases.

C. Radiolocalization of Tumors (Tumor Imaging)

MAb can be used in the diagnosis of malignant tumors by tumor imaging. Radiolabeled antibody, when injected into the patient, homes in on the tumor and localizes within it (Pressman and Korngold, 1953). The label is then detected by external scanning or scintigraphy. Conventional antisera to CEA, AFP, and chorionic gonadotrophin have been used in immunodetection of tumors (Scheinberg *et al.*, 1982; Solter *et al.*, 1982). In principle, an MAb to any antigen present on tumor cells in relatively greater abundance than on normal cells could be used for tumor imaging. The application of radioimmunodetection is particularly appropriate when a tumor marker detectable in the blood indicates the presence of tumor, but the site of tumor is unknown (Goldenberg *et al.*, 1981). In practice, a nonspecific antibody with a different radiolabel is also injected, but does not specifically localize in the tumor; rather, it reveals the vascularization. These values are subtracted from those with the specific antibody to give localization of the specific antibody corrected for vascularization differences in different tissues (Goldenberg *et al.*, 1981).

Much knowledge about tumor imaging with MAb has been accumulated in rodent model systems, in which external scintigraphy can be compared and confirmed with immunohistological techniques. Experiments with rodent tumors in rodents have achieved a 39- to 478-fold increase in labeling with specific antibody compared to normal tissues, nonspecific antibody, or antibody to antigenically different cells (Houston *et al.*, 1980; Levine *et al.*, 1980; Key *et al.*,

1983; Solter *et al.*, 1982; Scheinberg and Strand, 1983). Tumor imaging at any time depended on the rate of clearance of MAb from the circulation and non-target tissues, as well as the rate of uptake, accretion, and residence time in tumors. All these variables are affected by vascular support and tumor size, as well as by antibody affinity. Targeting was rapid for tumor-specific antibodies, and optimal images were obtained early, 6–24 hr after antibody injection, within the $t_{1/2}$ of the antibody in blood. Bound antibody was rapidly catabolized and cleared in some cases by internalization of membrane-bound immunoglobulin. The isotype class of the MAb used affected the $t_{1/2}$ in the blood, but not the targeting and imaging. Antibody localization was dependent on the vascular anatomy of the tumor. Use of the more rapidly cleared F(ab)$_2$ minimized exposure and allowed for more rapid imaging.

Preclinical studies with human tumors have compared MAb with conventional antisera, and investigated accretion in tumors and clearance from serum of MAb. Several investigators have localized xenografts of human tumors in nude or immunosuppressed mice using antibodies to CEA (Hedin *et al.*, 1982b; Wahl *et al.*, 1983) or to cell surface antigens (Moshakis *et al.*, 1981; Herlyn *et al.*, 1983). Antibodies were labeled with ^{125}I or ^{131}I, and MAb localized 3- to 10-fold better than conventional antisera, sometimes facilitating localization without subtraction for the vascularization background. Bivalent F(ab)$_2$ fragments were again superior for imaging, facilitating clearance without affecting accretion. Liposomally entrapped (Begent *et al.*, 1982) or free (Goldenberg, 1983) second antibody also facilitated clearance of first antibody. Sears *et al.* (1982b) used surgical specimens of human colon for MAb perfusion and radioimmunolocalization *ex vivo*.

Rat (Smedley *et al.*, 1983), mouse (Mach *et al.*, 1981; Epenetos *et al.*, 1982b; Farrands *et al.*, 1982; Larson *et al.*, 1983), and human (Phillips *et al.*, 1983) MAb have been used to localize ovarian, breast, and colorectal carcinomas, gliomas, melanomas, and other tumors in patients. Monoclonal anti-CEA gave imaging results similar to those of polyclonal CEA (Mach *et al.*, 1981). Anti-mouse antibodies were detected in about half of the patients to whom mouse antibodies were administered (Farrands *et al.*, 1982; Larson *et al.*, 1983). No toxicity related to the anti-mouse immunoglobulins was observed, but the $t_{1/2}$ of subsequent antibody doses was decreased from 22 to 1 hr, with increased liver uptake and less marked tumor uptake (Larson *et al.*, 1983). Smedley *et al.* (1983) used MAb to colorectal carcinoma membranes to localize metastatic carcinoma in 13 of 16 colorectal cancer patients and three of four breast cancer patients; localized areas of uptake corresponded with known areas of disease. Larson *et al.* (1983) investigated metastatic melanoma in six patients using MAb to the p97 melanoma-associated antigen. All patients had positive scans, and 22 of 25 (88%) lesions larger than 1.5 cm were localized using injections of 1 mg of ^{131}I-labeled MAb. Epenetos *et al.* (1982b) used two MAb to tumor-associated antigens also present on the membranes of milk fat globules to detect primary and metastatic ovarian, breast, and gastrointestinal neoplasms in 20 patients. Some lesions detected by scintigraphy were not detectable by ultrasonography and X ray. Tumors became visible 3 min to 18 hr after injection of labeled antibody. On average, 0.6% of the injected amount of radiolabel localized in tumors.

If the suspected sites for tumor localization or metastasis are lymph nodes, delivery of MAb to the lymphatics by interstitial or subcutaneous injection, rather than by intravenous injection, may speed up localization with a lower antibody dose (Weinstein et al., 1982; Parker et al., 1983). Many of the problems of differential tissue vascularization and the side effects of circulating antigen, including deposition of antigen–antibody complexes in the kidney, can be avoided. Weinstein et al. (1982) were able to label <1 mg of tissue, with less antibody bound by the entire liver than by the draining popliteal node, which accounted for 32% of the dose absorbed within 2 hr of injection into the footpads. Injection into several subcutaneous sites could effectively deliver antibody to most of the lymphatic system.

As with immunohistological methods, radioimmunodetection of cancer using MAb is likely to be improved by using mixtures of MAb or "engineered polyclonal antibodies" that react with different determinants on the same antigen, different antigens on the same cells, or heterogeneous cell populations in the tumor (Goldenberg, 1983). Use of mixtures of two MAb for scintigraphic localization of colorectal and thyroid cancers has already been reported (Lumbroso et al., 1983; Chatal et al., 1983).

IV. THERAPEUTIC USES OF MONOCLONAL ANTIBODIES

Much of the work on MAb to tumor-associated antigens is aimed at the development of a new therapeutic modality: the use of MAb as the "magic bullet" envisioned by Ehrlich (see Davies, 1981). Cancer therapy using MAb is just beginning, but many of the principles and methods are already becoming clear. Clinical use of antibodies requires that they be highly specific and available in large amounts at high titer: these are precisely the qualities of MAb.

MAb can cause lysis or removal of tumor cells to which they bind by antibody-dependent cellular cytotoxity (Herlyn et al., 1979, 1980), complement-mediated cell lysis (Shouval et al., 1982), or opsonization, which promotes removal of antibody-coated cells by the reticuloendothelial system (Prentice et al., 1982). Chemotherapeutic drugs (Arnon and Sela, 1982; Baldwin et al., 1983) can be conjugated to MAb for targeting or encapsulated in lipsomes coupled to antibodies (Leserman et al., 1980, 1981), as can various toxins (Olsnes, 1981;

Thorpe and Ross, 1982) that have the advantage of being effective at levels of very few molecules per cell. Antibodies can also be used to bind to cell surfaces and receptors to change the activity of the cells (Trowbridge and Domingo, 1981), or conjugated to biological response modifiers such as interferon (Baldwin *et al.*, 1983). They thus could be used for immunomodulation (Evans *et al.*, 1981; Gilman *et al.*, 1983). Various factors influence the therapeutic efficiency of antibody treatment (Neville *et al.*, 1982; Ritz and Schlossman, 1982), including specificity and efficiency of binding to antigen, antibody distribution, sequestration and clearance when administered *in vivo,* antigenic modulation on the cells, presence of circulating antigen, and development of antibodies to determinants on the antibodies used for therapy. Although viruses in the MAb preparations used for therapy have been considered a potential hazard (Bartal *et al.*, 1982; Crawford *et al.*, 1983a), little toxicity associated with MAb therapy has been observed (Ritz and Schlossman, 1982).

A. *Ex Vivo* Treatment of Bone Marrow for Transplantation

Autologous and allogeneic bone marrow transplantations are being used to allow high-dose treatment regimens that would be lethal without bone marrow rescue. The therapeutic efficacy of allogeneic marrow transplantation, used especially for patients with leukemia, is decreased by graft-versus-host disease (GVHD), which is responsible for much of the toxicity associated with allogeneic transplantation and is fatal in 80% of cases when severe (Slavin and Santos, 1973). Nevertheless, a graft-versus-host response may also produce a significant antileukemic effect (Weiden *et al.*, 1981). The efficacy of high-dose therapy and autologous marrow transplantation is undermined by the presence of tumor cells in the bone marrow collected and saved for transplantation. The potential role for MAb in transplantation is the removal of tumor cells from autologous marrow and removal of the cells causing GVHD from allogeneic marrow. Alternatively, positive selection for the pluripotent stem cells needed for engraftment could be accomplished if MAb specific for stem cells were to be produced. Methodologies that could be used for positive selection include growth factor-coupled MAb (Block and Bothwell, 1983), magnetic microsphere-coupled MAb (Poynton *et al.*, 1983), and catalase-coupled MAb followed by H_2O_2 treatment (Basch *et al.*, 1983).

1. *Removal of T Cells from Allogeneic Transplants*

Although there may be three distinct and separable components to the graft-versus-host reaction defined in a mouse model system, at least two, and possibly all three, are T-cell mediated, and treatment with anti-T antibodies reduced fatalities by 85% (OKunewick *et al.*, 1982a,b). Treatment with antithymocyte globulin or anti-T-cell MAb can be prophylactically effective *in vivo* for elimination of circulating T cells by opsonization and removal by the reticuloendothelial system (Cosimi *et al.*, 1981; Rodt *et al.*, 1981, 1983; Chatenoud *et al.*, 1983). However, treatment of the marrow *in vitro* with MAb before transplant is the method of choice. Most of the MAb currently available are mouse MAb that may not work efficiently in humans *in vivo,* and treatment with mouse MAb may lead to the production of human anti-mouse antibodies. Moreover, the efficacy of the treatment can be monitored *in vitro*. Prentice *et al.* (1982) incubated allogeneic bone marrow with 1 mg/ml of OKT3, MAb that react with T cells, before marrow infusion into 17 transplant recipients. The treated marrow, including T cells, was transplanted, and opsonized T cells were slowly removed, apparently by the reticuloendothelial system. The incidence of GVHD was reduced to 18% (3 of 17), from 79% (11 of 14) for a similar group of patients with leukemia who received untreated allogeneic marrow. Sharp *et al.* (1983) investigated some of the parameters of T-cell removal from bone marrow using rabbit complement-mediated lysis with MAb to T cells *in vitro*. T cells were reduced from 6.5% of the nucleated cells to less than 1%, while stem cells forming colonies containing granulocytes and macrophages were not depleted, and in fact formed larger numbers of colonies *in vitro*. Therefore, removal of T cells from marrow for allogeneic transplantation can reduce the incidence of graft-versus-host disease, without affecting the ability of the transplanted marrow to repopulate the host.

2. Removal of Tumor Cells from Autologous Transplants

High-dose, whole-body chemotherapy and radiation therapy with autologous marrow rescue are emerging as accepted treatment modalities for metastatic solid tumors as well as for leukemia. Since 70–80% of patients with acute leukemia can be induced into complete morphological and clinical remission, and yet only 15–20% of these patients remain disease free for more than 5 years, the remission marrow of patients with leukemia that is stored for later autologous transplantation can be assumed to contain some leukemia cells (Keating *et al.*, 1980). These leukemia cells cannot be detected by standard morphological criteria but may be detectable by special methods (Hittelman *et al.*, 1983; Davis *et al.*, 1983a; Dicke *et al.*, 1983). Similarly, the use of MAb to tumor-associated and lineage-specific markers for diagnosis has also led to an increased detection of micrometastases of solid tumor cells in the marrow (Dearnaley *et al.*, 1981). Thus, MAb used to detect tumor cells may also be used in purging the marrow of tumor cells before infusion (reviewed by Poynton and Reading, 1983).

In addition to MAb-dependent complement-mediated lysis of tumor cells contaminating bone marrow (Buckman *et al.*, 1982; Kaizer *et al.*, 1982; Ritz *et al.*,

1982; Bast *et al.*, 1983; Baumgartner *et al.*, 1983a; Levy and Miller, 1983a), toxin-coupled MAb (Raso *et al.*, 1982; Filipovich *et al.*, 1983; Jansen *et al.*, 1983) and magnetic microsphere-coupled MAb (Poynton *et al.*, 1983) have been used to purge tumor cells from marrow.

In vitro marrow purging allows highly active rabbit complement to be added to the cell–antibody mixture; human complement is not as effective as rabbit complement (Bast *et al.*, 1983). Complement-fixing MAb specific for leukemia cells (Ritz *et al.*, 1982; Bast *et al.*, 1983), T cells (Kaizer *et al.*, 1982; Levy and Miller, 1983a), non-Hodgkin's lymphoma (Baumgartner *et al.*, 1983a,b), and breast and bladder carcinomas (Buckman *et al.*, 1982) have been used to lyse tumor cells specifically in the presence of marrow cells. Normal progenitor stem cells measured by colony formation in agar and methylcellulose were unaffected, and hematopoietic recovery was not delayed. Although it is still too early to evaluate the long-term therapeutic efficiency of this approach, six of eight patients with leukemia (Ritz *et al.*, 1982; Levy and Miller, 1983a) and four of five patients with lymphoma (Baumgartner *et al.*, 1983a,b; Levy and Miller, 1983a) have continued in remission for up to 20 mo and more. A 2-log decrease in tumor cells, present at concentrations up to 2×10^7 cells/ml in the presence of up to a 100-fold excess of normal bone marrow cells (up to 10^8 cells/ml), could be obtained under optimum conditions using three treatments of 30 min each (Bast *et al.*, 1983).

Only a fraction of the MAb that are potentially useful for cancer therapy is able to bind complement. For this reason, other methods for removal of tumor cells from marrow for transplantation have been developed. MAb have been conjugated to toxins (e.g., diphtheria toxin and ricin) to prepare immunotoxins with high specificity and potent cytotoxicity (Krolick *et al.*, 1980; Youle and Neville, 1980). Unlike drugs, even a few molecules of these toxins can effectively kill cells, since they act catalytically instead of stoichiometrically (Olsnes and Pihl, 1981; Olsnes, 1981). Immunotoxins can selectively kill 99–100% of their target cells (Gilliland *et al.*, 1980; Houston and Nowinski, 1981; Jansen *et al.*, 1982; Neville and Youle, 1982; Thorpe and Ross, 1982). In the presence of nontarget cells, antibody–toxin conjugates can exhibit specific cytotoxicity over a concentration range of 5 logs (Jansen *et al.*, 1983). Ricin and diphtheria toxins are composed of two polypeptide chains: chain A for toxicity and chain B normally used for lectin-type binding (Olsnes and Pihl, 1981). Since the B chain of ricin binds to galactose-containing receptors, this binding can be blocked by the addition of lactose (Youle and Neville, 1980). Alternatively, the A chain alone can be conjugated to antibodies. MAb conjugates with both ricin subunits have been shown to be more active although less selective (Neville and Youle, 1982). Different MAb may facilitate the entry of toxins into cells in different ways (Gilliland *et al.*, 1980), however, and the faster rates of cell kill achieved with MAb–ricinAB conjugates may be important with some antibodies, especially those with low affinities (Neville and Youle, 1982; Jansen et al., 1983). The parameters affecting toxicity and specificity of MAb–ricinA conjugates for human tumor cells in the presence of normal bone marrow cells have been investigated (Raso et al., 1982; Gorin et al., 1983; Jansen et al., 1983). The addition of NH_4Cl to lyse red blood cells potentiated specific killing of tumor cells at 10^{-10} to 10^{-13} M, whereas normal stem cells were not affected by up to 10^{-7} M. The method was effective at total cell concentrations up to 10^7 cells/ml. The bivalent $F(ab')_2$ conjugate was 70-fold better than the monovalent $F(ab)$; the increase was thought to be related to the bivalent's ability to induce modulation of the surface antigen and internalization of the antibody–toxin conjugates. In mouse model systems in which even one tumor cell can be fatal, injection of up to 10^4 antibody–ricin-treated tumor cells gave rise to tumors in only 3 of 20 animals (Krolick et al., 1982).

MAb can also be conjugated to magnetic compounds to remove tumor cells physically from bone marrow cells, thus circumventing such problems as toxicity and need for internalization that are observed with complement treatment or MAb conjugated to drugs or toxins. Methods for magnetic separation have been developed particularly for in vitro bone marrow purging. MAb conjugated to colloidal cobalt have been used to remove leukemia cells from bone marrow (Poynton et al., 1983; Poynton and Reading, 1983). The treatment and separation procedure required 3 hr and was used at a cell concentration of 10^8 cells/ml, of which 1–60% were antibody reactive before separation. Removal of antibody-reactive cells was effective over a 2-log range (limits of detection), stem cell toxicity could not be demonstrated, and four patients exhibited rapid engraftment with no toxicity. Kemshead et al. (1983b) used a panel of six MAb specific for a neuroblastoma cell line and developed a procedure to remove neuroblastoma cells from bone marrow. MAb conjugated to magnetic polystyrene spheres were used to remove 97–99% of the antibody-reactive cells without damage to normal stem cells. Engraftment after purging was observed in two of two patients from whose marrow neuroblastoma cells were removed using this procedure.

The results of bone marrow purging are promising, although the long-term therapeutic efficacy of this approach has yet to be evaluated.

B. Serotherapy

Passive immunization against tumor cells by infusion of MAb may decrease the population of tumor cells by antibody-dependent cellular cytotoxicity, complement-mediated cell lysis, or increased removal of opsonized cells by the reticuloendothelial system. The relative contribution of the various mechanisms is not known. In syngeneic mouse model systems, marked therapeutic effects and some cures have been observed, especially if the animals were treated when the tumor burden was low (Bernstein et al., 1980a; Kirch and Hammerling, 1981; Kennel et al., 1983). Vollmers and Birchmeier (1983) have recently described the use of MAb to the mouse B_{16} melanoma that blocked adhesion of the melanoma cells to plastic dishes *in vitro* and abolished metastatic lung colonization *in vivo*. MAb to cell surface glycolipids were also effective in suppressing tumor growth, and in one animal that developed a tumor, the tumor had a lower quantity of antigen, suggesting either antigenic modulation or selection of a low antigenic variant (Young and Hakomori, 1981). Therapy with IgG antibodies was more effective than with IgM antibodies and IgG2a antibodies better than IgG1, IgG2b, and IgG3 (Herlyn *et al.*, 1980; Bernstein *et al.*, 1980b; Kirch and Hammerling, 1981), although the reasons for this are not clear. In general, *in vitro* effectiveness exceeded *in vivo* effectiveness: antibody to the murine Thy-1 antigen blocked GVHD when incubated with marrow cells *in vitro*, but did not work *in vivo* in spite of high complement-fixing and cytolytic activity *in vitro*, longer *in vivo* half-life than rabbit antithymocyte globulin, and demonstrable binding to target cells (Thierfelder *et al.*, 1983). One particularly disturbing observation was that although therapy with MAb Lyt 2 suppressed the growth of the ERLD murine leukemia, it enhanced the growth of the EL 4 leukemia (Kirch and Hammerling, 1981). Thus, since the mechanisms involved in passive serotherapy are not well understood, some preclinical studies to avoid deleterious effects are required.

Two types of preclinical models have been described. Johnson and Shin (1983) used MAb that reacted with a normal human differentiation antigen on acute myelogenous leukemia cells and some undifferentiated, but not mature, normal myelomonocytic cells. The differentiation antigen is also found on the corresponding cells in rats. The antibody is an IgM, and it lyses leukemia cells *in vitro* in the presence of complement. Tumor growth was suppressed in rats challenged with 10^2 to 10^3 rat leukemia cells, and no side effects were observed. This study emphasizes the utility of MAb to antigens that also appear on normal cells, but not on normal stem cells. Other investigators have studied therapy of human tumors in nude mice and reported inhibition of tumor growth (Herlyn *et al.*, 1980; Herlyn and Koprowski, 1982; Shouval *et al.*, 1982).

There are now reports (reviewed by Levy and Miller, 1983a) of passive MAb serotherapy of 24 patients with leukemia or lymphoma (reviewed by Ritz and Schlossman, 1982), four patients with gastrointestinal tumors (Sears *et al.*, 1982c), and one patient with glioma (Watson *et al.*, 1983). Responses have been seen, and some problems affecting therapeutic efficacy have been defined. To date, all reported therapeutic trials have used mouse MAb, usually IgG2a, with the exception of the study of Watson *et al.* (1983), in which human MAb were used.

Nadler *et al.* (1980c) reported the treatment of a patient with diffuse, poorly differentiated, lymphocytic lymphoma with Ab89, an IgG2a that is specifically active against tumor cells *in vitro* according to complement-mediated cellular cytotoxicity and macrophage adherence tests. Two courses consisting of a total dose of 2 g were administered 1 mo apart. No free antibody could be detected in the serum at any time, which was thought to be a result of circulating tumor antigen. After each infusion, a transient decrease in circulating tumor cells and the rapid appearance of circulating dead cells suggested complement-dependent lysis, but ^{51}Cr-labeled, MAb-coated tumor cells were cleared slowly, suggesting reticuloendothelial system clearance by the liver. No toxicity was noted, even though the 2 g of antibody is above the normal range for development of serum sickness (Fisher *et al.*, 1982); however, the immune system of the patient may have been severely compromised. After each antibody infusion, a transient decrease in creatinine clearance was observed, consistent with deposition of immune complexes in the kidney, but returned to normal in 24 hr.

Eight patients with cutaneous T-cell lymphoma (Miller and Levy, 1981; Levy and Miller, 1983a) and eight with T-cell leukemia (Miller *et al.*, 1981; Levy and Miller, 1983a) were treated with MAb to normal differentiation antigens that also appear on tumor cells. Partial remissions were achieved by six of eight patients with lymphoma. One patient with lymphoma tolerated 17 treatments over 10 weeks with up to 20 mg MAb without toxicity and showed a good response of cutaneous lesions, but antibody-reactive cells persisted and complete remission was not achieved. The patients with leukemia received doses of up to 50 mg each. Transient reductions in white blood cell counts were observed in some patients, but not all; no lasting clinical benefit was observed, and cell counts returned to pretreatment levels in 24 hr. Moreover, although no circulating free antigen was detected in the serum of one patient before treatment, it was detected after each treatment, accompanied by a transient decline in creatinine clearance. Cutaneous pain, dyspnea, urticaria, and sporadic coagulopathy were observed in one patient each; otherwise no toxicity was reported. Anti-mouse MAb antibodies were observed in half the patients, but no evident toxicity was associated with them; however, renewed growth of the tumor in a patient who had obtained a partial remission was related to the appearance of anti-mouse antibodies.

MAb serotherapy has been used to treat four patients with non-T-cell acute lymphoblastic leukemia (Ritz *et al.*, 1981a,b). The J5 antibody to the common acute lymphoblastic leukemia (cALL) antigen was used. Patients were treated with multiple intravenous injections. Rapid, yet transient, declines of up to 90% of circulating leukemia blasts were observed, but elimination of bone marrow blasts was not. Leukemia cells were coated *in vivo* with J5 MAb and with complement C3, yet human complement could not lyse J5-coated cells *in vitro*, so clearance by the reticuloendothelial system may have been involved in the decrease in circulating blasts. Antigenic modulation on the blast cells was also apparent: before treatment with MAb, the circulating blasts were J5 positive, but most blasts after treatment were J5 negative, even though their numbers were at pretreatment levels. *In vitro* studies using J5-positive cell lines also showed antigenic modulation (Ritz *et al.*, 1980b).

Dillman *et al.* (1982a,b) have used T101 MAb, an antibody to a 65-kilodalton T-cell differentiation antigen, to treat two patients with end stage chronic lymphocytic leukemia. These MAb are cytolytic for leukemia cells *in vitro* with rabbit complement although not with human complement, and are not active in tests of antibody-dependent cellular cytotoxicity, when normal peripheral blood lymphocytes are used as effectors. One or three doses of antibody up to 12 mg/dose were administered. Levels of MAb in the sera were highest at the end of the infusion, but not detectable 2–4 hr later. After each treatment, the number of circulating cells exhibited a transient decrease, returning to surpass pretreatment levels. T101 MAb bound rapidly to, and saturated the binding sites of, the leukemia cells *in vivo*, but serum complement levels did not change. No evidence for free circulating antigen or antigenic modulation was obtained. Toxicity from which the patients subsequently recovered was associated with MAb infusion: the first patient developed an anaphylactoid reaction after the third (12 mg) dose, and the second patient experienced hypotension and dyspnea, rigors, and fever after the first (10 mg) dose.

The most successful application of therapy with MAb was reported by Miller *et al.* (1982a), who treated a patient with a nodular, poorly differentiated B-cell lymphoma using anti-idiotype IgG2b MAb reactive with the immunoglobulin on the surface of the lymphoma cells (Hatzubai *et al.*, 1981). Low levels (3.5 µg/ml) of idiotype protein in the form of an IgM pentamer were present in the patient's serum before MAb treatment. Their concentration correlated with the tumor burden, which was progressively increasing at the time MAb therapy began. Plasmapheresis before therapy to remove idiotype protein decreased the level to 0.75 µg/ml for 12 hr, after which time the idiotype level returned to baseline. Eight doses of MAb, totaling 0.5 g (up to 150 mg/dose), were administered over a 4-week period. Doses ≥15 mg dramatically decreased circulating idiotype protein, concomitant with the appearance of anti-idiotype MAb in the serum. Following the sixth dose (150 mg), serum idiotype became and remained undetectable, concomitant with a 50% reduction in tumor volume index. MAb were demonstrably bound to tumor cells in lymph nodes *in vivo*, but antigenic sites were not fully saturated. Therapy with MAb was discontinued after eight doses, the tumor continued to regress, and the patient has remained in remission (13+ mo). Anti-idiotype MAb were detectable for 3 weeks after the last antibody dose. No toxicity was associated with MAb therapy, and no anti-mouse antibody was detected. Complement-mediated cytolysis was not thought to be involved in tumor response, since a lytic effect with human complement could not be demonstrated *in vitro*, nor was any change in serum complement levels detected. The authors suggested the anti-idiotype MAb may have inhibited the proliferation of the B-cell lymphoma by a regulatory mechanism. Foon (1982) suggested the response may have been due to the removal of the stem cells for the malignant transformation, which may have represented only a small proportion of the lymphoma cells that bound MAb. Miller *et al.* (1982b) responded that B-cell tumors are renewed from pre-B cells, which lack surface immunoglobulins, and therefore would not react with anti-idiotype antibodies, citing work of Kubagawa *et al.* (1979).

One of the MAb that suppressed growth of human gastrointestinal tumors in nude mice (Herlyn *et al.*, 1980), mediated lysis of colorectal carcinoma cells *in vitro* by both human and mouse effector cells (Herlyn *et al.*, 1979), and specifically bound to tumor cells in perfused resected colons (Sears *et al.*, 1982b), has been investigated in phase I clinical trials of treatment for gastrointestinal tumors (Sears *et al.*, 1982c). Four patients with metastatic carcinoma were treated prior to tumor resection. Three received single intravenous MAb doses of 15, 150, and 180 mg. The fourth patient received four intravenous doses (15 mg–200 mg), plus autologous peripheral blood mononuclear cells preincubated with 67 mg MAb. Mouse MAb were detectable in the serum of all patients for 2 to 40 days after treatment. Circulating MAb were able to bind to cultured human carcinoma cells. The therapeutic effect of MAb was evaluable only in the fourth patient, because the other three patients required immediate resection. Antigen recognized by MAb was detected on sections of the primary gastric tumor and in liver and bone metastases. Although levels of CEA were normal, high levels of a circulating tumor antigen, identified as a monosialoganglioside, were detected using other MAb (Koprowski *et al.*, 1981; Magnani *et al.*, 1981), and remained high throughout therapy. This antigen was also detected on sections of the primary gastric tumor and the liver metastases, but not the bone metastasis. Three days after the infusion of the MAb–mononuclear cell mixture, resected hepatic metastases showed marked necrosis, with infiltration of the necrotic area by mononuclear cells, but sections from the bone metastasis biopsied on day 14 did not. Ultrasound examination 3 weeks after therapy with MAb showed a decrease in size of hepatic metastases with a change in echogenic characteristics; although there was no histological evidence for destruction of the bone metastasis, it apparently became smaller. Anti-mouse immunoglobulins were observed in three of four patients. Patients given one dose of antibody exhibited no immediate or delayed side effects. The patient given repeated doses complained of bronchospasm during the final dose, and therapy was discontinued. The patient exhibited no signs of serum sickness over the following 2 weeks.

Watson *et al.* (1983) have devised a subcutaneous culture chamber for continuous infusion of MAb. The chamber, containing hybridoma cells, was inserted into the upper anterior abdominal wall of a patient with recurrent glioma, and the kinetics of release of human MAb from the hybridoma cells in the chamber was followed. The MAb produced had previously been shown by tumor imaging to localize in the tumor (Phillips *et al.*, 1983). Prelabeled MAb were released from the cells in the chamber into the bloodstream over a 3-day period. No infection, toxicity, or inflammation around the chamber was observed (for over 3 mo). No therapeutic effect was reported.

In summary, MAb for tumor therapy have been administered to 29 patients; 28

patients have received mouse MAb. The total number of doses ranged from 1 to 17, the total antibody received from 15 mg to 2 g, the size of single doses from 1 to 1500 mg. Response was not evaluated in four patients. One complete remission was achieved by a patient treated with anti-idiotype MAb; six of eight patients with cutaneous T-cell lymphoma achieved a partial remission; and a decrease in tumor mass in some sites was achieved by one evaluable patient treated with MAb to colorectal carcinoma cells. Most patients with leukemia or lymphoma, treated with MAb to differentiation antigens, demonstrated transiently decreased circulating tumor cells. Six patients exhibited transient symptoms of toxicity associated with antibody infusion; no serum sickness or persistent toxicity was observed. Anti-mouse antibody was observed in about half of the patients.

C. Targeting of Drugs, Toxins, and Radionuclides

Since antibodies by themselves do not kill tumor cells, therapy with MAb alone requires the adequate functioning of host systems for complement-mediated cytotoxicity, antibody-dependent cellular cytotoxicity, or removal by the reticuloendothelial system. These host immune functions may be severely impaired, particularly in a patient who has been heavily treated with radiation and chemotherapy. However, MAb can be used as carriers of drugs, toxins, or radionuclides. Such immunotoxins depend on the specificity of the MAb to bind specifically to tumor cells and on the action of the drug, toxin, or radionuclide for cytotoxicity, and are therefore not dependent on the function of the patient's immune system. Therefore, *in vivo* therapy with immunotoxins combines the targeting aspects of MAb used in diagnostic radiolocalization (Section III,C) and toxicity aspects independent of the host's immune system, as in purging of tumor cells from bone marrow for autologous transplantation (Section IV,A,2). The use of MAb immunotoxins as therapeutic agents has not yet been reported in patients, but many aspects have been defined in animal model systems.

Drugs that exhibit toxicity for tumor cells when administered alone have been coupled to MAb for more specific delivery to target cells. Arnon and Sela (1982) coupled daunomycin to an antitumor antibody using a dextran bridge. After conjugation, the drug retained 12–86% of its cytotoxicity, and the antibody retained 30–70% of its binding activity. In mouse model systems both monoclonal and polyclonal antibody–drug conjugates gave higher specific localization of drug to the tumor than to nontumor tissues, and therapeutic effects were observed when conventional antibody–drug complexes were used (Dullens *et al.*, 1979; Tsukada *et al.*, 1982). When MAb–drug complexes were used, cytotoxicity could be demonstrated *in vitro* and drug was shown to enter cells *in vivo*, but the therapeutic effects were unremarkable.

Mew *et al.* (1983) have described the successful use of MAb–hematoporphyrin conjugates in a mouse tumor model system. This photodrug is activated by visible light, and the cytotoxic effect is mediated by the production of single oxygen atoms, which have a short reactive distance. MAb are used to target the hematoporphyrin, and exposure to light can be controlled until the conjugates are specifically localized in surface tumors.

It may be that an insufficient quantity of active drug is targeted to the cells using MAb-drug conjugates. One way of increasing the amount of drug that can be targeted is to encapsulate the drug in lipsomes and link the liposomes to antibodies covalently. *In vitro* tests using antibody-coupled liposomes have been described (Leserman *et al.*, 1980, 1981; Harsch *et al.*, 1981; Bragman *et al.*, 1983), although use of this method *in vivo* has not been reported.

Yet another means of increasing the toxicity of immunotoxins is to use toxins that are effective even when only a few molecules per cell are bound. Therefore, conjugates of antibodies with ricin or diphtheria toxin have been prepared. Such conjugates have been shown to be active both *in vivo* and *in vitro* (Blythman *et al.*, 1981; Jansen *et al.*, 1982, 1983; Krolick *et al.*, 1982; Raso *et al.*, 1982; Thorpe and Ross, 1982; Thorpe *et al.*, 1982).

Although the use of drugs or toxins conjugated to antibodies avoids the necessity of participation by the host immune system to accomplish tumor cell kill, cytotoxicity does depend on internalization of the immunotoxins by the cells (Leserman *et al.*, 1981; Thorpe and Ross, 1982), so that the amount of antibody conjugate bound may not be proportional to activity observed. The capping and internalization required may not occur with some antibodies or with insufficient numbers of antibodies bound to cells. Insufficient cross-linking of surface components to initiate capping may result. Cross-linking of surface molecules may also be inhibited by circulating antigen. A possible means of overcoming this limitation would be to use radionuclides for immunoradiotherapy, designing these agents to deposit their energy within a few cell diameters and within the available time when antibodies are bound to tumor cells (Order *et al.*, 1980, 1981). This approach has resulted in successful therapy of tumors in animal models (Scheinberg and Strand, 1982; De Nardo *et al.*, 1983) and can soon be expected to be utilized in patients.

Levy and Miller (1983a) have also pointed out that MAb that are directly cytotoxic may also prevent the formation of anti-MAb, since their toxicity would also be likely to be expressed against the relevant antibody-forming B cells of the patient.

D. Immunological Manipulation

Antithymocyte globulin has been widely administered to patients receiving transplanted organs to ablate or reduce the immune response that would result in graft rejection. MAb specific for antigens present on individual lymphocyte cell types, which perform specific roles in the immune system, could be used to modulate various immune responses. In addition, antibodies to other growth-promoting "factors" or hormones, as well as to the cellular receptors to which these molecules bind, could be used to modify biologically the growth and activity of tumor cells.

MAb to T-cell subsets can block T-cell-mediated reactions *in vitro* (Engleman *et al.*, 1981; Evans *et al.*, 1981) and *in vivo* (Giorgi *et al.*, 1983; Jonker *et al.*, 1983b; Lems *et al.*, 1983). Waldor *et al.* (1983), for example, used anti-Ia antibodies to suppress antibody formation to soluble acetylcholine receptor administered to patients. Such an approach might be of use in blocking the production of anti-mouse antibodies in treated patients. Anti-Ia MAb inhibit interleukin synthesis and T-cell proliferation (Gilman *et al.*, 1983). Drebin *et al.* (1983) used monoclonal anti-IJ antibodies therapeutically in a mouse tumor model system to inhibit the activation of suppressor T cells by the tumor. Alternatively, T-cell activities can be augmented using MAb. MAb against an antigen-specific helper factor have been shown to augment T-cell helpers, leading to enhanced antibody production *in vitro* (James *et al.*, 1983). Anti-idiotype MAb may be particularly valuable in regulating the proliferation of individual clones of lymphocytes (Lampson and Levy, 1979; Hatzubai *et al.*, 1981; Auchincloss *et al.*, 1983), and indeed the remarkable therapeutic effect achieved with MAb reactive with the idiotype of the antibodies on the surface of tumor cells of a patient with lymphoma may have been due to modulation of the growth control mechanisms of these cells (Miller *et al.*, 1982a). MAb to the transferrin receptor have also been used to modulate cell growth (Trowbridge and Domingo, 1981).

E. Factors Influencing Therapeutic Efficiency

It is clear from the foregoing discussion that many factors will influence the therapeutic efficacy of any treatment strategy using MAb. The consideration of these factors suggests future directions for research.

Some of the factors influencing efficacy of therapy with MAb are related to properties of the individual antibodies used. The most obvious requirement for MAb-mediated tumor cytotoxicity is specificity of the antibody for the tumor cells. Even this requirement is not absolute, however, since antibodies to normal differentiation antigens have been used effectively for therapy in animal model systems (Shouval *et al.*, 1982; Johnson and Shin, 1983) and in patients (Miller and Levy, 1981). The complete remission obtained by a patient with lymphoma (Miller *et al.*, 1982a) resulted from therapy with anti-idiotype MAb, which are highly specific for a single clone of cells. The rule seems to be that treatment with tumor-reactive MAb can be therapeutically effective if the killing of normal cells bearing the antigen is not toxic. Specificity may also be obtained by methods utilizing a combination of MAb that target to cells bearing unique combinations of antigens (Bragman *et al.*, 1983) or by using antibodies with dual specificities (Raso, 1982).

Mixtures of two monoclonal antibodies have been reported to be more effective than either antibody alone in localization and in therapy. *In vitro*, mixtures of antibodies to different epitopes on the same antigen bind in a cooperative fashion to yield increased affinity (Ehrlich *et al.*, 1982; Ehrlich and Moyle, 1983; Moyle *et al.*, 1983). Mizuguchi *et al.* (1982) demonstrated that two distinct MAb to tetanus toxin were required to give efficient neutralization *in vivo*. Jonker *et al.* (1983a) reported that two MAb to helper T cells were required to modify the immune response to a graft in monkeys. Use of two MAb to different epitopes on a prostate tumor-associated antigen resulted in more antibody endocytosis by the cells than either MAb used alone (Webb *et al.*, 1983); increased endocytosis of antibody could result in more efficient intracellular delivery of drugs or toxins. However, endocytosis may be deleterious to therapeutic efficacy of MAb if nonconjugated MAb are removed from the cell surface, causing antigenic modulation of their bound antigen and the failure of cytolytic mechanisms dependent on cell surface antigen–antibody complexes (Ritz *et al.*, 1982; Chatenoud *et al.*, 1983).

The class and subclass of MAb, the species from which the MAb were produced, and whether intact MAb or F(ab) fragments are used will also affect the antitumor responses that they can mediate (Herlyn and Koprowski, 1982), their *in vivo* half-life (Sears *et al.*, 1982c), and their ability to induce endocytosis (Baldwin *et al.*, 1981) and an anti-MAb response (Chatenoud *et al.*, 1983; Jaffers *et al.*, 1983).

Other factors influencing the efficiency of therapy with MAb are related to properties of the tumor. Tumor burden (Thorpe and Ross, 1982), size of lesions (Buckman *et al.*, 1982), and location (Sears *et al.*, 1982c) may influence efficacy. Cells in small lesions, or micrometastases, may be the most susceptible to therapy with MAb. The method of antibody administration can also be optimized for tumor location, such as subcutaneous injection of MAb to direct them to draining lymph nodes that might include micrometastases (Weinstein *et al.*, 1982).

One of the most important properties of tumor cells that influence efficacy of antibody therapy is the heterogeneity of cell surface antigens (Albino *et al.*, 1981), which may lead to emergence of MAb-resistant antigen-negative tumors (Young and Hakomori, 1981). Antigenic modulation caused by binding of MAb and resulting in antigen endocytosis (MacLean *et al.*, 1982; Sears *et al.*, 1982c; Webb *et al.*, 1983; Wikstrand *et al.*, 1983) and antigen shedding into the circulation (Nadler *et al.*, 1980c; Miller *et al.*, 1981) are also important.

The efficacy of therapy with MAb is also influenced by host factors, such as sufficient effector cells to remove MAb-coated tumor cells or the ability of the patient to respond to foreign antibodies used in therapy with anti-MAb (Levy and Miller, 1983a).

F. Viruses in MAb Preparations Used for Therapy

There is some concern about the presence of viruses in preparations of hybridoma-produced mouse (Bartal *et al.*, 1982; Weiss, 1982; Huppert *et al.*, 1983) and human (Kozbor and Roder, 1983) MAb. Noninfectious A-type virus particles and C-type particles characteristic of retroviruses, which are infectious for human cells in culture, are produced by murine hybridomas. However, there is no evidence that people become infected by these viruses or that they are pathogenic in humans. Typical procedures for antibody purification (Section II,A,4) can also be expected to inactivate and remove infectious virus. Human retroviruses have not yet been seen in human fusion partners; yet a human retrovirus has been identified (Poiesz *et al.*, 1980).

Human lymphoblastoid cell lines are EBV positive (Yokochi *et al.*, 1982; Kozbor and Roder, 1983), and EBV transformation of patient lymphocytes is a promising method for human MAb production (Section II,B,3). Although infectious virus particles have not been detected in human MAb preparations, antibody purification should remove or inactivate any that were there. Crawford *et al.* (1983a) have addressed this problem directly and concluded that human MAb will be safe to use, since 80–90% of adults in Western populations have already been exposed to EBV, and EBV exposure by whole-blood transfusion or in antibodies for injection prepared from pooled human serum is not considered to be dangerous enough to warrant screening of blood or antibody preparations for EBV.

V. CONCLUSIONS

The production and use of MAb will be a significant advance in clinical oncology. All functions for which conventional antisera are currently used will be accomplished by MAb as the MAb become available, because of their reproducibility, specificity, and unlimited supply. Human MAb will become increasingly important in diagnosis, since they may recognize a broader spectrum of tumor antigens than murine antibodies, and in therapy, since they are expected to be less immunogenic. Mixtures of monoclonal antibodies of defined specificities, engineered polyclonal antibodies, will be increasingly used. New MAb and new methods of production, detection, and delivery will continue to add to the armamentarium the oncologist uses to detect and treat human malignancies.

Acknowledgments

We thank Christopher L. Reading and Walter N. Hittelman for reviewing the manuscript, Susan K. Fowler for verifying the bibliographical information, and Josephine J. Neicheril for expert secretarial assistance. This work was supported by Grants CA-28153 and CA-34783 from the National Cancer Institute, National Institutes of Health.

REFERENCES

Abrahamson, C. S., Kersey, J. H., and Le Bien, T. W. (1981). A monoclonal antibody (BA-1) reactive with cells of human B lymphocyte lineage. *J. Immunol.* **126**, 83–88.

Accolla, R. S., Carrel, S., and Mach, J.-P. (1980). Monoclonal antibodies specific for carcinoembryonic antigens and produced by two hybrid cell lines. *Proc. Natl. Acad. Sci. U.S.A.* **77**, 563–566.

Aisenberg, A. C., and Wilkes, B. M. (1980). Unusual human lymphoma phenotype defined by monoclonal antibodies. *J. Exp. Med.* **152**, 1126–1131.

Aisenberg, A. C., and Wilkes, B. M. (1982). Lymph node T cells in Hodgkin's disease: Analysis of suspensions with monoclonal antibody and rosetting techniques. *Blood* **59**, 522–527.

Albino, A. P., Lloyd, K. O., Houghton, A. N., Oettgen, H. F., and Old, L. J. (1981). Heterogeneity in surface antigen and glycoprotein expression of cell lines derived from different melanoma metastases of the same patient. *J. Exp. Med.* **154**, 1764–1778.

Anderson, K. C., Park, E. K., Bates, M. P., Leonard, R. C. F., Hardy, R., Schlossman, S. F., and Nadler, L. M. (1983). Antigens on human plasma cells identified by monoclonal antibodies. *J. Immunol.* **130**, 1132–1138.

Anonymous (1979). Monoclonal antibodies: Clinical potential of a growth industry. *JAMA, J. Am. Med. Assoc.* **242**, 2161–2163.

Aota, F., Chang, D., Hill, N. O., and Khan, A. (1983). Monoclonal antibody against myeloid leukemia cell line (KG-1). *Cancer Res.* **43**, 1093–1096.

Armitage, R. J., Worman, C. P., Mills, K. H. G., and Cawley, J. C. (1983). A B-cell proliferation with aberrant true E-rosette formation: A sequential study with a panel of monoclonal antibodies and other surface markers. *Scand. J. Haematol.* **30**, 211–217.

Arnon, R., and Sela, M. (1982). *In vitro* and *in vivo* efficacy of conjugates of daunomycin with antitumor antibodies. *Immunol. Rev.* **62**, 5–27.

Ashall, F., Bramwell, M. E., and Harris, H. (1982). A new marker for human cancer cells. I. The Ca antigen and Ca1 antibody. *Lancet* **ii**, 1–6.

Astaldi, G. C. B., Janssen, M. C., Lansdorp, P., Willems, C., Zeijlemaker, W. P., and Oosterhof, F. (1980). Human endothelial culture supernatant (HECS): A growth factor for hybridomas. *J. Immunol.* **125**, 1411–1414.

Atkinson, B. F., Ernst, C. S., Herlyn, M., Steplewski, Z., Sears, H. F., and Koprowski, H. (1982). Gastrointestinal cancer-associated antigen in immunoperoxidase assay. *Cancer Res.* **42**, 4820–4823.

Auchincloss, H., Jr., Bluestone, J. A., and Sachs, D. H. (1983). Antiidiotypes against anti-H-2 monoclonal antibodies. V. *In vivo* antiidiotype treatment induces idiotype-specific helper T-cells. *J. Exp. Med.* **157**, 1273–1286.

Auerbach, R., Alby, L., Grieves, J., Joseph, J., Lindgren, C., Morrissey, L. W., Sidky, Y. A., Tu, M., and Watt, S. L. (1982). Monoclonal antibody against angiotensin-converting enzyme: Its use as a marker for murine bovine and human endothelial cells. *Proc. Natl. Acad. Sci. U.S.A.* **79**, 7891–7895.

Baldwin, R. W., Embleton, M. J., and Price, M. R. (1981). Monoclonal antibodies specifying human tumour-associated antigens and their potential for therapy. *Mol. Aspects Med.* **4**, 329–368.

Baldwin, R. W., Embleton, M. J., and Pimm, M. V. (1983). Monoclonal antibodies for radioimmunodetection of tumours and for targeting. *Bull. Cancer* **70**, 132–136.

Ball, E. D., Graziano, R. F., and Fanger, M. W. (1983). A unique antigen expressed on myeloid cells and acute leukemia blast cells defined by a monoclonal antibody. *J. Immunol.* **130**, 2937–2941.

Bankert, R. B., Des Soye, D., and Powers, L. (1980). Antigen promoted cell fusion: Antigen-coated myeloma cells fuse with antigen-reactive spleen cells. *Transplant. Proc.* **12**, 443–446.

Bartal, A. H., Feit, C., Erlandson, R., and Hirshant, Y. (1982). The presence of viral particles in hybridoma clones secreting monoclonal antibodies. *N. Engl. J. Med.* **306**, 1423.

Basch, R. S., Berman, J. W.,and Lakow, E. (1983). Cell separation using positive immunoselective techniques. *J. Immunol. Methods* **56**, 269–280.

Bast, R. C., Jr., Feeney, M., Lazarus, H., Nadler, L. M., Colvin, R. B., and Knapp, R. C. (1981). Reactivity of a monoclonal antibody with human ovarian carcinoma. *J. Clin. Invest.* **68**, 1331–1337.

Bast, R. C., Jr., Ritz, J., Lipton, J. M., Feeney, M., Sallan, S. E., Nathan, D. G., and Schlossman, S. F. (1983). Elimination of leukemic cells from human bone marrow using monoclonal antibody and complement. *Cancer Res.* **43**, 1389–1394.

Battifora, H., and Trowbridge, I. S. (1983). A monoclonal antibody useful for the differential diagnosis between malignant lymphoma and nonhematopoietic neoplasms. *Cancer* **51**, 816–821.

Baumgartner, C., Brun del Re, G., Bucher, U., Forster, H. K., Hirt, A., Imback, P., Luthy, A., Morell, A., Odavic, R., and Wagner, H. P. (1983a). Autologous bone marrow transplantation for stage IV abdominal non-Hodgkin's lymphoma: *In vitro* marrow purging with the monoclonal antibody anti-Y 29/55 and complement. *Exp. Hematol.* **11** *S13,* 169.

Baumgartner, C., Brun del Re, G., Bucher, U., Forster, H. K., Hirt, A., Imbach, P., Luthy, A., Morell, A., Odavic, R., and Wagner, H. P. (1983b). Autologous bone marrow transplantation (ABMT) for advanced abdominal non-Hodgkin's lymphoma (NHL) after *in vitro* purging with anti-Y 29/55 monoclonal antibody and complement. *Exp. Hematol.* **11** *S14,* 6.

Bazin, H. (1982). Production of rat monoclonal antibodies with the LOU rat non-secreting IR 983 F myeloma cell line. *Protides Biol. Fluids* **29**, 615–618.

Begent, R. H. J., Green, A. J., Bagshawe, K. D., Jones, B. E., Keep, P. A., Searle, F., Jewkes, R. F., Barratt, G. M., and Ryman, B. E. (1982). Liposomally entrapped second antibody improves tumour imaging with radiolabelled (first) antitumour antibody. *Lancet* **ii**, 739–742.

Bellet, D., Schlumberger, M., Bidart, J. M., Assicot, M., Caillou, B., Motte, P., Vignal, A., and Bohuon, C. (1983). Production and *in vitro* utilization of monoclonal antibodies to human thyroglobulin. *J. Clin. Endocrinol. Metab.* **56**, 530–533.

Bernard, A., Boumsell, L., Reinherz, E. L., Nadler, L. M., Ritz, J., Coppin, H., Richard, Y., Valensi, F., Dausset, J., Flandrin, G., Lemerle, J., and Schlossman, S. F. (1981). Cell surface characterization of malignant T cells from lymphoblastic lymphoma using monoclonal antibodies: Evidence for phenotypic differences between malignant T cells from patients with acute lymphoblastic leukemia and lymphoblastic lymphoma. *Blood* **57**, 1105–1110.

Bernengo, M. G., Lisa, F., Puiatti, P., Meregalli, M., Berruto, G., and Zina, G. (1983). T-Cell subsets in melanoma patients evaluated by anti-T-cell monoclonal antibodies. *Thymus* **5**, 223–233.

Bernstein, I. D., Tam, M. R., and Nowinski, R. C. (1980a). Mouse leukemia: Therapy with monoclonal antibodies against a thymus differentiation antigen. *Science* **207**, 68–71.

Bernstein, I. D., Nowinski, R. C., Tam, M. R., McMaster, B., Houston, L. L., and Clark, E. A. (1980b). Monoclonal antibody therapy of mouse leukemia. *In* "Monoclonal Antibodies:

Hybridomas: A New Dimension in Biological Analyses'' (R. H. Kennett, T. J. McKearn, and K. B. Bechtol, eds.), pp. 275–291. Plenum, New York.

Bettelheim, P., Paietta, E., Majdic, O., Gadner, H., Schwarzmeier, J., and Knapp, W. (1982). Expression of a myeloid marker on TdT-positive acute lymphocytic leukemic cells: Evidence by double-fluorescence staining. *Blood* **60**, 1392–1396.

Beverley, P. (1983). Monoclonal antibodies and human leucocyte antigens. *Immunol. Today* **4**, 61–62.

Bishop, J. M. (1982). Retroviruses and cancer genes. *Adv. Cancer Res.* **37**, 1–32.

Block, T., and Bothwell, M. (1983). Use of iron- or selenium-coupled monoclonal antibodies to cell-surface antigens as a positive selection system for cells. *Nature (London)* **301**, 342–344.

Blythman, H. E., Casellos, P.,Gros, O., Gros, P., Jansen, F. K., Paolucci, F., Pau, B., and Vidal, H. (1981). Immunotoxins: Hybrid molecules of monoclonal antibodies and a toxin subunit specifically kill tumour cells. *Nature (London)* **290**, 145–146.

Boucheix, C., Perrot, J.-Y., Mirshahi, M., Bernadou, A., and Rosenfeld, C. (1983). A rapid method for detection of membrane antigens by immunofluorescence and its application to screening hybridoma antibodies. *J. Immunol. Methods* **57**, 145–150.

Bradstock, K. F., Janossy, G., Pizzolo, G., Hoffbrand, A. V., McMichael, A., Pilch, J. R., Milstein, C., Beverley, P., and Bollum, F. J. (1980). Subpopulations of normal and leukemic human thymocytes: An analysis with the use of monoclonal antibodies. *JNCI, J. Natl. Cancer Inst.* **65**, 33–42.

Bragman, K. S., Heath, T. D., and Papahadjopoulos, D. (1983). Simultaneous interaction of monoclonal antibody-targeted liposomes with two receptors on K562 cells. *Biochim. Biophys. Acta* **730**, 187–195.

Breard, J., Reinherz, E. L., Kung, P. C., Goldstein, G., and Schlossman, S. F. (1980). A mono-clonal antibody reactive with human peripheral blood monocytes. *J. Immunol.* **124**, 1943–1948.

Brenner, B. G., Jothy, S., Shuster, J., and Fuks, A. (1982). Monoclonal antibodies to human lung tumor antigens demonstrated by immunofluorescence and immunoprecipitation. *Cancer Res.* **42**, 3187–3192.

Brockhaus, M., Magnani, J. L., Blaszczyk, M., Steplewski, Z., Koprowski, H., Karlsson, K. A., Larson, G., and Ginsburg, V. (1981). Monoclonal antibodies directed against the human Le[b] blood-group antigen. *J. Biol. Chem.* **256**, 13223–13225.

Brockhaus, M., Magnani, J. L., Herlyn, M., Blaszczyk, M., Steplewski, Z., Koprowski, H., and Ginsburg, V. (1982). Monoclonal antibodies directed against the sugar sequence of lacto-*N*-fucopentaose III are obtained from mice immunized with human tumors. *Arch. Biochem. Biophys.* **217**, 647–651.

Brodin, T., Olsson, L., and Sjogren, H.-O. (1983). Cloning of human hybridoma, myeloma and lymphoma cell lines using enriched human monocytes as feeder layer. *J. Immunol. Methods* **60**, 1–7.

Brodsky, F. M., Parham, P., Barnstable, C. J., Crumpton, M. J., and Bodmer, W. F. (1979). Monoclonal antibodies for analysis of the HLA system. *Immunol. Rev.* **47**, 3–61.

Brooks, D. A., Beckman, I., Bradley, J., McNamara, P. J., Thomas, M. E., and Zola, H. (1980). Human lymphocyte markers defined by antibodies derived from somatic cell hybrids. I. A hybridoma secreting antibody against a marker specific for human B lymphocytes. *Clin. Exp. Immunol.* **39**, 477–485.

Brown, D. T., and Moore, M. (1982). Monoclonal antibodies against two human lung carcinoma cell lines. *Br. J. Cancer* **46**, 794–801.

Brown, J. M. (1983). Detection of a human sarcoma-associated antigen with monoclonal antibodies. *Cancer Res.* **43**, 2113–2120.

Brown, J. P., Wright, P. W., Hart, C. E., Woodbury, R. G., Hellstrom, K. E., and Hellstrom, I.

(1980). Protein antigens of normal and malignant human cells identified by immunoprecipitation with monoclonal antibodies. *J. Biol. Chem.* **255**, 4980–4983.

Brown, N. A. (1982). Prospects for human monoclonal antibodies: A critical perspective. *Yale J. Biol. Med.* **55**, 297–303.

Buckman, R., Shepherd, V., Coombes, R. C., McIlhinney, R. A. J., Patel, S., and Neville, A. M. (1982). Elimination of carcinoma cells from human bone marrow. *Lancet* **ii**, 1428–1430.

Bumol, T. F., Chee, D. O., and Resifeld, R. A. (1982). Immunochemical and biosynthetic analysis of monoclonal antibody-defined melanoma associated antigen. *Hybridoma* **1**, 283–292.

Burchell, J., Durbin, H., and Taylor-Papadimitriou, J. (1983). Complexity of expression of antigenic determinants recognized by monoclonal antibodies HMFG-1 and HMFG-2, in normal and malignant human mammary epithelial cells. *J. Immunol.* **13**, 508–513.

Burnett, R. A., Deery, A. R. S., Adamson, M. R., Liddle, C., Thomas, M., and Roberts, G. H. (1983). Evaluation of Ca1 antibody in pleural biopsy material. *Lancet* **i**, 1158.

Burtin, P., and Nardelli, J. (1983). Monoclonal antibodies against human solid tumors. *Bull. Cancer* **70**, 108–112.

Busch, H., Gyorkey, F., Busch, R. K., Davis, F. M., Gyorkey, P., and Smetana, K. (1979). A nucleolar antigen found in a broad range of human malignant tumor specimens. *Cancer Res.* **39**, 3024–3030.

Cairncross, J. G., Mattes, M. J., Beresford, H. R., Albino, A. P., Houghton, A. N., Lloyd, K. O., and Old, L. J. (1982). Cell surface antigens of human astrocytoma defined by mouse monoclonal antibodies: Identification of astrocytoma subsets. *Proc. Natl. Acad. Sci. U.S.A.* **79**, 5641–5645.

Cambon-de-Mouzon, A., and Olsson, L. (1983). Human monoclonal antibodies (HuMAbs) against cell membrane antigens. *Transplant. Proc.* **15**, 220–224.

Carrel, S., Accolla, R. S., Carmagnola, A. L., and Mach, J.-P. (1980). Common human melanoma-associated antigen(s) detected by monoclonal antibodies. *Cancer Res.* **40**, 2523–2528.

Carter, R. L., Foster, C. S., Dinsdale, E. A., and Pittam, M. R. (1983). Perineural spread by squamous carcinomas of the head and neck: A morphological study using antiaxonal and antimyelin monoclonal antibodies. *J. Clin. Pathol.* **36**, 269–275.

Ceriani, R. L., Sasaki, M., Sussman, H., Ward, W. M., and Blank, E. W. (1982). Circulating human mammary epithelial antigens in breast cancer. *Proc. Natl. Acad. Sci. U.S.A.* **79**, 5420–5424.

Chan, M. M., Tada, N., Kimura, S., Hoffmann, M. K., Miller, R. A., Stutman, O., and Hammerling, U. (1983). Characterization of T lymphocyte subsets with monoclonal antibodies: Discovery of a distinct marker, Ly-m22, of T suppressor cells. *J. Immunol.* **130**, 2075–2078.

Chapman, C. M., Allhoff, E. P., Proppe, K. H., and Prout, G. R., Jr. (1983). Use of monoclonal antibodies for the localization of tissue isoantigens A and B in transitional cell carcinoma of the upper urinary tract. *J. Histochem. Cytochem.* **31**, 557–561.

Chatal, J. F., Bourdoiseau, M., Fumoleau, P., Douillard, J. Y., Kremer, M., Curtet, C., and Le Mevel, B. (1983). Utilisation d'anticorps monoclonaux radio-marqués pour la détection scintigraphique des cancers colorectaux humains. *Bull. Cancer* **70**, 103–107.

Chatenoud, L., Baudrihaye, M. F., Chkoff, N., Kreis, H., and Bach, J. F. (1983). Immunologic follow-up of renal allograft recipients treated prophylactically by OKT3 alone. *Transplant. Proc.* **15**, 643–645.

Chee, D. O., Yonemoto, R. H., Leong, S. P. L., Richards, G. F., Smith, V. R., Klotz, J. L., Goto, R. M., Gascon, R. L., and Drushella, M. M. (1982). Mouse monoclonal antibody to a melanoma–carcinoma-associated antigen synthesized by a human melanoma cell line propagated in serum-free medium. *Cancer Res.* **42**, 3142–3147.

Chiorazzi, N., Wasserman, R. L., and Kunkel, H. G. (1982). Use of Epstein–Barr virus-transformed B cell lines for the generation of immunoglobulin producing human B cell hybridomas. *J. Exp. Med.* **156**, 930–935.

Choe, B. K., Lillehoj, H. S., Dong, M. K., Gleason, S., Barron, M., and Rose, N. R. (1982). Characterization of antigenic sites of human prostatic acid phosphatase. *Ann. N. Y. Acad. Sci.* **390**, 16–26.

Clarke, S. M., Merchant, D. J., and Starling, J. J. (1982). Monoclonal antibodies against a soluble cytoplasmic antigen in human prostatic epithelial cells. *Prostate* **3**, 203–214.

Clement, L. T., Lehmeyer, J. E., and Gartland, G. L. (1983). Identification of neutrophil subpopulations with monoclonal antibodies. *Blood* **61**, 326–332.

Cleveland, W. L., Wood, I., and Erlanger, B. F. (1983). Routine large-scale production of monoclonal antibodies in a protein-free culture medium. *J. Immunol. Methods* **56**, 221–234.

Colcher, D., Hand, P. H., Nuti, M., and Schlom, J. (1981). A spectrum of monoclonal antibodies reactive with human mammary tumor cells. *Proc. Natl. Acad. Sci. U.S.A.* **78**, 3199–3203.

Cooper, H. S. (1982). Peanut lectin-binding sites in large bowel carcinoma. *Lab. Invest.* **47**, 383–390.

Cosimi, A. B., Burton, R. C., Colvin, R. B., Goldstein, G., Delmonico, F. L., La Quaglia, M. P., Tolkoff-Rubin, N., Rubin, R. H., Herrin, J. T., and Russell, P. S. (1981). Treatment of acute renal allograft rejection with OKT3 monoclonal antibody. *Transplantation* **32**, 535–539.

Cote, R. J., Morrissey, D. M., Houghton, A. N., Beattie, E. J., Jr., Oettgen, H. F., and Old, L. J. (1983). Generation of human monoclonal antibodies reactive with cellular antigens. *Proc. Natl. Acad. Sci. U.S.A.* **80**, 2026–2030.

Crawford, D. H., Huehns, E. R., and Epstein, M. A. (1983a). Therapeutic use of human monoclonal antibodies. *Lancet* **i**, 1040.

Crawford, D. H., Barlow, M. J., Harrison, J. F., Winger, L., and Huehns, E. R. (1983b). Production of human monoclonal antibody to rhesus D antigen. *Lancet* **i**, 386–388.

Croce, C. M., Linnenbach, A., Hall, W., Steplewski, Z., and Koprowski, H. (1980). Production of human hybridomas secreting antibodies to measles virus. *Nature (London)* **288**, 488–489.

Cuttitta, F., Rosen, S., Gazdar, A. F., and Minna, J. D. (1981). Monoclonal antibodies that demonstrate specificity for several types of human lung cancer. *Proc. Natl. Acad. Sci. U.S.A.* **78**, 4591–4595.

Daar, A. S., and Fabre, J. W. (1983). The membrane antigens of human colorectal cancer cells: Demonstration with monoclonal antibodies of heterogeneity within and between tumors and of anomalous expression of HLA-DR. *Eur. J. Cancer Clin. Oncol.* **19**, 209–220.

Damjanov, I., and Knowles, B. B. (1983). Biology of disease: Monoclonal antibodies and tumor-associated antigens. *Lab. Invest.* **48**, 510–525.

Damjanov, I., Fox, N., Knowles, B. B., Solter, D., Lange, P. H., and Fraley, E. E. (1982). Immunohistochemical localization of murine stage-specific embryonic antigens in human testicular germ cell tumors. *Am. J. Pathol.* **108**, 225–230.

Davies, T. (1981). Magic bullets. *Nature (London)* **289**, 12–13.

Davis, F. M., Gyorkey, F., Busch, R. K., and Busch, H. (1979). Nucleolar antigen found in several human tumors but not in the non-tumor tissues studied. *Proc. Natl. Acad. Sci. U.S.A.* **76**, 892–896.

Davis, F. M., Dicke, K. A., Jagannath, S., and Rao, P. N. (1983a). Detection of leukemic cell colonies in agar plates by immunostaining for human malignancy-associated nucleolar antigen. *J. Immunol. Methods* **58**, 349–357.

Davis, F. M., Tsao, T. Y., Fowler, S. K., and Rao, P. N. (1983b). Monoclonal antibodies to mitotic cells. *Proc. Natl. Acad. Sci. U.S.A.* **80**, 2926–2930.

Dearnaley, D. P., Sloane, J. P., Ormerod, M. G., Steele, K., Coombes, R. C., Clink, H. M. D., Powles, T. J., Ford, H. T., Gazet, J. C., and Neville, A. M. (1981). Increased detection of mammary carcinoma cells in marrow smears using antisera to epithelial membrane antigen. *Br. J. Cancer* **44**, 85–90.

De Nardo, S. J., Hines, H. H., Erickson, K. L., and De Nardo, G. L. (1983). The evaluation of radiolabeled monoclonal antibody parameters necessary for cancer immunoradiotherapy. *In*

"Rational Basis for Chemotherapy" (B. A. Chabner, ed.), pp. 379–387. Liss, New York.

Deng, C., El-Awar, N., Cicciarelli, J., Terasaki, P. I., Billing, R., and Lagasse, L. (1981). Cytotoxic monoclonal antibody to a human leiomyosarcoma. *Lancet* **i,** 403–405.

Deng, C.-T., Terasaki, P., Chia, J., and Billing, R. (1982). Monoclonal antibody specific for human T acute lymphoblastic leukaemia. *Lancet* **i,** 10–11.

Diamond, B., and Scharff, M. D. (1982). Monoclonal antibodies. *JAMA, J. Am. Med. Assoc.* **248,** 3165–3169.

Diamond, B. A., Yelton, D. E., and Scharff, M. D. (1981). Monoclonal antibodies: A new technology for producing serologic reagents. *N. Engl. J. Med.* **304,** 1344–1349.

Dicke, K. A., Tindle, S. E., Davis, F. M., and Reading, C. L. (1982). Elimination of myeloid leukemic cells in human bone marrow after treatment with monoclonal antibodies to cell surface determinants. *In* "Differentiation and Function of Hematopoietic Cell Surfaces" (V. T. Marchesi and R. C. Gallo, eds.), pp. 283–292. Alan R. Liss, New York.

Dicke, K. A., Tindle, S. E., Davis, F. M., Jagannath, S., Tucker, S., Lilien, M., van Leeuwen, P., Verma, D. S., and Vellekoop, L. (1983). Leukemic cell colony formation in soft agar by bone marrow cells from untreated acute leukemia patients. *Exp. Hematol.* **11,** 341–350.

Dillman, R. O., Shawler, D. L., Sobol, R. E., Collins, H. A., Beauregard, J. C., Wormsley, S. B., and Royston, I. (1982a). Murine monoclonal antibody therapy in 2 patients with chronic lymphocytic leukemia. *Blood* **59,** 1036–1045.

Dillman, R. O., Sobol, R. E., Collins, H., Beauregard, J., and Royston, I. (1982b). T101 monoclonal antibody therapy in chronic lymphocytic leukemia. *In* "Hybridomas in Cancer Diagnosis and Treatment" (M. S. Mitchell and H. F. Oettgen, eds.), pp. 151–171. Raven, New York.

Dimitriu-Bona, A., Burmester, G. R., Waters, S. J., and Winchester, R. J. (1983). Human mononuclear phagocyte differentiation antigens. I. Patterns of antigenic expression on the surface of human monocytes and macrophages defined by monoclonal antibodies. *J. Immunol.* **130,** 145–152.

Dippold, W. G., Lloyd, K. O., Li, L. T. C., Ikeda, H., Oettgen, H. F., and Old, L. J. (1980). Cell surface antigens of human malignant melanoma: Definition of six antigenic systems with mouse monoclonal antibodies. *Proc. Natl. Acad. Sci. U.S.A.* **77,** 6114–6118.

Drebin, J. A., Waltenbaugh, C., Schatten, S., Benacerraf, B., and Greene, M. I. (1983). Inhibition of tumor growth by monoclonal anti-I-J antibodies. *J. Immunol.* **130,** 506–509.

Dulbecco, R., Unger, M., Bologna, M., Battifora, H., Syka, P., and Okada, S. (1981). Cross-reactivity between Thy-1 and a component of intermediate filaments demonstrated using a monoclonal antibody. *Nature (London)* **292,** 772–774.

Dullens, H. F., De Weger, R. A., Vennegoor, C., and Den Otter, W. (1979). Anti-tumour effect of chlorambucil-antibody complexes in a murine melanoma system. *Eur. J. Cancer* **15,** 69–75.

Edwards, P. A. W. (1981). Some properties and applications of monoclonal antibodies. *Biochem. J.* **200,** 1–10.

Edwards, P. A. W., Foster, C. S., and McIlhinney, R. A. J. (1980). Monoclonal antibodies to teratomas and breast. *Transplant. Proc.* **12,** 398–402.

Edwards, P. A. W., Smith, C. M., Munro Neville, A., and O'Hare, M. J. (1982). A human-human hybridoma system based on a fast growing mutant of the ARH-77 plasma cell leukaemia-derived line. *Eur. J. Immunol.* **12,** 641–648.

Ehrlich, P. H., and Moyle, W. R. (1983). Cooperative immunoassays: Ultrasensitive assays with mixed monoclonal antibodies. *Science* **221,** 279–281.

Ehrlich, P. H., Moyle, W. R., Moustafa, Z. A., and Canfield, R. E. (1982). Mixing two monoclonal antibodies yields enhanced affinity for antigen. *J. Immunol.* **128,** 2709–2713.

Eisenbarth, G. S., Linnenbach, A., Jackson, R., Scearce, R., and Croce, C. M. (1982). Human hybridomas secreting anti-islet autoantibodies. *Nature (London)* **300**, 264–267.

Embleton, M. J., Gunn, B., and Baldwin, R. W. (1981). Monoclonal antibodies against human osteogenic sarcoma cells. *Br. J. Cancer* **43**, 568–569. (Abstr.)

Engleman, E. G., Benike, C. J., Glickman, E., and Evans, R. L. (1981). Antibodies to membrane structures that distinguish suppressor/cytotoxic and helper T lymphocyte subpopulations block the mixed leukocyte reaction in man. *J. Exp. Med.* **154**, 193–198.

Epenetos, A. A., Canti, G., Taylor-Papadimitriou, J., Curling, M., and Bodmer, W. F. (1982a). Use of two epithelium-specific monoclonal antibodies for diagnosis of malignancy in serous effusions. *Lancet* **ii**, 1004–1006.

Epenetos, A. A., Mather, S., Granowska, M., Nimmon, C. C., Hawkins, L. R., Britton, K. E., Shepherd, J., Taylor-Papadimitriou, J., Durbin, H., Malpas, J. S., and Bodmer, W. F. (1982b). Targeting of iodine-123-labelled tumour-associated monoclonal antibodies to ovarian, breast, and gastrointestinal tumours. *Lancet* **ii**, 999–1004.

Epstein, A. L., and Clevenger, C. V. (1984). Identification of nuclear antigens in human cells by immunofluorescence, immunoelectron microscopy, and immunobiochemical methods using monoclonal antibodies. *In* "Recent Advances in Non-Histone Chromosomal Protein Research" (I. Bekhor, ed.), CRC Press, Boca Raton, Florida (in press).

Evans, R. L., Wall, D. W., Platsoucas, C. D., Siegal, F. P., Fikrig, S. M., Testa, C. M., and Good, R. A. (1981). Thymus-dependent membrane antigens in man: Inhibition of cell-mediated lympholysis by monoclonal antibodies to T_{H2} antigen. *Proc. Natl. Acad. Sci. U.S.A.* **78**, 544–548.

Falk, K.-E., Karlsson, K.-A., Larson, G., Thurin, J., Blaszczyk, M., Steplewski, Z., and Koprowski, H. (1983). Mass spectrometry of a human tumor glycolipid antigen being defined by mouse monoclonal antibody NS-19-9. *Biochem. Biophys. Res. Commun.* **110**, 383–391.

Farrands, P. A., Pimm, M. V., Embleton, M. J., Perkins, A. C., Hardy, J. D., Baldwin, R. W., and Hardcastle, J. D. (1982). Radioimmunodetection of human colorectal cancers by an anti-tumor monoclonal antibody. *Lancet* **ii**, 397–400.

Fazekas de St. Groth, S. (1983). Automated production of monoclonal antibodies in a cytostat. *J. Immunol. Methods* **57**, 121–136.

Fazekas de St. Groth, S., and Scheidegger, D. (1980). Production of monoclonal antibodies: Strategy and tactics. *J. Immunol. Methods* **35**, 1–21.

Feder, M., Jonak, Z. L., Smith, A. A., Glick, M. C., and Kennett, R. H. (1983). Wandering around the cell surface–monoclonal antibodies against human neuroblastoma and leukemia cell surface antigens. *In* "Hybridomas and Cellular Immortality" (J. P. Allison and B. H. Tom, eds.), pp. 145–158, Plenum Press, New York.

Filipovich, A. H., Quinones, R., Vallera, D., and Kersey, J. H. (1983). T lymphocyte depletion of human bone marrow *in vitro* for prevention of graft vs. host disease (GVHD) in allogeneic bone marrow transplantation (BMT). *Exp. Hematol.* **11** *S14*, 188.

Finan, P. J., Wight, D. G. D., Lennox, E. S., Sacks, S. H., and Bleehen, N. M. (1983). Human blood group isoantigen expression on normal and malignant gastric epithelium studied with anti-A and anti-B monoclonal antibodies. *JNCI, J. Natl. Cancer Inst.* **70**, 679–685.

Fisher, R. I., Silver, B. A., Vanhaelen, C. P., Jaffe, E. S., and Cossman, J. (1982). Objective regressions of T- and B-cell lymphomas in patients following treatment with anti-thymocyte globulin. *Cancer Res.* **42**, 2465–2469.

Flotte, T. J., Springer, T. A., and Thorbecke, G. J. (1983). Dendritic cell and macrophage staining by monoclonal antibodies in tissue sections and epidermal sheets. *Am. J. Pathol.* **111**, 112–124.

Foa, R., Cappio, F. C., Campana, D., Fierro, M. T., Bergui, L., Giubellino, M. C., and Lusso, P.

(1983). Relevance of monoclonal antibodies in the diagnosis of unusual T-cell acute lympho-blastic leukemia. *Scand. J. Haematol.* **30,** 303–307.

Foon, K. A. (1982). Treatment of B-cell lymphoma with monoclonal anti-idiotype antibody. *N. Engl. J. Med.* **307,** 686.

Foon, K. A., Schroff, R. W., and Gale, R. P. (1982). Surface markers on leukemia and lymphoma cells. Recent advances. *Blood* **60,** 1–19.

Forster, H. K., Gudat, F. G., and Obrecht, J. P. (1981). Cells of human B leukemias express a lymphoid tissue-specific B lymphocyte antigen. *In* "The Immune System" (C. M. Steinberg and I. Lefkovits, eds.) pp. 425–430. Karger, Basel.

Forster, H. K., Gudat, F. G., Girard, M.-F., Albrecht, R., Schmidt, J., Ludwig, C., and Obrecht, J.-P. (1982). Monoclonal antibody against a membrane antigen characterizing leukemic human B-lymphocytes. *Cancer Res.* **42,** 1927–1934.

Foster, C. S. (1982). Lymphocyte hybridomas. *Cancer Treat. Rev.* **9,** 59–84.

Foster, C. S., Edwards, P. A. W., Dinsdale, E. A., and Neville, A. M. (1982a). Monoclonal antibodies to the human mammary gland. I. Distribution of determinants in non-neoplastic mammary and extra-mammary tissues. *Virchows Arch. A. Pathol. Anat.* **394,** 279–293.

Foster, C. S., Dinsdale, E. A., Edwards, P. A. W., and Neville, A. M. (1982b). Monoclonal antibodies to human mammary gland. II. Distribution of determinants in breast carcinomas. *Virchows Arch. A. Pathol. Anat.* **394,** 295–305.

Fox, P. C., Berenstein, E. H., and Siraganian, R. P. (1981). Enhancing the frequency of antigen-specific hybridomas. *Eur. J. Immunol.* **11,** 431–434.

Fox, P. C., Berenstein, E. H., and Siraganian, R. P. (1982). Techniques for enhancing the yield of antigen-specific hybridomas. *In* "Hybridomas in Cancer Diagnosis and Treatment" (M. S. Mitchell and H. F. Oettgen, eds.), pp. 15–18. Raven, New York.

Frankel, A. E., Chu, T. M., Rouse, R. V., Wang, M. C., and Herzenberg, L. A. (1982). Mono-clonal antibodies to a human prostate antigen. *Cancer Res.* **42** 3714–3718.

Funderud, S., Lindmo, T., Ruud, E., Marton, P. F., Langholm, R., Folling Elgjo, R., Vaage, S., Lie, S., and Godal, T. (1983). Delineation of subsets in human B-cell lymphomas by a set of monoclonal antibodies raised against B lymphoma cells. *Scand. J. Immunol.* **17,** 161–169.

Galfre, G., and Milstein, C. (1981). Preparation of monoclonal antibodies: strategies and pro-cedures. *In* Methods in Enzymology (J. J. Langone, ed.), Vol. 73B, pp. 3–46. Academic Press, New York.

Galfre, G., Howe, S. C., Milstein, C., Butcher, G. W., and Howard, J. C. (1977). Antibodies to major histocompatibility antigens produced by hybrid cell lines. *Nature (London)* **266,** 550–552.

Galfre, G., Milstein, C., and Wright, B. (1979). Rat × rat hybrid myelomas and a monoclonal anti-Fd portion of mouse IgG. *Nature (London)* **277,** 131–133.

Garcia-Perez, A., and Smith, W. L. (1983). Use of monoclonal antibodies to isolate cortical collect-ing tubule cells: AVP induces PGE release. *Am. J. Physiol.* **244,** C211–C220.

Gatter, K. C., and Mason, D. Y. (1982). The use of monoclonal antibodies for histopathologic diagnosis of human malignancy. *Semin. Oncol.* **9,** 517–525.

Gefter, M. L., Margulies, D. H., and Scharff, M. D. (1977). A simple method for polyethylene glycol-promoted hybridization of mouse myeloma cells. *Somatic Cell Genet.* **3,** 231–236.

Ghetie, V., and Moraru, I. (1983). Preparation and applications of multivalent antibodies with dual specificity. *In* "Methods in Enzymology" (J. J. Langone and H. Van Vunakis, eds.), Vol. 92E, pp. 523–543. Academic Press, New York.

Giacomini, P., Ng, A. K., Kantor, R. R. S., Natali, P. G., and Ferrone, S. (1983). Double determinant immunoassay to measure a human high-molecular-weight melanoma-associated antigen. *Cancer Res.* **43,** 3586–3590.

Gilliland, D. G., Steplewski, Z., Collier, R. J., Mitchell, K. F., Chang, T. H., and Koprowski, H. (1980). Antibody-directed cytotoxic agents: Use of monoclonal antibody to direct the action of toxic A chains to colorectal carcinoma cells. *Proc. Natl. Acad. Sci. U.S.A.* **77,** 4539–4543.

Gilman, S. C., Rosenberg, J. S., and Feldman, J. D. (1983). Inhibition of interleukin synthesis and T cell proliferation by a monoclonal anti-Ia antibody. *J. Immunol.* **130**, 1236–1240.

Giorgi, J. V., Burton, R. C., Barrett, L. V., Delmonico, F. L., Goldstein, G., and Cosimi, A. B. (1983). Immunosuppressive effect and immunogenicity of OKT11A monoclonal antibody in monkey allograft recipients. *Transplant. Proc.* **15**, 639–642.

Glassy, M. C., Handley, H., Astarita, R., Strayer, D., Lowe, D. H., and Royston, I. (1983). The use of lymphocytes isolated from regional draining lymph nodes of cancer patients to generate human monoclonal antibodies. *Proc. Am. Assoc. Cancer Res.* **24**, 223. (Abstr.)

Glode, M. L., Epstein, A., and Smith, C. G. (1981). Reduced γ-cystathionase protein content in human malignant leukemia cell lines as measured by immunoassay with monoclonal antibody. *Cancer Res.* **41**, 2249–2254.

Goding, J. W. (1980). Antibody production by hybridomas. *J. Immunol. Methods* **39** *S1*, 285–308.

Goldenberg, D. M. (1983). Tumor imaging with monoclonal antibodies. *J. Nucl. Med.* **24**, 360–362.

Goldenberg, D. M., Neville, A. M., Carter, A. C., Go, V. L. W., Holyoke, E. D., Isselbacher, K. J., Schein, P. S., and Schwartz, M. (1981). CEA (carcinoembryonic antigen): Its role as a marker in the management of cancer. *J. Cancer Res. Clin. Oncol.* **101**, 239–242.

Gooi, H. C., Thorpe, S. J., Hounsell, E. F., Rumpold, H., Draft, D., Forster, O., and Feizi, T. (1983). Marker of peripheral blood granulocytes and monocytes of man recognized by two monoclonal antibodies VEP8 and VEP9 involves the trisaccharide 3-fucosyl-*N*-acetyllactosamine. *Eur. J. Immunol.* **13**, 306–312.

Gorin, N. C., Douay, L., Jansen, F. K., Voisin, G. A., Baillou, C., Najam, A., and Duhamel, G. (1983). Preclinical study of immunotoxin T101: Absence of cytotoxicity against hemopoietic progenitor stem cells. Application to *in vitro* therapy prior to autologous bone marrow transplantation. *Exp. Hematol.* **11** *S14,* 6.

Greaves, M. F. (1981). Analysis of the clinical and biological significance of lymphoid phenotypes in acute leukemia. *Cancer Res.* **41**, 4752–4766.

Habeshaw, J. A., Bailey, D., Stansfeld, A. G., and Greaves, M. F. (1983). The cellular content of non-Hodgkin lymphomas: A comprehensive analysis using monoclonal antibodies and other surface marker techniques. *Br. J. Cancer* **47**, 327–351.

Hakomori, S. (1983). Tumor-associated glycolipid antigens defined by monoclonal antibodies. *Bull. Cancer* **70**, 118–126.

Hancock, W. W., and Atkins, R. C. (1983). Monoclonal antibodies to human glomerular cells: A marker for glomerular epithelial cells. *Nephron* **33**, 83–90.

Hancock, W. H., Becker, G. J., and Atkins, R. C. (1982). A comparison of fixatives and immunohistochemical techniques for use with monoclonal antibodies to cell surface antigens. *Am. J. Clin. Pathol.* **78**, 825–831.

Hansen, R. S., and Beavo, J. A. (1982). Purification of two calcium/calmodulin-dependent forms of cyclic nucleotide phosphodiesterase by using conformation-specific monoclonal antibody chromatography. *Proc. Natl. Acad. Sci. U.S.A.* **79**, 2788–2792.

Hansson, G. C., Karlsson, K.-A., Larson, G., McKibbin, J. M., Blaszczyk, M., Herlyn, M., Steplewski, Z., and Koprowski, H. (1983). Mouse monoclonal antibodies against human cancer cell lines with specificities for blood group and related antigens. Characterization by antibody binding to glycosphingolipids in a chromatogram binding assay. *J. Biol. Chem.* **258**, 4091–4097.

Harsch, M., Walther, P., and Weder, H. G. (1981). Targeting of monoclonal antibody-coated liposomes to sheep red blood cells. *Biochem. Biophys. Res. Commun.* **103**, 1069–1076.

Haskell, C. M., Buchegger, F., Schreyer, M., Carrel, S., and Mach, J.-P. (1983). Monoclonal antibodies to carcinoembryonic antigen: Ionic strength as a factor in the selection of antibodies for immunoscintigraphy. *Cancer Res.* **43**, 3857–3864.

Hatzubai, A., Maloney, D. G., and Levy, R. (1981). The use of a monoclonal anti-idiotype antibody to study the biology of a human B cell lymphoma. *J. Immunol.* **126**, 2397–2402.

Hawkes, R., Niday, E., and Gordon, J. (1982). A dot-immunobinding assay for monoclonal and other antibodies. *Anal. Biochem.* **119**, 142–147.

Hedin, A., Hammarstrom, S., and Larsson, A. (1982a) Specificities and binding properties of eight monoclonal antibodies against carcinoembryonic antigen. *Mol. Immunol.* **19**, 1641–1648.

Hedin, A., Wahren, B., and Hammarstrom, S. (1982b). Tumor localization of CEA-containing human tumors in nude mice by means of monoclonal anti-CEA antibodies. *Int. J. Cancer* **30**, 547–552.

Hedin, A., Carlsson, L., Berglund, A., and Hammarstrom, S. (1983). A monoclonal antibody-enzyme immunoassay for serum carcinoembryonic antigen with increased specificity for carcinomas. *Proc. Natl. Acad. Sci. U.S.A.* **80**, 3470–3474.

Hengartner, H., Luzzati, A. L., and Schreier, M. (1978). Fusion of *in vitro* immunized lymphoid cells with X63Ag8. *Curr. Top. Microbiol. Immunol.* **81**, 92–99.

Herlyn, D., and Koprowski, H. (1982). Monoclonal antibodies against solid human tumors inhibit tumor growth in nude mice. *Hybridoma* **1**, 206.

Herlyn, D. M., Steplewski, Z., Herlyn, M. F., and Koprowski, H. (1980). Inhibition of growth of colorectal carcinoma in nude mice by monoclonal antibody. *Cancer Res.* **40**, 717–721.

Herlyn, D., Powe, J., Alavi, A., Mattis, J. A., Herlyn, M., Ernst, C., Vaum, R., and Koprowski, H. (1983). Radioimmunodetection of human tumor xenografts by monoclonal antibodies. *Cancer Res.* **43**, 2731–2735.

Herlyn, M., Steplewski, Z., Herlyn, D., and Koprowski, H. (1979). Colorectal carcinoma-specific antigen: Detection by means of monoclonal antibodies. *Proc. Natl. Acad. Sci. U.S.A.* **76**, 1438–1442.

Herlyn, M., Sears, H. F., Steplewski, Z., and Koprowski, H. (1982). Monoclonal antibody detection of a circulating tumor-associated antigen. I. Presence of antigen in sera of patients with colorectal, gastric, and pancreatic carcinoma. *J. Clin. Immunol.* **2**, 135–140.

Hittelman, W. N., Davis, F. M., and Keating, M. J. (1983). Implications of premature chromosome condensation findings in human leukemia. *In* "Cancer: Etiology and Prevention" (R. G. Crispen, ed.), pp. 1–20. Elsevier, New York.

Hosoi, S., Nakamura, T., Higashi, S., Yamamuro, T., Toyama, S., Shinomiya, K., and Mikawa, H. (1982). Detection of human osteosarcoma-associated antigen(s) by monoclonal antibodies. *Cancer Res.* **42**, 654–659.

Houston, L. L., and Nowinski, R. C. (1981). Cell-specific cytotoxicity expressed by a conjugate of ricin and murine monoclonal antibody directed against thy 1.1. antigen. *Cancer Res.* **41**, 3913–3917.

Houston, L. L., Nowinski, R. C., and Bernstein, I. D. (1980). Specific *in vivo* localization of monoclonal antibodies directed against the thy 1.1 antigen. *J. Immunol.* **125**, 837–843.

Huang, L. C., Brockhaus, M., Magnani, J. L., Cuttitta, F., Rosen, S., Minna, J. D., and Ginsburg, V. (1983a). Many monoclonal antibodies with an apparent specificity for certain lung cancers are directed against a sugar sequence found in lacto-*N*-fucopentaose III. *Arch. Biochem. Biophys.* **220**, 318–320.

Huang, L. C., Civin, C. I., Magnani, J. L., Shaper, J. H., and Ginsburg, V. (1983b). My-1, the human myeloid-specific antigen detected by mouse monoclonal antibodies, is a sugar sequence found in lacto-*N*-fucopentaose III. *Blood* **61**, 1020–1023.

Huppert, J., Lyon, M., and Brochier, J. (1983). Viral particles in monoclonal antibodies preparations. *Presse Med.* **12**, 702.

Imai, K., Molinaro, G. A., and Ferrone, S. (1980). Monoclonal antibodies to human melanoma-associated antigens. *Transplant. Proc.* **12**, 380–383.

Irie, R. F., Sze, L. L., and Saxton, R. E. (1982). Human antibody to OFA-I, a tumor antigen, produced *in vitro* by Epstein-Barr virus-transformed human B-lymphoid cell lines. *Proc. Natl. Acad. Sci. U.S.A.* **79**, 5666–5670.

Jaffers, G. J., Colvin, R. B., Cosimi, A. B., Giorgi, J. V., Goldstein, G., Fuller, T. C., Kurnick, J. T., Lillehei, C., and Russell, P. S. (1983). The human immune response to murine OKT3 monoclonal antibody. *Transplant. Proc.* **15**, 646–648.

James, R. F. L., Kontiainen, S., Maudsley, D. J., Culbert, E. J., and Feldman, M. (1983). A monoclonal antibody against antigen-specific helper factor augments T-cell help. *Nature (London)* **301**, 160–163.

Janckila, A. J., Stelzer, G. T., Wallace, J. H., and Yam, L. T. (1983). Phenotype of the hairy cells of leukemic reticuloendotheliosis defined by monoclonal antibodies. *Am. J. Clin. Pathol.* **79**, 431–437.

Jansen, F. K., Blythman, H. E., Carriere, D., Casellas, P., Gros, O., Gros, P., Laurent, J. C., Paolucci, F., Pau, B., Poncelet, P., Richer, G., Vidal, H., and Voisin, G. (1982). Immunotoxins: Hybrid molecules combining high specificity and potent cytotoxicity. *Immunol. Rev.* **62**, 185–216.

Jansen, F. K., Blythman, H. E., Carriere, D., Casellas, P., Hellstrom, I., Hellstrom, K. E., Gros, O., Gros, P., Laurent, J.-C., Poncelet, P., Richer, G., Royston, I., Vidal, H., and Voisin, G. A. (1983). Immunotoxins with high specific cytotoxicity in human tumor model systems. *Proc. Am. Assoc. Cancer Res.* **24**, 228. (Abstr.)

Johnson, P. M., Cheng, H. M., Molloy, C. M., Stern, C. M. M., and Slade, M. B. (1981). Human trophoblast-specific surface antigens identified using monoclonal antibodies. *Am. J. Reprod. Immunol.* **1**, 246–254.

Johnson, R. J., and Shin, H. S. (1983). Monoclonal antibody against a differentiation antigen on human leukemia cells: Cross-reactivity with rat leukemia and suppression of rat leukemia *in vivo*. *J. Immunol.* **130**, 2930–2936.

Jonak, Z. L., Kennett, R. H., and Bechtol, K. B. (1982). Detection of neuroblastoma cells in human bone marrow using a combination of monoclonal antibodies. *Hybridoma* **1**, 349–368.

Jonker, M., Malissen, B., van Vreeswijk, W., Mawas, C., Goldstein, G., Tax, W., and Balner, H. (1983a). *In vivo* application of monoclonal antibodies specific for human T cell subsets permits the modification of immune responsiveness in rhesus monkeys. *Transplant. Proc.* **15**, 635–650.

Jonker, M., Goldstein, G., and Balner, H. (1983b). Effects of *in vivo* administration of monoclonal antibodies specific for human T cell subpopulations of the immune system in a rhesus monkey model. *Transplantation* **35**, 521–526.

Kaizer, H., Levy, R., Brovall, C., Civin, C. I., Fuller, D. J., Hsu, S. H., Leventhal, B. G., Miller, R. A., Milvenan, E. S., Santos, G. W., and Wharam, M. D. (1982). Autologous bone marrow transplantation in T-cell malignancies: A case report involving *in vitro* treatment of marrow with pan-T-cell monoclonal antibody. *J. Biol. Response Modifiers* **1**, 233–243.

Kammer, K. (1983). Monoclonal antibodies to influenza A virus FMI (HINI) proteins require individual conditions for optimal reactivity in binding assays. *Immunology* **48**, 799–808.

Kasai, K., Koshiba, H., Ishii, Y., and Kikuchi, K. (1983). A monoclonal antibody defining human B cell differentiation antigen (HLB-1 Antigen). *Microbiol. Immunol.* **27**, 51–64.

Kearney, J. F., Radbruch, A., Liesegang, B., and Rajewsky, K. (1979). A new mouse myeloma cell line that has lost immunoglobulin expression but permits the construction of antibody-secreting hybrid cell lines. *J. Immunol.* **123**, 1548–1550.

Keating, M. J., Smith, T. L., Gehan, E. A., McCredie, K. B., Bodey, G. P., Spitzer, G., Hersh, E., Gutterman, J., and Freireich, E. J. (1980). Factors related to length of complete remission in adult acute leukemia. *Cancer* **45**, 2017–2029.

Kemshead, J. T., Fritschy, J., Goldman, A., Malpas, J. S., and Pritchard, J. (1983a). Use of panels of monoclonal antibodies in the differential diagnosis of neuroblastoma and lymphoblastic disorders. *Lancet* **i**, 12–14.

Kemshead, J. T., Gibson, F. J., Ugelstad, J., and Rembaum, A. (1983b). A flow system for the *in vitro* separation of tumour cells from bone marrow using monoclonal antibodies and magnetic microspheres. *Proc. Am. Assoc. Cancer Res.* **24**, 217. (Abstr.)

Kennel, S. J., Lankford, T., and Flynn, K. M. (1983). Therapy of a murine sarcoma using syngeneic monoclonal antibody. *Cancer Res.* **43**, 2843–2847.

Kennett, R. H. (1979). Cell fusion. In "Methods in Enzymology" (W. B. Jakoby and H. Pastan, eds.), Vol. 58, pp. 345–359. Academic Press, New York.

Kennett, R. H., and Gilbert, F. (1979). Hybrid myelomas producing antibodies against a human neuroblastoma antigen present on fetal brain. *Science* **203**, 1120–1121.

Kennett, R. H., Denis, K. A., Tung, A. S., and Klinman, N. R. (1978). Hybrid plasmacytoma production: Fusions with adult spleen cells, monoclonal spleen fragments, neonatal spleen cells, and human spleen cells. *Curr. Top. Microbiol. Immunol.* **81**, 77–91.

Kersey, J. H., LeBien, T. W., Abramson, C. S., Newman, R., Sutherland, R., and Greaves, M. (1981). p24: A human leukemia-associated and lympho-hemopoietic progenitor cell surface structure identified with monoclonal antibody. *J. Exp. Med.* **153**, 726–731.

Kessler, S. W. (1975). Rapid isolation of antigens from cells with a staphylococcal protein A-antibody adsorbent: Parameters of the interactions of antibody-antigen complexes with protein A. *J. Immunol.* **115**, 1617–1624.

Key, M. E., Bexhard, M. I., Hoyer, L. C., Foon, K. A., Oldham, R. K., and Hanna, M. G., Jr. (1983). Guinea pig line 10 hepatocarcinoma model for monoclonal antibody serotherapy: *In vivo* localization of a monoclonal antibody in normal and malignant tissues. *J. Immunol.* **130**, 1451–1457.

Kirch, M. E., and Hammerling, U. (1981). Immunotherapy of murine leukemias by monoclonal antibody. I. Effect of passively administered antibody on growth of transplanted tumor cells. *J. Immunol.* **127**, 805–810.

Klinman, N. R., and Press, J. L. (1975). The B cell specificity repertoire: its relationship to definable subpopulations. *Transplant. Rev.* **24**, 41–83.

Knowles, D. M., and Halper, J. P. (1982). Human T-cell malignancies: Correlative clinical, histopathologic, immunologic, and cytochemical analysis of 23 cases. *Am. J. Pathol.* **106**, 187–203.

Kohler, G. (1976). Frequency of precursor cells against the enzyme β-galactosidase. An estimate of the BALB/c strain antibody repertoire. *Eur. J. Immunol.* **6**, 340–347.

Kohler, G., and Milstein, C. (1975). Continuous cultures of fused cells secreting antibody of predefined specificity. *Nature (London)* **256**, 495–497.

Kohler, G., and Milstein, C. (1976). Derivation of specific antibody-producing tissue culture and tumor lines by cell fusion. *Eur J. Immunol.* **6**, 511–519.

Koprowski, H., Steplewski, Z., Herlyn, D., and Herlyn, M. (1978). Study of antibodies against human melanoma produced by somatic cell hybrids. *Proc. Natl. Acad. Sci. U.S.A.* **75**, 3405–3409.

Koprowski, H., Steplewski, Z., Mitchell, K., Herlyn, M., Herlyn, D., and Fuhrer, P. (1979). Colorectal carcinoma antigens detected by hybridoma antibodies. *Somatic Cell Genet.* **5**, 957–972.

Koprowski, H., Sears, H. F., Herlyn, M., and Steplewski, Z. (1981). Specific antigen in serum of patients with colon carcinoma. *Science* **212**, 53–55.

Kozbor, D., and Roder, J. C. (1983). The production of monoclonal antibodies from human lymphocytes. *Immunol. Today* **4**, 72–79.

Kozbor, D., Lagarde, A. E., and Roder, J. C. (1982). Human hybridomas constructed with antigen-specific Epstein-Barr virus-transformed cell lines. *Proc. Natl. Acad. Sci. U.S.A.* **79**, 6651–6655.

Krausz, T. J., van Noorden, S., and Evans, D. J. (1983). Experience of the Oxford tumour marker. *Lancet* **i**, 1097.

Kreth, H. W., and Williamson, A. R. (1973). The extent of diversity of anti-hapten antibodies in inbred mice: Anti-NIP (4-hydroxy-5-iodo-3-nitro-phenacetyl) antibodies in CBA/H mice. *Eur. J. Immunol.* **3**, 141–147.

Krolick, K. A., Villemez, C., Isakson, P., Uhr, J. W., and Vitetta, E. S. (1980). Selective killing of normal or neoplastic B cells by antibodies coupled to the A chain of ricin. *Proc. Natl. Acad. Sci. U.S.A.* **77**, 5419–5423.

Krolick, K. A., Uhr, J. W., and Vitetta, E. S. (1982). Selective killing of leukaemia cells by antibody-toxin conjugates: Implications for autologous bone marrow transplantation. *Nature (London)* **295**, 604–605.

Kubagawa, H., Vogler, L. B., Capra, J. D., Conrad, M. E., Lawton, A. R., and Cooper, M. D. (1979). Studies on the clonal origin of multiple myeloma. *J. Exp. Med.* **150**, 792–807.

Kung, P. C., Goldstein, G., Reinherz, E. L., and Schlossman, S. F. (1979). Monoclonal antibodies defining distinctive human T cell surface antigens. *Science* **206**, 347–349.

Kupchik, H. Z., Zurawski, V. R., Hurrell, J. G. R., Zamcheck, N., and Black, P. H. (1981). Monoclonal antibodies to carcinoembryonic antigen produced by somatic cell fusion. *Cancer Res.* **41**, 3306–3310.

Lampson, L. A., and Levy, R. (1979). A role for clonal antigens in cancer diagnosis and therapy. *JNCI, J. Natl. Cancer Inst.* **62**, 217–219.

Larson, S. M., Brown, J. P., Wright, P. W., Carrasquillo, J. A., Hellstrom, I., and Hellstrom, K. E. (1983). Imaging of melanoma with I-131-labeled monoclonal antibodies. *J. Nucl. Med.* **24**, 123–129.

Lebacq, A.-M., and Bazin, H. (1983). Obtention of rat monoclonal antibodies reactive with human leukaemic lymphoblasts. *Bull. Cancer* **70**, 93–95.

Lee, C. L., Li, C. Y., Jou, Y. H., Murphy, G. P., and Chu, T. M. (1982). Immunochemical characterization of prostatic acid phosphatase with monoclonal antibodies. *Ann. N. Y. Acad. Sci.* **390**, 52–61.

Lehmann, F.-G., and Wegener, T. (1979). Alpha-fetoprotein in liver cirrhosis. II. Early detection of hepatoma. *In* "Carcinoembryonic Proteins. I." (F.-G. Lehmann, ed.), pp. 233–-245. Elsevier, Amsterdam.

Lems, S. P. M., Tax, W. J. M., Capel, P. J. A., and Koene, R. A. P. (1983). Immune regulation by monoclonal antibodies: Failure to enhance mouse skin allografts. *J. Immunol.* **131**, 86–91.

Lerner, R. A. (1982). Tapping the immunological repertoire to produce antibodies of predetermined specificity. *Nature (London)* **299**, 592–596.

Leserman, L. D., Barbet, J., Kourilsky, F., and Weinstein, J. N. (1980). Targeting to cells of fluorescent liposomes covalently coupled with monoclonal antibody or protein A. *Nature (London)* **288**, 602–604.

Leserman, L. D., Machy, P., and Barbet, J. (1981). Cell-specific drug transfer from liposomes bearing monoclonal antibodies. *Nature (London)* **293**, 226–228.

Levine, G., Ballou, B., Reiland, J., Solter, D., Gumerman, L., and Hakala, T. (1980). Localization of I-131-labeled tumor-specific monoclonal antibody in the tumor-bearing BALB/c mouse. *J. Nuclear Med.* **21**, 570–573.

Levy, R., and Dilley, J. (1978). Rescue of immunoglobulin secretion from human neoplastic lymphoid cells by somatic cell hybridization. *Proc. Natl. Acad. Sci. U.S.A.* **75**, 2411–2415.

Levy, R., and Miller, R. A. (1983a). Tumor therapy with monoclonal antibodies. *Fed. Proc., Fed. Am. Soc. Exp. Biol.* **42**, 2650–2656.

Levy, R., and Miller, R. A. (1983b). Biological and clinical implications of lymphocyte hybridomas: Tumor therapy with monoclonal antibodies. *Annu. Rev. Med.* **34**, 107–116.

Levy, R., Dilley, J., Fox, R. I., and Warnke, R. (1979). A human thymus–leukemia antigen defined by hybridoma monoclonal antibodies. *Proc. Natl. Acad. Sci. U.S.A.* **76**, 6552–6556.

Light, P. A., Foster, J. P., Felton, T., Eckert, H., and Tovey, K. C. (1983). Molecular hetero-geneity of chorionic gonadotropin in some testicular cancer patients. *Lancet* **i,** 1284.

Lillehoj, H.-S., Choe, B.-K., and Rose, N. R. (1982). Monoclonal anti-human prostatic acid phosphatase antibodies. *Mol. Immunol.* **19,** 1199–1202.

Lin, J. J.-C., and Queally, S. A. (1982). A monoclonal antibody that recognizes Golgi-associated protein of cultured fibroblast cells. *J. Cell Biol.* **92,** 108–112.

Lin, M. F., Lee, C., and Chu, T. M. (1983). Simple assay for serum prostatic acid phosphatase with specific monoclonal antibody. *Clin. Chim. Acta* **130,** 263–267.

Lindholm, L., Holmgren, J., Svennerholm, L., Fredman, P., Nilsson, O., Persson, B., Myrvold, H., and Lagergard, T. (1983). Monoclonal antibodies against gastrointestinal tumor-associated antigens isolated as monosialogangliosides. *Int. Arch. Allergy App. Immunol.* **71,** 178–181.

Liskay, R. M., and Patterson, D. (1978). Selection of somatic cell hybrids between HGPRT⁻ and APRT⁻ cells. *Methods Cell Biol.* **20,** 355–360.

Liszka, K., Majdic, O., Bettelheim, P., and Knapp, W. (1981). A monoclonal antibody (VIL-A1) reactive with common acute lymphatic leukemia (CALL) cells. *In* "Leukemia Markers" (W. Knapp, ed.), pp. 61–64. Academic Press, New York.

Littlefield, J. W. (1964). Selection of hybrids from mating of fibroblasts *in vitro* and their presumed recombinants. *Science* **145,** 709–710.

Locker, D., and Motta, G. (1983). Detection of antibody secreting hybridomas with diazobenzylox-ymethyl paper: An easy, sensitive, and versatile assay. *J. Immunol. Methods* **59,** 269–275.

Lockhart, C. G., Stinson, R. S., Margraf, H. W., Parker, C. W., and Philpott, G. W. (1980). Production of anti-carcinoembryonic antigen (CEA) antibody by somatic cell hybridization. *Fed. Proc., Fed. Am. Soc. Exp. Biol.* **39,** 928.

Luben, R. A. Brazeau, P., Bohlen, P., and Guillemin, R. (1982). Monoclonal antibodies to hypo-thalamic growth hormone-releasing factor with picomoles of antigen. *Science* **218,** 887–889.

Lumbroso, J., Berche, C., Mach, J.-P., Rougier, P., Aubry, F., Buchegger, F., Lasser, P., Parmen-tier, C., and Tubiana, M. (1983). Utilisation en tomoscintigraphie d'anticorps monoclonaux radio-marqués pour la détection chez l'homme des cancers digestifs et des cancers medullaires de la thyroide. *Bull. Cancer* **70,** 96–102.

Luzzati, A. L., Hengartner, H., and Schreier, M. H. (1977). Induction of plaque-forming cells in cultured human lymphocytes by combined action of antigen and EB virus. *Nature (London)* **269,** 419–420.

McEver, R. P., Baenziger, N. L., and Majerus, P. W. (1980). Isolation and quantitation of the platelet membrane glycoprotein deficient in thrombasthenia using a monoclonal hybridoma antibody. *J. Clin. Invest.* **66,** 1311–1318.

McGee, J. O'D., Woods, J. C., Ashall, F., Bramwell, M. E., and Harris, H. (1982). A new marker for human cancer cells. 2. Immunohistochemical detection of the Ca antigen in human tissues with the Ca1 antibody. *Lancet* **ii,** 7–10.

McGregor, J. L., Brochier, J., Wild, F., Follea, G., Trzeciak, M.-C, James, E., Dechavanne, M., McGregor, L., and Clemetson, K. J. (1983). Monoclonal antibodies against platelet membrane glycoproteins. Characterization and effect on platelet function. *Eur. J. Biochem.* **131,** 427–436.

Mach, J.-P., Buchegger, F., Forni, M., Ritschard, J., Berche, C., Lumbroso, J.-D., Schreyer, M., Girardet, C., Accolla, R. S., and Carrel, S. (1981). Use of radiolabelled monoclonal anti-CEA antibodies for the detection of human carcinomas by external photoscanning and tomoscin-tigraphy. *Immunol. Today* **2,** 239–249.

McKenzie, I. F. C., and Zola, H. (1983). Monoclonal antibodies to B cells. *Immunol. Today* **4,** 10–15.

McLaughlin, P. J., Cheng, H. M., Slade, M. B., and Johnson, P. M. (1982). Expression on cultured human tumour cells of placental trophoblast membrane antigens and placental alkaline phosphatase defined by monoclonal antibodies. *Int. J. Cancer* **30**, 21–26.

McLaughlin, P. J., Gee, H., and Johnson, P. M. (1983). Placental-type alkaline phosphatase in pregnancy and malignancy plasma: Specific estimation using a monoclonal antibody in a solid phase enzyme immunoassay. *Clin. Chim. Acta* **130**, 199–209.

MacLean, G. D., Seehafer, J., Shaw, A. R. E., Kieran, M. W., and Longenecker, B. M. (1982). Antigenic heterogeneity of human colorectal cancer cell lines analyzed by a panel of monoclonal antibodies. I. Heterogeneous expression of Ia-like and HLA-like antigenic determinants. *JNCI, J. Natl. Cancer Inst.* **69**, 357–363.

McMichael, A. J., and Bastin, J. M. (1980). Clinical applications of monoclonal antibodies. *Immunol. Today* **1**, 56–61.

McMichael, A. J., and Fabre, J. W., eds. (1982). "Monoclonal Antibodies in Clinical Medicine." Academic Press, New York.

McMichael, A. J., Pilch, J. R., Galfre, G., Mason, D. Y., Fabre, J. W., and Milstein, C. (1979). A human thymocyte antigen defined by a hybrid myeloma monoclonal antibody. *Eur. J. Immunol.* **9**, 205–210.

Magnani, J. L., Brockhaus, M., Smith, D. F., Ginsburg, V., Blaszczyk, M., Mitchell, K. F., Steplewski, Z., and Koprowski, H. (1981). A monosialoganglioside is a monoclonal antibody-defined antigen of colon carcinoma. *Science* **212**, 55–56.

Magnani, J. L., Nilsson, B., Brockhaus, M., Zopf, D., Steplewski, Z., Koprowski, H., and Ginsburg, V. (1982). A monoclonal antibody-defined antigen associated with gastrointestinal cancer is a ganglioside containing sialylated lacto-*N*-fucopentaose II. *J. Biol. Chem.* **257**, 14365–14369.

Mannoni, P., Janowska-Wieczorek, A., Turner, A. R., McGann, L., and Turc, J.-M. (1982). Monoclonal antibodies against human granulocytes and myeloid differentiation antigens. *Hum. Immunol.* **5**, 309–323.

Martin, P. J., Giblett, E. R., and Hansen, J. A. (1982). Phenotyping human leukemic T-cell lines: Enzyme markers, surface antigens, and cytogenetics. *Immunogenetics (N. Y.)* **15**, 385–398.

Mazauric, T., Mitchell, K. F., Letchworth, G. J., III, Koprowski, H., and Steplewski, Z. (1982). Monoclonal antibody-defined human lung cell surface protein antigens. *Cancer Res.* **42**, 150–154.

Medrano, L., Cesarini, J.-P., Daveau, M., Phillips, J., Salazar, G., Fontaine, M., Phillips, T., Viza, D., and Prunieras, M. (1983). Anti-melanoma hybridoma antibodies against partially purified melanoma antigen. *Eur. J. Cancer Clin. Oncol.* **19**, 153–161.

Menard, S., Tagliabne, E., Canevari, S., Fossati, G., and Colnaghi, M. I. (1983). Generation of monoclonal antibodies reacting with normal and cancer cells of human breast. *Cancer Res.* **43**, 1295–1300.

Metzgar, R. S., Gaillard, M. T., Levine, S. J., Tuck, F. L., Bossen, E. H., and Borowitz, M. J. (1982). Antigens of human pancreatic adenocarcinoma cells defined by murine monoclonal antibodies. *Cancer Res.* **42**, 601–608.

Mew, D., Wat, C.-K., Towers, G. H. N., and Levy, J. G. (1983). Photoimmunotherapy treatment of animal tumors with tumor-specific monoclonal antibody-hematoporphyrin conjugates. *J. Immunol.* **130**, 1473–1477.

Miller, G., and Lipman, M. (1973). Release of infectious Epstein-Barr virus by transformed marmoset leukocytes. *Proc. Natl. Acad. Sci. U.S.A.* **70**, 190–194.

Miller, R. A., and Levy, R. (1981). Response of cutaneous T cell lymphoma to therapy with hybridoma monoclonal antibody. *Lancet* **ii**, 226–230.

Miller, R. A., Maloney, D. G., McKillop, J., and Levy, R. (1981). *In vivo* effects of murine hybridoma monoclonal antibody in a patient with T-cell leukemia. *Blood* **58**, 78–86.

Miller, R. A., Maloney, D. G., Warnke, R., and Levy, R. (1982a). Treatment of B-cell lymphoma with monoclonal anti-idiotype antibody. *N. Engl. J. Med.* **306**, 517–522.

Miller, R. A., Maloney, D. G., and Levy, R. A. (1982b). Reply to letter "Treatment of B-cell lymphoma with monoclonal anti-idiotype antibody." *N. Engl. J. Med.* **307**, 686–687.

Mills, K. H. G., and Cawley, J. C. (1983). Abnormal monoclonal antibody-defined helper/suppressor T-cell subpopulations in multiple myeloma: Relationship to treatment and clinical stage. *Br. J. Haematol.* **53**, 271–275.

Milstein, C., and Lennox, E. (1980). The use of monoclonal antibody techniques in the study of developing cell surfaces. *Curr. Top. Dev. Biol.* **14**, 1–32.

Minna, J. D., Cuttitta, F., Rosen, S., Bunn, P. A., Jr., Carney, D. N., Gazdar, A. F., and Krasnow, S. (1981). Methods for production of monoclonal antibodies with specificity for human lung cancer cells. *In vitro* **17**, 1058–1070.

Mitchell, K. F., Fuhrer, J. P., Steplewski, Z., and Koprowski, H. (1980). Biochemical characterization of human melanoma cell surfaces: Dissection with monoclonal antibodies. *Proc. Natl. Acad. Sci. U.S.A.* **77**, 7287–7291.

Mitchell, K. F., Fuhrer, J. P., Steplewski, Z., and Koprowski, H. (1981). Structural characterization of the "melanoma-specific" antigen detected by monoclonal antibody 691 I 5 NU-4-B. *Mol. Immunol.* **18**, 207–218.

Mitchell, K. F., Steplewski, Z., and Koprowski, H. (1982). Hybridoma antibodies specific for human tumor antigens. *In* "Monoclonal Hybridoma Antibodies: Techniques and Applications" (J. G. R. Hurrell, ed.), pp. 151–168. CRC Press, Boca Raton, Florida.

Mitchell, M. S., and Oettgen, H. F., eds. (1982). "Hybridomas in Cancer Diagnosis and Treatment." Raven, New York.

Mizuguchi, J., Yoshida, T., Sato, Y., Nagaoka, F., Kondo, S., and Matuhasi, T. (1982). Requirement of at least two distinct monoclonal antibodies for efficient neutralization of tetanus toxin *in vivo. Naturwissenschaften* **69**, 597–598.

Morgan, A. C., Jr., and McIntyre, R. F. (1983). Monoclonal antibodies to human melanoma-associated antigens: An amplified enzyme-linked immunosorbent assay for the detection of antigen, antibody and immune complexes. *Cancer Res.* **43**, 3155–3159.

Morgan, A. C., Jr., Galloway, D. R., and Resifeld, R. A. (1981). Production and characterization of monoclonal antibody to a melanoma-specific glycoprotein. *Hybridoma* **1**, 17–36.

Moshakis, V., McIlhinney, R. A. J., Raghavan, D., and Neville, A. M. (1981). Monoclonal antibodies to detect human tumours: An experimental approach. *J. Clin. Pathol.* **34**, 314–319.

Moyle, W. R., Lin, C., and Corson, R. L. (1983). Quantitative explanation for increased affinity shown by mixtures of monoclonal antibodies: Importance of a circular complex. *Mol. Immunol.* **20**, 439–452.

Mulshine, J. L., Cuttitta, F., Bibro, M., Fedorko, J., Fargion, S., Little, C., Carney, D. N., Gazdar, A. F., and Minna, J. D. (1983). Monoclonal antibodies that distinguish non-small cell from small cell lung cancer. *J. Immunol.* **131**, 497–502.

Murakami, H., Masui, H., Sato, G. H., Sueoka, N., Chow, T. P., and Kano-Sueoka, T. (1982). Growth of hybridoma cells in serum-free medium: Ethanolamine is an essential component. *Proc. Natl. Acad. Sci. U.S.A.* **79**, 1158–1162.

Nadler, L. M., Stashenko, P., Hardy, R., and Schlossman, S. F. (1980a). A monoclonal antibody defining a lymphoma-associated antigen in man. *J. Immunol.* **125**, 570–577.

Nadler, L. M., Reinherz, E. L., Weinstein, H. J., D'Orsi, C. J., and Schlossman, S. F. (1980b). Heterogeneity of T-cell lymphoblastic malignancies. *Blood* **55**, 806–810.

Nadler, L. M., Stashenko, P., Hardy, R., Kaplan, W. D., Button, L. N., Kufe, D. W., Antman, K. H., and Schlossman, S. F. (1980c). Serotherapy of a patient with a monoclonal antibody directed against a human lymphoma-associated antigen. *Cancer Res.* **40**, 3147–3154.

Nadler, L. M., Ritz, J., Hardy, R., Pesando, J. M., and Schlossman, S. F. (1981a). A unique cell surface antigen identifying lymphoid malignancies of B cell origin. *J. Clin. Invest.* **67,** 134–140.

Nadler, L. M., Stashenko, P., Hardy, R., van Agthoven, A., Terhorst, C., and Schlossman, S. F. (1981b). Characterization of a human B-cell-specific antigen (B2) distinct from B1. *J. Immunol.* **126,** 1941–1947.

Nadler, L. M., Stashenko, P., Hardy, R., Tomaselli, K. J., Yunis, E. J., Schlossman, S. F., and Pesando, J. M. (1981c). Monoclonal antibody identifies a new Ia-like (p29,34) polymorphic system linked to the HLA-D/DR region. *Nature (London)* **290,** 591–593.

Naiem, M., Gerdes, J., Abdulaziz, Z., Sunderland, C. A., Allington, M. J., Stein, H., and Mason, D. Y. (1982). The value of immunohistological screening in the production of monoclonal antibodies. *J. Immunol. Methods* **50,** 145–160.

Naiem, M., Gerdes, J., Abdulaziz, Z., Stein, H., and Mason, D. Y. (1983). Production of a monoclonal antibody reactive with human dendritic reticulum cells and its use in the immunohistological analysis of lymphoid tissue. *J. Clin. Pathol.* **36,** 167–175.

Naritoku, W. Y., and Taylor, C. R. (1982). A comparative study of the use of monoclonal antibodies using three different immunohistochemical methods: An evaluation of monoclonal and polyclonal antibodies against human prostatic acid phosphatase. *J. Histochem. Cytochem.* **30,** 253–260.

Neville, D. M., Jr., and Youle, R. J. (1982). Monoclonal antibody-ricin or ricin A chain hybrids: Kinetic analysis of cell killing for tumor therapy. *Immunol. Rev.* **62,** 75–91.

Neville, A. M., Foster, C. S., Moshakis, V., and Gore, M. (1982). Monoclonal antibodies and human tumor pathology. *Hum. Pathol.* **13,** 1067–1081.

Nigg, E. A., Walter, G., and Singer, S. J. (1982). On the nature of cross reactions observed with antibodies directed to defined epitopes. *Proc. Natl. Acad. Sci. U.S.A.* **79,** 5939–5943.

Nilsson, K., Scheirer, W., Merten, O. W., Ostberg, L., Liehl, E., Katinger, H. W. D., and Mosbach, K. (1983). Entrapment of animal cells for production of monoclonal antibodies and other biomolecules. *Nature (London)* **302,** 629–630.

Nowinski, R., Berglund, C., Lane, J., Lostrum, M., Bernstein, I., Young, W., Hakomori, S.-I, Hill, L., and Cooney, M. (1980). Human monoclonal antibody against Forssman antigen. *Science* **210,** 537–539.

Nunez, G., Ugolini, V., Capra, J. D., and Stastny, P. (1982). Monoclonal antibodies against human monocytes. II. Recognition of two distinct cell surface molecules. *Scand. J. Immunol.* **16,** 515–523.

Nuti, M., Teramoto, Y. A., Mariani-Costantini, R., Horan Hand, P., Colcher, D., and Schlom, J. (1982). A monoclonal antibody (B72.3) defines patterns of distribution of a novel tumor-associated antigen in human mammary carcinoma cell populations. *Int. J. Cancer* **29,** 539–545.

Oi, V. T., and Herzenberg, L. A. (1980). Immunoglobulin-producing hybrid cell lines. *In* "Selected Methods in Cellular Immunology" (B. B. Mishell and S. M. Shiigi, eds.), pp. 351–372. Freeman, San Francisco, California.

OKunewick, J. P., Meredith, R. F., Raikow, R. B., Buffo, M. J., and Jones, D. L. (1982a). Possibility of three distinct and separable components to fatal graft-vs-host reaction. *Exp. Hematol.* **10,** 277–291.

OKunewick, J. P., Meredith, R. F., Braunschweiger, P. G., Buffo, M. J., Jones, D. L., and Beschorner, W. E. (1982b). Definition and prevention of graft-versus-host disease with the use of monoclonal antibodies. *Exp. Hematol.* **10** *S12,* 12–22.

Old, L. J. (1981). Cancer immunology: The search for specificity. *Cancer Res.* **41,** 361–375.

Olsnes, S. (1981). Directing toxins to cancer cells. *Nature (London)* **290,** 84.

Olsnes, S., and Pihl, A. (1981). Chimaeric toxins. *Pharmacol. Ther.* **15**, 355–381.

Olsson, L. (1983). Monoclonal antibodies in clinical immunobiology. Derivation, potential and limitations. *Allergy* **38**, 145–154.

Olsson, L., and Kaplan, H. S. (1980). Human-human hybridomas producing monoclonal antibodies of predefined antigenic specificity. *Proc. Natl. Acad. Sci. U.S.A.* **77**, 5429–5431.

Olsson, L., and Kaplan, H. S. (1983). Human-human monoclonal antibody-producing hybridomas-technical aspects. *In* "Methods in Enzymology" (J. J. Langone and H. Van Vunakis, eds.), Vol. 92E, pp. 3–16. Academic Press, New York.

Olsson, L., Kronstrom, H., Cambon-De Mouzon, A., Honsik, C., Brodin, T., and Jakobsen, B. (1983). Antibody producing human-human hybridomas. I. Technical aspects. *J. Immunol. Methods* **61**, 17–32.

Order, S. E., Klein, J. L., Ettinger, D., Alderson, P., Siegelman, S., and Leichner, P. (1980). Phase I–II study of radiolabeled antibody integrated in the treatment of primary hepatic malignancies. *Int. J. Radiat. Oncol., Biol. Phys.* **6**, 703–710.

Order, S. E., Klein, J. L., and Leichner, P. K. (1981). Antiferritin IgG antibody for isotopic cancer therapy. *Oncology* **38**, 154–160.

Osband, M., Cavagnaro, J., and Kupchik, H. Z. (1982). Successful production of human-human hybridoma IgG antibodies against Rh(D) antigen. *Blood* **60** *S1,* 81a. (Abstr.)

Paiva, J., Damjanov, I., Lange, P. H., and Harris, H. (1983). Immunohistochemical localization of placental-like alkaline phosphatase in testis and germ-cell tumors using monoclonal antibodies. *Am. J. Pathol.* **111**, 156–165.

Pallesen, G., Jepsen, F. L., Hastrup, J., Ipsen, A., and Hvidberg, N. (1983). Experience with the Oxford tumour marker (Ca1) in serous fluids. *Lancet* **i**, 1326.

Papsidero, L. D., Croghan, G. A., O'Connell, M. J., Valenzuela, L. A., Nemoto, T., and Chu, T. M. (1983). Monoclonal antibodies (F36/22 and M7/105) to human breast carcinoma. *Cancer Res.* **43**, 1741–1747.

Pardue, R. L., Brady, R. C., Perry, G. W., and Dedman, J. R. (1983). Producton of monoclonal antibodies against calmodulin by *in vitro* immunization of spleen cells. *J. Cell Biol.* **96**, 1149–1154.

Park, S. S., Fujino, T., West, D., Guengerich, F. P., and Gelboin, H. V. (1982). Monoclonal antibodies that inhibit enzyme activity of 3-methyl-cholanthrene-induced cytochrome P-450. *Cancer Res.* **42**, 1798–1808.

Parker, R. J., Weinstein, J. N., Stellar, M. A., Hwang, K. M., Covell, D. G., Sieber, S. M., Keenan, A. M., and Key, M. E. (1983). Monoclonal antibodies in the lymphatics: Selective delivery to lymph nodes containing solid tumor metastases. *Proc. Am. Assoc. Cancer Res.* **24**, 210. (Abstr.)

Parks, D. R., Bryan, V. M., Oi, V. T., and Herzenberg, L. A. (1979). Antigen-specific identification and cloning of hybridomas with a fluorescence-activated cell sorter. *Proc. Natl. Acad. Sci. U.S.A.* **76**, 1962–1966.

Parsa, I., Sutton, A. L., Chen, C. K., and Delbridge, C. (1982). Monoclonal antibody for identification of human duct cell carcinoma of pancreas. *Cancer Lett. (Shannon, Irel.)* **17**, 217–222.

Pearson, T. W., and Anderson, N. L. (1983). Use of high resolution 2-dimensional gel electrophoresis for analysis of monoclonal antibodies and their specific antigens. *In* Methods in Enzymology (J. Langone and H. Van Vunakis, eds.), Vol. 92E, pp. 196–220, Academic Press, New York.

Perri, R. T., Royston, I., LeBien, T. W., and Kay, N. E. (1983). Chronic lymphocytic leukemia progenitor cells carry the antigens T65, BA-1, and Ia. *Blood* **61**, 871–875.

Phillips, J., Alderson, T., Sikora, K., and Watson, J. (1983). Localisation of malignant glioma by a radiolabelled human monoclonal antibody. *J. Neurol., Neurosurg. Psychiatry* **46**, 388–392.

Pizzolo, G., Sloane, J., Beverley, P., Thomas, J. A., Bradstock, K. F., Mattingly, S., and Janossy, G. (1980). Differential diagnosis of malignant lymphoma and non-lymphoid tumors using monoclonal antileucocyte antibody. *Cancer* **46**, 2640–2647.

Poiesz, B. J., Ruscetti, F. W., Gazdar, A. F., Bunn, P. A., Minna, J. D., and Gallo, R. C. (1980). Detection and isolation of type C retrovirus particles from fresh and cultured T-cell lymphoma. *Proc. Natl. Acad. Sci. U.S.A.* **77**, 7415–7419.

Poynton, C. H., and Reading, C. L. (1984). Monoclonal antibodies: A review of some of the possibilities for cancer therapy. *Exp. Biol.* **43**, 13–33.

Poynton, C. H., Dicke, K. A., Culbert, S., Frankel, L. S., Jagannath, S., and Reading, C. L. (1983). Immunomagnetic removal of CALLA positive cells from human bone marrow. *Lancet* **i**, 524.

Prentice, H. G., Blacklock, H. A., Janossy, G. Bradstock, K. F., Skeggs, D., Goldstein, G., and Hoffbrand, A. V. (1982). Use of anti-T-cell monoclonal antibody OKT3 to prevent acute graft-versus-host disease in allogeneic bone-marrow transplantation for acute leukaemia. *Lancet* **i**, 700–703.

Pressman, D., and Korngold, L. (1953). The *in vivo* localization of anti-Wagner-osteogenic-sarcoma antibodies. *Cancer* **6**, 619–623.

Raso, V. (1982). Antibody mediated delivery of toxic molecules to antigen-bearing target cells. *Immunol. Rev.* **62**, 93–117.

Raso, V., Ritz, J., Basala, M., and Schlossman, S. F. (1982). Monoclonal antibody-ricin A chain conjugate selectively cytotoxic for cells bearing the common acute lymphoblastic leukemia antigen. *Cancer Res.* **42**, 457–464.

Reading, C. L. (1982). Theory and methods for immunization in culture and monoclonal antibody production. *J. Immunol. Methods* **53**, 261–291.

Reading, C. L. (1983). Procedures for *in vitro* immunization and monoclonal antibody production. *In* "Hybridomas and Cellular Immortality" (J. P. Allison and B. H. Tom, eds.), pp. 235–250. Plenum Press, New York.

Reinherz, E. L., Kung, P. C., Goldstein, G., Levey, R. H., and Schlossman, S. F. (1980). Discrete stages of human intrathymic differentiation: Analysis of normal thymocytes and leukemic lymphoblasts of T-cell lineage. *Proc. Natl. Acad. Sci. U.S.A.* **77**, 1588–1592.

Reisfeld, R. A., Galloway, D., Imai, K., Ferrone, S., and Morgan, A. C. (1980). Molecular profiles of human melanoma associated antigens. *Fed. Proc., Fed. Am. Soc. Exp. Biol.* **39**, 351.

Ritz, J., and Schlossman, S. F. (1982). Utilization of monoclonal antibodies in the treatment of leukemia and lymphoma. *Blood* **59**, 1–11.

Ritz, J., Pesando, J. M., Notis-McConarty, J., Lazarus, H., and Schlossman, S. F. (1980a). A monoclonal antibody to human acute lymphoblastic leukemia antigen. *Nature (London)* **283**, 583–585.

Ritz, J., Pesando, J. M., Notis-McConarty, J., and Schlossman, S. F. (1980b). Modulation of human acute lymphoblastic leukemia antigen induced by monoclonal antibody *in vitro*. *J. Immunol.* **125**, 1506–1514.

Ritz, J., Pesando, J. M., Notis-McConarty, J., Clavell, L. A., Sallan, S. E., and Schlossman, S. F. (1981a). Use of monoclonal antibodies as diagnostic and therapeutic reagents in acute lymphoblastic leukemia. *Cancer Res.* **41**, 4771–4775.

Ritz, J., Pesando, J. M., Sallan, S. E., Clavell, L. A., Notis-McConarty, J., Rosenthal, P., and Schlossman, S. F. (1981b). Serotherapy of acute lymphoblastic leukemia with monoclonal antibody. *Blood* **58**, 141–152.

Ritz, J., Bast, R. C., Jr., Clavell, L. A., Hercend, T., Sallan, S. E., Lipton, J. M., Feeney, M., Nathan, D. G., and Schlossman, S. F. (1982). Autologous bone-marrow transplantation in

CALLA-positive acute lymphoblastic leukemia after *in vitro* treatment with J5 monoclonal antibody and complement. *Lancet* **ii**, 60–63.

Robbins, D. S., and Fudenberg, H. H. (1983). Human lymphocyte subpopulations in metastatic neoplasia—six years later. *N. Engl. J. Med.* **308**, 1595–1597.

Rodt, H., Kolb, H. J., Netzel, B., Haas, R. J., Wilms, K., Gotze, Ch. B., Link, H., and Thierfelder, S. (1981). Effect of anti-T-cell globulin on GVHD in leukemic patients treated with BMT. *Transplant. Proc.* **13**, 257–261.

Rodt, H., Thierfelder, S., and Kummer, U. (1983). Effect of monoclonal antibodies on GVHD in minor and MHC-incompatible mouse models. *Transplant. Proc.* **15**, 1472–1476.

Rosen, A., Persson, K., and Klein, G. (1983). Human monoclonal antibodies to a genus-specific chlamydial antigen, produced by EBV-transformed B cells. *J. Immunol.* **130**, 2899–2902.

Rotblat, F., Goodall, A. H., O'Brien, D. P., Rawlings, E., Middleton, S., and Tuddenham, E. G. D. (1983). Monoclonal antibodies to human procoagulant factor VIII. *J. Lab. Clin. Med.* **101**, 736–746.

Royston, I., Majda, J. A., Baird, S. M., Meserve, B. L., and Griffiths, J. C. (1980). Human T-cell antigens defined by monoclonal antibodies: The 65,000-dalton antigen of T-cells (T65) is also found on chronic lymphocytic leukemia cells bearing surface immunoglobulin. *J. Immunol.* **125**, 725–731.

Ruiter, D. J., Bhan, A. K., Harrist, T. J., Sober, A. J., and Mihm, M. C., Jr. (1982). Major histocompatibility antigens and mononuclear inflammatory infiltrate in benign nevomelanocytic proliferations and malignant melanoma. *J. Immunol.* **129**, 2808–2815.

Rumpold, H., Kraft, D., Obexer, G., Radaszkiewicz, T., Majdic, O., Bettelheim, P., Knapp, W., and Bock, G. (1983). Phenotypes of human large granular lymphocytes as defined by monoclonal antibodies. *Immunobiology* **164**, 51–62.

Russell, P. J., Doolan, T. J., Webb, J., and Carr, G. A. (1983). Membrane antigens of human cells of the monocyte/macrophage lineage studied with monoclonal antibodies. *Pathology* **15**, 45–52.

Sanchez-Madrid, F., Szklut, P., and Springer, T. A. (1983). Stable hamster–mouse hybridomas producing IgG and IgM hamster monoclonal antibodies of defined specificity. *J. Immunol.* **130**, 309–312.

Saunders, G. C. (1979). Art of solid-phase immunoassay including selected protocols. *In* "Immunoassays: Clinical Laboratory" (R. M. Nakamura, W. R. Dito, and E. S. Tucker III, eds.), pp. 99–118. Alan R. Liss, New York.

Scheinberg, D. A., and Strand, M. (1982). Leukemic cell targeting and therapy by monoclonal antibody in a mouse model system. *Cancer Res.* **42**, 44–49.

Scheinberg, D. A., and Strand, M. (1983). Kinetic and catabolic considerations of monoclonal antibody targeting in erythroleukemic mice. *Cancer Res.* **43**, 265–272.

Scheinberg, D. A., Strand, M., and Gransow, O. A. (1982). Tumor imaging with radioactive metal chelates conjugated to monoclonal antibodies. *Science* **215**, 1511–1513.

Schlom, J., Wunderlich, D., and Teramoto, Y. A. (1980). Generation of human monoclonal antibodies reactive with human mammary carcinoma cells. *Proc. Natl. Acad. Sci. U.S.A.* **77**, 6841–6845.

Schlom, J., Colcher, D., Teramoto, Y. A., Horan Hand, P., Nuti, M., Austin, F., Mariani, R., and Wunderlich, D. (1982). Generation and characterization of murine and human monoclonal antibodies reactive with human mammary tumor cells. *In* "Hybridomas in Cancer Diagnosis and Treatment" (M. S. Mitchell and H. F. Oettgen, eds.), pp. 213–214. Raven, New York.

Schmitz, H. E., Atassi, H., and Atassi, M. Z. (1982). Production of monoclonal antibodies with preselected submolecular binding specificities to protein determinants. *Mol. Immunol.* **19**, 1699–1702.

Schnegg, J. F., Diserens, A. C., Carrel, S., Accolla, R. S., and Tribolet, N. (1981). Human glioma-associated antigens detected by monoclonal antibodies. *Cancer Res.* **41**, 1209–1213.

Schneider, M. D., and Eisenbarth, G. S. (1979). Transfer plate radioassay using cell monolayers to detect anti-cell surface antibodies synthesized by lymphocyte hybridomas. *J. Immunol. Methods* **29**, 331–342.

Sears, H. F., Herlyn, M., Del Villano, B., Steplewski, Z., and Koprowski, H. (1982a). Monoclonal antibody detection of a circulating tumor-associated antigen. II. A longitudinal evaluation of patients with colorectal cancer. *J. Clin. Immunol.* **2**, 141–149.

Sears, H. F., Herlyn, D., Herlyn, M., Steplewski, Z., Gratzinger, P., and Koprowski, H. (1982b). *Ex vivo* perfusion of human colon with monoclonal anticolorectal cancer antibodies. *Cancer* **49**, 1231–1235.

Sears, H. F., Mattis, J., Herlyn, D., Hayry, P., Atkinson, B., Ernst, C., Steplewski, Z., and Koprowski, H. (1982c). Phase-I clinical trial of monoclonal antibody in treatment of gastrointestinal tumours. *Lancet* **i**, 762–765.

Seon, B. K., Negoro, S., and Barcos, M. P. (1983). Monoclonal antibody that defines a unique human T-cell leukemia antigen. *Proc. Natl. Acad. Sci. U.S.A.* **80**, 845–849.

Sharon, J., Morrison, S. L., and Kabat, E. A. (1979). Detection of specific hybridoma clones by replica immunoadsorption of their secreted antibodies. *Proc. Natl. Acad. Sci. U.S.A.* **76**, 1420–1424.

Sharp, T. G., Sachs, D. H., Fauci, A. S., Messerschmidt, G. L., and Rosenberg, S. A. (1983). T-cell depletion of human bone marrow using monoclonal antibody and complement-mediated lysis. *Transplantation* **35**, 112–120.

Shevinsky, L. H., Knowles, B. B., Damjanov, I., and Solter, D. (1982). Monoclonal antibody to murine embryos defines a stage-specific embryonic antigen expressed on mouse embryos and human teratocarcinoma cells. *Cell* **30**, 697–705.

Shoenfeld, Y., Hsu-Lin, S. C., Gabriels, J. E., Silberstein, L. E., Furie, B. C., Furie, B., Stollar, B. D., and Schwartz, R. S. (1982). Production of autoantibodies by human–human hybridomas. *J. Clin. Invest.* **70**, 205–208.

Shouval, D., Shafritz, D. A., Zurawski, V. R., Jr., Isselbacher, K. J., and Wands, J. R. (1982). Immunotherapy in nude mice of human hepatoma using monoclonal antibodies against hepatitis B virus. *Nature (London)* **298**, 567–569.

Shulman, M., Wilde, C. D., and Kohler, G. (1978). A better cell line for making hybridomas secreting specific antibodies. *Nature (London)* **276**, 269–270.

Sikora, K. (1982). Monoclonal antibodies in oncology. *J. Clin. Pathol.* **35**, 369–375.

Sikora, K., and Wright, R. (1981). Human monoclonal antibodies to lung cancer antigens. *Br. J. Cancer* **43**, 696–700.

Sikora, K., Alderson, T., Phillips, J., and Watson, J. V. (1982). Human hybridomas from malignant gliomas. *Lancet* **i**, 11–14.

Sikora, K., Alderson, T., Ellis, J., Phillips, J., and Watson, J. (1983). Human hybridomas from patients with malignant disease. *Br. J. Cancer* **47**, 135–145.

Silver, L. M., and Elgin, S. C. R. (1979). Immunofluorescent analysis of chromatin structure in relation to gene activity: A speculative essay. *Curr. Top. Biol.* **13**, 71–88.

Simpson, H. W., Candlish, W., Liddle, C., McGregor, F. M., Mutch, F., and Tinklen, B. (1983). Experience of the Oxford tumour marker. *Lancet* **i**, 1097.

Siraganian, R. P., Fox, P. C., and Berenstein, E. H. (1983). Methods of enhancing the frequency of antigen-specific hybridomas. *In* "Methods in Enzymology" (J. J. Langone and H. Van Vunakis, eds.), 92E, pp. 17–26. Academic Press, New York.

Skubitz, K. M., Zhen, Y., and August, J. T. (1983). A human granulocyte-specific antigen characterized by use of monoclonal antibodies. *Blood* **61**, 19–26.

Slaughter, C. A., Coseo, M. C., Cancro, M. P., and Harris, H. (1981). Detection of enzyme polymorphism by using monoclonal antibodies. *Proc. Natl. Acad. Sci. U.S.A.* **78,** 1124–1128.

Slavin, R. E., and Santos, G. W. (1973). The graft versus host reaction in man after bone marrow transplantation: Pathology, pathogenesis, clinical features, and implication. *Clin. Immunol. Immunopathol.* **1,** 472–498.

Smedley, H. M., Finan, P., Lennox, E. S., Ritson, A., Takei, F., Wraight, P., and Sikora, K. (1983). Localisation of metastatic carcinoma by a radiolabelled monoclonal antibody. *Br. J. Cancer* **47,** 253–259.

Solter, D., and Knowles, B. B. (1978). Monoclonal antibody defining a stage-specific mouse embryonic antigen (SSEA-1). *Proc. Natl. Acad. Sci. U.S.A.* **75,** 5565–5569.

Solter, D., Ballou, B., Reilan, J., Levine, G., Hakala, T. R., and Knowles, B. B. (1982). Radioimmunodetection of tumors using monoclonal antibodies. *In* "Hybridomas in Cancer Diagnosis and Treatment" (M. S. Mitchell and H. F. Oettgen, eds.), pp. 241–244. Raven, New York.

Sorg, C., Bruggen, J., Suter, L., and Brocker, E.-B. (1983). Monoclonal antibodies against human malignant melanoma. *Bull. Cancer* **70,** 113–117.

Soule, H. R., Linder, E., and Edgington, T. S. (1983). Membrane 126-kilodalton phosphoglycoprotein associated with human carcinomas identified by a hybridoma antibody to mammary carcinoma cells. *Proc. Natl. Acad. Sci. U.S.A.* **80,** 1332–1336.

Srikumaran, S., Guidry, A. J., and Goldsby, R. A. (1983). Bovine × mouse hybridomas that secrete bovine immunoglobulin G_1. *Science* **220,** 522–524.

Staines, N. A., and Lew, A. M. (1980). Review. Whither monoclonal antibodies? *Immunology* **40,** 287–293.

Stamatoyannopoulos, G., Farquhar, M., Lindsley, D., Brice, M., Papayannopoulou, Th., and Nute, P. E. (1983). Monoclonal antibodies specific for globin chains. *Blood* **61,** 530–539.

Stashenko, P., Nadler, L. M., Hardy, R., and Schlossman, S. F. (1980). Characterization of a human B lymphocyte-specific antigen. *J. Immunol.* **125,** 1678–1685.

Steinitz, M., and Klein, G. (1980). EBV-transformation of surface IgA-positive human lymphocytes. *J. Immunol.* **125,** 194–196.

Steinitz, M., Klein, G., Koskimies, S., and Makel, O. (1977). EB-virus-induced B lymphocyte cell lines producing specific antibody. *Nature (London)* **269,** 420–422.

Steinitz, M., Seppala, I., Eichmann, K., and Klein, G. (1979). Establishment of a human lymphoblastoid cell line with specific antibody production against group A streptococcal carbohydrate. *Z. Immunitaetsforsch.* **156,** 41–47.

Steinitz, M., Izak, G., Cohen, S., Ehrenfeld, M., and Flechner, I. (1980). Continuous production of monoclonal rheumatoid factor by EBV-transformed lymphocytes. *Nature (London)* **287,** 443–445.

Steplewski, Z., Herlyn, M., Herlyn, D., Clark, W. H., and Koprowski, H. (1979). Reactivity of monoclonal anti-melanoma antibodies with melanoma cells freshly isolated from primary and metastatic melanoma. *Eur. J. Immunol.* **9,** 94–96.

Steplewski, Z., Chang, T. H., Herlyn, M., and Koprowski, H. (1981). Release of monoclonal-antibody defined-antigens by human colorectal carcinoma and melanoma cells. *Cancer Res.* **41,** 2723–2727.

Steplewski, Z., Mitchell, K. F., and Koprowski, H. (1982). Biological studies of antimelanoma monoclonal antibodies. *In* "Melanoma Antigens and Antibodies" (R. Reisfeld and S. Ferrone, eds.), pp. 365–380. Plenum, New York.

Stocker, J. W., Trucco, M. M., Jacot-Guillarmod, H., and Ceppellini, R. (1978). Analytical potential of monoclonal antibodies in the detection of cell surface antigens. *In* "Current Trends in Tumour Immunology" (S. Ferrone, S. Gorini, R. B. Herberman, and R. A. Reisfeld, eds.), pp. 219–231. Garland STPM Press, New York.

Stocker, J. W., and Heusser, C. H. (1979). Methods for binding cells to plastic: Application to a solid-phase radioimmunoassay for cell-surface antigens. *J. Immunol. Methods* **26**, 87–95.

Tabin, C. J., Bradley, S. M., Bargmann, C. I., and Weinberg, R. A. (1982). Mechanism of activation of a human oncogene. *Nature (London)* **300**, 143–152.

Taggart, R. T., and Samloff, I. M. (1983). Stable antibody-producing murine hybridomas. *Science* **219**, 1228–1230.

Talle, M. A., Rao, P. E., Westberg, E., Allegar, N., Makowski, M., Mittler, R. S., and Goldstein, G. (1983). Patterns of antigenic expression on human monocytes as defined by monoclonal antibodies. *Cell Immunol.* **78**, 83–99.

Taparowsky, E., Suard, Y., Fasano, O., and Wigler, M. (1982). Activation of the T24 bladder carcinoma transforming gene is linked to a single amino acid change. *Nature (London)* **300**, 762–765.

Teramoto, Y. A., Mariani, R., Wunderlich, D., and Schlom, J. (1982). The immunohistochemical reactivity of a human monoclonal antibody with tissue sections of human mammary tumors. *Cancer* **50**, 241–249.

Thierfelder, S., Hoffmann-Fezer, G., Rodt, H., Doxiadis, I., Eulitz, M., and Kummer, V. (1983). Antilymphocyte antibodies and marrow transplantation. VI. Absence of immunosuppression *in vivo* after injection of monoclonal antibodies blocking graft-versus-host reactions and humoral antibody formation *in vitro*. *Transplantation* **35**, 249–254.

Thompson, C. H., Jones, S. L., Pihl, E., and McKenzie, I. F. C. (1983). Monoclonal antibodies to human colon and colorectal carcinoma. *Br. J. Cancer* **47**, 595–605.

Thompson, J. J., Herlyn, M. F., Elder, D. E., Clark, W. H., Steplewski, Z., and Koprowski, H. (1982a). Expression of DR-antigens in freshly frozen human tumors. *Hybridoma* **1**, 161–168.

Thompson, J. J., Herlyn, M. F., Elder, D. E., Clark, W. H., Steplewski, Z., and Koprowski, H. (1982b). Use of monoclonal antibodies in detection of melanoma associated antigens in intact human tumors. *Am. J. Pathol.* **107**, 357–361.

Thorgeirsson, S. S., Sanderson, N., Park, S. S., and Gelboin, H. V. (1983). Inhibition of 2-acetylaminofluorene oxidations by monoclonal antibodies specific to 3-methylcholanthrene-induced rat liver cytochrome P450. *Carcinogenesis* **4**, 639–641.

Thorpe, P. E., and Ross, W. C. J. (1982). The preparation and cytotoxic properties of antibody–toxin conjugates. *Immunol. Rev.* **62**, 119–158.

Thorpe, P. E., Mason, D. W., Brown, A. N. F., Simmonds, S. J., Ross, W. C. J., Cumber, A. J., and Forrester, J. A. (1982). Selective killing of malignant cells in a leukemic rat bone marrow using an antibody–ricin conjugate. *Nature (London)* **297**, 594–596.

Thurlow, P. J., and McKenzie, I. F. C. (1983). Monoclonal antibodies in clinical medicine. *Aust. N. Z. J. Med.* **13**, 91–100.

Tilden, A. B., Abo, T., and Balch, C. M. (1983). Suppressor cell function of human granular lymphocytes identified by the HNK-1 (Leu 7) monoclonal antibody. *J. Immunol.* **130**, 1171–1175.

Towbin, H., Staehelin, T., and Gordon, J. (1979). Electrophoretic transfer of proteins from polyacrylamide gels to nitrocellulose sheets: Procedure and some applications. *Proc. Natl. Acad. Sci. U.S.A.* **76**, 4350–4354.

Trojanowski, J. Q., and Lee, V. M.-Y. (1983). Anti-neurofilament monoclonal antibodies: Reagents for the evaluation of human neoplasms. *Acta Neuropath.* **59**, 155–158.

Trowbridge, I. S. (1978). Interspecies spleen-myeloma hybrid producing monoclonal antibodies against mouse lymphocyte surface glycoprotein, T200. *J. Exp. Med.* **148**, 313–323.

Trowbridge, I. S., and Domingo, D. L. (1981). Anti-transferrin receptor monoclonal antibody and toxin-antibody conjugates affect growth of human tumour cells. *Nature (London)* **294**, 171–173.

Trucco, M. M., Stocker, J. W., and Ceppellini, C. (1978). Monoclonal antibodies against human lymphocyte antigens. *Nature (London)* **273**, 666–668.

Tsang, V. C. W., Peralta, J. M., and Simons, A. R. (1983). Enzyme-linked immunoelectrotransfer blot techniques (EITB) for studying the specificities of antigens and antibodies separated by gel electrophoresis. *In* "Methods in Enzymology" (J. J. Langone and H. Van Vunakis, eds.), Vol. 92E, pp. 377–391. Academic Press, New York.

Tsu, T. T., and Herzenberg, L. A. (1980). Solid-phase radioimmune assays. *In* "Selected Methods in Cellular Immunology" (B. B. Mishell and S. M. Shiigi, eds.), pp. 373–397. Freeman, San Francisco, California.

Tsukada, Y., Bischof, W. K.-D., Hibi, N., Hirai, H., Hurwitz, E., and Sela, M. (1982). Effect of a conjugate of daunomycin and antibodies to rat α-fetoprotein on the growth of α-fetoprotein-producing tumor cells. *Proc. Natl. Acad. Sci. U.S.A.* **79**, 621–625.

Tsung, Y.-K., Milunsky, A., and Alpert, E. (1980). Derivation and characterization of monoclonal hybridoma antibody specific for human alpha-fetoprotein. *J. Immunol. Methods* **39**, 363–368.

Uchanska-Ziegler, B., Wernet, P., and Ziegler, A. (1981). Monoclonal antibodies against human lymphoid and myeloid antigens: AMML cells as immunogen. *In* "Leukemia Markers" (W. Knapp, ed.), pp. 243–246. Academic Press, New York.

Underwood, P. A., Kelly, J. F., Harman, D. F., and MacMillan, H. M. (1983). Use of protein A to remove immunoglobulins from serum in hybridoma culture media. *J. Immunol. Methods* **60**, 33–45.

Uotila, M., Engvall, E., and Ruoslahti, E. (1980). Monoclonal antibodies to human alphafetoprotein. *Mol. Immunol.* **17**, 791–794.

Vainchenker, W., Deschamps, J. F., Bastin, J. M., Guichard, J., Titeux, M., Breton-Gorius, J., and McMichael, A. J. (1982). Two monoclonal antiplatelet antibodies as markers of human megakaryocyte maturation: Immunofluorescent staining and platelet peroxidase detection in megakaryocyte colonies and *in vivo* cells from normal and leukemic patients. *Blood* **59**, 514–521.

van der Reijden, H. J., van Wering, E. R., van de Rijn, J. M., Melief, C. J. M., van't Veer, M. B., Behrendt, H., and von dem Borne, A. E. G. Kr. (1983). Immunological typing of acute lymphoblastic leukemia. *Scand. J. Haematol.* **30**, 356–366.

Ved Brat, S. S., Hammerling, U., Hardy, W. D., Jr., Borenfreund, E., and Prensky, W. (1980). Monoclonal antibodies: Detection of transformation-related antigens. *Cold Spring Harbor Symp. Quant. Biol.* **44**, 715–720.

Venuta, S., Mertelsmann, R., Welte, K., Feldman, S. P., Wang, C. Y., and Moore, M. A. S. (1983). Production and regulation of interleukin-2 in human lymphoblastic leukemias studied with T-cell monoclonal antibodies. *Blood* **61**, 781–789.

Vollmers, H. P., and Birchmeier, W. (1983). Monoclonal antibodies inhibit the adhesion of mouse B16 melanoma cells *in vitro* and block lung metastasis *in vivo*. *Proc. Natl. Acad. Sci. U.S.A.* **80**, 3729–3733.

Wahl, R. L., Parker, C. W., and Philpott, G. W., (1983). Improved radioimaging and tumour localization with monoclonal F (ab')$_2$. *J. Nucl. Med.* **24**, 317–325.

Waldor, M. K., Sriram, S., McDevitt, H. O., and Steinman, L. (1983). *In vivo* therapy with monoclonal anti-I-A antibody suppresses immune responses to acetylcholine receptor. *Proc. Natl. Acad. Sci. U.S.A.* **80**, 2713–2717.

Ware, J. L., Paulson, D. F., Parks, S. F., and Webb, K. S. (1982). Production of monoclonal antibody α PR03 recognizing a human prostatic carcinoma antigen. *Cancer Res.* **42**, 1215–1222.

Warnke, R. A., and Link, M. P. (1983). Identification and significance of cell markers in leukemia and lymphoma. *Annu. Rev. Med.* **34**, 117–131.

Watson, J. D., and Crick, F. H. C. (1953). Molecular structure of nucleic acids. A structure for deoxyribose nucleic acids. *Nature (London)* **171**, 737–738.

Watson, J. V., Alderson, T., Sikora, K., and Phillips, J. (1983). Subcutaneous culture chamber for continuous infusion of monoclonal antibodies. *Lancet* **i**, 99–100.

Webb, K. S., Ware, J. L., Parks, S. F., Briner, W. H., and Paulson, D. F. (1983). Monoclonal antibodies to different epitopes on a prostate tumor-associated antigen: Implications for immunotherapy. *Cancer Immunol. Immunother.* **14**, 155–166.

Weiden, P. L., Sullivan, K. M., Flourney, N., Storb, R., and Thomas, E. D. (1981). Antileukemic effect of chronic graft-versus-host disease. *N. Engl. J. Med.* **304**, 1529–1533.

Weinstein, J. N., Parker, R. J., Keenan, A. M., Dower, S. K., Morse, H. C., III, and Sieber, S. M. (1982). Monoclonal antibodies in the lymphatics: Toward the diagnosis and therapy of tumor metastases. *Science* **218**, 1334–1337.

Weiss, R. A. (1982). Retroviruses produced by hybridomas. *N. Engl. J. Med.* **307**, 1587.

Wiels, J., Fellous, M., and Tursz, T. (1981). Monoclonal antibody against a Burkitt lymphoma-associated antigen. *Proc. Natl. Acad. Sci. U.S.A.* **78**, 6485–6488.

Wikstrand, C. J., Bigner, S. H., and Bigner, D. D. (1983). Demonstration of complex antigenic heterogeneity in a human glioma cell line and eight derived clones by specific monoclonal antibodies. *Cancer Res.* **43**, 3327–3334.

Williams, A. F., Galfre, G., and Milstein, C. (1977). Analysis of cell surfaces by xenogeneic myeloma-hybrid antibodies: Differentiation antigens of rat lymphocytes. *Cell* **12**, 663–673.

Williams, L. K., Sullivan, A., McIlhinney, R. A. J., and Neville, A. M. (1982). A monoclonal antibody marker of human primitive endoderm. *Int. J. Cancer* **30**, 731–738.

Wilson, B. S., Ruberto, G., and Ferrone, S. (1983). Immunochemical characterization of a human high molecular weight–melanoma associated antigen identified with monoclonal antibodies. *Cancer Immunol. Immunother.* **14**, 196–201.

Winchester, R., Toguchi, T., Szer, I., Burmester, G., Lo Galbo, P., Cuttner, J., Capra, J. D., and Nunez-Roldan, A. (1983). Association of susceptibility to certain hematopoietic malignancies with the presence of Ia alloderminants distinct from the DR series: Utility of monoclonal antibody reagents. *Immunol. Rev.* **70**, 155–166.

Witte, P. L., and Ber, R. (1983). Improved efficiency of hybridoma ascites production by intra-splenic inoculation in mice. *JNCI, J. Natl. Cancer Inst.* **70**, 575–577.

Woodbury, R. G., Brown, J. P., Yeh, M.-Y., Hellstrom, I., and Hellstrom. K. E. (1980). Identification of a cell surface protein, p97, in human melanomas and certain other neoplasms. *Proc. Natl. Acad. Sci.* **77**, 2183–2186.

Woods, J. C., Spriggs, A. I., Harris, H., and McGee, J. O.'D. (1982). A new marker for human cancer cells. 3. Immunocytochemical detection of malignant cells in serous fluids with the Ca1 antibody. *Lancet* **ii**, 512–515.

Worman, C. P., Brooks, D. A., Hogg, N., Zola, H., Beverley, P. C. L., and Cawley, J. C. (1983). The nature of hairy cells—a study with a panel of monoclonal antibodies. *Scand. J. Haematol.* **30**, 223–226.

Wunderlich, D., Teramoto, Y. A., Alford, C., and Scholm, J. (1981). The use of lymphocytes from axillary lymph nodes of mastectomy patients to generate human monoclonal antibodies. *Eur. J. Cancer* **17**, 719–730.

Yarmush, M. L., Gates, F. T., III, Weisfogel, D. R., and Kindt, T. J. (1980). Identification and characterization of rabbit–mouse hybridomas secreting rabbit immunoglobulin chains. *Proc. Natl. Acad. Sci. U.S.A.* **77**, 2899–2903.

Yeh, M.-Y., Hellstrom, I., Brown, J. P., Warner, G. A., Hansen, J. A., and Hellstrom, K. E. (1979). Cell surface antigens of human melanoma identified by monoclonal antibody. *Proc. Natl. Acad. Sci. U.S.A.* **76**, 2927–2931.

Yeh, M.-Y., Hellstrom, I., Abe, K., Hakomori, S., and Hellstrom, K. E. (1982). A cell-surface antigen which is present in the ganglioside fraction and shared by human melanomas. *Int. J. Cancer* **29**, 269–275.

Yelton, D. E., and Scharff, M. D. (1981). Monoclonal antibodies: A powerful new tool in biology and medicine. *Annu. Rev. Biochem.* **50,** 657–680.

Yokochi, T., Holly, R. D., and Clark, E. A. (1982). B lymphoblast antigen (BB-1) expressed on Epstein–Barr virus-activated B cell blasts, B lymphoblastoid cell lines, and Burkitt's lymphomas. *J. Immunol.* **128,** 823–827.

Youle, R. J., and Neville, D. M., Jr. (1980). Anti-Thy 1.2 monoclonal antibody linked to ricin is a potent cell-type-specific toxin. *Proc. Natl. Acad. Sci. U.S.A.* **77,** 5483–5486.

Young, W. W., and Hakomori, S.-I. (1981). Therapy of mouse lymphoma with monoclonal antibodies to glycolipid: Selection of low antigenic variants *in vivo. Science* **211,** 487–489.

Young, W. W., Johnson, H. S., Tamura, Y., Karlsson, K.-A., Larson, G., Parker, J. M. R., Khare, D. P., Spohr, U., Baker, D. A., Hindsgaul, O., and Lemieux, R. U. (1983). Characterization of monoclonal antibodies specific for the Lewis a human blood group determinant. *J. Biol. Chem.* **258,** 4890–4894.

Zola, H., and Brooks, D. (1982). Techniques for the production and characterization of monoclonal hybridoma antibodies. *In* "Monoclonal Hybridoma Antibodies: Techniques and Applications" (J. G. R. Hurrell, ed.), pp. 1–57. CRC Press, Boca Raton, Florida.

Zola, H., McNamara, P. J., Moore, H. A., Smart, I. J., Brooks, D. A., Beckman, I. G. R., and Bradley, J. (1983). Maturation of human B lymphocytes—Studies with a panel of monoclonal antibodies against membrane antigens. *Clin. Exp. Immunol.* **52,** 655–664.

3

Inhibitors of Polyamine Biosynthesis as Antitumor and Antimetastatic Agents

PRASAD S. SUNKARA AND
NELLIKUNJA J. PRAKASH
Merrell Dow Research Institute
Cincinnati, Ohio

I.	Introduction	94
II.	Polyamine Biosynthesis	94
III.	Polyamine Catabolism	96
IV.	Polyamines in Growth and Development	97
V.	Polyamines and Differentiation	98
VI.	Polyamines and Cell Cycle	100
VII.	Polyamine Biosynthesis in Normal and Transformed Cells	100
	A. Polyamine Synthesis during Viral-Induced Transformation	100
	B. Polyamine Synthesis during Chemical Carcinogenesis	101
	C. Polyamines in Experimental Animal Tumors	102
	D. Polyamines in Clinical Cancer	102
VIII.	Inhibitors of Polyamine Biosynthesis	103
	A. DL-α-Difluoromethylornithine	103
	B. Inhibition of Cell Growth by Inhibitors of Polyamine Biosynthesis	106
	C. Effect of Inhibition of Polyamine Synthesis on Cell Cycle Traverse of Normal and Transformed Cells	107
	D. Effect of Combinations of DFMO and Cytotoxic Agents on the Growth of Tumor Cells in Culture	108
IX.	Activity of DFMO against Experimental Tumors	109
	A. Inhibition of Chemical Carcinogenesis	109
	B. Monotherapy of Experimental Tumors with DFMO	110
	C. Combination Chemotherapy with DFMO and Other Antineoplastic Agents	111
	D. Inhibition of Tumor Metastases by DFMO	113

93

Novel Approaches to Cancer Chemotherapy
Copyright © 1984 by Academic Press, Inc.
All rights of reproduction in any form reserved.
ISBN 0-12-676980-X

X. DFMO and Clinical Cancer.................................. 116
XI. Summary 117
    References 117

I. INTRODUCTION

The naturally occurring polyamines, putrescine, spermidine, and spermine, are ubiquitous in eukaryotic organisms. The structural formulas for these physiological cations are shown in Figure 1. Although the discovery of spermine as precipitating crystals by Leeuwenhoek in human semen dates back to 1677 (Mann, 1964), a critical role for these amines has been reocgnized only since specific inhibitors of polyamine-biosynthetic enzymes became available in the last decade (Abdel-Monem, 1974; Metcalf *et al.* 1978). A number of studies have suggested that polyamines play an important role in cell proliferation and differentiation (Janne *et al.,* 1978; Sunkara and Rao, 1981; Heby, 1981; Pegg and McCann, 1982).

In this review we will examine the role of polyamines in rapid cell growth and transformation. In addition, the biochemical and pharmacological consequences of inhibiting polyamine biosynthesis by DL-α-difluoromethylornithine (DFMO), a specific inhibitor of ornithine decarboxylase (ODC), and the potential therapeutic use of this inhibitor as an antitumor and antimetastatic agent are also described in some detail.

II. POLYAMINE BIOSYNTHESIS

The biosynthetic pathways leading to polyamines have been reviewed extensively (Morris and Fillingame, 1974; Tabor and Tabor, 1976; Pegg and

$$H_2N\text{-}CH_2\text{-}CH_2\text{-}CH_2\text{-}CH_2\text{-}NH_2$$

Putrescine

$$H_2N\text{-}CH_2\text{-}CH_2\text{-}CH_2\text{-}NH\text{-}CH_2\text{-}CH_2\text{-}CH_2\text{-}CH_2\text{-}NH_2$$

Spermidine

$$H_2N\text{-}CH_2\text{-}CH_2\text{-}CH_2\text{-}NH\text{-}CH_2\text{-}CH_2\text{-}CH_2\text{-}CH_2\text{-}NH\text{-}CH_2\text{-}CH_2\text{-}CH_2\text{-}NH_2$$

Spermine

Fig. 1. The structural formulas of naturally occurring polyamines.

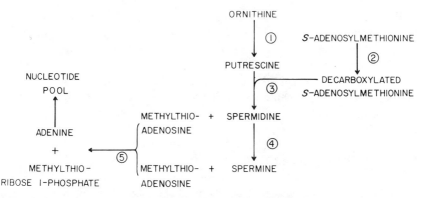

Fig. 2. Biochemical aspects of polyamines in mammalian tissues. The enzymes involved in the biosynthetic pathway are (1) ornithine decarboxylase, (2) S-adenosylmethionine decarboxylase, (3) spermidine synthase, (4) spermine synthase, (5) methylthioadenosine phosphorylase.

Williams-Ashman, 1981). The following overview is intended to give the reader a necessary basis to understand the rationale behind the biological activities of specific inhibitors of polyamine biosynthesis.

L-Ornithine and S-adenosyl-L-methionine are the primary precursors of poly-amines in mammalian cells. Arginase, a widely distributed extrahepatic enzyme of the urea cycle, converts arginine to ornithine. Arginine can therefore be thought of as a precursor in the polyamine-biosynthetic pathway. The biosynthetic pathway of polyamines in animal cells is summarized in Fig. 2.

Ornithine decarboxylase, a pyridoxal phosphate-dependent enzyme, catalyzes the formation of putrescine from ornithine. This reaction appears to be an important step in the polyamine-biosynthetic pathway. ODC is present in very small amounts in quiescent normal cells and tissues. A dramatic increase in enzyme activity occurs during the early phase of cell growth as a result of exposure to trophic stimuli such as hormones, drugs, and growth factors (Janne *et al.*, 1978; Russel, 1981). Mammalian ODC turns over rapidly with an apparent half-life of 15 to 20 min and has the shortest half-life of any mammalian enzyme known so far.

The synthesis of higher polyamines spermidine and spermine is catalyzed by spermidine synthase and spermine synthase, respectively. These enzymes catalyze the transfer of propylamine group from decarboxylated S-adenosyl-L-methionine to putrescine and spermidine, respectively. Decarboxylation of S-adenosylmethionine is carried out by the enzyme adenosylmethionine decarboxylase (SAMDC). Mammalian SAMDC has pyruvate covalently linked to the enzyme as a prosthetic group. SAMDC activity also fluctuates rapidly upon growth stimulation by hormones or growth factors.

The other product of the aminopropyltransferase reaction is 5'-methylthioadenosine (MTA). MTA is produced in stoichiometric amounts with the polyamines, but it is rapidly degraded to adinine and 5'-methylthioribose 1-phosphate by the enzyme methylthioadenosine phosphorylase (Williams-Ashman *et al.*, 1982). The adenine is rapidly converted to AMP by adenine phosphoribosyltransferase, and the 5'-methylthioribose 1-phosphate is convered back to methionine (Trackman and Abeles, 1983). MTA phosphorylase is a ubiquitous enzyme. Mutant cell lines lacking this enzyme excrete the MTA into the medium.

III. POLYAMINE CATABOLISM

It is well established that the conversion of spermine to spermidine and spermidine to putrescine takes place in mammalian cells (Holtta, 1977). The pathways of interconversion and degradation of polyamines are depicted in Fig. 3. The enzymes spermidine-N^1-acetyltransferase and polyamine oxidase are involved in these interconversion reactions. The first enzyme converts spermidine and spermine to N^1-acetylspermidine and N^1-acetylspermine, respectively, in the presence of acetyl-CoA (Pegg *et al.*, 1981). These acetylated polyamines are better substrates than the parent polyamines for the enzyme (polyamine oxidase). Polyamine oxidase catalyzes the conversion of these acetylated polyamines to *N*-

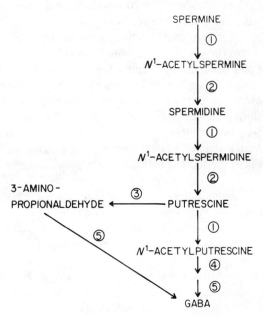

Fig. 3. Catabolism of polyamines. The enzymes involved are (1) N^1-acetyltransferase, (2) polyamine oxidase, (3) diamine oxidase, (4) putrescine, *N*-acetyltransferase, (5) monoamine oxidase.

acetyl propionaldehyde and putrescine or spermidine depending on the substrate (Bolkenius and Seiler, 1981; Seiler *et al.,* 1981). The catabolism of putrescine takes place via two reactions. One is oxidative deamination catalyzed by diamine oxidase, and the other involves the initial conversion of putrescine to *N*-acetyl-putrescine by the enzyme putrescine acetyltransferase (acetyl-CoA:putrescine *N*-acetyltransferase) (Seiler and Al-Therib, 1974). Amine oxidase (copper-containing) (diamine oxidase) catalyzes the formation of γ-aminobutyraldehyde (GABA) (Seiler, 1981) from putrescine; γ-aminobutyraldehyde is subsequently oxidized to Δ^1-pyrroline.

The activities of the catabolic enzymes diamine oxidase and polyamine oxidase were found to be elevated during rapid cell growth in normal and transformed cells (Quash *et al.,* 1979). However, at confluence the levels of diamine oxidase were lower in transformed than in normal cells (Quash *et al.,* 1979). Increase in ODC activity and decrease in diamine oxidase levels may be responsible for the elevation of the putrescine levels in many transformed cell lines (Gazdar *et al.,* 1976; Bachrach *et al.,* 1974; Don *et al.,* 1975). Studies by Sunkara *et al.* (1981b) indicated that the relative rates of polyamine synthesis were high during mitosis and G_1 phases but decreased rapidly and reached the lowest levels during the S phase; however, the concentrations of polyamines, particularly those of spermidine and spermine, were highest during S phase. Since polyamines are assumed to play a role in DNA synthesis (Krokan and Erikson, 1977; Knutson and Morris, 1978), one would expect a high rate of polyamine synthesis during the S phase; however, the observed rate of polyamine synthesis during the S phase was one-tenth of that during mitosis or the G_1 phase, suggesting that the turnover rate of polyamines is very high during the mitosis and G_1 phases and the lowest during the S phase. Accordingly, the diamine oxidase activity was high during mitosis and late G_1, and low during the S phase of the cell cycle. These observations indicate that the cell could maintain adequate levels of polyamines for DNA synthesis by modulating both biosynthetic and catabolic rates (Sunkara *et al.,* 1981b).

IV. POLYAMINES IN GROWTH AND DEVELOPMENT

Early work on polyamines suggested that they play an important role in cell proliferation and differentiation. The patterns of changes in cellular polyamine content were found to be temporally related to proliferative as well as developmental processes. The recent availability of specific inhibitors of polyamine biosynthesis has made it possible to delineate the physiological functions of the polyamines in growth and development of eukaryotic cells. The initial studies on developing chick embryos (Raina, 1963; Caldarera *et al.,* 1965) clearly demonstrated a strong correlation between the polyamine concentrations, protein, and

RNA content. The activities of ODC and SAMDC also peaked during embryonic development in African clawed frog, *Xenopus laevis* (Russell, 1970), and fetal development in mammals (Snyder *et al.*, 1970; Russell, 1970). The ODC and polyamine levels were also found to increase during rodent embryogenesis (Guha and Janne, 1976; Fozard *et al.*, 1980). Heby and Emanuelsson (1978) reported that de novo synthesis of putrescine is essential for nucleolar formation in early embryos of polychete *Ophryotrocha,* and inhibition of its synthesis by α-methylornithine, a competitive inhibitor of ODC, results in the arrest of embryonic development. Fozard *et al.* (1980) have reported that inhibition of ODC by DL-α-difluoromethylornithine during mammalian embryogenesis resulted in the arrest of embryonic development. A rapid increase in ODC and accumulation of putrescine was observed during meiotic maturation of amphibian (*Xenopus laevis*) oocytes induced either by progesterone or human chorionic gonadotrophin. Inhibition of putrescine accumulation by DFMO resulted in inhibition of oocyte matruation (Sunkara *et al.*, 1981a).

A rapid increase in hepatic ODC activity was one of the earliest biochemical changes observable after partial hepatectomy in the rat (Russell and Snyder, 1968; Janne and Raina, 1968). This was followed by an increase in putrescine concentration, reaching peak levels by about 4 hr. Prevention of this increase by the use of inhibitors of polyamine biosynthesis retarded rat liver regeneration (Poso and Janne, 1976; Poso and Pegg, 1982). Similar increases in ODC activity and polyamine levels were observed during renal and cardiac hypertrophy (Brandt *et al.*, 1972; Russell *et al.*, 1971b; Krelhaus *et al.*, 1976; Sogani *et al.*, 1972). However, thyroxin-induced cardiac hypertrophy was not blocked by DFMO even after complete inhibition of increase in the polyamine levels (Pegg, 1981). Bartolome *et al.* (1980) reported that DFMO did attenuate isoproterenol-induced cardiac hypertrophy, suggesting a difference in the requirements of polyamines by different agents eliciting cardiac hypertrophy.

The molecular mechanism of hormone stimulation of ODC during cellular growth is not yet clear (Kaye *et al.*, 1971; Kobayashi *et al.*, 1971; Cohen *et al.*, 1970; Nureddin, 1977). Based on the parallel increase in the ODC and cyclic AMP-dependent protein kinase activities after hormonal stimulation of growth, it has been proposed by Russell *et al.* (1976) that the induction of ODC results from a stimulation of protein kinase by cAMP. This hypothesis remains to be substantiated by direct experimental evidence.

V. POLYAMINES AND DIFFERENTIATION

There is ample evidence to suggest that polyamines play an important role in mammalian cell differentiation. The studies by Oka and co-workers (1981) have shown that spermidine is an essential requirement for milk protein synthesis, a differentiated function in mammary glands. Casein and α-lactalbumin synthesis can be blocked by inhibiting spermidine synthesis. These authors have also shown that increased synthesis of putrescine is needed for mammary cell growth and spermidine is essential for milk protein production.

Friend erythroleukemia cells in culture can be induced to differentiate by compounds such as dimethyl sulfoxide and hexamethylene bisacetamide. These agents were shown to enhance polyamine synthesis. Inhibitors of polyamine biosynthesis prevented the differentiation stimulated by the inducers, and this inhibition could be reversed by exogeneously added polyamines, suggesting a possible role for polyamines in Friend erythroleukemia cell differentiation (Gazitt and Friend, 1980). Similar increases in polyamine levels were observed by agents inducing terminal differentiation in human HL-60 promyelocytic leukemia cells. However, induction of differentiation in HL-60 was not affected by inhibitors of polyamine synthesis (Huberman *et al.*, 1981; Luk *et al.*, 1982).

Verma and Sunkara (1982) reported an enhanced polyamine synthesis during colony-stimulating factor-induced proliferation and differentiation of human granulocyte–macrophage progenitor cells. Furthermore, inhibition of polyamine biosynthesis by DFMO resulted in an inhibition of differentiation that could be reversed easily by an exogenous supply of putrescine, suggesting an essential role for polyamines during granulopoietic differentiation. Requirement for polyamines during differentiation has been reported in a number of model systems. For example, matrix-induced endochondrial bone differentiation (Rath and Reddi, 1981), differentiation of rabbit costal chondrocytes (Takano *et al.*, 1981), differentiation of 3T3-L1 fibroblasts into adipocytes (Bethell and Pegg, 1981), and differentiation of L6 myoblasts into myotubes (Erwin *et al.*, 1982).

In certain model systems, inhibition of polyamine synthesis was shown to induce differentiation. Chen *et al.* (1982) have reported that cAMP-induced neuroblastoma cell differentiation is accompanied by a decrease in ODC and polyamines. Further, they have also shown that DFMO potentiates the neuroblastoma cell differentiation at suboptimal concentrations of dibutyryl-cAMP.

Depletion of polyamines in Cloudman melanoma cells was reported to result in the expression of melanin synthesis, a differentiated biochemical characteristic of these cells (Kepyaho and Janne, 1983). In this model, treatment of cells with DFMO resulted in an increase in the activity of tyrosinase and stimulation of melanogenesis. Exogenous putrescine reversed the DFMO-induced increase in tyrosinase activity in these cells. However, the melanin-stimulating hormone-induced increase in tyrosinase activity and melanogenesis was not reversed by exogenous putrescine. Studies in our laboratory with B_{16} melanoma, both *in vitro* and *in vivo*, also indicated that polyamine depletion by DFMO resulted in an enhanced tyrosinase activity followed by an increase in the melanin content.

The foregoing experimental data indicate that inhibition of polyamine biosynthesis results in either a stimulatory or an inhibitory effect on cellular differentiation depending on the model studied. These studies suggest that the expression of differentiated function following DFMO treatment could be merely an effect secondary to growth inhibition by DFMO. The exact molecular mechanisms by which these polycations exert their effect on cellular differentiation remain to be elucidated.

VI. POLYAMINES AND CELL CYCLE

The stimulation of cell growth both *in vitro* and *in vivo,* and the associated increase in the rate of polyamine biosynthesis prompted a number of investigators to study the fluctuations in the activities of biosynthetic enzymes (ODC and SAMDC) during the cell cycle. The earliest studies by Friedman *et al.* (1972) using synchronized Chinese hamster (DON) cells indicated three peaks of ODC activity: one during mitosis, the second during G_1-S transition, and the third during late S phase. However, synchronized Chinese hamster ovary (CHO) cells exhibited only two peaks of activity for both ODC and SAMDC, which coincided with mitosis and G_1-S transition (Russell and Stambrook, 1975; Heby *et al.,* 1976). The fluctuations in level of enzyme activity were associated with the changes in the concentration of polyamines, especially putrescine and spermidine, in a number of cell systems studied (Russell and Stambrook, 1975; Sunkara *et al.,* 1977, 1981b; McCann *et al.,* 1975; Mamont *et al.,* 1976). As mentioned earlier, the turnover rate of polyamine is high during mitosis and late G_1, and lowest in the S phase. Diamine oxidase, one of the catabolic enzymes, also showed high activity in mitosis and late G_1, and low activity during S phase of the cell cycle (Sunkara *et al.,* 1981b). These studies suggest that the cellular requirement for polyamines for DNA synthesis in S phase is attained by increasing the biosynthesis and also by lowering the catabolism of these amines.

VII. POLYAMINE BIOSYNTHESIS IN NORMAL AND TRANSFORMED CELLS

A. Polyamine Synthesis during Viral-Induced Transformation

Bachrach and co-workers (Don *et al.,* 1975) have employed the virus-induced transformation of primary cultures of chick fibroblasts as a model to study the role of polyamines in neoplastic growth. Infection of chick embryos with oncogenic viruses resulted in an enhanced accumulation of putrescine and spermidine, while infection with a variety of nononcogenic viruses did not show any effect. A temperature-sensitive mutant of Rous sarcoma virus caused an increase in the cellular polyamine content at 37°C, but not at the nonpermissive temperature of 42°C. This observation suggests that the enhanced polyamine synthesis is a result of virus-induced transformation but not of viral multiplication, since the virus multiplies equally well at both temperatures but induces transformation only at the permissive temperature (Don and Bachrach, 1975). An early stimulation of ODC was seen in chick embryo fibroblasts infected with Rous sarcoma virus and in 3T3 cells infected with murine sarcoma virus (Don *et al.*, 1975; Gazdar *et al.*, 1976). The increase in the putrescine synthesis may be due to either stabilization of ODC (Bachrach, 1976) or a decrease in the activity of the catabolic enzyme, diamine oxidase. It is of interest to determine whether the changes in the enzyme activities are the primary effect of transformation or secondary to some general inhibition of proteolysis resulting from transformation. The studies just described clearly demonstrate a specific association between the increase in polyamine synthesis and viral-induced cell transformation.

B. Polyamine Synthesis during Chemical Carcinogenesis

The most widely used system for studying the role of polyamines in chemical carcinogenesis is the mouse skin tumor model. The induction of skin tumors in mice involves two phases, initiation and promotion. Initiation is achieved by a single subcarcinogenic dose of a variety of chemicals, followed by promotion with the repeated application of certain phorbol esters (Boutwell, 1977). A single application of promoting agents, but not their nonpromoting analogs, resulted in a transient stimulation of ODC and SAMDC activities (O'Brien *et al.*, 1975; Yuspa *et al.*, 1976). Nonpromoting but hyperplastic agents had little or no effect on epidermal ODC activity, ruling out the possibility that the increase is due to general enhancement of protein synthesis (O'Brien *et al.*, 1975). Furthermore, the inhibition of skin tumor promotion by a number of retinoids closely correlated with their ability to inhibit the induction of ODC (Verma and Boutwell, 1977). The induction of ODC and increase in putrescine concentration were also seen in mouse epidermis exposed to UV radiation (Seiler and Knodgen, 1979a).

In the model system of diaminoazobenzene-induced liver carcinogenesis, Scalabrino *et al.* (1978) observed that liver ODC and SAMDC activities increased in a bimodal fashion. The first peak of activity, observed 1 mo after initiation of the carcinogenic diet, was followed by a second peak 3 mo later. Thereafter, the activity remained elevated until the tumors began to appear. The levels of putrescine also remained high during hepatocarcinogenesis. These changes in the enzymes appear to be specific to the liver, since the hepatocarcinogenic diet produced a marked drop in the activity of ODC in the kidneys. Administration of a single dose of liver carcinogen, diethylnitrosamine, to rats resulted in a rapid increase in ODC activity within 3 hr after carcinogen administration. ODC remained elevated for 7 days (Olsen and Russell, 1979). The foregoing studies clearly demonstrated an increase in polyamine biosynthesis during chemical carcinogenesis.

C. Polyamines in Experimental Animal Tumors

The earliest studies of polyamine synthesis in animal tumors were performed with Ehrlich ascites carcinoma cells grown in the peritoneal cavities of mice (Siimes and Janne, 1967; Bachrach et al., 1967). The concentration of spermidine was found to be rather high compared with that found in regenerating rat liver (Siimes and Janne, 1967; Russell and Snyder, 1968). The changes in tumor polyamine levels, especially those of cellular putrescine and ODC, showed a close correlation with tumor cell multiplication (Anderson and Heby, 1972).

Williams-Ashman and co-workers (1972, 1973) performed a systematic study to correlate the concentration of polyamines with the growth rate of various transplantable hepatomas. Their studies with several hepatomas having widely different growth rates revealed that, in general, the concentration of putrescine and the ODC activity of the tumor cells were substantially higher in tumor cells than in normal rat liver. Further, putrescine was approximately 10-fold higher in the most rapidly growing hepatomas. The concentration of spermidine was also found to be elevated. In contrast, very little change was observed in the concentration of spermine in tumor cells.

Marton and Heby (1974) observed high levels of putrescine, spermidine, and their biosynthethic enzymes in the peripheral part of the brain when a chemically induced brain tumor was transplanted into the brain. High concentrations of putrescine were observed in nitrosoethylurea-induced rat gliomas (Seiler et al., 1975). Kremzner and co-workers (1970) had found that the concentration of putrescine in human brain tumors was severalfold higher than in normal human brain. A sixfold increase in ODC activity was observed in transplanted mouse L1210 leukemia than in normal mouse liver 4 days after implantation (Russell and Levy, 1971).

D. Polyamines in Clinical Cancer

The presence of polyamines in high concentrations in neoplastic tissues suggests that increased amounts of these compounds may be found in extracellular body fluids. Russell and co-workers (1971a) reported that urinary excretion of polyamines was considerably greater in leukemia, lymphoma, and solid tumor patients than in healthy persons with nonmalignant diseases. Since then, several laboratories have been engaged in the measurement of polyamine levels from different body fluids and red blood cells as biochemical markers for human malignancies (Marton et al., 1976; Rennert et al., 1977; Nishioka and Romsdahl, 1974; Takami *et al.*, 1979). This topic was extensively reviewed by Savory and Shipe (1975), Bachrach (1976), and Janne *et al.* (1978). In general, it appears that polyamine levels in body fluids are of little or no value in the diagnosis of cancer (Waalkes *et al.*, 1975; Raina and Janne, 1975). However, in certain cases, such as suspected brain tumors, polyamine determinations may be of value when applied in conjunction with other diagnostic techniques (Marton, 1981). In contrast, there is ample evidence to suggest that polyamine determinations could be useful in assessing tumor response to chemotherapy (Russell, 1977) and the prognosis of certain tumors (Cohen, 1977).

VIII. INHIBITORS OF POLYAMINE BIOSYNTHESIS

The ubiquitous occurrence of polyamines, their association with nucleic acids, and accumulation of these polycations in rapidly dividing cells stimulated considerable research into the design of specific inhibitors of polyamine-biosynthetic enzymes. It is not altogether surprising that early efforts were focused on inhibitors of ODC, the rate-limiting enzyme. Several substrate analogs were synthesized as potential competitive inhibitors of the enzyme (Table I), and a considerable body of information about the enzyme and the role of polyamines was accumulated by employing these inhibitors. However, the rebound of the enzyme activity when the inhibitor was removed from the system rendered these competitive inhibitors unsatisfactory for the pharmacological manipulation of polyamines *in vivo*. The availability of DFMO (Fig. 4), a suicide inhibitor of ODC, made it possible to obtain a sustained ODC inhibition and a decrease in putrescine and spermidine concentrations *in vivo,* by either oral or systemic administration to animals. Since then a number of other substrate and product analogs with specific and irreversible inhibitory activity have been made (Sjoerdsma and Schechter, 1983), with the aim of obtaining a more potent and longer-acting compound than DFMO (Table I).

A. DL-α-Difluoromethylornithine

DL-α-Difluoromethylornithine (Fig. 4) is a potent and specific irreversible inhibitor of ornithine decarboxylase (Bey, 1978; Metcalf *et al.*, 1978). According to the scheme of Metcalf *et al.* (1978), DFMO binds to the enzyme and an aldimine is formed between the α-amino group of the inhibitor and the aldehyde group of pyridoxal 5′-phosphate, followed by decarboxylation of the ornithine analog. The enzyme is then inactivated through alkylation of a hypothetical nucleophilic residue located at, or close to, the active site (Metcalf *et al.*, 1978). The apparent dissociation constant for the enzyme–inhibitor complex is about 40 $\mu M,$ and the half-life of inactivation about 3 min. The inhibition is irreversible,

TABLE I

Inhibitors of Polyamine Biosynthesis

Target enzyme	Inhibitor	Mechanism of action	References
Ornithine decarboxylase (ODC)	Substrate analogs		
	(a) DL-α-Hydrazinoornithine	Reversible and competitive	Harik and Snyder, 1973; Inoue *et al.*, 1975
	(b) DL-α-Methylornithine	Reversible and competitive	Abdel-Monem *et al.*, 1974; O'Leary and Herreid, 1978
	(c) DL-α-Hydrazino-α-methylornithine	Reversible and competitive	Abdel-Monem *et al.*, 1975
	(d) *trans*-3-Dehydro-DL-ornithine	Reversible and competitive	Relyea and Rando, 1975
	(e) DL-α-Difluoromethylornithine	Catalytic irreversible	Metcalf *et al.*, 1978
	(f) α-Monofluoromethylornithine	Catalytic irreversible	Metcalf *et al.*, 1978
	(g) Dehydro-α-difluoromethylornithine	Catalytic irreversible	Bey *et al.*, 1983
	(h) Dehydro-α-monofluoromethylornithine	Catalytic irreversible	Bey *et al.*, 1983
	(i) α-Acetylenic ornithine	Catalytic irreversible	Metcalf *et al.*, 1978
	(j) α-Vinylornithine	Catalytic irreversible	Metcalf *et al.*, 1978
	Product analogs		
	(k) *trans*-1,4-Diamino-2-butene	Reversible and competitive	Relyea and Rando, 1975
	(l) 1,4-Diaminobutanone	Reversible and competitive	Stevens *et al.*, 1978
	(m) 5-Hexyne-1,4-diamine	Catalytic irreversible	Metcalf *et al.*, 1978
	(n) *trans*-Hex-2-en-5-yne-1,4-diamine	Catalytic irreversible	Metcalf *et al.*, 1978
	(o) Homologous diamines with 3–12 C atoms (1,3-diaminopropane to 1,12-diamino-dodecane)	Indirect, e.g., by induction of ODC-inhibitory protein (ODC antizyme)	Poso and Janne, 1976; McCann *et al.*, 1980

Enzyme	Inhibitor	Mechanism	Reference
	(p) 1,3-Diamino-2-propanol	Indirect	Piik et al., 1978
	(q) α-Monofluoromethylputrescine	Catalytic irreversible	Metcalf et al., 1978
	(r) α-Difluoromethylputrescine	Catalytic irreversible	Metcalf et al., 1978
	(s) Dehydro-α-monofluoromethylputrescine	Catalytic irreversible	Bey et al., 1983
	(t) Dehydro-α-difluoromethylputrescine	Catalytic irreversible	Bey et al., 1983
	(u) α-Acetylenic putrescine	Catalytic irreversible	Metcalf et al., 1978
	(v) Dehydroacetylenic putrescine	Catalytic irreversible	Metcalf et al., 1978
	(w) δ-Methylacetylenic putrescine	Catalytic irreversible	Metcalf et al., 1978
	(x) (R,R)-δ-methylacetylinic putrescine	Catalytic irreversible	Metcalf et al., 1978
	(y) α-Vinylputrescine	Catalytic irreversible	Metcalf et al., 1978
S-Adenosylmethionine decarboxylase (SAMDC)	(a) Methylglyoxalbis(guanylhydrazone); 1,1'-[(methylethanediylidene)dinitrilo]diguanidine; (MGBG)	Reversible and competitive with respect to the substrate (S-adenosyl-L-methionine)	Williams-Ashman and Schenone, 1972; Corti et al., 1974, Dave et al., 1978
	(b) 1,1'-[Methylethanediylidene(dinitrilo)]bis(3-aminoguanidine); (MBAG)	Initially reversible and competitive with respect to the substrate, but subsequently irreversible	Pegg, 1978
	(c) S-Adenosyl-DL-2-methylmethionine	Reversible and competitive with respect to the substrate	Wang et al., 1980; Pankaskie and Abdel-Monem, 1980
Spermidine synthase	α,ω-Diamines with 3–12 C atoms (1,5-diaminopentane is most active)	Reversible and competitive with respect to one of the substrates (putrescine)	Hibasami and Pegg, 1978
	S-Adenosyl-3-thio-1,8-diaminooctane (ADODATO)	Transition state analog	Tang et al., 1980
	Dicyclohexylamine	Competitive	Hibasami et al., 1980
Spermine synthase	α,ω-Diamines with 3–12 C atoms (1,3-diaminopropane and 1,5-diaminopentane are most active)	Reversible and competitive with respect to one of the substrates (spermidine)	Hibasami and Pegg, 1978

$$
\underset{\underset{NH_2}{|}}{\overset{\overset{CHF_2}{|}}{H_2N(CH_2)_3 - C - COOH}}
$$

Fig. 4.   The structural formula of DL-α-difluoromethylornithine.

because no enzyme activity could be recovered after extensive dialysis. This inactivation of ODC by DFMO can be protected by L-ornithine, suggesting that the action of the inhibitor is active site directed.

DFMO was shown to inhibit ODC, to decrease intracellular putrescine and spermidine concentrations, and to inhibit cell growth in a number of cells in culture (Mamont *et al.*, 1978; Sunkara *et al.*, 1980; Sidenfield *et al.*, 1980; Luk *et al.*, 1981) and in animal tumors *in vivo* (Prakash *et al.*, 1978, 1980; Marton *et al.*, 1981; Sunkara *et al.*, 1982, 1983b). DFMO also showed contragestational activity (Fozard *et al.*, 1980) and antiprotozoal activity (Bacchi *et al.*, 1980; McCann *et al.*, 1981; Sjoerdsma, 1981; Sjoerdsma and Schechter, 1983) because of its interference with polyamine metabolism.

DFMO has been generally well tolerated by experimental animals. Single oral doses of 5 g/kg had no apparent adverse effects on mice. Administration of a total daily dose of 4 g/kg for 4 weeks to mice and rats did not slow their normal weight gain, and no organ toxicity was found. The only side effect seen was diarrhea in rats, which was easily reversible when the administration of the drug was stopped (Koch-Weser *et al.*, 1981). Since DFMO seems to be a highly specific inhibitor, the rest of the chapter is mainly devoted to the antitumor and antimetastatic activities of DFMO, and the status of this drug in the clinical treatment of cancer.

B. Inhibition of Cell Growth by Inhibitors of Polyamine Biosynthesis

The initial studies on the correlation of polyamine levels and rapid cell proliferation indicated a requirement for polyamines in DNA snythesis and cell proliferation. A search for specific inhibitors of polyamine biosynthesis was initiated to clarify the exact role of polyamines in cell growth. Initially a number of ornithine analogs like α-hydrazinoornithine (Johansson and Skinner, 1973; Harik and Snyder, 1973) and α-methylornithine (Abdel-Monem *et al.*, 1974) were made. These compounds are reversible competitive inhibitors of ODC. Although they were effective in inhibiting the accumulation of polyamines (Inoue *et al.*, 1975; Mamont *et al.*, 1976; Heby *et al.*, 1978; Sunkara *et al.*, 1979a,b), their effects were easily reversible *in vivo*.

The availability of DL-α-difluoromethylornithine, an irreversible catalytic inhibitor of ODC, made it possible to confirm the role of polyamines in rapid cell

proliferation in a number of systems. The initial studies indicated antiproliferative activity of DFMO against HTC cells, L1210 leukemia cells, and MA-160
human prostatic adenoma cells grown in cell culture (Mamont *et al.*, 1978).
These inhibitory effects were completely reversible by the addition of exogenous
putrescine and spermidine. Antiproliferative effects of DFMO were confirmed in
a number of other cells like human embryo fibroblasts (Holtta *et al.*, 1979),
concanavalin A-stimulated lymphocytes (Seyfried and Morris, 1979), HeLa cells
(Sunkara *et al.*, 1980), Ehrlich ascites carcinoma cells (Oredsson *et al.*, 1980),
and 9L rat gliosarcoma cells (Sidenfield *et al.*, 1980). The earlier studies indicated that DFMO was a cytostatic agent. However, several observations with
human small-cell carcinoma cells (Luk *et al.*, 1981), HeLa (Sunkara *et al.*,
1983a), and mouse B_{16} melanoma (Sunkara *et al.*, 1983b) indicated that DFMO
is cytotoxic to certain cells in culture. In the case of small-cell lung carcinoma
cells, polyamine depletion induced by DFMO was followed by pronounced cell
loss and rapid decrease in viability. In the cases of HeLa and B_{16} melanoma
cells, a decrease in plating efficiency was found. Further, B_{16} melanoma seemed
to be more sensitive, and an increase in the cytotoxicity (as determined by the
plating efficiency), reaching about 80% of the cell survival over the control at the
end of 7 days, was observed in the DFMO-treated cultures (Sunkara *et al.*,
1984b). These results indicate that DFMO is a cytostatic or cytotoxic agent
depending on the cell line employed.

C. Effect of Inhibition of Polyamine Synthesis on Cell Cycle Traverse of Normal and Transformed Cells

The cell cycle-specific fluctuations in polyamine levels, especially a peak in
late G_1, and the requirement for polyamines for optimal rates of DNA replication, indicate that these physiological cations may play an important role in the
traverse of cells through G_1 into S phase (Otani *et al.*, 1974; Fillingame *et al.*,
1975). Seyfried and Morris (1979) found that DFMO inhibited DNA replication
in activated lymphocytes without altering the number of cells in S phase. Harada
and Morris (1981) employed α-methylornithine in CHO cells and found that the
longer doubling times in inhibitor-treated cells was due to increase in the length
of G_1 and S phases. Heby and Anderson (1980) found an accumulation of Erlich
ascites cells in S and G_2 phases of the cell cycle when treated with α-methylornithine or methylglyoxal bis(guanylhydrazone) (MGBG). In fact, several studies
indicate that inhibition of polyamine biosynthesis by MGBG in a number of
normal cells like WI-38, rat embryo, mouse 3T3, and human skin fibroblasts
(PA_2) causes an arrest of these cells in G_1 phase (Boynton *et al.*, 1976; Rupniak
and Paul, 1980; Sunkara *et al.*, 1979a). This arrest is easily reversed with
spermidine or spermine. However, treatment of transformed cells (HeLa,
SV-3T3, and CHO) with MGBG or DFMO results in the arrest of a majority of

cells in S phase (Rupniak and Paul, 1978; Sunkara *et al.*, 1981c). We treated exponentially growing normal (human skin fibroblast line PA_2), mouse 3T3 (W1-38), and transformed (HeLa, SV-3T3, 2RA) cells with MGBG (40 μM) or DFMO (2.5 mM) for 48 or 96 hr, respectively. At the end of this period, cell cycle analysis was performed according to the premature chromosome condensation (PCC) method (Rao *et al.*, 1977). The results indicated that inhibition of putrescine and spermidine synthesis resulted in a G_1 block in normal cells, whereas a majority of transformed cells were arrested in S phase. These data suggested that a specific polyamine-requiring process exists in G_1 and was necessary for entry of cells into S period. Normal cells recognized this control signal and stopped in G_1. However, transformed cells did not recognize the polyamine limitation or restriction, and continued to progress through the cell cycle; a majority of them entered S phase but failed to complete DNA synthesis and were thus arrested in S pahse. This differential effect of inhibition of polyamine biosynthesis on the cell cycle traverse of normal and transformed cells was exploited to kill transformed cells preferentially in combination with other S-phase-specific anticancer drugs.

Rupniak and Paul (1980) showed that a combination MGBG and hydroxyurea can preferentially kill transformed SV-3T3 cells over normal 3T3 cells. By pretreating proliferating cultures of 3T3 and SV-3T3 cells with MGBG, and subsequently treating the cultures with hydroxyurea, an S-phase-specific cytotoxic drug, they obtained highly selective killing of the still cycling transformed SV-3T3 cells. In contrast, normal 3T3 cells were protected from the cytotoxic effects of hydroxyurea by virtue of their MGBG-induced growth arrest in the insensitive G_1 phase. Our studies also indicated that the use of an S-phase-specific drug like Ara-C (1-β-D-arabinofuranosylcytosine) following DFMO treatment resulted in a synergistic killing of tumor cells (HeLa and 2RA) (Sunkara *et al.*, 1980, 1981c). However, the normal human diploid fibroblasts (WI-38) did not suffer the cytotoxic effects of Ara-C, since they were arrested in G_1 phase as a result of the DFMO treatment. The effect of DFMO on the cell cycle traverse seems to depend also on the cell line studied. Oredsson *et al.* (1983) observed that DFMO did not block 9L brain tumor cells in any particular phase of the cell cycle, and, in fact, DFMO pretreatment seemed to reduce Ara-C toxicity. These observations indicated that the effect of the inhibitors of polyamine synthesis might vary from cell to cell and also with the duration of treatment with the inhibitor.

D. Effect of Combinations of DFMO and Cytotoxic Agents on the Growth of Tumor Cells in Culture

Several studies have indicated the usefulness of DFMO in potentiating the cytotoxicity of other antitumor agents in a number of cell systems grown in culture (Sunkara *et al.*, 1980; 1981c; Marton, 1981; Sunkara *et al.*, 1983a,b;

Kingsnorth *et al.*, 1983b). Most of these studies were based on rational approaches. As discussed earlier, we exploited the differential cell cycle response of normal and tumor cells to DFMO and showed that we could preferentially kill the tumor cells both *in vitro* (Sunkara *et al.*, 1980, 1981c) and *in vivo* (Prakash and Sunkara, 1983) by a combination of DFMO and S-phase-specific drug Ara-C. Kingsnorth *et al.* (1983b) reported the potentiation of the antiproliferative effect of 5-fluorouracil against human adenocarcinoma cells by DFMO. Marton and his co-workers (1981) have found that DFMO enhanced the cytotoxicity of 1,3-bis(2-chloroethyl)-1-nitrosourea (BCNU) in rat 9L gliosarcoma cells in culture. Other results from their laboratory also suggest that polyamine depletion by DFMO modifies the DNA structure and conformation and might sensitize the 9L cells to nitrosoureas (Hung *et al.*, 1983). Oredsson *et al.* (1982) observed that pretreatment of 9L cells with DFMO reduced the cytotoxicity of *cis*-platinum. Sidenfield *et al.* (1981) reported that pretreatment of 9L cells with DFMO did not potentiate the X-ray-induced cell kill. These results clearly suggest that the effects of DFMO seem to vary with the companion cytotoxic agent used.

Janne and his colleagues (Alhonen-Hongisto *et al.*, 1980; Seppanen *et al.*, 1981) observed that uptake of MGBG, a cytotoxic polyamine antimethabolite, was enhanced after pretreatment of Ehrlich ascites cells. This enhanced uptake was also associated with increased cytotoxicity. Sunkara *et al.* (1983a) also observed a three- to fourfold increase in MGBG uptake and corresponding cytotoxicity of MGBG to HeLa cells following DFMO pretreatment. We have observed that mouse type I interferon potentiated the cytotoxic activity of DFMO to B_{16} melanoma cells grown in culture (Sunkara *et al.*, 1983b).

The foregoing studies in cell cultures laid the foundation for the investigations to determine the usefulness of DFMO as an antitumor agent, either by itself or in combination with other cytotoxic agents in experimental tumors, and, eventually, in the treatment of human cancers.

IX. ACTIVITY OF DFMO AGAINST EXPERIMENTAL TUMORS

A. Inhibition of Chemical Carcinogenesis

Oral administration of 7,12-dimethylbenz[*a*]anthracene (DMBA) to female rats induced mammary cancers; a majority of these tumors were estrogen dependent (Huggins *et al.*, 1959) and slow growing (Pearson and Manni, 1978). Oral administration of DFMO beginning on day 30 after the carcinogen was given had a dramatic inhibitory effect on the frequency of appearance of tumors as well as on the number of tumors per animal (Fozard and Prakash, 1982). At autopsy on day 105 following the dose of DMBA, all animals in the untreated group had at least one tumor, whereas 6 of 20 animals in the DFMO-treated group were tumor free. The range of the tumor weight in the treated group was 0–200 mg, whereas in the untreated group numerous tumors weighing 200–600 mg and 400–600 mg were observed. In this study, the animals received DFMO only between days 30 and 73 post-DMBA administration, indicating that the drug is effective in suppressing tumor development even when administered after the onset of tumor initiation. Not surprisingly, the compound had a marginal effect on the growth of established tumors that were, in general, very slow growing and low in ODC activity. DFMO was reported to inhibit significantly the development of colon tumors induced by dimethylhydrazine in rats (Kingsnorth *et al.*, 1983a). In this model, ODC inhibition and decreases in tissue concentrations of putrescine and spermidine in the affected organ, namely the colon, could be demonstrated following administration of DFMO.

The two-step skin carcinogenesis reported in mice (Mottram, 1944; Berenblum and Shubik, 1944) has been extensively employed as a model for chemical carcinogenesis because of the ease with which biochemical events pertaining to initiation or induction can be studied (Boutwell, 1964; Verma *et al.*, 1982). The induction of ODC and subsequent accumulation of putrescine appear to play an important role in the development of tumors in this model (weeks *et al.*, 1982; O'Brien, 1976). Both topical and systemic administration of DFMO were found to inhibit ODC and subsequent accumulation of putrescine and spermidine in the skin following the application of tumor promoter in a dose-dependent manner (Takigawa *et al.*, 1982). These biochemical changes were accompanied by a striking inhibition of carcinogenesis. Significantly, the effect of DFMO on promoter-induced hyperplasia and DNA synthesis was less striking than its effect on ODC and polyamine accumulation. The drug was also without effect on the induction of dark basal keratinocytes (Weeks *et al.*, 1982) or ultraviolet light-induced skin hyperplasia (Seiler and Knodgen, 1979a). These experimental observations indicate that DFMO may have applications as a chemopreventative agent against cancer.

B. Monotherapy of Experimental Tumors with DFMO

Early studies with L1210 leukemia in mice (Prakash *et al.*, 1978) showed antitumor activity when the compound was administered systemically on a frequent schedule. The increase in survival time observed was 23% compared to untreated controls. Subsequent work with the same tumor model, but with DFMO administered in the drinking water, indicated that only a marginal increase in survival time was attainable with larger oral doses despite significant decreases in intracellular tumor putrescine and spermidine concentrations (Prakash and Sunkara, 1983; Bartholeyns and Koch-Weser, 1982). However, when administered in the drinking water, the compound inhibited EMT_6 solid tumor growth in mice by 80% by day 35 compared to untreated controls (Prakash *et al.*,

1980). Extensive work with a variety of other experimental tumor models has indicated that, in general, the compound as a single agent is moderately effective in bringing about substantial reduction in tumor burden (Fozard and Koch-Weser, 1982; Sjoerdsma and Schechter, 1983), even when the therapy is initiated during the early stages of tumor growth.

Among the several experimental tumors studied to date, the B_{16} melanotic melanoma in mice was found to be most sensitive to the antiproliferative activity of DFMO. Greater than 80% inhibition of tumor growth was observed when the drug was given orally (Sunkara et al., 1983a). Inhibition of growth and depletion of polyamines in this tumor by DFMO were accompanied by the induction of the enzyme tyrosinase and also accumulation of melanin (Sunkara et al., 1984b), indicating that at least in this tumor model, inhibition of polyamine biosynthesis brings about other biochemical changes characteristic of differentiated function. Induction of differentiated biochemical functions by DFMO has also been reported in Cloudman S91 melanoma cells in culture (Kapyaho and Janne, 1983). Although melanoma in humans constitutes only 1–2% of the total cancer incidence, the virulence and the poor chemotherapeutic response observed render this disease an extremely difficult one to manage clinically. The fairly nontoxic nature of DFMO and its effectiveness as a single agent against B_{16} melanoma and the unique biochemical changes observed offer a strong impetus for clinical studies with the compound against human melanomas.

A study on the viability of human small-cell lung carcinoma cells during polyamine depletion by DFMO indicates that these cells are unable to maintain structural integrity during prolonged polyamine starvation and eventually die under sustained polyamine deprivation (Luk et al., 1981). This study appears to be the first to report clear in vitro cytotoxicity for DFMO toward a mammalian cell. Established human small-cell variant lung carcinoma implants in athymic nude mice were later reported to respond successfully to oral therapy with DFMO (Luk et al., 1983). These experimental results raise the possibility that this durg could also provide beneficial therapeutic effects against this malignancy in humans.

C. Combination Chemotherapy with DFMO and Other Antineoplastic Agents

Extensive in vitro and in vivo studies and also available pharmacokinetic and toxicological data on the DFMO (Fozard and Koch-Weser, 1982; Sjoerdsma and Schechter, 1983) suggest that the chemotherapeutic potential of the compound can best be exploited by combining it with appropriate cytotoxic agents. Early studies with DFMO and cyclophosphamide against EMT_6 solid tumor in mice showed only an additive antitumor effect (Prakash et al., 1980). Subsequently, this combination was shown to be effective in suppressing the growth of established DMBA-induced tumor in rats even though the tumors were not very responsive to monotherapy with either of the two agents alone (Fozard and Prakash, 1982). This combination was also reported to provide synergistic anti-tumor activity in a rat prostate tumor model (Heston et al., 1982). Synergistic antitumor activity was reported with DFMO in combination with Adriamycin or vindesine against L1210 leukemia, hepatoma solid tumor in rats, and EMT$_6$ solid tumor in mice (Bartholeyns and Koch-Weser, 1981). In these studies, the selection of the cytotoxic drugs was arbitrary and was primarily based on the premise that DFMO is likely to provide at least an additive therapeutic effect by delaying the recovery of the tumor cells from the cytotoxic drug-induced injury.

Studies with two other DNA-reactive drugs and DFMO demonstrated that synergistic or even antagonistic therapeutic effects could be expected depending on the cytotoxic agent selected. Thus, synergistic therapeutic effects were observed with BCNU and DFMO against 9L rat brain tumor (Marton et al., 1981), whereas mutual antagonism was reported with DFMO and cis-platinum against 9L tumor cells (Oredsson et al., 1982). Clearly, it would be highly desirable to be able to select combinations, based on biochemical and pharmacological findings, which are likely to provide synergistic or at least additive antitumor effects. The usefulness of sister chromatid exchange assay was reported in predicting the synergistic or antagonistic effects of DNA-reactive cytotoxin agents in combination with DFMO (Tofilron et al., 1982). Extensive further work is needed to test the reliability of this procedure in ascertaining the suitability of cytotoxic agents for combination protocols with DFMO.

The differential effect of polyamine depletion on cell cycle traverse of normal and transformed cells (Rupniak and Paul, 1980; Sunkara et al., 1981b), as described earlier, has been the basis for the rational design of therapeutic protocols involving DFMO and phase-specific cytotoxic drugs in a murine leukemia model (Prakash and Sunkara, 1983). Preferential accumulation of L1210 tumor cells in S phase compared to normal bone marrow cells was also observed when DFMO was administered to mice. Therapeutic synergism with a combination of DFMO and Ara-C could be demonstrated in this tumor model when Ara-C administration was timed to coincide with the maximum differential accumulation of tumor cells in S phase (Prakash and Sunkara, 1983). Ideally, in human neoplasia with relatively high growth rates, namely, leukemias and lymphomas, polyamine limitation might lead to their selective accumulation in S phase priming them for a synergistic cell kill by S-phase-specific cytotoxic drugs such as Ara-C and hydroxyurea.

Sequential therapy with DFMO and MGBG is another example of a combination regimen arrived at primarily on the basis of biochemical and pharmacological studies with the two compounds. The structural analogy with spermidine and also the observation that in vivo antineoplastic activity could partially be reversed by exogenous spermidine (Mihich, 1963) indicate some degree of polyamine antagonism for MGBG. Polyamines and MGBG were also reported to share a common cellular transport system (Dave and Caballeri, 1973). These experimental observations led Janne and colleagues to pretreat tumor cells with DFMO to deplete intracellular polyamines and subsequently expose these cells to MGBG, an experimental manipulation that led to a three- to fourfold increase in the uptake of MGBG into the tumor cells (Alhonen-Hongesto et al., 1980). DFMO pretreatment was later reported to potentiate the antitumor activity of MGBG against L1210 leukemia (Burchenal et al., 1981). Work in our laboratory (Sunkara et al., 1983b) employing L1210 leukemia in mice showed that polyamine depletion in L1210 cells by DFMO resulted in a two- to threefold increase in the accumulation of MGBG into tumor cells. The extent of MGBG uptake correlated inversely with intracellular spermidine concentration. Spermidine was also found to be a more potent inhibitor of MGBG uptake than putrescine in this system. A distinct synergistic increase in survival time was also observed with a combination of DFMO and MGBG in this tumor model.

Finally, the report on the efficacy of DFMO in combination with interferon in suppressing the growth of subcutaneous B_{16} melanomas in mice (Sunkara et al., 1983a) is indicative of the potential for effective therapeutic protocols involving combinations of polyamine-biosynthetic inhibitors and immunomodulators. Although the dose of interferon employed in the study was insufficient to provide any significant antitumor effect, the combination of DFMO and interferon resulted not only in pronounced synergistic antitumor effect but also tumor eradication in some animals (Fig. 5). Work in our laboratory showed that the DFMO–interferon combination was equally effective against Lewis lung (3LL) carcinoma, a tumor with poor therapeutic response to either DFMO or interferon therapy alone. In addition, another immunomodulatory peptide, tuftsin, was also found to be very effective in suppressing B_{16} melanoma growth in mice (Sunkara et al., 1984a). The doses of DFMO, interferon, or tuftsin employed in these preliminary studies stress the need for further studies into the mechanism of therapeutic synergism involving DFMO and immunomodulators.

D. Inhibition of Tumor Metastases by DFMO

Although a vast amount of literature presented in the earlier sections of the chapter indicates an important role for polyamines in tumor cell growth, there is no information available on the role of these cations in the process of tumor metastases. We have examined the effect of DFMO on the growth and pulmonary metastasis of 3LL tumor in mice (Sunkara et al., 1982; Bartholeyns, 1983). The Lewis lung tumor of C57BL mice provides an excellent experimental model for studying tumor metastases. The primary tumor grows rapidly at the inoculation site and metastasizes to lungs in about 3 weeks after tumor transplantation, and these pulmonary foci can easily be counted.

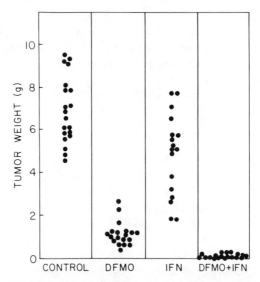

Fig. 5. Effects of DFMO and interferon (IFN) on B$_{16}$ melanoma growth in C57BL mice. The experimental details and the data were obtained from Sunkara *et al.* (1983a). All the animals (C57BL mice) were inoculated with 10^5 B$_{16}$ melanoma cells subcutaneously at the interscapular region on day 0. Treatment groups as were as follows: (1) control, normal drinking water; (2) DFMO, 2% in drinking water starting day 1; (3) interferon (IFN), 1000 U/mouse sc on alternate days for 10 doses starting day 2; and (4) DFMO plus interferon. Each point represents tumor weight in an individual mouse. Note that in group 4 there was no detectable tumor in 4 of 20 animals. (Reprinted with permission from Sjoerdsma and Schechter, 1983.)

The results of our study showed that administration of DFMO to animals bearing tumors resulted in a 69% and a 75% decrease in the intracellular levels of putrescine and spermidine in the primary tumor, respectively, without any change in the spermine concentrations (Fig. 6). The decreased polyamine levels were also associated with a 43% inhibition of tumor growth. Inhibition of polyamine biosynthesis as a result of DFMO administration not only inhibited growth of the primary tumor but also dramatically decreased the secondary pulmonary metatases by 79%, with 25% of the animals showing no visible metastases (Table II). Further, this inhibition of tumor growth and metastases could be reversed by simultaneous administration of putrescine to the animals (Fig. 6 and Table II). Administration of putrescine to animals receiving DFMO did not result in any significant elevation of tumor putrescine concentrations, although spermidine concentrations were substantially elevated compared to tumors from animals that received DFMO alone. The lack of any effect on tumor putrescine concentration following exogenous putrescine administration to DFMO-treated animals is most likely due to its rapid conversion to spermidine. Since polyamine depletion in tumor cells leads to an increase of SAMDC (S-adenosyl-L-methio-

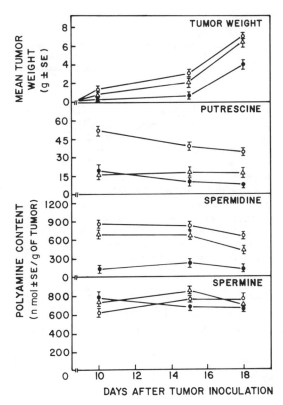

Fig. 6. Effect of DFMO on the growth and polyamine levels of Lewis lung tumor (3LL) in mice. Tumors were induced in C57BL/6J mice by sc injection of 1×10^6 viable 3LL cells/mouse in the intrascapular region. DFMO was administered in the drinking water as a 2% aqueous solution (approximately 3 g/kg/day). Putrescine was administered ip at a dose of 100 mg/kg/day. This experimental protocol is the same as that shown in Table II. Points represent mean ± SEM ($n = 20$). ○, Untreated animals; ●, DFMO treated; △, DFMO + putrescine-treated animals. (Reprinted with permission from Sunkara *et al.*, 1982.)

nine decarboxylase), the rate-limiting enzyme involved in the conversion of putrescine to spermidine, DFMO treatment is likely to facilitate the conversion of exogenous putrescine to spermidine in the solid tumor employed in the study. Essentially similar results were obtained by Bartholeyns (1983).

The novel finding of the metastases study is that inhibition of polyamine biosynthesis resulted in a decrease in the spread of the tumor cells to lungs. The fact that the inhibition of metastases could be reversed by simultaneous administration of putrescine suggests that polyamines may play a role not only in tumor growth (Prakash *et al.*, 1980; Marton *et al.*, 1981; Sunkara *et al.*, 1983a,b) but also in the process of tumor metastases. Although the mechanism by which

TABLE II

Effect of DFMO on Growth and Pulmonary Metastases of Lewis Lung
(3LL) Carcinoma in Mice[a,b]

Treatment	Tumor weight[c] (g)	Inhibition (%)	Number of animals showing visible metastases	Metastatic foci[c]	Inhibition (%)
Control	7.01 ± 0.39	—	20/20	21.38 ± 5.8	—
DFMO	4.01 ± 0.46**	43	15/20	4.60 ± 1.43**	79
DFMO + putrescine	6.54 ± 0.72*	7	20/20	24.80 ± 5.10*	0

[a]Reprinted with permission from Sunkara et al., 1982.
[b]1×10^6 3LL tumor cells per animal were injected sc at the intrascapular region. DFMO was administered as 2% aqueous solution as the sole drinking fluid (approximately 3 g/kg/day). Putrescine 100 mg/kg was given ip daily starting day 1–18. At the end of 18 days the animals were sacrificed, tumors were excised and weighed, and pulmonary metastases were determined.
[c]Mean ± SE; $n = 20$. *Not significant; **significant at $p < .01$.

DFMO inhibits tumor metastases is not yet clear, one can envisage that the depletion of cellular polyamines in the primary tumor could have affected (1) the invasion of the tumor cells into the lymphatics or blood vessels, (2) their transport into distant organs, and (3) the establishment of a microenvironment unfavorable to the growth of pulmonary metastases (Poste and Fidler, 1980).

Several studies suggest that DFMO might affect the second phase in the metastatic process. We found that administration of DFMO did not inhibit the spread of the metastatic cells from the primary tumor. However, their transportation to the distant organs and establishment into pulmonary metastases was inhibited (P. S. Sunkara and A. L. Rosenberger, unpublished data). These results indicate that DFMO and other specific inhibitors of polyamine synthesis merit consideration as potential therapeutic agents in the clinical management of metastasis.

X. DFMO AND CLINICAL CANCER

Phase I tolerance studies with DFMO in the United States and abroad have just been completed. The initial data indicate that DFMO is well tolerated with no serious toxicity (Sjoerdsma and Schechter, 1983; Abeloff et al., 1983). Thrombocytopenia, anemia, and hearing loss have been reported, with reversal upon stopping the drug. Tolerance by the intravenous route was better than by the oral route, with diarrhea tending to limit dosage in the latter case. Doses as high as 20 to 30 g intravenously daily for several days, and 7.5 to 15 g in divided dosage daily for 0.5 to 6 mo, have been well tolerated by individual patients. Phase II clinical studies with DFMO in combination with leukocyte interferon or MGBG are in progress.

XI. SUMMARY

Based on the available experimental evidence, it appears that polyamines play an important role in the proliferation of normal and transformed cells. Although the requirement for polyamines for DNA replication is well established, the molecular events in which the polyamines are essential are yet to be determined. DL-α-Difluoromethylornithine, a specific irreversible inhibitor of ornithine decarboxylase, has proved to be important in understanding the role of polyamines in cell proliferation and differentiation. DFMO has shown interesting antitumor activities in a number of experimental tumors either administered alone or in combination with other cytotoxic agents. Currently DFMO is in phase II clinical trials in combination with leukocyte interferon against melanoma in the United States, and it will be of interest to see whether this exciting compound will gain a place in the fight against cancer and other proliferative diseases.

REFERENCES

Abdel-Monem, M. M., Newton, N. E., and Weeks, C. E. (1974). Inhibitors of polyamine biosynthesis. I. α-Methyl-(+)-ornithine, an inhibitor of ornithine decarboxylase. *J. Med. Chem.* **17**, 447–451.

Abdel-Monem, M. M., Newton, N. E., and Weeks, C. E. (1975). Inhibitors of polyamine biosynthesis. 3(±) 5-Amino-2-hydrazino-2-methyl pentanoic acid, an inhibitor of ornithine decarboxylase. *J. Med. Chem.* **18**, 945–948.

Abeloff, M. D., Slavik, M., Luk, G., Griffin, C., Hermann, I., Blanc, O., Sjoerdsma, A., and Baylin, S. (1983). Phase I trial and pharmacokinetic studies of oral α-difluoromethyl ornithine (DFMO). *Proc. Am. Soc. Clin. Oncol.* **2**, 22.

Alhonen-Hongisto, L., Seppanen, P., and Janne, J. (1980). Intracellular putrescine and spermidine deprivation induces increased uptake of the natural polyamines and methylglyoxal bis (guanyl hydrazone). *Biochem. J.* **192**, 941–945.

Anderson, G., and Heby, O. (1972). Polyamine and nucleic acid concentration in Ehrlich ascites carcinoma cells and liver of tumor-bearing mice at various stages of tumor growth. *JNCI J. Natl. Cancer Inst.* **48**, 165–172.

Bacchi, C. J., Nathan, H. N., Hutner, S. H., McCann, P. P., and Sjoerdsma, A. (1980). Polyamine metabolism: A potential therapeutic target in trypanosomes. *Science* **210**, 332–334.

Bachrach, U. (1976). Polyamines as chemical markers of malignancy. *Ital. J. Biochem.* **25**, 77–93.

Bachrach, U., Bekierkunst, A., and Abzug, S. (1967). The occurrence of putrescine, spermidine and spermine in Ehrlich ascites cells. *Isr. J. Med. Sci.* **3**, 474–477.

Bachrach, U., Son, S., and Wiener, H. (1974). Polyamines in normal and in virus-transformed chick embryo fibroblasts. *Cancer Res.* **34**, 1577–1580.

Bartholeyns, J. (1983). Treatment of metastatic Lewis lung carcinoma with DL-α-difluoromethyl ornithine. *Eur. J. Cancer Clin. Oncol.* **19**, 567–572.

Bartholeyns, J., and Koch-Weser, J. (1981). Effects of α-difluoromethylornithine alone and combined with adriamycin or vindesine on L1210 leukemia in mice, EMT_6 solid tumor in mice and HTC solid tumors in rats. *Cancer Res.* **41**, 5158–5161.

Bartolome, J., Huguenard, J., and Slotkin, T. A. (1980). Role of ornithine decarboxylase in cardiac growth and hypertrophy. *Science* **210**, 793–794.

Berenblum, I., and Shubik, P. (1944). The role of croton oil application associated with a single painting of a carcinogen in tumour induction of the mouse's skin. *Br. J. Cancer* **1**, 378–382.

Bethell, D. R., and Pegg, A. E. (1981). Polyamines are needed for the differentiation of 3T3-L1 fibroblasts into adipose cells. *Biochem. Biophys. Res. Commun.* **102**, 272–278.

Bey, P. (1978). Substrate-induced irreversible inhibition of α-amino acid decarboxylases. Application to glutamate, aromatic L-α-amino acid and ornithine decarboxylases. *In* "Enzyme-Activated Irreversible Inhibitors" N. Seiler, M. J. Jung, and J. Koch-Weser, eds.), pp. 27–41. Elsevier Amsterdam.

Bey,P., Gerhart, F., Van Dorsselaer, V., and Danzin, C. (1983). α-Fluoro methyl-dehydro-ornithine and putrescine analogues as irreversible inhibitors (EC 4.1.1.17). *J. Med. Chem.* **26**, 1551–1556.

Bolkenius, F. N., and Seiler, N. (1981). Acetylderivatives as intermediates in polyamine catabolism. *Int. J. Biochem.* **13**, 287–292.

Boutwell, R. K. (1964). Some biological aspects of skin carcinogenesis. *Prog. Exp. Tumor Res.* **4**, 207–250.

Boutwell, R. K. (1977). The role of the induction of ornithine decarboxylase in tumor promotion. *In* "Origins of Human Cancer" (H. H. Hiatt, J. D. Watson, and J. A. Winsten, eds.), pp. 773–783. Cold Spring Harbor Lab., Cold Spring Harbor, New York.

Boynton, A. L., Whitfield, J. F., and Isaacs, R. J. (1976). A possible involvement of polyamines in the initiation of DNA synthesis by human W138 and mouse BABL/3T3 cells. *J. Cell. Physiol.* **89**, 481–488.

Brandt, J. T., Pierre, D. A., and Fauston, N. (1972). Ornithine decarboxylase activity and polyamine synthesis during kidney hypertrophy. *Biochim. Biophys. Acta* **279**, 184–193.

Burchenal, J. H., Lokys, L., Smith, R., Cartmell, S., and Warrel, R. (1981). Potentiation of methylglyoxal-bis-(guanylhydrazone) by α-difluoromethyl ornithine, stilbamidine, and pentamidine. *Proc. Am. Assoc. Cancer Res.* **22**, 230.

Caldarera, C. M., Barbiroli, B., and Moruzzi, G. (1965). Polyamines and nucleic acids during development of the chick embryo. *Biochem. J.* **97**, 94–88.

Chen, K. P., Nau, D., and Liu, A. Y-C. (1982). Effects of inhibitors of ornithine decarboxylase on the differentiation of mouse neuroblastoma cells. *Cancer Res.* **43**, 2812–2818.

Cohen, S., O'Malley, B. W., and Stastny, M. (1970). Estrogenic induction of ornithine decarboxylase *in vivo* and *in vitro*. *Science* **170**, 336–338.

Corti, A., Dave, C., Williams-Ashman, H. G., Mihich, E., and Schenone, A. (1974). Specific inhibition of enzymatic decarboxylation of *S*-adenosyl methionine by methyl glyoxal bis (guanyl hydrazone) and related substances. *Biochem. J.* **139**, 351–357.

Dave, C., and Caballeri, L. (1973). Studies on the uptake of methylglyoxal bis (guanylhydrazone) [CH_3-G]) and spermidine (Spd) in mouse leukemia L1210 sensitive and resistant to CH_3-G. *Fed. Proc. Fed. Am. Soc. Exp. Biol.* **32**, 763.

Dave, C., Patnak, S. N., and Porter, C. W. (1978). Studies on the mechanism of cytotoxicity of methyl glyoxal bis (guanylhydrazone) in cultured L1210 cells. *Adv. Polyamine Res.* **1**, 200–218.

Don, S., and Bachrach, U. (1975). Polyamine metabolism in normal and virus-transformed chick embryo fibroblasts. *Cancer Res.* **35**, 3618–3622.

Don, S., Wiener, H., and Bachrach, U. (1975). Specific increase in polyamine levels in chick embroy cells transformed by Rous sarcoma virus. *Cancer Res.* **35**, 194–198.

Erwin, B. G., Ewton, D. Z., Florini, J. R., and Pegg, A. E. (1983). Polyamine depletion inhibits the differentiation in L6 myoblast cells. *Biochem. Biophys. Res. Commun.* **114**, 944–949.

Fillingame, R. H., Jorstad, C. M., and Morris, D. R. (1975). Increased cellular levels of spermidine or spermine are required for optimal DNA synthesis in lymphocytes activated by concanavalin A. *Proc. Natl. Acad. Sci. U.S.A.* **72**, 4042–4045.

Fozard, J. R., and Koch-Weser, J. (1982). Pharmacological consequences of inhibition of polyamine biosynthesis with DL-α-difluoromethylornithine. *Trends Pharmacol. Sci.* **3**, 107–110.

Fozard, J. R., and Prakash, N. J. (1982). Effects of DL-α-difluoromethylornithine, an irreversible inhibitor of ornithine decarboxylase on rat mammary tumour induced by 7,12-dimethylbenz[a]-anthracene. *Nauyn-Schmiedebergs Arch. Pharmakol.* **320**, 72–77.

Fozard, J. R., Part, M. L., Prakash, N. J., Grove, J., Schechter, P. J., Sjoersma, A., and Koch-Weser, J. (1980). L-Ornithine decarboxylase: An essential role in early mammalian embryogenesis. *Science* **208**, 505–508.

Friedman, S. J., Bellantone, R. A., and Canellakis, E. (1972). Ornithine decarboxylase activity in synchronously growing DON C cells. *Biochim. Biophys. Acta* **261**, 188–193.

Gazdar, A. F., Stull, H. B., Kilton, L. J., and Bachrach, U. (1976). Increased ornithine decarboxylase activity in murine sarcoma virus infected cells. *Nature (London)* **262**, 696–698.

Gazitt, Y., and Friend, C. (1980). Polyamine biosynthetic enzymes in the induction and inhibition of differentiation in Friend erythroleukemia cells. *Cancer Res.* **40**, 1727–1732.

Guha, S. K., and Janne, J. (1976). The synthesis and accumulation of polyamines in reproductive rgans of the rat during pregnancy. *Biochim. Biophys. Acta* **437**, 244–252.

Harada, J. J., and Morris, D. R. (1981). Cell cycle parameters of Chinese hamster ovary cells during exponential polyamine-limited growth. *Mol. Cell. Biol.* **1**, 594–599.

Harik, S. I., and Snyder, S. H. (1973). Ornithine decarboxylase: Inhibition by α-hydrazinoornithine. *Biochim. Biophys. Acta* **327**, 501–509.

Heby, O. (1981). Role of polyamines in the control of cell proliferation and differentiation. *Differentiation (Berlin)* **19**, 1–20.

Heby, O., and Andersson, G. (1980). Polyamines and the cell cycle. *In* "Polyamines in Biomedical Research" (J. M. Gaugas, ed.), pp. 17–34. Wiley, New York.

Heby, O., and Emanuelsson, H. (1978). Possible involvement of putrescine in nucleolar formation in early embryos. *Cell Tissue Res.* **194**, 103–114.

Heby, O., Gray, J. R., Llindl, P. A., Marton, L. J., and Wilson, C. B. (1976). Changes in L-ornithine decarboxylase activity during the cell cycle. *Biochem. Biophys. Res. Commun.* **71**, 99–105.

Heby, O., Andersson, G. and Gray, J. W. (1978). Interference with S and G1 phase progression by polyamine synthesis inhibitors. *Exp. Cell Res.* **111**, 461–464.

Heston, W. D. W., Fair, W. R., and Kadmon, D. (1982). Growth inhibition of a prostate tumor by α-difluoromethylornithine and by cyclophosphamide. *Cancer Lett. (Shannon, Irel.)* **16**, 71–79.

Hibasami, H., and Pegg, A. E. (1978). Differential inhibition of mammalian aminopropyltransferase activities. *Biochem. Biophys. Res. Commun.* **81**, 1398–1405.

Hibasami, H., Tanaka, M., Nagai, J., and Ikeda, T. (1980). FEBS Lett. **116**, 99–101.

Holtta, E. (1977). Oxidation of spermidine and spermine in rat liver: Purification and properties of polyamine oxidase. *Biochemistry* **16**, 91–100.

Holtta, E., Janne, J., and Hovi, T. (1979). Suppression of the formation of polyamines and macromolecules by DL-α-difluoromethylornithine and methylglyoxal bis(guanylhydrazone) in phytohaemagglutinin-activated human lymphocytes. *Biochem. J.* **178**, 109–117.

Huberman, E., Weeks, C., Heirmann, A., Callihan, M., and Slaga, T. (1981). Alterations in polyamine levels induced by phorbol diesters and other agents that promote differentiation in human promyelocytic leukemia cells. *Proc. Natl. Acad. Sci. U.S.A.* **78**, 1062–1066.

Huggins, C., Briziarelli, G., and Sutton, H. (1959). Rapid induction of mammary carcinoma in the rat and the influence of hormones on tumors. *J. Exp. Med.* **109**, 25–42.

Hung, D. T., Marton, L. J., Deen, D. F., and Shafer, R. H. (1983). Depletion of intracellular polyamines may alter DNA conformation in 9L rat brain tumor cells. *Science* **221**, 368–370.

Inoue, H., Kato, Y., Takigawa, M., Adachi, K., and Takeda, Y. (1975). Effect of DL-α-hydrazine-δ-amino-valeric acid, an inhibitor of ornithine decarboxylase, on polyamine metabolism in isoproterenol-stimulated mouse parotid glands. *J. Biochem (Tokyo)* **77**, 879–893.

Janne, J., and Raina, A. (1968). Stimulation of spermidine synthesis in the regenerating rat liver: Relation to increased ornithine decarboxylase activity. *Acta Chem. Scand.* **22**, 1349–1351.

Janne, J., Poso, H., and Raina, A. (1978). Polyamines in rapid growth and cancer. *Biochim. Biophys. Acta* **473**, 241–293.

Johansson, J., and Skinner, W. A. (1973). α-Hydrazino-ornithine and precursors. U.S. Patent No. 3,754.027. *Chem. Abstr.* **79**, 137504.

Kaye, A. M., Icekson, I., and Lindner, H. R. (1971). Stimulation by estrogens of ornithine and S-adenosylmethionine decarboxylases in the immature rat uterus. *Biochim. Biophys. Acta* **252**, 150–159.

Kepzaho, K., and Janne, J. (1983). Stimulation of melanotic expression in murine melanoma cells exposed to polyamine antimetabolites. *Biochem. Biophys. Res. Commun.* **113**, 8–23.

Kingsnorth, A. N., King, W. W., McCann, P. P., Diekema, K. A., Ross, J. S., and Malt, R. A. (1983a). Inhibition of ornithine decarboxylase with α-difluoromethylornithine: Reduced incidence of dimethylhydrazineinduced colonic tumors in mice. *Cancer Res.* **43**, 2545–2549.

Kingsnorth, A. N., Russell, W. E., McCann, P. P., Diekema, K. and Malt, R. A. (1983b). Effects of α-difluoromethylornithine and 5-fluorouracil on the proliferation of a human colon adenocarcinoma cell line. *Cancer Res.* **43**, 4035–4038.

Knutson, J. C., and Morris, D. R. (1978). Cellular polyamine depletion reduces DNA synthesis in isolated lymphocyte nuclei. *Biochim. Biophys. Acta* **520**, 291–301.

Kobayashi, Y., Kupelian, J., and Maudsley, D. V. (1971). Ornithine decarboxylase stimulation in rat ovary by luteinizing hormone. *Science* **172**, 379–380.

Koch-Weser, J., Schechter, P. J., Bey, P., Danzin, C., Fozard, J. R., Jung, M. J., Mamont, P. S., Prakash, N. J., Seiler, N., and Sjoerdsma, A. (1981). Potential of ornithine decarboxylase inhibitors as therapeutic agents. *In* "Polyamines in Biology and Medicine" (D. R. Morris and L. J. Marton, eds.), pp. 437–453. Dekker, New York.

Krelhaus, W., Gibson, L., and Harris, P. (1976). The effects of hypoxia, hypertrophy and diet on rat myocardial ornithine carboxylase activity. *Recent Adv. Stud. Card. Struct. Metabo.* **7**, 85–90.

Kremzner, L. T., Barrett, R. E., and Terrano, J. J. (1970). Polyamine metabolism in the central and peripheral nervous system. *Ann. N. Y. Acad. Sci.* **171**, 735–748.

Krokan, H., and Erikson, A. (1977). DNA synthesis in HeLa cells and isolated nuclei after treatment with an inhibitor of spermidine synthesis, methyl glyoxal bis(guanylhydrazone). *Eur. J. Biochem.* **72**, 501–508.

Luk, G. D., Goodwin, G., Marton, L. J., and Baylin, S. G. (1981). Polyamines are necessary for the survival of human small-cell lung carcinoma in culture. *Proc. Natl. Acad. Sci. U.S.A.* **78**, 2355–2358.

Luk, G. D., Civin, C. I., Weissman, R. M., and Baylin, S. B. (1982). Ornithine decarboxylase: Essential in proliferation but not in differentiation of human promyelocytic leukemia cells. *Science* **216**, 75–77.

Luk, G. D., Abeloff, M. D., Griffin, C. A., and Baylin, S. B. (1983). Successful treatment with DL-α-difluoromethylornithine in established human small cell variant lung carcinoma implant in athymic mice. *Cancer Res.* **43**, 4239–4243.

McCann, P. O., Tardif, C., Mamont, P. S., and Schuber, F. (1975). Biphasic induction of ornithine decarboxylase and putrescine levels in growing HTC cells. *Biochem. Biophys. Res. Commun.* **64**, 335–341.

McCann, P. P., Tardif, C., Pegg, A. E., and Diekema, K. (1980). The dual action of the non-physiological diamines 1,3-diaminopropane and cadaverine on ornithine decaroxylase of HTC cells. *Life Sci.* **26**, 2003–2010.

McCann, P. O., Bacchi, C. J., Clarkson, A. B., Seed, J. R., Nathan, H. C., Amole, B. O., Hutner, S. H., and Sjoerdsma, A. (1981). Further studies on difluoromethylornithine in African trypanosomes. *Med. Biol.* **59**, 434–440.

Mamont, P. S., Bohlen, P., McCann, P. P., Bey, P., Schuber, F., and Tardif, C. (1976). α-Methyl ornithine, a potent competitive inhibitor of ornithine decarboxylase, blocks proliferation of rat hepatoma cells in culture. *Proc. Natl. Acad. Sci. U.S.A.* **73**, 1626–1630.

Mamont, P. S., Duchesne, M. C., Grove, J., and Bey, P. (1978). Antiproliferative properties of DL-α-difluoromethylornithine in cultured cells. A consequence of the irreversible inhibition of ornithine decarboxylase. *Biochem. Biophys. Res. Commun.* **81**, 58–66.

Mann, T. (1964). "The Biochemistry of Semen and of the Male Reproductive Tract." Methuen, London.

Marton, L. J. (1981). Polyamines and brain tumors: Relationship to patient monitoring and therapy. *Adv. Polyamine Res.* **3**, 425–430.

Marton, L. J., and Heby, O. (1974). Polyamine metabolism in tumor, spleen and liver of tumor-bearing rats. *Int. J. Cancer* **13**, 619–628.

Marton, L. J., Heby, O., Levin, V. A., Lubich, W. P., Crafts, D. C., and Wilson, C. B. (1976). The relationship of polyamines in cerebrospinal fluid to the presence of central nervous system tumors. *Cancer Res.* **36**, 973–977.

Marton, L. J., Levin, V. A., Hervatin, S. J., Koch-Weser, J., McCann, P. P., and Sjoerdsma, A. (1981). Potentiation of the antitumor therapeutic effects of 1,3-bis(2-chloroethyl)-1-nitro-sourea by α-difluoromethyl ornithine, an ornithine decarboxylase inhibitor. *Cancer Res.* **41**, 4436–4431.

Metcalf, B. W., Bey, P., Danzin, C., Jung, M. J., Casara, P., and Vevert, J. P. (1978). Catalytic irreversible inhibition of mammalian ornithine decarboxylase (E.C.4.1.1.17) by substrate and product analogues. *J. Am. Chem. Soc.* **100**, 2551–2553.

Mihich, E. (1963). Prevention of the antitumor activity of methylglyoxal-bis-(guanylhydrazone) (CH$_3$-G) by spermidine. *Pharmacologist* **5**, 270.

Morris, D. R. and Fillingame, R. H. (1974). Regulation of amino acid decarboxylation. *Annu. Rev. Biochem.* **43**, 303–325.

Mottram, J. C. (1944). Developing factor in experimental blastogenesis. *J. Pathol. Bacteriol.* **56**, 181–187.

Nishioka, K., and Romsdahl, M. M. (1974). Elevation of putrescine and spermidine in sera of patients with solid tumors. *Clin. Chim. Acta* **57**, 155–161.

Nureddin, A. (1977). Ovarian ornithine decarboxylase induction: A specific and rapid *in vivo* bioassay of LH. *Biochem. Med.* **17**, 67–79.

O'Brien, T. G. (1976). The induction of ornithine decarboxylase as an early, possibly obligatory, event in mouse skin carcinogenesis. *Cancer Res.* **36**, 2644–2653.

O'Brien, T. G., Simsiman, R. C., and Boutwell, R. K., (1975). Induction of the polyamine-biosynthetic enzymes in mouse epidermis and their specificity for tumor promotion. *Cancer Res.* **35**, 2426–2433.

Oka, T., Perry, J. W., Takemoto, T., Sakai, T., Terada, N., and Inoue, H. (1981). The multiple regulatory roles of polyamines in the hormonal induction of mammary gland development. *Adv. Polyamine Res.* **3**, 309–320.

O'Leary, M. H., and Herreid, R. M. (1978). Mechanism of inactivation of ornithine decarboxylase by β-methylornithine. *Biochemistry* **17**, 1010–1014.

Olson, J. W., and Russell, D. H. (1979). Prolonged induction of hepatic ornithine decarboxylase and its relation to cyclic adenosine 3′5′-monophosphate dependent protein kinase activation after a single administration of diethylnitrosamine. *Cancer Res.* **39**, 3074–3079.

Oredsson, S., Anehus, S., and Heby, O. (1980). Irreversible inhibition of the early increase in ornithine decarboxylase activity following growth stimulation is required to block Ehrlich ascites tumor cell proliferation in culture. *Biochem. Biophys. Res. Commun.* **94**, 151–158.

Oredsson, S. M., Deen, D. F., and Marton, L. J. (1982). Decreased cytotoxicity of cis-diaminodichloro platinum(II) by α-difluoromethylornithine after depletion of polyamines in 9L rat brain tumor cells *in vitro*. *Cancer Res.* **42**, 1296–1299.

Oredsson, S. M., Gray, J. W., Deen, D. F., and Marton, L. J. (1983). Decreased cytotoxicity of 1-β-D-arabinofuranosylcytosine to 9L rat brain tumor cells pretreated with α-difluoromethylornithine *in vitro*. *Cancer Res.* **43**, 2541–2644.

Otani, S., Mizoguchi, Y., Matsui, I., and Morisawa, S. (1974). Inhibition of DNA synthesis by methyl-glyoxal bis(guanylhydrazone) during lymphocyte transformation. *Mol. Biol. Rep.* **1**, 431–436.

Pankaskie, M., and Abdel-Monem, M. M. (1980). Inhibitors of polyamine biosynthesis. 8. Irreversible inhibition of mammalian *S*-adenosylmethionine decarboxylase by substrate analogs. *J. Med. Chem.* **23**, 121–127.

Pearson, O. H., and Manni, A. (1978). Hormonal control of breast cancer growth in women and rats. *Curr. Top. Exp. Endocrinol.* **3**, 75–92.

Pegg, A. E. (1978). Inhibition of mammalian *S*-adenosylmethionine decarboxylase activity by 1-1′-[methylethaneidylidene dinitrilo]-bis-(3-aminoguanidine). *J. Biol. Chem.* **253**, 539–542.

Pegg, A. E. (1981). Effect of α-difluoromethylornithine on cardiac polyamine content and hypertrophy. *J. Mol. Cell. Cardiol.* **13**, 881–888.

Pegg, A. E., and McCann, P. P. (1982). Polyamine metabolism and function: A review. *Am. J. Physiol.* **243**, C212–C221.

Pegg, A. E., and Williams-Ashman, H. G. (1981). Biocynthesis of putrescine. *In* "Polyamines in Biology and Medicine" (D. R. Morris and L. J. Marton, eds.), pp. 3–42. Dekker, New York.

Pegg, A. E., Hibasami, H., Matsui, I., and Bethell, D. R. (1981). Formation and interconversion of putrescine and spermidine in mammalian cells. *Adv. Enzyme Regul.* **19**, 427–451.

Piik, K., Poso, H., and Janne, J. (1978). Reversible inhibition of rat liver regeneration by 1,3-diamino-2-propanol, an inhibitor of ornithine decarboxylase. *FEBS Lett.* **89**, 307–312.

Prakash, N. J., and Sunkara, P. S. (1983). Combination chemotherapy involving α-difluoromethylornithine and 1-β-D-arabinofuranosylcytosine in murine L1210 leukemia. *Cancer Res.* **43**, 3192–3196.

Prakash, N. J., Schechter, P. J., Grove, J., and Koch-Weser, J. (1978). Effect of α-difluoromethylornithine, an enzyme-activated irreversible inhibitor of ornithine decarboxylase, on L1210 leukemia in mice. *Cancer Res.* **38**, 3059–3062.

Prakash, N. J., Schechter, P. J., Mamont, P. S., Grove, J., Koch-Weser, J., and Sjoerdsma, A. (1980). Inhibition of EMT6 tumor growth by interference with polyamine biosynthesis; effects of α-difluoromethylornithine, an irreversible inhibitor of ornithine decarboxylase. *Life Sci.* **26**, 181–194.

Poso, H., and Janne, J. (1976). Inhibition of polyamine accumulation and deoxyribonucleic acid synthesis in regenerating rat liver. *Biochem. J.* **158**, 485–488.

Poso, H., and Pegg, A. E. (1982). Effect of α-difluoromethylornithine on polyamine and DNA synthesis in regenerating rat liver: Reversal of inhibition of DNA synthesis by putrescine. *Biochim. Biophys. Acta* **696**, 179–186.

Poste, G., and Fidler, J. (1980). The pathogenesis of cancer metastasis. *Nature (London)* **283**, 139–146.

Quash, G., Keolouangkhot, T., Gazzolo, L., Ripoll, H., and Saez, S. (1979). Diamine oxidase and polyamine oxidase activities in normal and transformed cells. *Biochem. J.* **177**, 275–282.

Raina, A. (1963). Studies on the determination of spermidine and spermine and their metabolism in the developing chick embryo. *Acta Physiol. Scand., Suppl.* **218**, 1–81.

Raina, A., and Janne, J. (1975). Physiology of the natural polyamines putrescine, spermidine and spermine. *Med. Biol.* **53**, 121–147.

Rao, P. N., Wilson, B., and Puck, T. T. (1977). Premature chromosome condensation and cell cycle analysis. *J. Cell. Physiol.* **91**, 131–141.

Rath, N. C., and Reddi, A. H. (1981). Changes in polyamines, RNA synthesis, and cell proliferation during matrix-induced cartilage, bone, and bone marrow development. *Dev. Biol.* **82**, 211–216.

Relyea, N., and Rando, R. R. (1975). Potent inhibition of ornithine decarboxylase by β-unsaturated substrate analogs. *Biochem. Biophys. Res. Commun.* **67**, 392–402.

Rennert, O. M., Lawson, D. L., Shukla, J. B., and Miale, T. D. (1977). Cerebrospinal fluid polyamine monitoring in central nervous system leukemia. *Clin. Chim. Acta* **75**, 365–369.

Rupniak, H. T., and Paul, D. (1978). Inhibition of spermidine and spermine synthesis leads to growth arrest of rat embryo fibroblasts in G_1. *J. Cell. Physiol.* **94**, 161–170.

Rupniak, H. T., and Paul, D. (1980). Selective killing of transformed cells by exploitation of their defective cell cycle control by polyamines. *Cancer Res.* **40**, 293–297.

Russell, D. H. (1970). Discussion: Putrescine and spermidine biosynthesis in growth and development. *Ann. N. Y. Acad. Sci.* **171**, 772–782.

Russell, D. H. (1977). Clinical relevance of polyamines as biochemical markers of tumor kinetics. *Clin. Chem.* **23**, 22–27.

Russell, D. H. (1981). Ornithine decarboxylase: Transcriptional induction by trophic harmones via a cAMP and cAMP dependent protein kinase pathway. *In* "Polyamines in Biology and Medicine" (D. R. Morris and L. J. Marton, eds.), pp. 109–125. Dekker, New York.

Russell, D. H., and Levy, C. C. (1971). Polyamine accumulation and biosynthesis in a mouse L1210 leukemia. *Cancer Res.* **31**, 248–251.

Russell, D. H., and Snyder, S. H. (1968). Amine synthesis in rapidly growing tissues: Ornithine decarboxylase activity in regenerating rat liver, chick embryo and various tumors. *Proc. Natl. Acad. Sci. U.S.A.*, **60**, 1420–1427.

Russell, D. H., and Stambrook, P. J. (1975). Cell cycle specific fluctuations in adenosine 3':5'-cyclic monophosphate and polyamines of Chinese hamster cells. *Proc. Natl. Acad. Sci. U.S.A.* **72**, 1482–1486.

Russell, D. H., Levy, C. C., Schimpff, S. C., and Hawk, I. A. (1971a). Urinary polyamines in cancer patients. *Cancer Res.* **31**, 1555–1558.

Russell, D. Hl., Shiverick, K. T., Hamrell, B. B., and Alpert, N. R. (1971b). Polyamine synthesis during initial phases of stress-induced cardiac hypertrophy. *Am. J. Physiol.* **221**, 1287–1291.

Russell, D. H., Byus, C. V., and Manen, C. A. (1976). Proposed model of major sequential biochemical events of a trophic response. *Life Sci.* **19**, 1297–1306.

Savory, J., and Shipe, J. R. (1975). Serum and urine polyamines in cancer. *Ann. Clin. Lab. Sci.* **5**, 110–114.

Scalabrino, G., Poso, H., Holtta, E., Hannonen, P., Kallio, A., and Janne, J. (1978). Synthesis and accumulation of polyamines in rat liver during chemical carcinogenesis. *Int. J. Cancer* **21**, 239–245.

Seiler, N. (1981). Turnover of polyamines. *In* "Polyamines in Biology and Medicine" (D. R. Morris and L. J. Marton, eds.), pp. 169–182, Dekker, New York.

Seiler, N., and Al-Therib, M. J. (1974). Putrescine catabolism in mammalian brain. *Biochem. J.* **144**, 29–35.

Seiler, N., and Knodgen, B. (1979a). Effects of ultraviolet light on epidermal polyamine metabolism. *Biochem. Med.* **21**, 168–181.

Seiler, N., and Knodgen, B. (1979b). Determination of the naturally occurring monoacetyl derivatives of di- and polyamines. *J. Chromatogr.* **164**, 155–168.

Seiler, N. S., Lamberty, U., and Al-Therib, J. J. (1975). Acetyl-coenzyme A: 1,4-Diaminobutane *N*-acetyl-transferase: Activity in rat brain during development, in experimental brain tumours and in brains of fish of different metabolic activity. *J. Neurochem.* **24**, 797–800.

Seppanen, P., Alhonen-Hongisto, L., and Janne, J. (1981). Polyamine deprivation induced enhanced uptake of methylglyoxal bis(guanylhydrazone) by tumor cells. *Biochim. Biophys. Acta* **674**, 169–177.

Seyfried, C. E., and Morris, D. R. (1979). Relationship between inhibition of polyamine biosynthesis and DNA replication in activated lymphocytes. *Cancer Res.* **39**, 4861–4867.

Sidenfield, J., Deen, D. F., and Marton, L. J. (1980). Depletion of intracellular polyamine content does not alter the survival of 9L rat brain tumor cells after X-irradiation. *Int. J. Radiat. Biol.* **38**, 223–229.

Sidenfield, J., Gray, J. W., and Marton, L. J. (1981). Depletion of 9L rat brain tumor cell polyamine content by treatment with DL-α-difluoromethylornithine inhibits proliferation and the G1 to S transition. *Exp. Cell Res.* **131**, 209–216.

Siimes, M., and Janne, J. (1967). Polyamines and their biosynthesis in Ehrlich ascites cells. *Acta Chem. Scand.* **21**, 815–817.

Sjoerdsma, A. (1981). Suicide enzyme inhibitors as potential drugs. *Clin. Pharmacol. Ther.* **30**, 3–22.

Sjoerdsma, A., and Schechter, P. J. (1983). Chemotherapeutic implications of polyamine biosynthesis inhibition. *Clin. Pharmacol. Ther.* **35**, 287–300.

Snyder, S. H., Kreuz, D. S., Medina, V. J., and Russell, D. H. (1970). Polyamine synthesis and turnover in rapidly growing tissues. *Ann. N. Y. Acad. Sci.* **171**, 749–771.

Sogani, R. K., Matsushita, S., Mueller, J. F., and Raben, M. S. (1972). Stimulation of ornithine decarboxylase activity in rat tissues by growth hormone and by serum growth factor from rats infected with spargana of *Spirometra mansonoides*. *Biochim. Biophys. Acta* **279**, 377–386.

Stevens, L., McKinnon, I. M., Turner, R. M., and North, M. J. (1978). The effects of 1,4-diamino butanone on polyamine metabolism in bacteria, a cellular slime mould and rat tissues. *Biochem. Soc. Trans.* **6**, 407–409.

Sunkara, P. S., and Rao, P. N. (1981). Differential cell cycle response of normal and transformed cells to polyamine limitation. *Adv. Polyamine Res.* **3**, 347–356.

Sunkara, P. S., Rao, P. N., and Nishioka, K. (1977). Putrescine biosynthesis in mammalian cells: Essential for DNA synthesis but not for mitosis. *Biochem. Biophys. Res. Commun.* **74**, 1125–1133.

Sunkara, P. S., Pargac, M. B., Nishioka, K., and Rao, P. N. (1979a). Differential effects of inhibition of polyamine biosynthesis on cell cycle traverse and structure of the prematurely condensed chromosomes of normal and transformed cells. *J. Cell. Physiol.* **98**, 451–458.

Sunkara, P. S., Rao, P. N., Nishioka, K., and Brinkley, B. R. (1979b). Role of polyamines in cytokinesis of mammalian cells. *Exp. Cell Res.* **119**, 63–68.

Sunkara, P. S., Fowler, S. K., Nishioka, K., and Rao, P. N. (1980). Inhibition of polyamine biosynthesis by α-difluoromethylornithine potentiates the cytotoxic effects of arabinosylcytosine in HeLa cells. *Biochem. Biophys. Res. Commun.* **95**, 423–430.

Sunkara, P. S., Wright, D. A., and Nishioka, K. (1981a). An essential role for putrescine biosynthesis during meiotic maturation of amphibian oocytes. *Dev. Biol.* **87**, 351–355.

Sunkara, P. S., Ramakrishna, S., Nishioka, K., and Rao, P. N. (1981b). The relationship between levels and rates of synthesis of polyamines during mammalian cell cycle. *Life Sci.* **28**, 1497–1506.

Sunkara, P. S., Fowler, S. K., and Nishioka, K. (1981c). Selective killing of transformed cells in combination with inhibitors of polyamine biosynthesis and S-phase specific drugs. *Cell Biol. Int. Rep.* **5**, 991–997.

Sunkara, P. S., Prakash, N. J., and Rosenberger, A. L. (1982). An essential role for polyamines in tumor metastases. *FEBS Lett.* **150**, 397–399.

Sunkara, P. S., Prakash, N. J., Mayer, G. D., and Sjoerdsma, A. (1983a). Tumor suppression with a combination of α-difluoromethylornithine and interferon. *Science* **219**, 851–853.

Sunkara, P. S., Prakash, N. J., Chang, C. C., and Sjoerdsma, A. (1983b). Cytotoxicity of methylglyoxal bis(guanyl hydrazone) in combination with α-difluoromethylornithine against HeLa cells and mouse L1210 leukemia. *JNCI, J. Natl. Cancer Inst.* **40**, 505–509.

Sunkara, P. S., Prakash, N. J., and Nishioka, K. (1984a). Potentiation of antitumor activity of α-difluoromethylornithine by an immunomodulatory peptide, tuftsin. *Ann. N. Y. Acad. Sci.* **419**, 268–272.

Sunkara, P. S., Chang, C. C., and Prakash, N. J. (1984b). Inhibition of polyamine biosynthesis on the growth and differentiation of B16 melanoma *in vitro* and *in vivo. Cancer Res.* (submitted).

Tabor, C. W., and Tabor, H. (1976). 1,4-Diaminobutane (putrescine), spermidine and spermine. *Annu. Rev. Biochem.* **45**, 285–306.

Takami, H., Romsdahl, M. M., and Nishioka, K. (1979). Polyamines in blood cells as a cancer marker. *Lancet* **2** (8148), 912.

Takigawa, M., Verma, A. K., Simsiman, R. C., and Boutwell, R. K. (1982). Polyamine biosynthesis and skin tumor pormotion: Inhibition of 12-*O*-tetradecanoyl phorbol-13-acetate-promoted mouse skin tumor formation by the irreversible inhibitor or ornithine decarboxylase α-difluoromethylornithine. *Biochem. Biophys. Res. Commun.* **105**, 969–976.

Takona, T., Takigawa, M., and Suzuki, F. (1981). Role of polyamines in expression of the differentiated phenotype of chondrocytes in culture. *Med. Biol.* **59**, 423–427.

Tang, K. C., Pegg, A. E., and Coward, J. K. (1980). Specific and potent inhibition of spermidine synthase by the transition-state analog, *S*-adenosyl-3-thio-1,8-diaminooctane. *Biochem. Biophys. Res. Commun.* **96**, 1371–1377.

Tofilron, P. J., Ordesson, S. M., Dean, D. F., and Marton, L. J. (1982). Polyamine depletion influences drug-induced chromosomal damage. *Science* **217**, 1046–1048.

Trackman, P. C., and Abeles, R. H. (1983). Methionine synthesis from 5′-*S*-methylthioadenosine. Resolution of enzyme activities and identification of 1-phosopho-5-*S*-methylthioribulose. *J. Biol. Chem.* **258**, 6717–6720.

Verma, A. K., and Boutwell, R. K. (1977). Vitamin A acid (retinoic acid), a potent inhibitor of 12-α-tetradecanoyl-phorbol-13-acetate–induced ornithine decarboxylase activity in mouse epidermis. *Cancer Res.* **37**, 2196–2201.

Verma, D. S., and Sunkara, P. S. (1982). An essential role for polyamine biosynthesis during human granulopoietic differentiation. *Cancer Res.* **42**, 3046–3049.

Verma, A. K., Conrad, E. A., and Boutwell, R. K. (1982). Differential effects of retinoic acid and 7,8-benzoflavone on the induction of mouse skin tumors by the complete carcinogenesis process and by initiation promotion regimen. *Cancer Res.* **42**, 3519–3525.

Waalkes, T. P., Gehrke, C. W., Tormey, D. C., Zumwalt, R. W., Hueser, J. N., Kuo, K. C., Lakings, D. B., Ahmann, D. L., and Moertel, C. G. (1975). Urinary excretion of polyamines by patients with advanced malignancy. *Cancer Chemother. Rep.* **59**, 1103–1116.

Wang, T., Pankaskie, M. C., Foker, J. E., and Abdel-Monem, M. M. (1980). Inhibition of spermine biosynthesis and thymidine incorporation in concanavalin A transformed lymphocytes by *S*-adenosyl-(±)2-methyl methionine. *Biochem. Biophys. Res. Commun.* **94**, 85–92.

Weeks, C. E., Herrmann, A. L., Nelson, F. R., and Sloga, T. J. (1982). α-difluoromethylornithine, an irreversible inhibitor of ornithine decarboxylase, inhibits tumor promotor-induced polyamine accumulation and carcinogenesis in mouse skin. *Proc. Natl. Acad. Sci. U.S.A.* **79,** 6028–6032.

Williams-Ashman, H. G., and Schenone, A. (1972). Methyl glyoxal bis (guanylhydrazone) as a potent inhibitor of mammalian and yeast S-adenosyl methionine decarboxylases. *Biochem. Biophys. Res. Commun.* **46,** 288–295.

Williams-Ashman, H. G. Coppoc, G. L., and Weber, G. (1972). Imbalance in ornithine metabolism in hepatomas of different growth rates as expressed in formation of putrescine, spermidine, and spermine. *Cancer Res.* **32,** 1924–1932.

Williams-Ashman, H. G., Coppoc, G. L., Schenone, A., and Weber, G. (1973). Aspects of polyamine biosynthesis in normal and malignant eukaryotic cells. *In* "Polyamines in Normal and Neoplastic Growth" (D. H. Russell, ed.), pp. 181–197. Raven, New York.

Williams-Ashman, H. G., Seidenfeld, J., and Galletti, P. (1982). Trends in the biochemical pharmacology of 5'-deoxy-5'-methylthioadenosine. *Biochem. Pharmacol.* **31,** 277–288.

Yuspa, S. H., Lichti, U., Ben, T., Patterson, E., Hennings, H., Slaga, T. J., Colburn, N., and Kelsey, W. (1976). Phorbol esters stimulate DNA synthesis and ornithine decarboxylase activity in mouse epidermal cell cultures. *Nature (London)* **262,** 402–404.

4

Prostaglandin, Thromboxane, and Leukotriene Biosynthesis: Target for Antitumor and Antimetastatic Agents

KENNETH V. HONN

Department of Radiology,
and Department of Radiation Oncology
Wayne State University
Detroit, Michigan

LAWRENCE J. MARNETT

Department of Chemistry
Wayne State University
Detroit, Michigan

I.	Introduction: Arachidonic Acid Metabolism	128
II.	Modulators of Arachidonate Metabolism as Chemopreventative	
	Agents: Inhibition of Tumor Initiation	133
III.	Inhibition of Tumor Promotion.................................	135
IV.	Overview of the Metastatic Cascade............................	138
	Hemostatic Mechanisms and Metastasis	140
V.	Prostacyclin, Thromboxanes, and Tumor Cell Metastasis..........	141
	A. Prostacyclin Effects *in Vivo* and *in Vitro*	142
	B. Prostacyclin Effects on Platelet-Induced Tumor Cell Adhesion	
	in Vitro	143
	C. Prostacyclin Effects on Metastasis *in Vivo*	144
	D. Prostacyclin as an Endogenous Deterrent to Metastasis.........	145
	E. Effects of Agents That Stimulate or Synergize with Endogenous	
	Prostacyclin Production	146
VI.	Conclusion	152
	References	153

Novel Approaches to Cancer Chemotherapy
Copyright © 1984 by Academic Press, Inc.
All rights of reproduction in any form reserved.
ISBN 0-12-676980-X

I. INTRODUCTION: ARACHIDONIC ACID
METABOLISM

Prostaglandins (PG) and leukotrienes (LT) are generic names for two classes of lipids that possess diverse and potent biological activities. They are widespread in mammalian tissue, and they appear to be important regulators of cellular processes including growth, differentiation, and motility (Powles et al., 1982). The pathways of their biosynthesis are complex, but advances in biochemistry and pharmacology have made it possible to select individual pathways for stimulation or inhibition. Intensive ongoing investigation promises to expand the scope of selective pharmacological manipulation. This will provide significant opportunities for cancer chemoprevention and therapy for those who understand the pathways, consequences, and manipulation of prostaglandin and leukotriene biosynthesis.

Arachidonic acid serves as the substrate for two oxygenases in mammalian tissue (Fig. 1). Cyclooxygenase introduces two molecules of molecular oxygen into the carbon framework of arachidonate to generate the hydroperoxy endoperoxide, PGG_2 (Hamberg et al., 1974; Nugteren and Hazelhof, 1973). The hydroperoxy group is reduced by a peroxidase to an alcohol (Ohki et al., 1979). The hydroxy endoperoxide generated (PGH_2) is the branch point in biosynthesis (Hamberg and Samuelsson, 1973; Nugteren and Hazelhof, 1973). Its cyclic peroxy group is converted by isomerases to prostaglandins, thromboxanes, and prostacyclin (Yamamoto et al., 1980; Hamberg et al., 1975; Johnson et al., 1976). Although PGG_2 and PGH_2 have potent muscle-contracting and platelet-aggregating activity, they are usually metabolized so rapidly by isomerases that they are not important regulatory molecules. However, under conditions where the isomerases are inhibited—for example, inhibition of thromboxane (TX) synthase in platelets—significant quantities of PGH_2 can accumulate and exert biological effects (Aiken et al., 1981). Specific cell types do not contain all of the PGH_2-metabolizing enzymes. Rather, one or two isomerases are present in high abundance, and the others are present in low amounts or not at all. The balance of isomerizing enzymes is characteristic of the cell type and appears to be determined at the level of gene transcription.

Enzymes have been described and partially purified that catalyze the rearrangement of PGH_2 to PGE_2 and PGD_2 (Yamamoto et al., 1980). Both enzymes require reduced glutathione. Although an endoperoxide analog has been described that inhibits the conversion of PGH_2 to PGE_2, inhibitors of either enzyme are not generally available (Wlodawer et al., 1971). In fact, it would be experimentally very difficult to inhibit completely the formation of PGE_2 or PGD_2 even if a battery of specific inhibitors was available. This is because PGH_2 isomerizes spontaneously to both compounds in the absence of a catalyst (Hamberg and Samuelsson, 1973; Nugteren and Hazelhof, 1973). If the enzymatic conversion could be completely inhibited, significant nonenzymatic conversion would still occur. The conversion of PGH_2 to $PGF_{2\alpha}$ is a reduction that requires an electron source. Despite the discovery that several different naturally occurring compounds will reduce PGH_2 to $PGF_{2\alpha}$, an enzyme that catalyzes this reaction has never been described (Marnett and Bienkowski, 1977). $PGF_{2\alpha}$ is probably generated by reduction of PGH_2 *in vivo*, but a reductase has not been detected. Pyridine nucleotide-dependent dehydrogenases have been isolated and purified that catalyze the reversible reduction of PGE_2 and PGD_2 to $PGF_{2\alpha}$ (Lee and Levine, 1975). This indirect pathway also accounts for the formation of $PGF_{2\alpha}$ from arachidonic acid *in vivo* (Lee and Levine, 1974).

Thromboxane synthase catalyzes the rearrangement of PGH_2 to thromboxane A_2 (TXA_2) (Yoshimoto et al., 1977; Hammarstrom and Falardeau, 1977). This bicyclic acetal is the most potent stimulator of muscle contraction and platelet aggregation yet described (Hamberg et al., 1975). TXA_2 is very unstable to spontaneous hydrolysis ($t_{1/2}$ 1 min at 37°C). The hydrolysis product TXB_2 is stable but biologically inactive (Hamberg et al., 1975). Several excellent thromboxane synthase inhibitors are available for *in vitro* and *in vivo* animal testing (Gorman, 1983; Aiken, 1983). Prostacyclin synthase catalyzes the rearrangement of PGH_2 to prostacyclin (PGI_2) (DeWitt and Smith, 1983). In contrast to TXA_2, PGI_2 is a muscle relaxant and the most potent inhibitor of platelet aggregation known (Johnson et al., 1976). Similar to TXA_2, though, PGI_2 is unstable to spontaneous hydrolysis; its half-life is approximately 30 sec and the product, 6-keto-$PGF_{1\alpha}$, is inactive (Johnson et al., 1976). PGI_2 synthase is irreversibly inactivated by low concentrations of hydroperoxy, but not hydroxy, fatty acids (Moncada et al., 1976a). The antagonistic activities of TXA_2 and PGI_2 and the fact that they are derived from a common precursor provide a foundation for the evolution of regulatory mechanisms.

Prostaglandins do not function as classical circulating hormones. This is because of the rapid oxidation of the 15-hydroxyl group to inactive keto derivatives during pulmonary circulation (Samuelsson et al., 1971). Oxidation is catalyzed by 15-hydroxyprostaglandin dehydrogenase, and although Fig. 1 only illustrates its action on PGI_2, all of the cyclooxygenase-dependent metabolites of arachidonate are substrates for it. Inhibitors of the dehydrogenase have been described, and they may have important pharmacological effects by virtue of their ability to prolong the half-lives of the biologically active species (Wong et al., 1982).

The second major enzyme of arachidonic acid metabolism is lipoxygenase. Several different enzymes exist that introduces a single molecule of oxygen at separate positions of the arachidonate framework (Hamberg and Samuelsson, 1974; Borgeat et al., 1976; Narumiya et al., 1981). The isomeric hydroperoxy acids generated (HPETE's) are either reduced to hydroxy fatty acids (HETE's) by peroxidases or metabolized to epoxy derivatives (Bryant et al., 1982). The HPETE's and HETE's have moderate biological activities and are chemotactic

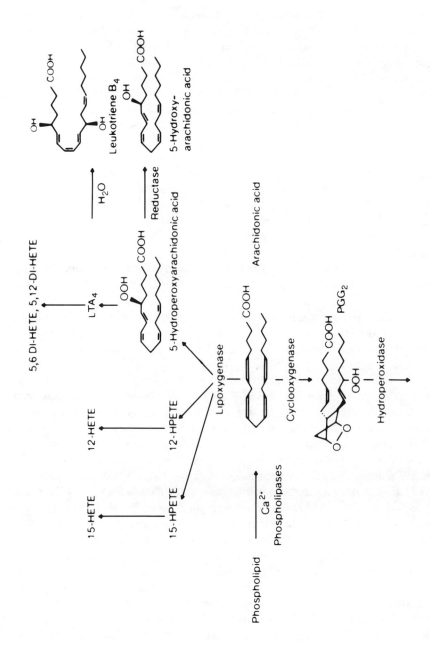

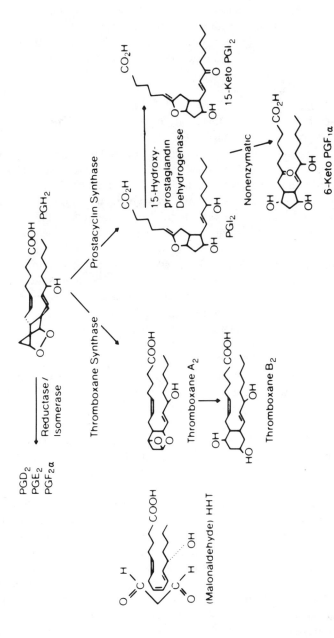

Fig. 1. Arachidonic acid metabolism via the lipoxygenase pathway resulting in hydroperoxy fatty acids and leukotrienes, and via the prostaglandin endoperoxide synthase (cyclooxygenase + hydroperoxidase) pathway resulting in prostaglandins (including prostacyclin) and thromboxanes. (Reproduced from Honn *et al.*, 1983a, with permission of Pergamon Press.)

131

for polymorphonuclear leukocytes (PMN's) (Goetzel *et al.*, 1979). There is evidence that 12-H(P)ETE plays an as yet undefined role in platelet aggregation (Goset and Lagarde, 1983). Since hydroperoxy fatty acids are irreversible inhibitors of prostacyclin synthase, the lipoxygenase pathway may play an important role in regulating the levels of PGI_2 by generating irreversible inhibitors of its synthesis. Since TXA_2 synthase is not particularly sensitive to hydroperoxide-dependent inactivation, modulation of the levels of HPETE's can have a dramatic effect on the balance of PGI_2 and TXA_2. The levels of HPETE can be altered by affecting either the lipoxygenases that catalyze HPETE synthesis or the peroxidases that catalyze HPETE reduction.

A particularly important hydroperoxy acid is 5-HPETE. This compound serves as the precursor to an epoxide named leukotriene A_4 (LTA_4) (Borgeat and Samuelsson, 1979). Since the epoxy group is α to a conjugated triene, it is unstable and subject to enzymatic as well as nonenzymatic metabolism (Borgeat and Samuelsson, 1979). Addition of water to the 12-position, one of the termini of the triene functionality, forms leukotriene B_4 (LTB_4), an extremely potent chemotactic agent for PMN's and tumor cells (R. R. Gorman, J. Dunn, and K. V. Honn, manuscript in preparation). Trans addition of glutathione to the 6-position of LTA_4 generates LTC_4, a potent constrictor of smooth muscle (Hammarstrom *et al.*, 1979). LTC_4 is metabolized by sequential digestion of the tripeptide residue of glutathione to form LTD_4 and LTE_4. LTB_4, LTC_4, and LTD_4 appear to be important mediators of inflammation and allergic hypersensitivity (Samuelsson, 1983). The enzymes that convert LTA_4 to LTB_4 and LTC_4 are epoxide hydrases and glutathione transferases, respectively. LTA_4 also undergoes nonenzymatic hydrolysis to 5,6- and 5,12-dihydroxy acids (Borgeat and Samuelsson, 1979). However, the geometry of the triene double bonds differs from that of LTB_4, and the nonenzymatically formed dihydroxy acids have little or no biological activity (Sirois *et al.*, 1981).

Regardless of the metabolites of arachidonate that are made in a given cell type, the rate-limiting step of the overall process is the release of arachidonic acid from cellular stores. The cyclooxygenase component of PGH synthase only oxidizes free arachidonic acid, the concentration of which is extremely low in most cells (Lands and Samuelsson, 1968; Vonkeman and Van Dorp, 1968). Stimulation of cellular phospholipase activity results in the release of significant amounts of free arachidonate that can serve as a substrate for prostaglandin and leukotriene biosynthesis. Many agents, including hormones, proteinases, tumor promoters, antigens, and ionophores, as well as mechanical and electrical stimulation activate phospholipase activity and cause the release of arachidonate (Galli *et al.*, 1978). Prostaglandin and leukotriene biosynthesis is therefore critically dependent on the interaction of surface-active stimuli with the plasma membrane. Steroidal antiinflammatory agents inhibit the release of arachidonate by stimulating the synthesis of a protein inhibitor of phospholipase (macrocortin or lipomodulin) (Flower and Blackwell, 1979; Hirata *et al.*, 1980).

Arachidonate oxygenation by PGH synthase is inhibited by a large number of compounds, many of which are nonsteroidal antiinflammatory agents (Robinson and Vane, 1974). Aspirin and indomethacin are classic irreversible inhibitors that have been widely employed *in vitro* and *in vivo*. However, a variety of inhibitors are available that differ in their mechanism of action. Some of these compounds may provide means to inhibit prostaglandin biosynthesis in animals without the limiting side effects of gastric irritation and renal toxicity. Compounds are also available that inhibit lipoxygenase-catalyzed oxidation of arachidonate. Although agents have been described that inhibit specific lipoxygenase isoenzymes *in vitro,* their specificity and inhibitory potency has not been defined completely *in vivo*. Since this is an area of intensive investigation in the pharmaceutical industry, it is anticipated that potent, specific lipoxygenase inhibitors will be available in the near future.

A common strategy in testing for the involvement of prostaglandins or leukotrienes in a particular physiological or pharmacological response is to determine the effects of steroids or aspirinlike drugs on the response. If inhibition is seen, then it is concluded that an arachidonate metabolite is involved. However, if no effect is seen it cannot be concluded that arachidonate metabolites are not involved. This is because inhibition of arachidonate oxygenation completely abolishes the formation of all metabolites. If two arachidonate metabolites with antagonistic activities balance the physiological response, lowering of both their levels may have no effect. Alternatively, a particular ratio of metabolites may be necessary for a given response, and disturbing this ratio may actually have an undesired effect. For example, TXA_2 is an important mediator of platelet aggregation; yet high doses of aspirin do not significantly protect against thrombosis. This is because high-dose aspirin also inhibits PGI_2 biosynthesis in arterial endothelial cells; PGI_2 normally functions to inhibit platelet aggregation. Thus, it is much better to employ specific modulators of enzymes that metabolize PGH_2 (e.g., TXA_2 synthase inhibitor) than to inhibit the formation of PGH_2 and therefore all its derivatives. Steroidal and nonsteroidal antiinflammatory agents can only be considered analogous to the coarse control of an amplifier.

II. MODULATORS OF ARACHIDONATE METABOLISM AS CHEMOPREVENTATIVE AGENTS: INHIBITION OF TUMOR INITIATION

The transformation of a normal cell to a cancer cell is a complex process that can be induced by viruses, radiation, or chemicals. A principal action of each of these agents is mutation or alteration of the rate of expression of specific genes. In the case of chemically induced cancers, there is evidence that most chemicals form covalent linkages to cellular DNA. Unless the adduct is removed by repair processes, the lesion causes the introduction of a permanent genetic mutation.

This irreversible step is called initiation, and evidence for its importance in carcinogenesis is provided by the correlation between mutagenicity and carcinogenicity that obtains for many chemicals (McCann and Ames, 1976). Most of the potent chemical carcinogens are not reactive enough to bind covalently to DNA. However, they can be metabolized by host enzymes to derivatives that are electrophilic and react with DNA. The conversion of an unreactive precarcinogen to a reactive ultimate carcinogen is termed metabolic activation and is responsible for the carcinogenicity of a majority of chemical carcinogens.

An important step in metabolic activation is oxidation (Miller, 1970; Heidelberger, 1975). For example, the polycyclic aromatic hydrocarbon benzo[a]pyrene (BP) is converted by oxygenation and hydration to dihydrodiol epoxides that represent its ultimate carcinogenic forms (Sims et al., 1974; Huberman et al., 1976; Jeffrey et al., 1977; Kapitulnik et al., 1978). The oxygenations are catalyzed by mixed-function oxidases that utilize NADPH as an electron source (Conney, 1982). Work from several laboratories indicates that the enzyme that converts arachidonic acid to PGH_2 (PGH synthase) may trigger the metabolic activation of chemical carcinogens (Marnett and Eling, 1983). PGH synthase contains two enzymatic activities on the same protein; the first is the cyclooxygenase that oxygenates arachidonate to PGG_2, and the second is a peroxidase that reduces PGG_2 to PGH_2 (Ohki et al., 1979). The peroxidase oxidizes a wide variety of endogenous and foreign compounds concomitant with reduction of PGG_2 (Marnett and Eling, 1983). Among the compounds oxidized are chemical carcinogens that require oxidative activation to express their carcinogenic potential such as polycyclic aromatic hydrocarbons, aromatic amines, aflatoxin, and nitrofurans. In the case of polycyclic hydrocarbons, PGH synthase catalyzes the oxidation of dihydrodiol metabolites of the parent hydrocarbons to the ultimate carcinogens, dihydrodiol epoxides (Marnett, 1981). This indicates that the peroxidase activity of PGH synthase can participate in metabolic activation, at least in vitro.

Several reports indicate that arachidonic acid-dependent carcinogen activation can occur in cellular systems and perhaps in vivo. Boyd et al. (1982) have reported that arachidonic acid stimulates the transformation of C3H10T½ mouse embryo fibroblasts by BP-7,8-diol, the immediate precursor to the diol epoxides. The increase in transformation in the presence of arachidonate correlates with an increase in the metabolism of BP-7,8-diol. The PGH synthase inhibitor indomethacin abolishes the increases in metabolism and transformation, indicating that the enhancing role of arachidonic acid is due to stimulation of oxidative metabolism of BP-7,8-diol. Reed et al. (1983) have reported a similar increase in BP-7,8-diol metabolism by arachidonic acid in hamster trachea and human bronchus. Amstad and Cerutti (1983) have reported that indomethacin, eicosatetraynoic acid (ETYA; a lipoxygenase inhibitor), and p-bromophenacyl bromide (a phospholipase inhibitor) lower the level of DNA adducts formed from aflatoxin in C3H10T½ fibroblasts. They suggest this is due to inhibition of arachidonic acid-dependent epoxidation of aflatoxin to its ultimate carcinogenic form. The inhibition of DNA adduct formation by the phospholipase inhibitor suggests that aflatoxin stimulates the release of arachidonate from phospholipid stores, which results in arachidonate oxygenation. In other words, aflatoxin triggers its own metabolic activation by PGH synthase.

One of the tissues where arachidonate-dependent metabolic activation may play an important role in carcinogenicity is the kidney. Renal blood flow is high—25% of cardiac output to a pair of organs that make up only 0.4% of body weight. The role of the kidney as an excretory organ may expose it to toxic metabolites, since selective concentration processes occur there. Furthermore, the distribution of drug-metabolizing enzymes is compartmentalized—mixed-function oxidase is highest in the cortex, intermediate in the outer medulla, and virtually undetectable in the inner medulla, whereas PGH synthase exhibits the opposite relative distribution. Zenser et al. (1979) have shown that arachidonic acid-dependent metabolism of the urinary bladder carcinogen benzidine occurs in anesthetized dogs. Benzidine in saline containing 100 μM arachidonate was injected into the renal pelvis through ureteral catheters. The catheters were clamped for 5 min, the clamps were released, and urine was collected for 30 min at 5-min intervals. At an initial concentration of 30 μM, approximately 30% of the benzidine was metabolized. No metabolism was observed using dogs that had been treated with the PGH synthase inhibitor, sodium meclofenamate, 30 min prior to retrograde perfusion.

Zenser and co-workers have detected arachidonic acid-dependent metabolism of urinary bladder carcinogens in microsomal preparations of bladder transitional epithelia. They have reported with Cohen that the PGH synthase inhibitor aspirin reduces by 50% the incidence of preneoplastic lesions and carcinomas induced by feeding the nitrofuran bladder carcinogen, N-[4-(5-nitro-2-furyl)-2-thiazolyl] formamide (FANFT) (Cohen et al., 1981). This is the first report of the inhibition of chemically induced cancer by an inhibitor of arachidonic acid-dependent metabolic activation. It suggests that PGH synthase inhibitors may be useful prophylactic agents against certain types of chemical carcinogenesis.

III. INHIBITION OF TUMOR PROMOTION

The development of chemically induced cancers is characterized by a prolonged latent period between the time of application of the carcinogen and the formation of a palpable tumor. In animal tests, this latent period can be shortened by the repeated administration of compounds called promoters (Berenblum and Shubik, 1947). One of the most potent promoters currently available is tetradecanoyl phorbol acetate (TPA) (Baird and Boutwell, 1971). In tumorigenesis studies in mouse skin, TPA not only shortens the latent period for tumor development but also reduces the total amount of the carcinogen that must be applied prior to promotion. Thus, a single nontoxic dose of an initiator, insufficient by itself to cause tumors during the normal lifetime of the animal, can produce a high yield of tumors if it is followed by twice-weekly applications of 5 to 20 nmol of TPA. TPA applied in the absence of an initiator does not cause tumors.

TPA administration to mouse skin *in vivo* or to cells in culture results in many different biochemical changes. One of these is the release of arachidonic acid from phospholipid stores (Levine, 1981). This may explain the potent inhibition of tumor promotion by antiinflammatory steroids (Schwarz *et al.*, 1977). Levine and Hassid (1977) first reported that TPA treatment causes an elevation of prostaglandin levels (PGE_2 and $PGF_{2\alpha}$) in MDCK (dog kidney) cells. The TPA effect was inhibited by indomethacin, indicating that the enhanced prostaglandin levels were the result of *de novo* synthesis. TPA treatment of cells prelabeled with radiolabeled arachidonic acid caused a release of arachidonic acid as well as PGE_2 and $PGF_{2\alpha}$. This suggests that TPA stimulates the release of arachidonic acid from cellular lipids. The non-tumor-promoting analog 4-phorbol didecanoate caused no stimulation of prostaglandin synthesis (Levine and Hassid, 1977).

Brune *et al.* (1978) published a structure–activity study that indicates a correlation exists between tumor-promoting activity in mouse skin and the ability of a series of diterpene esters to stimulate PGE_2 biosynthesis in macrophages. Terpenes of the tigliane, ingenane, and daphnane type that are potent promoters stimulate PGE_2 biosynthesis. The authors suggest that deacylation of cellular phospholipids with release of arachidonic acid may be one of the earliest events occurring in mouse skin following the application of a tumor promoter.

Verma *et al.* (1977) had previously shown that indomethacin, flufenamic acid, or aspirin applied to mouse skin prior to the application of TPA substantially depressed the induction of ornithine decarboxylase (ODC) activity by TPA. Inhibition of OCD inductions by prostaglandin endoperoxide synthase (PES) inhibitors was completely overcome by subsequent treatment with PGE_1 or PGE_2 but not $PGF_{2\alpha}$. Application of PGE_1 or PGE_2 to mouse skin in the absence of TPA caused no increase in ODC activity. These results suggest that prostaglandins play a role in TPA-dependent induction of ODC activity and hence tumor promotion, but that they are not themselves tumor promoters. Similar results have been reported with respect to the mitogenic action of TPA (Furstenberger and Marks, 1978; Furstenberger *et al.*, 1979). Indomethacin application to mouse skin inhibits TPA-induced stimulation of DNA synthesis and increases the number of mitotic figures. PGE_2 but not $PGF_2\alpha$ overcomes the indomethacin inhibition of DNA synthesis, although PGE_2 alone has no effect on DNA synthesis.

Prostaglandins are synthesized by mouse skin in response to treatment with TPA (Bresnick *et al.*, 1979; Ashendel and Boutwell, 1979). Bresnick and Boutwell's groups simultaneously reported that approximately a 10-fold increase in

PGE_2 and a 3-fold increase in $PGF_{2\alpha}$ concentration is observed 12 hr after the administration of TPA. The stimulated prostaglandin levels decrease rapidly and are followed by a second rise in PGE_2 concentration at 24 hr and in $PGF_{2\alpha}$ concentration at 72 hr (Ashendel and Boutwell, 1979).

Boutwell has extended his initial observations on the effects of nonsteroidal antiinflammatory agents on TPA-dependent induction of ODC activity in mouse skin (Verma et al., 1980). ODC induction was inhibited by PGH synthase inhibitors in this order: indomethacin > naproxen > flufenamic acid > aspirin. The maximal effect of indomethacin was observed if it was applied 2–5 hr before the application of TPA. Inhibition could be overcome by PGE_1, PGE_2, PGD_2, and the 6,9-thio analog of PGI_2 but not by $PGF_{1\alpha}$, $PGF_{2\alpha}$, 6-keto-$PGF_{1\alpha}$, or 20:4. Application of 280 nmol of indomethacin 5 hr before each application of TPA inhibited the formation of skin papillomas by 65% at 14 weeks following initiation by dimethylbenzanthracene (DMBA). These studies suggest that prostaglandins E_1, E_2, D_2, and I_2 play a role in induction of ODC activity by TPA, and that this may be an important component of the mechanism of skin tumor promotion.

In contrast to these results (obtained with female CD-1 mice), Fischer et al. (1980) have reported that indomethacin stimulates TPA-dependent promotion in female Sencar mice. The authors suggest that this may be due to the fact that indomethacin, by inhibiting PGH synthase, stimulates the flux of 20:4 through the lipoxygenase pathway, which produces hydroperoxy fatty acids. If hydroperoxy fatty acids also play a role in promotion, the stimulation of their formation by indomethacin might actually enhance tumorigenesis as is observed. Consistent with this, eicosatetraynoic acid, which inhibits both PGH synthase and lipoxygenase, inhibits tumor promotion in Sencar mice (Fischer et al., 1980). Nordihydroguaiaretic acid, a lipoxygenase inhibitor, is an effective inhibitor of TPA promotion in CD-1 mice (Nakadate et al., 1982). Curiously, arachidonic acid, but not linoleic acid, also inhibits promotion (Slaga et al., 1982).

All the studies in mouse skin suggest that arachidonate metabolites play a role in tumor production but are not themselves tumor promoters. Their role(s) in this multistep process is important, because it is possible to alter the tumor response significantly by administration of inhibitors of arachidonate release and oxygenation. These effects are not restricted to skin. Pollard and Luckert (1981a,b) have shown that indomethacin has profound inhibitory effects on tumorigenesis by dimethylhydrazine, methylazoxymethanol acetate, and dimethylnitrosamine acetate in the intestine. Administration of indomethacin (20 mg/liter) in the drinking water to Sprague–Dawley rats 7, 14, or 35 days after treatment with the carcinogens significantly reduces the number of animals with tumor and the number of tumors per animal induced at 20 weeks. Since methylazoxymethanol acetate and dimethylnitrosamine acetate are activated derivatives that do not require oxidative activation, and since all three compounds were completely cleared from rats prior to indomethacin treatment, the effects of indomethacin do not appear to be due to inhibition of tumor initiation. Rather, indomethacin appears to serve as an inhibitor of promotion. This implies that a metabolite of the cyclooxygenase pathway plays a major role in the promotional phase of chemically induced intestinal cancer. These observations may be related to the finding that indomethacin inhibits the development of tumors from microscopic lesions in the colon of Donryu rats and to several reports that indomethacin retards the growth of transplanted tumors (Kudo *et al.*, 1980 and references therein).

Diets containing high levels of polyunsaturated fats enhance the susceptibility of female rats to mammary carcinogenesis by chemicals (Carroll and Khor, 1975). The enhancing effect is believed to result from an effect of fat on the promotional phase of carcinogenesis. Carter *et al.* (1983) have reported that indomethacin administration to female Sprague–Dawley rats, previously initiated with DMBA, completely inhibits the stimulation of tumor promotion by high-fat diets (18% corn oil). No effect of indomethacin on the serum levels of corticosterone was detected in the high-fat-fed animals. Indomethacin did not decrease the size or number of mammary tumors in animals fed a normal fat diet (5% corn oil). These results suggest that a major part of the stimulatory effect of high-fat diets on mammary tumorigenesis by DMBA is mediated by prostaglandins and that PGH synthase inhibitors may be useful prophylactic agents against mammary carcinogenesis. Similar results have been reported by Kollmorgen *et al.* (1983).

High-fat diets also stimulate the growth of transplantable tumors (Hillyard and Abraham, 1979). Kollmorgen *et al.* (1984) have shown that the growth of a DMBA-induced mammary tumor transplanted into Wistar–Furth rats is enhanced by diets containing 10 or 20% stripped corn oil relative to diets containing either 2 or 5% corn oil. The tumor growth-promoting effects of 10 and 20% fat diets were completely inhibited in rats administered indomethacin orally (20 mg/liter). Treatment of the animals with indomethacin also inhibited tumor growth in rats fed diets containing 2 or 5% fat. It was proposed that the inhibitory effect of indomethacin was due to enhancement of the immune system.

IV. OVERVIEW OF THE METASTATIC CASCADE

A metastatic lesion represents the result of a series of sequential events in which neoplastic cells are released from a primary tumor and disseminated to secondary sites. This process has been termed the "metastatic cascade." It is an inefficient process, since only a small population of cells that detach from the primary tumor possess the necessary phenotypic characteristics to ensure their eventual survival (Fidler, 1978; Warren, 1981).

As discussed by Salsbury (1975), the mere presence of viable circulating tumor cells is not indicative of a poor prognosis. Therefore, successful arrest and/or adhesion and the factors (e.g., platelets, endothelial cell surface determinants, tumor cell surface determinants) that activate and/or enhance this process must be regarded as the most important events in hematogenous metastasis. Carcinomas were once believed to metastasize via the lymphatics, whereas malignant tumors of mesenchymal origin were believed to spread via the hematogenous route. This separation between the two systems of dissemination is probably an oversimplification. Hilgard *et al.* (1972) have noted that tumor cells initially injected into the lymphatics will reach the vascular system. Similar conclusions have been reached by others (Fisher and Fisher, 1967; del Regato, 1977), and there is now substantial evidence that malignant cells can pass freely between the lymphatics and blood vessels (Weiss, 1977; Fidler 1978). Although the presence of tumor cells in the circulatory system does not necessarily indicate a poor prognosis (Salsbury, 1975), it must be concluded that the use of the hematogenous route for the spread of malignant cells is an event that does occur at some point in the disease.

Once tumor cells have entered the circulatory system, factors that influence their arrest, attachment to endothelium or deendothelialized surfaces, and eventual extravasation assume paramount importance. Several factors have been found to influence the arrest and/or attachment of tumor cells, and investigators have correlated tumor cell surface properties with the malignant phenotype (Raz *et al.*, 1980; Irimura and Nicolson, 1981; Irimura *et al.*, 1981). Nicolson and co-workers (Irimura and Nicolson, 1981; Irimura *et al.*, 1981) have described a role for tumor cell surface sialogalactoproteins in their binding to endothelial cell monolayers, the endothelial extracellular matrix, and immobilized fibronectin. Others have also found a relationship between sialoglycoproteins and metastatic potential (Raz *et al.*, 1980; Vilarem *et al.*, 1981). Karpatkin and co-workers have demonstrated a correlation between tumor cell sialic acid content, induction of platelet aggregation, and spontaneous metastasis in derivatives of the polyoma-induced PW20 Wistar–Furth rat renal sarcoma line (Pearlstein *et al.*, 1980).

Malignant cells adhere to vascular endothelium and stimulate endothelial cell retraction and exposure of the underlying basal laminalike matrix, whereupon tumor cells migrate to the subendothelial matrix surface (Kramer and Nicolson, 1979, 1981; Kramer *et al.*, 1980; Zamora *et al.*, 1980). This net movement of metastatic cells to the subendothelial lamina may occur because of an adhesive gradient that occurs between the endothelial cell surface and the matrix (Kramer *et al.*, 1980; Nicolson *et al.*, 1981). Nicolson and co-workers demonstrated using the $B_{16}F_1$ and $B_{16}F_{10}$ metastatic variants that tumor cells attached slowly to endothelial cell monolayers while they attached rapidly to the isolated extracellular matrix (Kramer and Nicolson, 1981; Kramer *et al.*, 1980), suggesting that damaged or deendothelialized surfaces offer preferential attachment sites for circulating tumor cells.

The mechanism of tumor cell attachment is a matter of debate. Nicolson's group has suggested that fibronectin may mediate tumor cell attachment to the extracellular matrix (Kramer *et al.*, 1980). Nevertheless, Liotta and co-workers (Terranova *et al.*, 1982) demonstrated that metastatic tumor cells preferentially attach to type IV collagen and that this attachment was enhanced by laminin and blocked by antilaminin antibody. In addition to these specific factors, platelets and/or platelet-derived products enhance the attachment of tumor cells to cultured endothelial cells (K. V. Honn, unpublished observation) and isolated vessels in a Baumgartner perfusion apparatus (Marcum *et al.*, 1980).

Hemostatic Mechanisms and Metastasis

Patients with malignant neoplasms often demonstrate abnormalities in their blood coagulability (Goodnight, 1974; Zacharski *et al.*, 1979; Donati and Poggi, 1980; Edwards *et al.*, 1981; Rickles and Edwards, 1983). These abnormalities include thrombocytopenia (Brain *et al.*, 1970), a reduction in fibrinogen, and an increase in fibrin–fibrinogen degradation products (Rickles and Edwards, 1981). Tumor cells have been reported to possess both a platelet-activating material (Pearlstein *et al.*, 1979, 1980; Karpatkin *et al.*, 1980; Gasic *et al.*, 1978) and a procoagulant activity responsible for alterations in the fibrin–fibrinogen system (Curatolo *et al.*, 1979; Gordon *et al.*, 1975; Gordon and Cross, 1981). These hemostatic alterations have been linked to tumor cell metastasis (for review, see Karpatkin and Pearlstein, 1981). In addition, many tumor cells have been reported to shed membrane vesicles spontaneously (Black, 1980; Liepins and Hillman, 1981; Liepins and de Harven, 1982). These membrane vesicles have been correlated with metastatic potential in the $B_{16}F_1$, $B_{16}F_{10}$ system (Poste and Nicolson, 1980) and contain platelet-aggregatory (Gasic *et al.*, 1978; Cavanaugh *et al.*, 1983) and procoagulant activities (Dvorak *et al.*, 1981).

Gasic and co-workers (Gasic *et al.*, 1968) were the first to provide direct experimental evidence for a role of platelets in tumor cell metastasis. They had noted that pretreatment of mice with neuraminidase resulted in formation of fewer lung colonies following injection of TA3 ascites tumor cells. These results were found to be attributable to induction of thrombocytopenia in the host by neuraminidase (Gasic *et al.*, 1968). Similar antimetastatic effects were observed when thrombocytopenia was induced with antiplatelet antiserum. Additional evidence was provided by the fact that the antimetastatic effects of neuraminidase could be reversed by platelet infusion (Gasic *et al.*, 1968).

In a series of follow-up papers, Gasic and co-workers (Gasic *et al.*, 1973, 1976, 1978) demonstrated that numerous human and animal tumor cells and plasma membrane vesicles shed from tumor cells were capable of aggregating platelets *in vitro* with a concomitant stimulation of the release reaction (measured as [^{14}C]serotonin released from prelabeled platelets). Several other laboratories have confirmed the *in vitro* aggregation of platelets by both animal and human tumor cells and the induction of thrombocytopenia following i.v. injection of some tumor lines (Hilgard, 1973; Gastpar *et al.*, 1977; Paschen *et al.*, 1979; Hara *et al.*, 1980; Pearlstein *et al.*, 1980, 1981; Skolnik *et al.*, 1980; Bastida *et al.*, 1981; a review of the area can be found in Jamieson, 1982). However, most of these studies only provide circumstantial evidence that host platelets facilitate hematogenous metastasis.

Work from Karpatkin, Pearlstein, and co-workers (Pearlstein *et al.*, 1980) provides more direct evidence that a causal relationship exists. Using 10 cell lines derived from the polyoma virus-induced PW20 Wistar–Furth rat renal sarcoma, they examined the correlation between the ability of the tumor cells to metastasize spontaneously from subcutaneous sites in syngeneic hosts and their platelet-aggregating activity *in vitro*. A significant correlation between platelet aggregability and spontaneous metastasis was observed.

Despite the foregoing findings, the mechanism by which platelets enhance metastasis remains to be definitely established. Several suggestions appear in the literature and include protection against destruction by host cytotoxic macrophages and increased ability of tumor–platelet emboli to arrest in the microvasculature. The relevance to platelet enhancement of tumor cell metastasis of each of the mechanisms just suggested remains to be established. However, it is generally accepted that platelets enhance metastasis by facilitating processes that occur during tumor cell arrest and/or adhesion.

For the reasons just advanced, antiplatelet and/or anticoagulant therapy with agents such as heparin (Elias *et al.*, 1973), warfarin (Lione and Bosmann, 1978), and dipyridamole (Gastpar, 1977) have been attempted to reduce tumor metastasis. These results have been inconsistent to date, with the exception of warfarin (Maat and Hilgard, 1981).

V. PROSTACYCLIN, THROMBOXANES, AND TUMOR CELL METASTASIS

Compounds derived from arachidonic acid (PGI$_2$ and TXA$_2$; Fig. 1) have been demonstrated to have a profound but possibly not exclusive (Vargaftif *et al.*, 1981) role in platelet aggregation and normal hemostasis. In 1975, Hamberg *et al.* demonstrated the formation of TXA$_2$ from the endoperoxide intermediate PGH$_2$ (Fig. 1). Subsequently, platelet TXA$_2$ biosynthesis was found to be stimulated by numerous aggregating agents and was believed to be an absolute requirement for platelet aggregation (Gorman, 1979).

One year following the discovery of TXA$_2$, Vane and co-workers (Moncada *et al.*, 1976b) discovered PGI$_2$ as a transformation product of prostaglandin endoperoxides. Prostacyclin is produced by vascular tissue of all species so far tested

(Moncada and Vane, 1980) and is the main product of arachidonic acid metabolism in isolated vascular tissue. Prostacyclin is the most potent endogenous inhibitor of platelet aggregation yet discovered, being 30 to 40 times more potent than PGE_1 (Moncada and Vane, 1977) and 1000 times more potent than adenosine (Mullane *et al.*, 1979). In addition, PGI_2 can reverse secondary platelet aggregation *in vitro* (Moncada and Vane, 1980) and in the circulatory system of humans (Szczeklik *et al.*, 1978). It has been suggested that PGI_2 and TXA_2 play an antagonistic and pivotal role in the control of thrombosis centered on their bidirectional (PGI_2 increases, TXA_2 decreases) effect on platelet cAMP levels.

Honn *et al.* (1981) first proposed the hypothesis that the normal intravascular balance between PGI_2 and platelet arachidonic acid metabolites (i.e., TXA_2) could be altered by the presence of a primary tumor and/or circulating tumor cells and their membrane-shed vesicles. This hypothesis predicts that arachidonic acid metabolism by the tumor cell, platelet, and vessel wall is a fundamental determinant in the sum total of their interactions, and that PGI_2 may be a natural deterrent to metastasis. This hypothesis also predicts that agents affecting arachidonic acid metabolism by the platelet (decreased TXA_2) and/or vessel wall (increased PGI_2) would alter tumor cell metastasis.

A. Prostacyclin Effects *in Vivo* and *in Vitro*

Prostacyclin Effects on Tumor Cell-Induced Platelet Aggregation

In vitro, the addition of elutriated (Sloane *et al.*, 1981) tumor cells to human platelet-rich plasma (PRP) resulted in irreversible platelet aggregation after a short lag period of 0.5 to 1 min (Fig. 2). This aggregation was inhibited by PGI_2 in a dose-dependent manner with maximal inhibition observed at a PGI_2 dose of 10 ng/ml (Fig. 2). Tumor cell-induced platelet aggregation (TCIPA) may occur via three distinct mechanisms dependent on tumor type (Pearlstein *et al.*, 1981; Bastida *et al.*, 1982).

Therefore, PGI_2 was tested against a variety of tumor types. Complete inhibition of TCIPA with PGI_2 (10 ng/ml) was observed in the B_{16} amelanotic melanoma (Honn *et al.*, 1983c), 15091A mammary adenocarcinoma, and Lewis lung (3LL) carcinoma (Honn and Sloane, 1983, 1984; Menter *et al.*, 1984). In addition, platelet aggregation in response to shed plasma membrane vesicles spontaneously from 15091A cells (Gasic *et al.*, 1981) was also inhibited by 10 ng/ml PGI_2 (Cavanaugh *et al.*, 1983). PGI_2 was the most potent of the prostaglandins with respect to inhibition of TCIPA. Two additional prostaglandins (PGE_1 and PGD_2) known to inhibit platelet aggregation (Vane *et al.*, 1982) were 100 times less potent than PGI_2 in inhibiting Walker carcinosarcoma (W256)-induced platelet aggregation (Honn and Sloane, 1984). The stable metabolite of

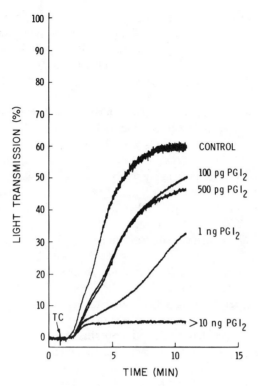

Fig. 2. Effect of PGI$_2$ on *in vitro* TCIPA (Walker 256 carcinosarcoma).

PGI$_2$, 6-keto-PGF$_{1\alpha}$, was only effective at supraphysiological doses (Honn and Sloane, 1984). In contrast, PGE$_2$ blocked the inhibitory effects of PGI$_2$ on TCIPA (Menter *et al.*, 1984).

B. Prostacyclin Effects on Platelet-Induced Tumor Cell Adhesion *in Vitro*

Fantone *et al.* (1982) have demonstrated that the adherence of Walker carcinosarcoma cells to plastic plates or nylon fibers can be stimulated by the tumor promoter phorbol myristate acetate and the chemotactic peptide fMet-Leu-Phe. Prostacyclin directly inhibited this increased adhesion; however, PGI$_2$ had no effect on basal (unstimulated) W256 cell adhesion (Fantone *et al.* 1982). Hara *et al.* (1980) reported that tumor cells will not aggregate washed platelets. However, the addition of a small amount (2% v/v) of platelet-poor plasma (PPP) restores a full aggregation response, suggesting an absolute requirement for a plasma factor during TCIPA (Hara *et al.*, 1980; Menter *et al.*, 1984). We have previously demonstrated that platelet–tumor cell adhesion can occur in the absence of overt platelet aggregation, and that this interaction results in alterations of the tumor cell surface topology (Honn et al., 1984). We therefore explored the possibility that platelets could enhance the adhesion of W256 cells under nonaggregatory (no PPP) and aggregatory (5% PPP v/v) conditions.

The adhesion of W256 cells to plastic plates was increased in the presence of washed rat platelets (Honn et al., 1984). This increase was variable with platelet preparation but ranged between 100 and 400%. An even larger increase (300–1400%) was observed if tumor cells were allowed to aggregate (addition of 5% PPP) with platelets. The addition of PGI_2 (30 μg/ml) completely prevented the increased adhesion under both aggregatory and nonaggregatory conditions. The PGI_2 effect was dose dependent both in the presence and absence of PPP, with a 40% decrease observed at 1 μg PGI_2/ml. Prostacyclin had no effect on basal (unstimulated) W256 cell attachment.

Rat platelets also enhanced the attachment of W256 cells to cultured rat endothelial cells, a response that can be blocked with PGI_2 (K. V. Honn, unpublished observation). These in vitro results suggest that platelets may increase tumor cell adhesion to endothelium in vivo and that PGI_2 may limit the formation of a stable tumor cell–endothelial cell interaction. Support for this concept can be derived from the experiments of Marcum et al. (1980), who utilized rabbit aortic segments in a standard Baumgartner perfusion chamber to study tumor cell (HUT 20)–platelet–endothelial cell and subendothelial interactions. Tumor cells and platelets were perfused in the presence of PGE_1 (30 μg/ml) or PGI_2 (50 ng/ml). Both agents totally inhibited TCIPA and the deposition of both tumor cells and platelets on the vascular surface.

C. Prostacyclin Effects on Metastasis in Vivo

We have previously reported that bolus iv injection of PGI_2 into mice reduced lung colony formation from tail vein-injected B_{16a} cells by $> 70\%$ and in combination with a phosphodiesterase inhibitor (theophylline) by $>93\%$ (Honn et al., 1981). Prostaglandins E_2, $F_{2\alpha}$, and the stable hydrolysis product of PGI_2, 6-keto-$PGF_{1\alpha}$, were ineffective (Honn et al., 1981). Prostaglandin D_2 is also antimetastatic, as reported by Stringfellow and Fitzpatrick (1979); however, we found PGD_2 to be less than one-third as effective as PGI_2 (Honn et al., 1981). These results correlate well with the effects of these various icosanoids on TCIPA (Honn et al., 1983a,b,c; Honn and Sloane, 1984; Menter et al., 1984).

Willmott et al. (1983) reported that the pretreatment of animals with the antiplatelet drug RA233 prior to tail vein injection of S-180 sarcoma cells resulted in enhanced extrapulmonary tumors. We demonstrated that PGI_2 does not significantly alter tumor cell distribution patterns using [^{125}I]deoxyuridine-labeled tumor cells. We found (Honn, 1983) that although some alteration of cell distribution may occur, these cells once released from the lung are not retained in the organ of secondary arrest (liver, spleen, etc.). In addition, there was no effect of PGI_2 on the initial entrapment of tumor cells in the lung following iv injection (Honn, 1983), which might be expected if the PGI_2 effect were due to vasodilation.

D. Prostacyclin as an Endogenous Deterrent to Metastasis

The foregoing results with exogenous PGI_2 demonstrate its efficacy as an antimetastatic agent. We have also proposed that the production of PGI_2 by the vascular endothelium is a natural deterrent to metastasis (Honn *et al.*, 1981). To test this hypothesis we perfused mice with a lipoxygenase product of arachidonic acid, 15-hydroperoxyeicosatetraenoic acid (15-HPETE), prior to tail vein injection of B_{16a} tumor cells. Hydroperoxy fatty acids in general are ($K_i \sim 10^{-7} M$) potent inhibitors of prostacyclin synthase (Salmon *et al.*, 1978). Little structural specificity is evident in the inhibition, since a number of isomeric hydroperoxides are equally effective (Salmon *et al.*, 1978). If mice were pretreated (approximately 20 min) with 15-HPETE (100–200 µg/animal) prior to tail vein injection of B_{16a} cells, 300–500% more pulmonary metastatic lesions were observed 26 days later (Fig. 3). Increased macroscopic tumors were also found in the liver and spleen of 15-HPETE-treated animals (Fig. 3). Infusion of 15-HPETE followed by PGI_2 plus theophylline significantly reduced the number of metastases compared to 15-HPETE infusion alone (Fig. 3).

Mehta and co-workers have provided clinical evidence that supports the concept that PGI_2 metabolism is affected in tumor-bearing patients. In a series of representative patients with malignant bone tumors, plasma concentrations of TXB_2 were within the range of age-matched controls; however, 6-keto-$PGF_{1\alpha}$ levels were markedly reduced (Mehta *et al.*, 1984). In addition, authentic PGI_2 incubated in plasma from patients with bone tumors demonstrated a significantly decreased biological $t_{1/2}$ compared to normal human plasma (Mehta, 1984). Mehta *et al.* (1983) reported that arterial PGI_2 production is decreased in patients with malignant bone tumors. Vessels removed from patients undergoing therapeutic resection of their tumor were incubated *in vitro* in the presence and absence of arachidonic acid. When *in vitro* basal or stimulated PGI_2 production (radioimmunoassay of 6-keto-$PGF_{1\alpha}$) was compared to vessels removed from non-tumor-bearing patients, a significant decrease was observed. Collectively these experimental and clinical results suggest that endogenous PGI_2 production may function as a natural deterrent to metastasis possibly by limiting tumor cell–platelet–vessel wall interactions. The clinical results also suggest that the "PGI_2–TXA_2 balance" is disrupted in patients with malignant disease.

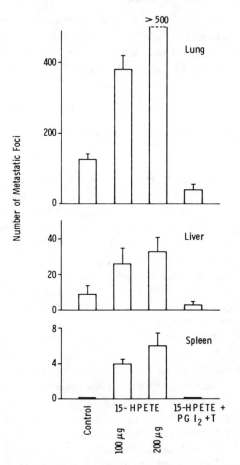

Fig. 3. Increased lung colony formation by B_{16a} cells due to prior administration of the PGI_2 synthase inhibitor, 15-HPETE. Exogenous PGI_2 reverses this effect. T, theophylline.

E. Effects of Agents That Stimulate or Synergize with Endogenous Prostacyclin Production

The use of PGI_2 as a clinical therapeutic entity is still in its infancy (Moncada, 1982), although several studies report therapeutic efficacy with PGI_2 infusion for advanced atherosclerotic lower limb peripheral vascular disease (Szczeklik *et al.*, 1979), peripheral artery disease (Szczeklik and Gryglewski, 1981), idiopathic pulmonary artery hypertension (Watkins *et al.*, 1980), coronary artery disease (Bergman *et al.*, 1981), and unstable angina (Hall and Dewar, 1981). Nevertheless, PGI_2 infusion is clinically impractical for use as an antimetastatic agent. We had originally proposed that long-lived analogs of PGI_2 could be used as antimetastatic agents (Honn *et al.*, 1981). Numerous analogs have been developed (Aristoff and Harrison, 1982; Hall and Dewar, 1981; Morton and Brokow, 1979; Nishiyama and Ohno, 1979; Pike and Bundy, 1982; Whittle *et al.*, 1980). Although some of these analogs have interesting and promising biological effects (Whittle *et al.*, 1980), none is more potent than native PGI_2, and the most effective of these must be administered by vascular infusion. We therefore propose that agents stimulating endogenous PGI_2 production and/or inhibiting its metabolism may be clinically useful as antimetastatic agents.

1. Agents That Alter PGI_2 Metabolism

One such compound, which may represent the prototype of a new class of pharmacologically active agents, is nafazatrom [Bay g 6575; 2,4-dihydro-5-methyl-2[-2-(2-naphthyloxy)ethyl]-3*H*-pyrazol-3-one]. Seuter *et al.* (1979) first reported significant antithrombotic activity of nafazatrom in several rat and rabbit models of experimental thrombosis. These authors reported that nafazatrom was devoid of direct effects on platelet thromboxane production, aggregation *in vitro* and *ex vivo*, and ADP- and collagen-induced platelet aggregation. Buchanan *et al.* (1982) have reinvestigated the antithrombotic effects of nafazatrom and reported no effects on venous thrombosis yet inhibition of arterial thrombosis. Differences in the model systems used for venous thrombosis could account for this discrepancy. In addition, Buchanan *et al.* (1982) reported that nafazatrom inhibited ADP-induced platelet aggregation *in vivo* and prolonged platelet survival time.

The mechanism(s) responsible for the antithrombotic effects of nafazatrom is a matter of current debate, which centers on nafazatrom's ability to stimulate vascular wall PGI_2 production or prolong its biological half-life. Vermylen *et al.* (1979) first presented evidence for increased PGI_2 production. Plasma obtained from human volunteers after ingestion of a single dose (1.2 g) of nafazatrom stimulated PGI_2 release from slices of rat aorta. Others also have reported increased PGI_2 production (Carreras *et al.*, 1980; Chamone *et al.*, 1981). Nafazatrom has now been reported to stimulate PGI_2 biosynthesis from arachidonic acid by ram seminal vesicle microsomes (Eling *et al.*, 1982; Marnett *et al.*, 1984), cultured endothelial cells, and B_{16a} cells (K. V. Honn, L. J. Marnett, and T. E. Eling, unpublished observation).

Three biochemical mechanisms have been proposed to explain the PGI_2-stimulating effects of nafazatrom. First, nafazatrom has been found to inhibit the cytosolic lipoxygenase (generation of HPETE) of B_{16a} cells (Honn and Dunn, 1982) as well as that of human and rabbit neutrophils (Busse *et al.*, 1982). Since vascular endothelial cells have been found to produce 12-HPETE by lipoxygenation of arachidonic acid (Herman *et al.*, 1979), and hydroperoxy fatty acid has been proposed as an endogenous regulator of PGI_2 biosynthesis, nafazatrom may interfere with PGI_2 synthase inhibition. Second, nafazatrom may act as a reducing cofactor for the hydroperoxidase activity of prostaglandin endoperoxide synthase (Eling *et al.*, 1982; Marnett *et al.*, 1984). Third, nafazatrom has been reported to inhibit the enzymatic degradation of PGI_2 to 15-keto-PGI_2 by 15-hydroxyprostaglandin dehydrogenase (Wong *et al.*, 1982). This is the major route of PGI_2 catabolism in the cat (Machleidt *et al.*, 1981) and human (Rosenkranz *et al.*, 1980). Any or all of these mechanisms would result in increased endogenous PGI_2 levels.

Nafazatrom has been evaluated for its antimetastatic activity against tail-vein-injected elutriated B_{16a} and 3LL tumor cells and found to inhibit lung colony formation by >70% (Honn and Sloane, 1984; Honn *et al.*, 1982, 1983b). In addition, this compound significantly reduces spontaneous pulmonary metastasis from subcutaneous B_{16a} and 3LL tumors (Honn *et al.*, 1982). Ambrus *et al.* (1982) have also reported antimetastatic activity of nafazatrom in three of four tumor lines tested. Collectively, these results point to significant antimetastatic properties of this PGI_2-enhancing agent.

2. Thromboxane Synthase Inhibitors

Thromboxane synthase inhibitors cause decreased platelet adhesion to injured vascular wall (Hall *et al.*, 1982) and increased platelet sensitivity to PGI_2 inhibition (Bertele *et al.*, 1982), presumably because the lower the platelet TXA_2 biosynthetic capability the lower the dose of PGI_2 required for inhibition of aggregation (Aiken *et al.*, 1981). In addition, TX synthase inhibitors have been reported to reorient platelet endoperoxide (PGH_2) metabolism toward PGI_2 biosynthesis by the vessel wall (Defreyn *et al.*, 1982). This hypothesis, originally termed the "steal hypothesis," was first proposed by Gryglewski *et al.* (1976). The hypothesis states that under conditions in which aggregating platelets are juxtaposed to the endothelium (in a narrow vessel lumen), platelet PGH_2 may be utilized by vessel wall PGI_2 synthase to augment basal PGI_2 production (Fig. 4). These results are consistent with the work of Needleman *et al.* (1979), which suggested that normally the "steal" of precursor by the vessel wall may not be an important pathway for PGI_2 biosynthesis. However, under conditions of a strong stimulus for platelet aggregation (i.e., circulating tumor cells), the selective blockade of TXA_2 synthase could drive platelet PGH_2 metabolism into PGI_2 biosynthesis by the vessel wall (Fig. 4). *In vivo* evidence for the "steal hypothesis" has been provided by the experiments of Aiken *et al.* (1981).

We had initially proposed that, in addition to PGI_2, TXA_2 synthase inhibitors would also function as antimetastatic agents (Honn *et al.*, 1982). This prediction was based on the working hypothesis that circulating tumor cells disrupt the intravascular balance between PGI_2 and TXA_2. We initially investigated a series of endoperoxide analogs that were thromboxane synthase inhibitors (Menter *et al.*, 1982; Honn *et al.*, i983b). One endoperoxide analog, TX synthase inhibitor U54701 (9,11-iminoepoxyprosta-5,13-dienoic acid; Fitzpatrick *et al.*, 1979),

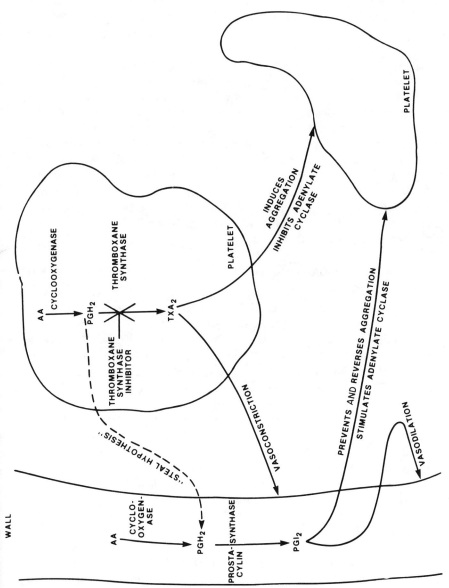

Fig. 4. The "steal hypothesis." See text for details. (Reproduced with permission of R. R. Gorman, Upjohn Co.)

completely inhibited TXA_2 production by human platelets in response to elutriated Lewis lung carcinoma cells concomitant with an inhibition of platelet aggregation (Honn et al., 1983b). However, W256 TCIPA was only inhibited 25% by a comparable dose of U54701, even though TXA_2 biosynthesis was almost completely inhibited (Honn et al., 1983b). Furthermore, TX synthase inhibitors that are imidazole derivatives [i.e., 1-(7-carboxyheptyl)imidazole] did not inhibit in vitro TCIPA even in the presence of inhibited platelet TXA_2 production. These aberrant results suggest that tumor cells can initiate platelet aggregation by a mechanism independent of TXA_2 biosynthesis (see discussion by Honn et al., 1983a). Nevertheless, both endoperoxide analogs and imidazole derivatives possess antimetastatic activity in vivo (Honn, 1983 and unpublished observations).

We propose that the discrepancy between lack of consistent inhibition of TCIPA by TX synthase inhibitors in vitro and their antimetastatic activity in vivo is due to the operation of the "steal hypothesis" in vivo. In vitro TCIPA may proceed by pathways independent of TXA_2 biosynthesis. Thus, the antimetastatic activity of TX synthase inhibitors in vivo may ultimately be due to augmented endogenous PGI_2 biosynthesis.

3. Calcium Channel Blocker Compounds

A number of vascular and myocardial disorders can be alleviated by inducing vasodilation with calcium channel blockers (CCB). Among them are vasospastic angina, acute myocradial infarction, arrhythmias, and pulmonary hypertension. For reviews, see Braunwald (1982), Henry (1982), Godfraind (1981), Pedersen (1981), and Flaim and Zelis (1981). In addition, CCB have been found to inhibit platelet aggregation (Ribeiro et al., 1980; Addonizio et al., 1980; Schmunk and Lefer, 1982). Therefore, we evaluated the effects of two CCB of the dihydropyridine class (nifedipine—Bay a 1040; and nimodipine—Bay e 9736) on TCIPA and spontaneous pulmonary metastasis of B_{16a}. Both compounds effected a dose-dependent inhibition of B_{16a} TCIPA over a dose range of 4 to 400 μg/ml (Honn et al., 1983d and unpublished observations). In addition, the platelet-stimulated adhesion of ^{125}I-Udr-labeled W256 cells to cultured rat endothelial cells was inhibited 60% with 40 μg/ml nimodipine (K. V. Honn and J. M. Onoda, unpublished observation). In vivo, the daily administration of nifedipine or nimodipine (80 mg/kg) to C57BL/6J mice bearing subcutaneous B_{16a} tumors inhibited spontenaous pulmonary metastasis >60% (nifedipine) and >80% (nimodipine) (K. V. Honn and J. M. Onoda, unpublished observation). We examined the possibility of a synergism between CCB and PGI_2 in inhibition of TCIPA in vitro. PGI_2 at a dose of 100 fg/ml does not significantly affect TCIPA induced by B_{16a} cells (Fig. 5). Similarly, nimodipine (1.5 μg/ml) only produces a 15% inhibition of TCIPA (Fig. 5). However, the combination of PGI_2 (100 fg/ml) plus nimodipine (1.5 μg/ml) results in a >50% inhibition of B_{16a}

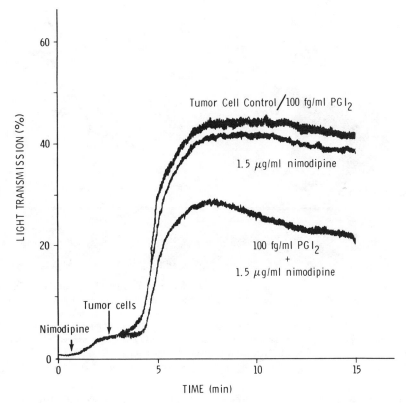

Fig. 5. Synergism between PGI_2 and the calcium channel blocker nimodipine on inhibition of platelet aggregation induced by B_{16a} cells.

TCIPA (Fig. 5). Although preliminary, these *in vitro* results suggest a possible synergism between CCB and PGI_2 for inhibition of tumor cell metastasis *in vivo*.

It is intuitive that for hematogenous metastasis to occur the tumor cell must arrest in the microvasculature and attach to the vessel wall prior to extravasation and growth into a metastatic focus. Indirect evidence supports the concept that tumor cells interact with platelets during this process as discussed earlier. The evidence just given suggests that the metabolism of arachidonic acid in the tumor cell, the platelet, and the vessel wall plays an essential role in the sum total of these interactions (Fig. 6).

Exogenous PGI_2 may function as an antimetastatic agent by inhibiting the association of the tumor cell with the vessel wall (Fig. 6). The interactions between the vessel wall and tumor cells or platelets may be inhibited by stimulation of platelet cAMP or tumor cell cAMP by exogenous PGI_2. Similarly, vessel

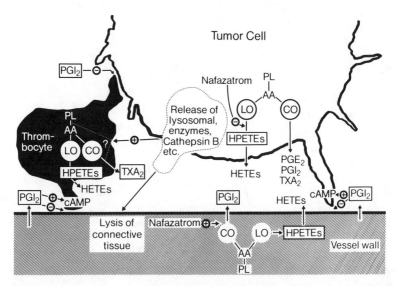

Fig. 6. Interactions among tumor cells, platelets (thrombocytes), and blood vessel wall. Direct interactions are possible between the platelet and the vessel wall, the tumor cell and vessel wall, and the platelet(s) and tumor cell(s). Any one or all of these interactions may enhance tumor cell arrest and metastasis. Prostacyclin may prevent attachment of tumor cell(s) to platelet(s) or to vessel wall. Pl, phospholipids; AA, arachidonic acid; CO, cyclooxygenase; LO, lipoxygenase; HPETEs, hydroperoxyeicosatetraenoic acids; HETEs, hydroxyeicosatetraenoic acids; PGI_2, prostacyclin; TXA_2, thromboxane A_2. (Reproduced from Honn *et al.*, 1983a, with permission of Pergamon Press.)

wall PGI_2 may serve as a natural deterrent to metastasis by inhibiting these interactions. A new class of antimetastatic agents are compounds that have the ability to stimulate endogenous PGI_2 production and/or prolong the half-life of PGI_2 (e.g., nafazatrom). A new proposal for the antimetastatic activity of TX synthase inhibitors ("steal hypothesis") may also center around enhanced endogenous PGI_2 production. Finally, a heretofore unsuspected class of pharmacological agents (CCB) are reported by us to have potent antimetastatic activity that may result in part from a synergism with PGI_2.

VI. CONCLUSION

This chapter demonstrates an involvement of arachidonic acid metabolites in various aspects of malignancy from transformation to metastasis. Modification of arachidonic acid metabolism has been demonstrated to alter tumor initiation, growth, and metastasis. The most spectacular results have been obtained with highly selective pharmacological manipulation. This is not surprising, since many products of arachidonic acid metabolism have been demonstrated to have opposing physiological effects (e.g., PGE_2 vs $PGF_{2\alpha}$ and PGI_2 vs TXA_2). This built-in reciprocal control suggests that all-or-none inhibitors (e.g., aspirin, ETYA) may be of little use or may even produce detrimental results. Alternatively, select manipulation of this complex pathway appears to hold more promise for the clinical chemotherapeutic therapy of cancer.

Acknowledgments

This investigation was supported by Grants CA-29405, CA-29997, GM-23642, and CA-22206 awarded by the National Institutes of Health, Department of Health and Human Services, and by American Cancer Society Grants BC-356 and BC-244, Miles Institute for Preclinical Pharmacology, and Bayer AG. Lawrence J. Marnett is a recipient of a Faculty Research Award, FRA-243, from the American Cancer Society.

REFERENCES

Addonizio, V. P., Fisher, C. A., and Edmunds, L. H. (1980). Effects of verapamil and nifedipine on platelet activation. *Circulation* **62,** 326 (Abstr.)

Aiken, J. W. (1983). Pharmacology of thromboxane synthetase inhibitors. *In* "Advances in Prostaglandin, Thromboxane, Leukotriene Research" (B. Samuelsson, R. Paoletti, and P. Ramwell, eds.), Vol. 11, pp. 253–258. Raven, New York.

Aiken, J. W., Shebuski, R. J., Miller, O. V., and Gorman, R. R. (1981). Endogenous prostacyclin contributes to the efficacy of a thromboxane synthetase inhibitor for preventing coronary artery thrombosis. *J. Pharmacol. Exp. Ther.* **219,** 299–308.

Ambrus, J. L., Ambrus, C. M., Gastpar, H., and Williams, P. (1982). Study of platelet aggregation *in vivo.* IX. Effects of nafazatrom on *in vivo* platelet aggregation and spontaneous tumor metastasis. *J. Med.* **13,** 35–47.

Amstad, P., and Cerutti, P. (1983). DNA binding of aflatoxin B_1 by co-oxygenation in mouse embryo fibroblasts C3H/10T½. *Biochem. Biophys. Res. Commun.* **112,** 1034–1040.

Aristoff, P. A., and Harrison, A. W. (1982). Synthesis of benzindene prostaglandins: A novel potent class of stable prostacyclin analogs. *Tetrahedon Lett.* **23,** 2067–2070.

Ashendel, C. L., and Boutwell, R. K. (1979). Prostaglandin E and F levels in mouse epidermis are increased by tumor-promoting phorbol esters. *Biochem. Biophys. Res. Commun.* **90,** 623–627.

Baird, W. M., and Boutwell, R. K. (1971). Tumor promoting activity of phorbol and four diesters of phorbol in mouse skin. *Cancer Res.* **31,** 1074–1079.

Bastida, E., Ordinas, A., and Jamieson, G. A. (1981). Idiosyncratic platelet responses to human tumor cells. *Nature (London)* **291,** 661–662.

Bastida, E., Ordinas, A., Giardina, S. L., and Jamieson, G. A. (1982). Differentiation of platelet-aggregating effects of human tumor cell lines based on inhibition studies with apyrase, hirudin and phospholipase. *Cancer Res.* **42,** 4348–4352.

Berenblum, I., and Shubik, P. (1947). A new, quantitative approach to the study of the stages of chemical carcinogenesis in the mouse skin. *Br. J. Cancer* **1,** 373–391.

Bergman, G., Daly, R., Atkinson, L., Rothman, M., Richardson, P. J., Jackson, G., and Jewitt, D. E. (1981). Prostacyclin: Haemodynamic and metabolic effects in patients with coronary artery disease. *Lancet* **1,** 569–572.

Bertele, V., Falanga, A., Roncaglioni, M. C., Cerletti, C., and de Gaetano, G. (1982). Thromboxane synthetase inhibition results in increased sensitivity to prostacyclin. *Thromb. Haemostasis* **47**, 294.

Black, P. H. (1980). Shedding from the cell surface of normal and cancer cells. *Adv. Cancer Res.* **32**, 75–199.

Borgeat, P., and Samuelsson, B. (1979). Arachidonic acid metabolism in polymorphonuclear leukocytes: An unstable intermediate in formation of dihydroxy acids. *Proc. Natl. Acad. Sci. U.S.A.* **76**, 3213–3217.

Borgeat, P., Hamberg, M., and Samuelsson, B. (1976). Transformation of arachidonic acid and homo-α-linolenic acid by rabbit polymorphonuclear leukocytes. *J. Biol. Chem.* **251**, 7816–7820.

Boyd, J. A., Barrett, J. C., and Eling, T. E. (1982). Prostaglandin endoperoxide synthetase-dependent cooxidation of (±)-*trans*-7.8-dihydroxy-7,8-dihydrobenzo[a]pyrene in C3H/10T½ clone 8 cells. *Cancer Res.* **42**, 2628–2632.

Brain, M. C., Azzopardi, J. G., Baker, L. R. I., Pinco, G. F., Roberts, P. D., and Dacie, J. V. (1970). Microangiopathic haemolytic anemia: The possible role of vascular lesions in pathogenesis. *Br. J. Haematol.* **18**, 183–193.

Braunwald, E. (1982). Mechanism of action of calcium-channel-blocking agents. *N. Engl. J. Med.* **307**, 1618–1627.

Bresnick, E., Neunier, P., and Lamden, M. (1979). Epidermal prostaglandins after topical application of a tumor promoter. *Cancer Letts. (Shannon, Irel.)* **7**, 121–125.

Brune, K., Kalin, H., Schmidt, R., and Hecker, E. (1978). Inflammatory, tumor initiating and promoting activities of polycyclic aromatic hydrocarbons and diterpene esters in mouse skin as compared with their prostaglandin releasing potency *in vitro*. *Cancer Letts. (Shannon Irel.)* **4**, 333–342.

Bryant, R. W., Simon, T. C., and Bailey, J. M. (1982). Role of glutathione peroxidase and hexose monophosphate shunt in the platelet lipoxygenase pathway. *J. Biol. Chem.* **257**, 14937–14943.

Buchanan, M. R., Blajchman, M., and Hirsch, J. (1982). Inhibition of arterial thrombosis and platelet function by nafazatrom. *Thromb. Res.* **28**, 157–170.

Busse, W. D., Mardin, M., Grutzmann, R., Dunn, J. R., Theodoreau, M., Sloane, B. F., and Honn, K. V. (1982). Nafazatrom (Bay g 6575): An inhibitor of cellular lipoxygenase. *Fed. Proc., Fed. Am. Soc. Exp. Biol.* **41**, 1717. (Abstr.)

Carreras, L. O., Chamone, D. A. F., Klerckx, P., and Vermylen, J. (1980). Decreased vascular prostacyclin (PGI$_2$) in diabetic rats. Stimulation of PGI$_2$ release in normal and diabetic rats by the antithrombotic compound Bay g 6575. *Thromb. Res.* **19**, 663–670.

Carroll, K. K., and Khor, H. T.(1975). Dietary fat in relation to tumorigenesis. *Prog. Biochem. Pharmacol.* **10**, 308–353.

Carter, C. A., Milholland, R. J., Shea, W., and Ip, M. M. (1983). Effect of the prostaglandin synthetase inhibitor indomethacin on 7,12-dimethylbenzanthracene-induced mammary tumorigenesis in rats fed different levels of fat. *Cancer Res.* **43**, 3559–3562.

Cavanaugh, P. G., Sloane, B. F., Bajkowski, A. S., Gasic, G. J., Gasic, T. B., and Honn, K. V. (1983). Involvement of a cathepin B-like cysteine proteinase in platelet aggregation induced by tumor cells and their shed membrane vesicles. *Clin. Exp. Metastasis* **1**, 297–307.

Chamone, D. A. F., van Damme, B., Carreras, L. D., and Vermylen, J. (1981). Increased release of vascular prostacyclin-like activity after long-term treatment of diabetic rats with Bay g 6575. *Haemostasis* **10**, 297–303.

Cohen, S. M., Zenser, T. V., Murasaki, G., Fukushima, S., Mattammal, M. B., Rapp, N. S., and Davis, V. V. (1981). Aspirin inhibition of *N*-[4-(5-nitro-α2-furyl)-2-thiagolyl] formamide-induced lesions of the urinary bladder correlated with inhibition of metabolism by bladder prostaglandin endoperoxide synthetase. *Cancer Res.* **41**, 3355–3359.

Conney, A. H. (1982). Induction of microsomal enzymes by foreign chemicals and carcinogens by polycyclic aromatic hydrocarbons. G. H. A. Clowes Memorial Lecture. *Cancer Res.* **42**, 4875–4917.

Curatolo, L., Colucci, M., Cambini, A. L., Poggi, A., Morasca, L., Donati, M. B., and Semeraro, N. (1)79). Evidence that cells from experimental tumours can activate coagulation factor X. *Br. J. Cancer* **40**, 228–233.

Defreyn, G., Deckmyn, H., and Vermyeln, J. (1982). A thromboxane synthetase inhibitor reorients endoperoxide metabolism in whole blood towards prostacyclin and prostaglandin E_2. *Thromb. Res.* **26**, 389–400.

del Regato, J. A. (1977). Pathways of metastatic spread of malignant tumors. *Semin. Oncol.* **4**, 33–38.

DeWitt, D. L., and Smith, W. L. (1983). Purification of prostacyclin synthase from bovine aorta by immunoaffinity chromatography. Evidence that the enzyme is a hemoprotein. *J. Biol. Chem.* **258**, 3285–3293.

Donati, M. B., and Poggi. A. (1980). Malignancy and haemostasis. *Br. J. Haematol.* **44**, 173–182.

Dvorak, H. F., Quay, S. C., Orenstein, N. S., Dvorak, A. M., Hahn, P., Bitzer, A. M., and Carvalho, A. C. (1981). Tumor shedding and coagulation. *Science* **212**, 923–924.

Edwards, R. L., Rickles, F. R., and Cronlund, M. (1981). Abnormalities of blood coagulation in patients with cancer. Mononuclear cell tissue factor generation. *J. Lab. Clin. Med.* **98**, 917–928.

Elias, E. G., Sepulveda, F., and Mink, I. B. (1973). Increasing the efficiency of cancer chemotherapy with heparin: Clinical study. *J. Surg. Oncol.* **5**, 189–193.

Eling, T. E., Honn, K. V., Busse, W. D., Seuter, F., and Marnett, L. J. (1982). Stimulation of PGI_2 biosynthesis by nafazatrom (Bay g 6575). *In* "Prostaglandins and Cancer" (T. J. Powles, R. S. Bockman, K. V. Honn, and P. Ramwell, eds.), pp. 783–787. Alan R. Liss, New York.

Fantone, J., Kunkel, S., and Varani, J. (1982). Inhibition of tumor cell adherence by prostaglandins. *In* "Prostaglandins and Cancer" (T. J. Powles, R. S. Bockman, K. V. Honn, and P. Ramwell, eds.), pp. 673–677. Alan R. Liss, New York.

Fidler, I. J. (1978). General considerations for studies of experimental cancer metastasis. *Methods Cancer Res.* **15**, 399–439.

Fischer, S. M., Gleason, G. L., Mills, G. D., and Slaga, T. J. (1980). Indomethacin enhancement of TPA tumor promotion in mice. *Cancer Letts (Shannon Irel.)* **10**, 343–350.

Fisher, E. R., and Fisher, B. (1967). Recent observations on concepts of metastasis.*Arch. Pathol.* **83**, 321–324.

Fitzpatrick, F., Bundy, G., Gorman, T., Honohan, R., McGuire, J., and Sun, F. (1979). 9,11-Iminoepoxyprosta-5,13-dienoic acid is a selective thromboxane A_2 synthetase inhibitor. *Biochim. Biophys. Acta* **573**, 238–244.

Flaim, S. F., and Zelis, R. (1981). Clinical use of calcium entry blockers. *Fed. Proc., Fed. Am. Soc. Exp. Biol.* **40**, 2877–2881.

Flower, R. J., and Blackwell, G. J. (1979). Anti-inflammatory steroids induce biosynthesis of a phospholipase A_2 inhibitor which prevents prostaglandin generation. *Nature (London)* **278**, 456–459.

Furstenberger, G., and Marks, F. (1978). Indomethacin inhibition of cell proliferation induced by the phorbol ester TPA is reversed by prostaglandin E_2 in mouse epidermis *in vivo*. *Biochem. Biophys. Res. Commun.* **84**, 1103–1111.

Furstenberger, G., deBravo, M., Berstch, S., and Marks, F. (1979). The effect of indomethacin on cell proliferation induced by chemical mechanical means in mouse epidermis *in vivo*. *Res. Commun. Chem. Pathol. Pharmacol.* **24**, 533–541.

Galli, C., Galli, G., and Porcellati, G., eds. (1978). Phospholipases and prostaglandins. *Adv. Prostaglandin Thromboxane Res.* 3, 206 pp.

Gasic, G. J., Gasic, T. B., and Stewart, C. C. (1968). Antimetastatic effects associated with platelet reaction. *Proc. Natl. Acad. Sci. U.S.A.* **61**, 46–52.

Gasic, G. J., Gasic, T. B., Galanti, N., Johnson, T., and Murphy, J. (1973). Platelet tumor-cell interactions in mice. The role of platelets in the spread of malignant disease. *Int. J. Cancer* **11**, 704–718.

Gasic, G. J., Koch, P. A. G., Hsu, B., Gasic, T. B., and Niewiarowski, S. (1976). Thrombogenic activity of mouse and human tumors: Effects on platelets, coagulation and fibrinolysis, and possible significance for metastasis. *Z. Krebsforsch.* **86**, 263–277.

Gasic, G. J., Boettiger, B., Catalfamo, J. L., Gasic, T. B., and Stewart, G. J. (1978). Aggregation of platelets and cell membrane vesiculation by rat cells transformed in vitro by Rous sarcoma virus. *Cancer Res.* **38**, 2950–2955.

Gasic, G. J., Catalfamo, J. L., Gasic, T. B., and Avdalovic, N. (1981). In vitro mechanism of platelet aggregation by purified plasma membrane vesicles shed by mouse 15091A tumor cells. *In* "Malignancy and the Hemostatic System" (M. B. Donati, J. F. Davidson, and S. Garattini, eds.), pp. 27–35. Raven, New York.

Gastpar, H. (1977). Platelet cancer cell interaction in metastasis formation: A possible therapeutic approach to metastasis prophylaxis. *J. Med.* **8**, 103–114.

Gastpar, H., Ambrus, J., and Thurber, L. E. (1977). Study of platelet aggregation in vivo. II. Effect of bencyclane on circulating metastatic tumor cells. *J. Med.* **8**, 53–56.

Godfraind, T. (1981). Mechanisms of action of calcium entry blockers. *Fed. Proc., Fed. Am. Soc. Exp. Biol.* **40**, 2866–2871.

Goetzl, E. J., Valone, F. H., Reinholt, U. N., and Gorman, R. R. (1979). Specific inhibition of the polymorphonuclear leukocyte chemotactic response to hydroxy-fatty acid metabolites of arachidonic acid by methyl ester derivatives. *J. Clin. Invest.* **63**, 1181–1186.

Goodnight, S. H. (1974). Bleeding and intravascular clotting in malignancy: A review. *Ann N. Y. Acad. Sci.* **230**, 271–288.

Gordon, S. G., and Cross, B. A. (1981). A factor X activating cysteine protease from malignant tissue. *J. Clin. Invest.* **67**, 1665–1671.

Gordon, S. G., Franks, J. J., and Lewis, B. (1975). Cancer procoagulant A: A factor X activating procoagulant from malignant tissue. *Thromb. Res.* **6**, 127–137.

Gorman, R. R. (1979). Modulation of human platelet function by prostacyclin and thromboxane A_2. *Fed. Proc., Fed. Am. Soc. Exp. Biol.* **38**, 83–88.

Gorman, R. R. (1983). Biology and biochemistry of thromboxane synthetase inhibitors. *In* "Advances in Prostaglandin, Thromboxane, and Leukotriene Research" (B. Samuelsson, R. Paoletti, and P. Ramwell, eds.), Vol. 11, pp. 235–240. Raven, New York.

Goset, M., and Lagarde, M. (1983). Stereospecific inhibition of PGH_2-induced platelet aggregation by lipoxygenase products of icosaenoic acids. *Biochem. Biophys. Res. Commun.* **112**, 878–883.

Gryglewski, R. J., Bunting, S., Moncada, S., Flower, R. J., and Vane, J. R. (1976). Arterial walls are protected against deposition of platelet thrombi by a substance (prostaglandin X) which they make from prostaglandin endoperoxides. *Prostaglandins* **12**, 685–713.

Hall, R. J. C., and Dewar, H. A. (1981). Safety of coronary arterial prostacyclin infusion. *Lancet* **1**, 949.

Hall, E. R., Chen, Y. C., Ho, T., and Wu, K. K. (1982). The reduction of platelet thrombi on damaged vessel wall by a thromboxane synthetase inhibitor in platelets. *Thromb. Res.* **27**, 501–511.

Hamberg, M., and Samuelsson, B. (1973). Detection and isolation of an endoperoxide intermediate in prostaglandin biosynthesis. *Proc. Natl. Acad. Sci. U.S.A.* **70**, 899–903.

Hamberg, M., and Samuelsson, B., (1974). Prostaglandin endoperoxides. Novel transformation of arachidonic acid in human platelets. *Proc. Natl. Acad. Sci. U.S.A.* **71**, 3400–3404.

Hamberg, M., Svensson, J., Wakabayashi, T., and Samuelsson, B. (1974). Isolation and structure of two prostaglandin endoperoxides that cause platelet aggregation. *Proc. Natl. Acad. Sci. U.S.A.* **71**, 345–349.

Hamberg, M., Svensson, J., and Samuelsson, B. (1975). Thromboxanes: A new group of biologically active compounds derived from prostaglandin endoperoxide. *Proc. Natl. Acad. Sci. U.S.A.* **72**, 2994–2998.

Hammarstrom, S., and Falardeau, P. (1977). Resolution of prostaglandin endoperoxide synthase and thromboxane synthase of human platelets. *Proc. Natl. Acad. Sci. U.S.A.* **74**, 3691–3695.

Hammarstrom, S., Murphy, R. C., Samuelsson, B., Clark, D. A., Mioskowski, C., and Corey, E. J. (1979). Structure of leukotriene C: Identification of the amino acid part. *Biochem. Biophys. Res. Commun.* **91**, 1266–1272.

Hara, Y., Steiner, M., and Baldini, M. G. (1980). Characterization of the platelet aggregating activity of tumor cells. *Cancer Res.* **40**, 1217–1222.

Heidelberger, C. (1975). Chemical carcinogensis. *Annu. Rev. Biochem.* **44**, 79–121.

Henry, P. D. (1982). Comparative pharmacology of calcium antagonists nifedipine, verapamil and diltiazime. *Am. J. Cardiol.* **46**, 1047–1058.

Herman, A. G., Claeys, M., Moncada, S., and Vane, J. R. (1979). Biosynthesis of prostacyclin (PGI$_2$) and 12L-hydroxy-5,8,10,14-eicosatetraenoic acid (HETE) by pericardium, pleura, peritoneum, and aorta of the rabbit. *Prostaglandins* **18**, 439–452.

Hilgard, P. (1973). The role of blood platelets in experimental metastases. *Br. J. Cancer* **28**, 429–435.

Hilgard, P., Beyerle, L., Hohage, R., Hiemeyer, V., and Kubler, M. (1972). The effect of heparin on the initial phase of metastasis formation. *Eur. J. Cancer* **8**, 347–352.

Hillyard, L. A., and Abraham, S. (1979). Effects of dietary polyunsaturated fatty acids on growth of mammary adenocarcinomas in mice and rats. *Cancer Res.* **39**, 4430–4437.

Hirata, F., Schiffman, E., Venkatasubramanian, K., Solomon, D., and Axelrod, J. (1980). A phospholipase A$_2$ inhibitory protein in rabbit neutrophils induced by glucocorticoids. *Proc. Natl. Acad. Sci. U.S.A.* **77**, 2533–2536.

Honn, K. V. (1983). Inhibition of tumor cell metastasis by modulation of the vascular prostacyclin/thromboxane A$_2$ system. *Clin. Exp. Metastasis* **1**, 103–114.

Honn, K. V., and Dunn, J. R. (1982). Nafazatrom (Bay g 6575) inhibition of tumor cell lipoxygenase activity and cellular proliferation. *FEBS Lett.* **139**, 65–68.

Honn, K. V., and Sloane, B. F. (1983). Prostacyclin, thromboxanes, and hematogenous metastasis. *In* "Advances in Prostaglandin, Thromboxane and Leukotriene Research" (B. Samuelsson, R. Paoletti, and P. Ramwell, eds.), Vol. 12, pp. 313–318. Raven, New York.

Honn, K. V., and Sloane, B. F. (1984). Prostaglandins in tumor cell metastasis. *In* "Basic Mechanisms and Clinical Treatment of Tumor Metastasis" (M. Torisu and T. Yoshida, eds.). Academic Press, New York (in press).

Honn, K. V., Cicone, B., and Skoff, A. (1981). Prostacyclin: A potent antimetastatic agent. *Science* **212**, 1270–1272.

Honn, K. V., Meyer, J., Neagos, G., Henderson, T., Westley, C., and Ratanatharathorm, V. (1982). Control of tumor growth and metastasis with prostacyclin and thromboxane synthetase inhibitors: Evidence for a new antitumor and antimetastatic agent (Bay g 6575). *In* "Interaction of Platelets and Tumor Cells" (G. A. Jamieson, ed.), pp. 295–331. Alan R. Liss, New York.

Honn, K. V., Busse, W. D., and Sloane, B. F. (1983a). Commentary. Prostacyclin and thromboxanes. Implications for their role in tumor cell metastasis. *Biochem. Pharmacol.* **32**, 1–11.

Honn, K. V., Menter, D., Cavanaugh, P. G., Neagos, G., Moilanen, D., Taylor, J. D., and Sloane, B. F. (1983b). A review of prostaglandins and the treatment of tumor metastasis. *Acta Clin. Belg.* **38**, 53–67.

Honn, K. V., Menter, D., Moilanen, D., Cavanaugh, P. G., Taylor, J. D., and Sloane, B. F. (1983c). Role of prostacyclin and thromboxanes in tumor cell-platelet-vessel wall interactions. *In* "Protective Agents in Cancer" (D. C. H. McBrien and T. F. Slater, eds.), pp. 57–79. Academic Press, New York.

Honn, K. V., Onoda, J. M., Diglio, C. A., and Sloane, B. F. (1983d). Calcium channel blockers: Potential antimetastatic agents. *Proc. Soc. Exp. Biol. Med.* **174,** 16–19.

Honn, K. V., Menter, D. G., Onoda, J. M., Taylor, J. D., and Sloane, B. F. (1984). Role of prostacyclin as a natural deterrent to hematogenous tumor metastasis. *In* "Cancer Invasion and Metastasis: Biologic and Therapeutic Agents" (G. L. Nicolson and L. Milas, eds.), pp. 361–388. Raven, New York.

Huberman, E., Sachs, L., Yang, S. K., and Gelboin, H. V. (1976). Identification of mutagenic metabolites of benzo[a]pyrene in mammalian cells. *Proc. Natl. Acad. Sci. U.S.A.* **73,** 607–611.

Irimura, T., and Nicolson, G. L. (1981). The role of glycoconjugates in metastatic melanoma blood-borne and arrest and cell surface properties. *J. Supramol. Struct. Cell. Biochem.* **17,** 325–336.

Irimura, T., Gonzalez, R., and Nicolson, G. L. (1981). Effects of tunicamycin on B16 metastatic melanoma cell surface glycoproteins and blood-borne arrest and survival properties. *Cancer Res.* **41,** 3411–3418.

Jamieson, G. A., ed. (1982). "Interaction of Platelets and Tumor Cells." Alan R. Liss, New York.

Jeffrey. A. M., Weinstein, I. B., Jennette, K. W., Grzeskowiak, K., Nakanishi, K., Harvey, R. G., Autrup, H., and Harris, C. (1977). Structure of benzo[a]pyrene-nucleic acid adducts formed in human and bovine bronchial explants. *Nature (London)* **269,** 348–350.

Johnson, R. A., Morton, D. R., Kinner, J. H., Gorman, R. R., McGuire, J. C., Sun, F. F., Whittaker, N., Bunting, S., Salmon, J., Moncada, S., and Vane, J. R. (1976). The chemical structure of prostaglandin X (prostacyclin). *Prostaglandins* **12,** 915–928.

Kapitulnik, J., Wislocki, P. G., Levin, W., Yagi, H., Jerina, D. M., and Conney, A. H. (1978). Tumorigenicity studies with diol-epoxides of benzo[a]pyrene which indicate that (±)-*trans*-7,8-dihydroxy-9,10-epoxy-7,8,9,10-tetrahydrobenzo[a]pyrene is an ultimate carcinogen in newborn mice. *Cancer Res.* **38,** 354–358.

Karpatkin, S., and Pearlstein, E. (1981). Role of platelets in tumor cell metastases. *Ann. Intern. Med.* **95,** 636–641.

Karpatkin, S., Smerling, A., and Pearlstein. E. (1980). Plasma requirement for the aggregation of rabbit platelets by an aggregating material derived from SV40-transformed 3T3 fibroblasts. *J. Lab. Clin. Med.* **96,** 994–1001.

Kollmorgen, G. M., King, M. M., Kosanke, S. D., and Do, C. (1983). Dietary fat and indomethacin influence growth of transplantable mammary tumors in rats. *Cancer Res.* **43,** 4714–4719.

Kollmorgen, G. M., Longley, R. E., Kosanke, S. D., Carpenter, M. P., and Loh, M. T. (1984). Dietary fat stimulates mammary tumor growth and inhibits immune responses. *In* "Modulation of Cancer" Karger, Basel (in press).

Kramer, R. H., and Nicolson, G. L. (1979). Interactions of tumor cells with vascular endothelial cell monolayers: A model for metastatic invasion. *Proc. Natl. Acad. Sci. U.S.A.* **76,** 5704–5706.

Kramer, R. H., and Nicolson, G. L. (1981). Invasion of vascular endothelial cell monolayers and underlying matrix by metastatic human cancer cells. *In* "International Cell Biology" (S. Schweiger, ed.), pp. 793–799. Springer-Verlag, Berlin and New York.

Kramer, R. H., Gonzalez, R., and Nicolson, G. L. (1980). Metastatic tumor cells adhere preferentially to the extracellular matrix underlying vascular endothelial cells. *Int. J. Cancer* **26,** 639–645.

Kudo, T., Narisawa, T., and Abo, S. (1980). Antitumor activity of indomethacin on methylazoxymethanol-induced large bowel tumors in rats. *Gann* **71,** 260–264.

Lands, W. E. M., and Samuelsson, B. (1968). Phospholipid precursors of prostaglandins. *Biochim. Biophys. Acta* **164,** 426–429.

Lee, S.-C., and Levine, L. (1974). Prostaglandin metabolism. Cytoplasmic reduced nicotinamide adenine dinucleotide phosphate-dependent and microsomal reduced nicotinamide adenine dinucleotide-dependent prostaglandin E 9-ketoreductase activities in monkey and pigeon tissues. *J. Biol. Chem.* **249,** 1369–1375.

Lee, S.-C., and Levine, L. (1975). Purification and regulatory properties of chicken heart prostaglandin E 9-ketoreductase. *J. Biol. Chem.* **250,** 4549–4555.

Levine, L. (1981). Arachidonic acid transformation and tumor production. *Adv. Cancer Res.* **35,** 49–79.

Levine, L., and Hassid, A. (1977). Effects of phorbol-12,13-diesters on prostaglandin production and phospholipase activity in canine kidney (MDCK) cells. *Biochem. Biophys. Res. Commun.* **79,** 477–484.

Liepins, A., and de Harven, E. (1982). Effects of cyclic nucleotides on the shedding of tumor cell surface molecules. *Exp. Cell Res.* **139,** 265–273.

Liepins, A., and Hillman, A. J. (1981). Shedding of tumor cell surface membranes. *Cell Biol. Int. Rep.* **5,** 15–26.

Lione, A., and Bosmann, H. B. (1978). The inhibitory effect of heparin and warfarin treatments on the intravascular survival of B16 melanoma cells in syngeneic C57 mice. *Cell Biol. Int. Rep.* **2,** 81–86.

Maat, B., and Hilgard, P. (1981). Anticoagulant and experimental metastases—evaluation of anti-metastatic effects in different model systems. *J. Cancer Res. Clin. Oncol.* **101,** 275–283.

McCann, J., and Ames, B. N. (1976). Detection of carcinogens as mutagens in the *Salmonella*/microsome test: Assay of 300 chemicals: Discussion. *Proc. Natl. Acad. Sci. U.S.A.* **73,** 950–954.

Machleidt, C., Forstermann, U., Anhut, H., and Hertting, G. (1981). Formation and elimination of prostacyclin metabolites in the cat in vivo as determined by radioimmunoassay of unextracted plasma. *Eur. J. Pharmacol.* **74,** 19–26.

Marcum, J. M., McGill, M., Bastida, E., Ordinas, A., and Jamieson, G. A. (1980). The interaction of platelets, tumor cells, and vascular subendothelium. *J. Lab. Clin. Med.* **96,** 1048–1053.

Marnett, L. J. (1981). Polycyclic hydrocarbon oxidation during prostaglandin biosynthesis. *Life Sci.* **29,** 531–546.

Marnett, L. J., and Bienkowski, M. J. (1977). Non-enzymatic reduction of prostaglandin H by lipoic acid. *Biochemistry* **16,** 4303–4307.

Marnett, L. J., and Eling, T. E. (1983). Cooxidation during prostaglandin biosynthesis: A pathway for the metabolic activation of xenobiotics. *Rev. Biochem. Toxicol.* **5,** 135–172.

Marnett, L. J., Siedlik, P. H., Ochs, R., Das, M., Honn, K. V., Warnock, R., Tainer, B., and Eling, T. E. (1984). Mechanism of the stimulation of prostaglandin H synthase and prostacyclin synthase by the antithrombotic and antimetastatic agent, nafazatrom. *Mol. Pharmacol.* (in press).

Mehta, P. (1984). Evidence for altered arachidonic acid metabolism in tumor metastasis. *In* "Hemostatic Mechanisms and Metastasis" (K. V. Honn and B. F. Sloane, eds.), pp. 223–243. Nijhoff, The Hague.

Mehta, P., Springfield, D., and Ostrowski, N. (1983). Arterial prostacyclin generation is decreased in patients with malignant bone tumors. *Cancer* **52,** 1297–1300.

Mehta, P., Gross, S., and Ostrowski, N. (1984). Plasma concentrations of thromboxanes and prostacyclin metabolites in patients with bone tumors. *Am. J. Ped. Hametol. Oncol.* (in press).

Menter, D., Neagos, G., Dunn, J., Palazzo, R., Tchen, T. T., Taylor, J. D., and Honn, K. V. (1982). Tumor cell induced platelet aggregation: Inhibition by prostacyclin, thromboxane A_2

and phosphodiesterase inhibitors. *In* "Prostaglandins and Cancer" (T. J. Powles, R. S. Bockman, K. V. Honn, and P. Ramwell, eds.), pp. 809–813. Alan R. Liss, New York.

Menter, D. G., Onoda, J. M., Taylor, J. D., and Honn, K. V. (1984). Effects of prostacyclin on tumor cell induced platelet aggregation. *Cancer Res.* **44,** 450–456.

Miller, J. A. (1970). Carcinogenesis by chemicals: An overview. G. H. A. Clowes Memorial Lecture. *Cancer Res.* **30,** 559–576.

Moncada, S. (1982). Biological importance of prostacyclin. *Br. J. Pharmacol.* **76,** 3–31.

Moncada, S., and Vane, J. R. (1977). The discovery of prostacyclin (PGX); a fresh insight into arachidonic acid metabolism. *In* "Biochemical Aspects of Prostaglandins and Thromboxanes" (N. Kharasch and J. Fried, eds.), pp. 155–177. Academic Press, New York.

Moncada, S., and Vane, J. R. (1980). Prostacyclin in the cardiovascular system. *Adv. Prostaglandin Thromboxane Res.* **6,** pp. 43–60.

Moncada, S., Gryglewski, R. J., Bunting, S., and Vane, J. R. (1976a). A lipid peroxide inhibits the enzyme in blood vessel microsomes that generates from prostaglandin endoperoxides the substance (prostaglandin X) which prevents platelet aggregation. *Prostaglandins* **12,** 715–733.

Moncada, S., Gryglewski, R. J., Bunting, S., and Vane, J. R. (1976b). An enzyme isolated from arteries transforms prostaglandin endoperoxides to an unstable substance that inhibits platelet aggregation. *Nature (London)* **263,** 663–665.

Morton, D. R., and Brokow, F. C. (1979). Total synthesis of 6a-carbaprostaglandin I_2 and related isomers. *J. Org. Chem.* **44,** 2880–2887.

Mullane, K. M., Dusting, G. J., Salmon, J. A., Moncada, S., and Vane, J. R. (1979). Biotransformation and cardiovascular effects of arachidonic acid in the dog. *Eur. J. Pharmacol.* **54,** 217–228.

Nakadate, T., Yamamoto, S., Iseki, H., Sonoda, S., Takemura, S., Ura, A., Hosoda, Y., and Kato, R. (1982). Inhibition of 12-0-tetradecanoylphorbol-13-acetate-induced tumor promotion by nordihydroguaiaretic acid, a lipoxygenase inhibitor, and *p*-bromophenacyl bromide, a phospholipase A_2 inhibitor. *Gann* **73,** 841–843.

Narumiya, S., Salmon, J. A., Cottee, F. H., Weatherby, B. C., and Flower, R. J. (1981). Arachidonic acid 15-lipoxygenase from rabbit peritoneal polymorphonuclear leukocytes. *J. Biol. Chem.* **256,** 9583–9592.

Needleman, P., Wyche, A., and Raz, A. (1979). Platelet and blood vessel arachidonate metabolism and interactions. *J. Clin. Invest.* **63,** 345–349.

Nicolson, G. L., Irimura, T., R. Gonzalez, and Ruoslahti, E. (1981). The role of fibronectin in adhesion of metastatic melanoma cells to endothelial cells and their basal lamina. *Exp. Cell Res.* **135,** 461–465.

Nishiyama, H., and Ohno, K. (1979). Synthesis of 6,7-dehydro-5-oxo-prostaglandin I_1: A stable analog of prostacyclin. *Tetrahedron Lett.* **36,** 3481–3484.

Nugteren, D. H., and Hazelhof, E. (1973). Isolation and properties of intermediates in prostaglandin biosynthesis. *Biochim. Biophys. Acta* **326,** 448–461.

Ohki, S., Ogino, N., Yamamoto, S., and Hayaishi, O. (1979). Prostaglandin hydroperoxidase, an integral part of prostaglandin endoperoxide synthetase from bovine vesicular gland microsomes. *J. Biol. Chem.* **254,** 829–836.

Paschen, W., Patscheke, H., and Worner, P. (1979). Aggregation of activated platelet with Walker 256 carcinoma cells. *Blut* **38,** 17–24.

Pearlstein, E., Cooper, L. B., and Karpatkin, S. (1979). Extraction and characterization of a platelet-aggregating material from SV 40-transformed mouse 3T3 fibroblasts. *J. Lab. Clin. Med.* **93,** 332–344.

Pearlstein, E., Salk, P. L., Yogeeswaran, G., and Karpatkin. S. (1980). Correlation between spontaneous metastatic potential, platelet-aggregating activity of cell surface extracts, and cell surface sialylation in 10 metastatic-varient derivatives of rat renal sarcoma cell line. *Proc. Natl. Acad. Sci. U.S.A.* **77**, 4336–4339.

Pearlstein, E., Ambrogio, C., Gasic, G., and Karpatkin, S. (1981). Inhibition of the platelet-aggregating activity of two human adenocarcinomas of the colon and an anaplastic murine tumor with a specific thrombin inhibitor, dansylarginine *N*-(3-ethyl-1,5-pentanediyl)amide. *Cancer Res.* **41**, 4535–4539.

Pedersen, O. L. (1981). Calcium blockade as a therapeutic principle in arterial hypertension. *Acta Pharmacol. Toxicol., Suppl. 2* **49**, 1–31.

Pike, J. E., and Bundy, G. L. (1982). Prostaglandin analogues. *In* "Prostaglandins and Cancer" (T. J. Powles, R. S. Bockman, K. V. Honn, and P. Ramwell, eds.), pp. 67–77. Alan R. Liss, New York.

Pollard, M., and Luckert, P. H. (1981a). Treatment of chemically-induced intestinal cancers with indomethacin (41142). *Proc. Soc. Exp. Biol. Med.* **167**, 161–164.

Pollard, M., and Luckert, P. H. (1981b). Effect of indomethacin on intestinal tumors induced by the acetate derivative of dimethylnitrosamine. *Science* **214**, 558–559.

Poste, G., and Nicolson, G. L. (1980). Arrest and metastasis of blood-borne tumor cells are modified by fusion of plasma membrane vesicles from highly metastatic cells. *Proc. Natl. Acad. Sci. U.S.A.* **77**, 399–403.

Powles, T. J., Bockman, R. S., Honn, K. V., and Ramwell, P. W., eds. (1982). "Prostaglandins and Cancer: First International Conference." Alan R. Liss, New York.

Raz, A., McLellan, W. L., Hart, I. R., Bucana, C. D., Hoyer, L. C., Sela, B. A., Dragsten, P., and Fidler, I. J. (1980). Cell surface properties of B16 melanoma variants with differing metastatic potential. *Cancer Res.* **40**, 1645–1651.

Reed, G. A., Grafstrom, R. C., Krauss, R. S., and Eling, T. E. (1983). Prostaglandin endoperoxide synthase-dependent cooxygenation of 7,8-dihydroxy-7,8-dihydrobenzol[*a*]pyrene in hamster trachea and human bronchus explants. *Proc. Am. Assoc. Cancer Res.* **24**, 80.

Ribeiro, L. G. T., Brandon, T. A., Horak, J. K., Solis, R. T., and Miller, R. (1980). Inhibition of platelet aggregation by verapamil: Further rationale for the use of calcium antagonists in coronary artery disease. *Circulation* **62**, 293. (Abstr.)

Rickles, F. R., and Edwards, R. L. (1983). Activation of blood coagulation in cancer: Trousseau's syndrome revisited. *Blood* **62**, 14–31.

Robinson, H. J., and Vane, J. R., eds. (1974). "Prostaglandin Synthetase Inhibitors—Their Effects on Physiological Functions and Pathological States." Raven, New York.

Rosenkranz, B., Fischer, C., Weimer, K. E., and Frolich, J. C. (1980). Metabolism of prostacyclin and 6-keto-prostaglandin $F_{1\alpha}$ in man. *J. Biol. Chem.* **255**, 10194–10198.

Salmon, J. A., Smith, D. R., Flower, R. S., Moncada, S., and Vane, J. R. (1978). Further studies on the enzymatic conversion of prostaglandin endoperoxide into prostacyclin by porcine aortic microsomes. *Biochem. Biophys. Acta* **523**, 250–262.

Salsbury, A. J. (1975). The significance of the circulating cancer cell. *Cancer Treat. Rev.* **2**, 55–72.

Samuelsson, B. (1983). Leukotrienes: Mediators of immediate hypersensitivity reactions and inflammation. *Science* **229**, 568–575.

Samuelsson, B., Granstrom, E., Green, K., and Hamberg, M. (1971). Metabolism of prostaglandins. *Ann. N. Y. Acad. Sci.* **180**, 138–163.

Schmunk, G. A., and Lefer, A. M. (1982). Anti-aggregatory actions of calcium channel blockers in cat platelets. *Res. Commun. Chem. Pathol. Pharmacol.* **35**, 179–187.

Schwarz, J. A., Viaje, A., Slaga, T. J., Yuspa, S. H., Hennings, H., and Lichti, U. (1977). Flucinolone acetonide: A potent inhibitor of skin tumor promotion and epidermal DNA synthesis. *Chem. Biol. Interact.* **17**, 331–347.

Seuter, F., Busse, W. D., Meng, K., Hoffmeister, F., Moller, E., and Horstmann, H. (1979). The antithrombotic activity of Bay g 6575. *Arzneim.-Forsch.* **29**, 54–59.

Sims, P., Grover, P. L., Swaisland, A., Pal, K., and Hewer, A. (1974). Metabolic activation of benzo[a]pyrene proceeds by a diolepoxide. *Nature (London)* **252**, 326–328.

Sirois, P., Roy, S., Borgeat, P., Picard, S., and Corey, E. J. (1981). Structural requirement for the action of leukotriene B_4 on the guinea-pig lung: Importance of double bond geometry in the 6,8,10-triene unit. *Biochem. Biophys. Res. Commun.* **99**, 385–390.

Skolnik, G., Alpsten, M., and Ivarsson, L. (1980). Studies on mechanisms involved in metastasis formation from circulating tumor cells. *J. Cancer Res. Clin. Oncol.* **97**, 249–256.

Slaga, T. J., Fischer, S. M., Weeks, C. E., Nelson, K., Mamrack, M., and Klein-Szanto, A. J. P. (1982). Specificity and mechanism(s) of promoter inhibitors in multistage promotion. In "Carcinogenesis. VII. Cocarcinogenesis and Biological Effects of Tumor Promoters" (E. Hecker, N. E. Fusenig, W. Kung, F. Marks, and H. W. Thielmann, eds.), pp. 19–34. Raven, New York.

Sloane, B. F., Dunn, J. R., and Honn, K. V. (1981). Lysosomal cathepsin B: Correlation with metastatic potential. *Science* **212**, 1151–1153.

Stringfellow, D. A., and Fitzpatrick, F. A. (1979). Prostaglandin D_2 controls pulmonary metastasis of malignant melanoma cells. *Nature (London)* **282**, 76–78.

Szczeklik, A., and Gryglewski, R. J. (1981). Treatment of vascular disease with prostacyclin. In "Clinical Pharmacology of Prostacyclin" (P. J. Lewis and J. O'Grady, eds.), pp. 159–167. Raven, New York.

Szczeklik, A., Gryglewski, R. J., Nizankowski, R., Musial, J., Pieton, R., and Mruk, J. (1978). Circulatory and anti-platelet effects of intravenous prostacyclin in healthy men. *Pharmacol. Res. Commun.* **10**, 545–556.

Szczeklik, A., Nizankowski, R., Skawinski, S., Szczeklik, J., Gluszko, P., and Gryglewski, R. J. (1979). Successful therapy of advanced arteriosclerosis obliterans with prostacyclin. *Lancet* **1**, 1111–1114.

Terranova, V. P., Liotta, L. A., Russo, R. G., and Martin, G. R. (1982). Role of laminin in the attachment and metastasis of murine tumor cells. *Cancer Res.* **42**, 2265–2269.

Vane, J. R., Bunting, S., and Moncada, S. (1982). Prostacyclin in physiology and pathophysiology. *Int.Rev. Exp. Pathol.* **23**, 161–207.

Vargaftif, B. B., Chignard, M., and Benveniste, J. (1981). Present concepts on the mechanism of platelet aggregation. *Biochem. Pharmacol.* **30**, 263–271.

Verma, A. K., Rice, H. M., and Boutwell, R. K. (1977). Prostaglandins and skin tumor promotion: Inhibition of tumor promoter-induced ornithine decarboxylase activity by inhibitors of prostaglandin synthesis. *Biochem. Biophys. Res. Commun.* **79**, 1160–1166.

Verma, A. K., Ashendel, C. L., and Boutwell, R. K. (1980). Inhibition by prostaglandin synthesis inhibitors of the induction of epidermal ornithine decarboxylase activity, the accumulation of prostaglandins, and tumor promotion caused by 12-0-tetradecanoylphorbol-13-acetate. *Cancer Res.* **40**, 308–315.

Vermylen, J., Chamone, D. A. F., and Verstraete, M. (1979). Stimulation of prostacyclin release from vessel wall by Bay g 6575, an antithrombic compound. *Lancet* **1**, 518–520.

Vilarem, M. J., Jouanneau, J., and Bourrillon. R. (1981). Differences in sialic acid contents of low cancer cells, high cancer cells and normal mouse lung counterparts. *Biochem. Biophys. Res. Commun.* **9**, 7–14.

Vonkeman, H., and Von Dorp, D. A. (1968). The action of prostaglandin synthetase on 2-arachidonyl-lecithin. *Biochim. Biophys. Acta* **164**, 430–432.

Warren, B. A. (1981). Cancer cell-endothelial reactions: The microinjury hypothesis and localized thrombosis in the formation of micrometastases. In "Malignancy and the Hemostatic System" (M. B. Donati, J. F. Davidson, and S. Garattini, eds.), pp. 5–26. Raven, New York.

Watkins, W. D., Peterson, M. B., Crone, R. K., Shannon, D. C., and Levine, L. (1980). Prostacyclin and prostaglandin E_1 for severe idiopathic pulmonary artery hypertension. *Lancet* **1**, 1083.

Weiss, L. (1977). A pathobiologic overview of metastasis. *Semin. Oncol.* **4**, 5–17.

Whittle, B. J. R., Moncada, S., Whiting, F., and Vane, J. R. (1980). Carbacyclin—A potent stable prostacyclin analogue for the inhibition of platelet aggregation. *Prostaglandins* **19**, 605–627.

Willmott, N., Malcolm, A., McLeod, T., Gracie, A., and Calman, K. C. (1983). Changes in anatomical distribution of tumour lesions and by platelet-active drugs. *Invasion Metastasis* **3**, 32–51.

Wlodawer, P., Samuelsson, B., Albonico, S. M., and Corey, E. J. (1971). Selective inhibition of prostaglandin synthetase by a bicyclo[2.2.1]hepene derivative. *J. Am. Chem. Soc.* **93**, 2815–2816.

Wong, P. Y.-K., Chao, P. H.-W., and McGiff, J. C. (1982). Nafazatrom (Bay g 6575), an antithrombotic and antimetastatic agent, inhibits 15-hydroxyprostaglandin dehydrogenase. *J. Pharmacol. Exp. Ther.* **223**, 757–760.

Yamamoto, S., Ohki, S., Ogino, N., Shimizu, T., Yoshimoto, T., Watanabe, K., and Hayaishi, O. (1980). Enzymes involved in the formation and further transformations of prostaglandin endoperoxides. *Adv. Prostaglandin Thromboxane Res.* **6**, 27–34.

Yoshimoto, T., Yamamoto, S., Okuma, M., and Hayaishi, O. (1977). Solubilization and resolution of thromboxane synthesizing system from microsomes of bovine blood platelets. *J. Biol. Chem.* **252**, 5871–5874.

Zacharski, L. R., Henderson, W. G., Rickles, F. R., Forman, W. B., Cornell, C. J., Forcier, R. J., Harrower, H. W., and Johnson, R. O. (1979). Rationale and experimental design for the VA cooperative study of anticoagulation (warfarin) in the treatment of cancer. *Cancer* **44**, 732–741.

Zamora, P. O., Danielson, K. G., and Hosick, H. L. (1980). Invasion of endothelial cell monolayers on collagen gels by cells from mammary tumor spheroids. *Cancer Res.* **40**, 4631–4639.

Zenser, T. V., Mattamal, M. B., Brown, W. W., and Davis, B. B. (1979). Co-oxygenation by prostaglandin cyclooxygenase from rabbit inner medulla. *Kidney Int.* **16**, 688–694.

5

Liposomes as a Drug Delivery System in Cancer Therapy

GEORGE POSTE

Smith Kline & French Laboratories
Philadelphia, Pennsylvania,
and Department of Pathology and Laboratory Medicine
University of Pennsylvania School of Medicine
Philadelphia, Pennsylvania

RICHARD KIRSH, AND PETER BUGELSKI

Smith Kline & French Laboratories
Philadelphia, Pennsylvania

I.	Introduction	166
II.	Liposomes	168
III.	Therapy of Experimental Animal Tumors Using Liposomes Containing Antineoplastic Drugs	172
IV.	Liposome Targeting	181
	Behavior of Liposomes Administered Intravenously: Implications for Drug Targeting	183
V.	Tumor Cell Heterogeneity and Cancer Therapy	198
	A. Variation in the Responsiveness of Tumor Cells to Antineoplastic Drugs	198
	B. Antigenic Heterogeneity of Tumor Cells and Antibody-Mediated Drug Targeting	199
VI.	Ligand-Directed Targeting of Liposomes within the Vascular Compartment	202
VII.	Passive Targeting of Liposome-Encapsulated Drugs to Mononuclear Phagocytes and Augmentation of Host Resistance to Tumors and Microorganisms	203
	A. Liposome-Encapsulated Immunomodulators and Macrophage-Mediated Destruction of Tumor Cells	204

Novel Approaches to Cancer Chemotherapy
Copyright © 1984 by Academic Press, Inc.
All rights of reproduction in any form reserved.
ISBN 0-12-676980-X

B. Liposomes and Antimicrobial Chemotherapy 207
C. Liposomes and Chemotherapy of Malignancies of the
   Mononuclear Phagocyte System.......................... 208
VIII. Physicochemical Targeting of Liposomes in Cancer Chemotherapy .. 208
IX. Liposomes and Drug Delivery to Lymph Nodes 210
X. Liposome Toxicity and Adverse Complications of Liposome Uptake
   by Mononuclear Phagocytes 212
A. Toxicity of the Liposomal Carrier 212
B. Toxicity Resulting from Altered Disposition of Liposome-
   Encapsulated Drugs...................................... 214
XI. Clinical Trials and Commercial Development of Liposomes as
   Drug Carriers 215
XII. Conclusions 219
   References 221

I. INTRODUCTION

Cancer therapy, and chemotherapy in particular, is entering a critical period. Notwithstanding the impressive gains made in the last 20 yr in the therapy of lymphoproliferative neoplasms and some solid tumors such as choriocarcinoma, Wilms' tumor, and testicular cancer, treatment of most solid malignant tumors and their metastases remains depressingly unsuccessful. The more common human malignancies arising in breast, lung, colon, and the prostate continue to resist therapy in the majority of patients, despite an assault by ever-growing combinations of drugs. The merits of current approaches to cancer chemotherapy are being challenged on several fronts. The first stems from subjective concern regarding whether the high cost of therapy and its adverse impact on the quality of life are justified by the results obtained. The second concern is more fundamental and questions whether the scientific rationale of certain approaches to chemotherapy, particularly single-agent therapy, is sound in the light of newer knowledge about the cellular composition of tumors, which reveals previously unimagined degrees of complexity and diversity in the therapeutic responses of different cell populations within the same tumor. Third, the relative lack of success of chemotherapy has stimulated research increasingly into alternative treatment modalities such as hyperthermia and biological response-modifying agents.

Two factors have contributed overwhelmingly to current deficiencies in the therapy of neoplastic disease. The first involves the extraordinary degree of cellular heterogeneity present in most solid tumors and their metastases. The coexistence within the same tumor of subpopulations of tumor cells that exhibit widely differing responses to a broad range of cancer treatments means that the only successful approach to therapy will be one that can circumvent this diversity and prevent emergence of tumor cells that are resistant to therapy. The second problem stems from the lack of selectivity of most anticancer drugs for tumor cells, resulting in significant destruction of normal cells and unacceptable toxicity to host tissues.

In any transitional period it is important to define a balance, so that effective strategies are not discarded and so that important new research opportunities are not stifled prematurely. In seeking new approaches for the chemotherapy of neoplastic disease, three different but nonexclusive strategies are being pursued. The first involves continuation of the many ongoing and painstaking clinical studies that seek to improve the effectiveness of existing drugs by exploring new drug combinations and different dosing regimens. Such studies are limited, however, by shortcomings inherent in the pharmacology of the agents available. The second strategy involves the search for new drugs with entirely novel pharmacological actions. Although the need for new drugs is obvious, the success of this quest is by no means guaranteed. The cellular and subcellular changes identified in tumor cells compared with their normal counterparts appear to be quantitative rather than qualitative, and the search for new targets for drug actions that are unique to tumor cells may be unrealistic. The fascinating observations on oncogenes have generated the inevitable hyperbole regarding a "breakthrough" that will lead to dramatic gains in cancer treatment (see Newmark, 1983). Even if future research reveals that such genes play a role in the initiation, progression, and/or metastasis of human tumors, it will be many years before drugs acting on these elements will be available for routine clinical use. This lengthy delay before new drugs could become available provides the rationale for the final strategy of improving the effectiveness of existing drugs using pharmaceutical techniques to alter drug disposition, kinetics, and dose–response relationships, and thus to achieve a higher therapeutic index. Drug delivery systems have been in the vanguard of this effort.

To be effective in cancer therapy, a targetable drug delivery system must at a minimum be capable of achieving selective localization at body sites where tumor cells reside and releasing drugs in an active form at a suitable rate to kill tumor cells while producing minimal effects on normal host cells. Ideally, normal host cells should be spared completely if the delivery system were capable of achieving "targeted" drug delivery to tumor cells. In the ultimate form of drug targeting, not only would the drug be delivered selectively to tumor cells, it would also be directed to specific intracellular sites to maximize its effectiveness.

The ability to target drugs to specific cells within the body has been one of the most sought-after goals in therapeutics. Ever since Paul Ehrlich (1906) foresaw the use of "bodies which possessed a particular affinity for a certain organ . . . as carriers by which to bring therapeutic active groups to the organ in question," considerable ingenuity has been devoted to the study of this challenging problem.

A wide variety of cellular, macromolecular, and particulate carriers have been investigated as potential drug delivery systems with the stated objective of improving cancer chemotherapy. These include erythrocytes, leukocytes, antibodies, nucleic acids, heat- or chemically denatured plasma proteins, and a diverse array of particulate carriers of differing sizes and biodegradability prepared from various polymeric materials including dextran, gelatin, agarose, cellulose, albumin, or phospholipids (for reviews, see Chien, 1982; Counsell and Ponland, 1982; Gregoriadis *et al.*, 1982a; Bruck, 1983; Levy and Miller, 1983; Tomlinson, 1983). Many have failed to fulfill their initial promise, but interest in drug delivery systems remains high in both academic and commercial laboratories. Among these systems, liposomes have attracted considerable interest, at least as judged by the number of published papers and patents issued concerning their potential value as a drug carrier.

This chapter presents a brief survey of the current status of liposomes as a vehicle for improving drug delivery in cancer therapy. Particular emphasis will be given to the problem of "targeting" liposomes to specific cell types and the importance of anatomical and physiological factors in influencing the behavior and disposition of liposomes administered by different routes.

II. LIPOSOMES

Liposomes are closed vesicles prepared from phospholipids comprising either one (unilamellar) or several lipid bilayers (multilamellar) surrounding an internal aqueous space or spaces. Their potential value as drug carriers stems from the ability to encapsulate water-soluble drugs within the aqueous interior or to incorporate hydrophobic drugs within the lipid bilayer(s). In addition, integral membrane proteins and antibody molecules can be covalently linked to the outer surface of liposomes either to serve as antigens for immunization or to interact with specific molecules on the surface of defined target cell types.

Methods for the preparation and characterization of liposomes of differing size and structure have been discussed at length in several reviews (Szoka and Papahadjopoulos, 1981; Hauser, 1982; Yatvin and Lelkes, 1982). The properties of liposomes prepared by different methods are summarized in Table I.

Very few of the methods listed in Table I were developed for the specific purpose of using liposomes as a drug delivery system. The majority of published work on liposome-mediated drug delivery *in vitro* and *in vivo* has been done with two classes of liposomes: small sonicated unilamellar vesicel liposomes (SUV) and large multilamellar vesicel liposomes (MLV). These classes of liposomes were developed in the 1960s as model membranes for analyzing the properties of lipid bilayers and have been adopted, largely without modification, for use in drug delivery. More attention is now being given to the design of liposomes as

TABLE I

Preparative Methods and Properties of Different Classes of Liposomes

Vesicle preparation[a]	Resulting vesicle[b]	Size range (average size, μm)	Encapsulation capacity (1 mol⁻¹ lipid)	Encapsulation efficiency[c]	Advantages	Disadvantages
Dispersion of lipid in H_2O: unsonicated dispersion of: (a) Neutral or isoelectric phospholipids	MLV		1–4	10–25	Simple and quick preparation	(1) Low encapsulation capacity (2) Heterogeneous population (3) Poorly characterized
(b) Acidic phospholipids	LUV with some MLV	0.1–2.0	1–7	10–15	Large encapsulation capacity	(1) Restricted to acidic phospholipid (2) Particle size dependent on ionic strength and nature of ion (3) Heterogeneous population
Reverse-phase evaporation	LUV	0.08–0.24 (0.16)		20–65	High encapsulation efficiency	Exposure of compounds to be encapsulated to organic solvent and ultrasonic irradiation
Ether infusion	LUV	0.07–0.19	8–20	—	(1) Large encapsulation capacity (2) Suitable for macromolecules	(1) Exposure of compounds to be encapsulated to organic solvents or high temperature (2) Heterogeneous (3) Low encapsulation efficiency

(*continued*)

TABLE I (*Continued*)

Vesicle preparation[a]	Resulting vesicle[b]	Size range (average size, μm)	Encapsulation capacity (1 mol^{-1} lipid)	Encapsulation efficiency[c]	Advantages	Disadvantages
Calcium-induced fusion	LUV	0.2–1.0	1–7	10–15	(1) Large encapsulation capacity (2) Suitable for macromolecules	(1) Restricted to acidic phospholipids (2) Heterogeneous (3) Particle size sensitive to environmental conditions
Ultrasonic irradiation	Mainly SUV + some residual MLV	0.02–0.05 (0.025)	0.2–1.5	0.1–1.0	—	(1) Low encapsulation capacity and efficiency (2) Heterogeneous mixture of SUV and MLV (3) Exclusion of molecules with M_r >40,000 (4) Contamination with metal from probe tip (5) Possible degradation of phospholipids and compounds to be encapsulated

Method	Vesicle type				Advantages	Retention of detergent(s) / Disadvantages
Removal of cholate (generally detergent) by dilution, dialysis, gel filtration, or specific binding	SUV	0.02–0.15	0.2–7.0	0.1–15.0	(1) Homogeneous population (2) Excellent reproducibility (3) Vesicle size can be varied between 0.02 and 0.1 μm depending on the phospholipid:cholate ratio	Retention of detergent(s)
Injection of ethanolic phospholipid solutions in H$_2$O or buffer	SUV + some aggregates of SUV	0.03–0.06	0.4–1.5	Not tested	—	(1) Heterogeneous (2) Resulting lipid dispersion is diluted
French press	SUV	0.02–0.06	0.2–4.5	Not tested	Method of preparation is applicable to large volumes of lipid dispersions	
Spontaneous vesiculation of phosphatidic acid dispersions or dispersions containing phosphatidic acid at pH >7	Mainly SUV and LUV + some MLV	SUV: 0.02–0.06 LUV: 0.06–0.50	0.2–1.5	10–30	(1) Simple and quick preparation (2) It is applicable to large volumes and hence large quantities of lipids (3) The surface charge density can be controlled and varied within a wide range	(1) Restricted to phosphatidic acid and mixtures of phospholipids with phosphatidic acid (2) Heterogeneous population of SUV and LUV

[a] Reproduced with permission from Hauser, 1982.

[b] Abbreviations used: MLV, multilamellar large vesicle(s); LUV, large unilamellar vesicle(s); SUV, small unilamellar vesicle(s).

[c] Defined as the percentage of the compound that becomes entrapped: the encapsulation efficiency depends on the lipid concentration, and the values presented refer to similar lipid concentrations at about 1–2% (w/v).

drug carriers, but significant methodological improvements in liposome preparation, homogeneity, drug encapsulation efficiency, and stability must occur before the full potential of liposomes as a drug delivery system can be realized. This is particularly true if liposomes are ever to be produced on a commercial scale for widespread clinical use (Section XI).

Selection of the appropriate liposome for drug delivery *in vivo* will depend on the proposed use. The more important factors to be considered are route of administration, dose, properties of the drug, efficiency of drug entrapment, liposome size and composition, tissue disposition, kinetics of clearance from the circulation if injected iv, and adverse effects caused by liposomes themselves or by changes in drug disposition or pharmacokinetics compared with conventional drug formulations. Also, when liposomes are not used immediately after their preparation, the stability of both drug and carrier must be evaluated (Section XI).

The factors influencing the efficiency of entrapment and retention of water-soluble and lipophilic or amphophilic drugs within liposomes of different size, composition, and structure (uni- or multilamellar), and their stability in various biological fluids have been discussed in detail in the proceedings of several symposia, and further review is redundant (Gregoriadis *et al.*, 1982a; Nicolau and Poste, 1983).

III. THERAPY OF EXPERIMENTAL ANIMAL TUMORS
USING LIPOSOMES CONTAINING
ANTINEOPLASTIC DRUGS

Considerable experimental work has been published in the last few years describing the effect of liposome-associated cytotoxic drugs administered by a variety of routes on the growth of experimental animal tumors of diverse histological origin (Table II). The data summarized in Table II reveal many examples in which liposomes containing antineoplastic drugs were equally or more effective than conventional (free) drug formulations in delaying tumor growth, reducing tumor burden, or prolonging host survival. A further attractive feature demonstrated in some studies is that significant antitumor activity could be achieved using significantly lower doses of liposome-associated drug, with resulting improvements in the therapeutic index and reduced host toxicity. A particularly notable example is the significant reduction in cardiotoxicity observed with liposome-entrapped doxorubicin (Adriamycin) compared with the free drug (Olson *et al.*, 1982; Rahman *et al.*, 1980, 1982; Forssen and Tokes, 1981, 1983; 1983; Gabizon *et al.*, 1982; Mayhew *et al.*, 1982).

Superficially, the results given in Table II seem impressive. In addition, when reinforced by speculation in many of the publications listed in Table II that selective targeting of liposomes to tumor cells via antibodies or other ligands would soon become feasible, it is perhaps not surprising that many investigators were attracted to this area of research. This optimism about liposome targeting in cancer therapy soon extended beyond scientific circles. Numerous magazine and newspaper articles and segments on TV science shows appeared in the late 1970s proclaiming that the demise of cancer as a clinical problem was imminent because of the ability of liposomes to home in on tumor cells like "guided missiles" or "smart bombs." (These are just two of many military metaphors used to convey the concept of drug targeting to the general public. Presumably Paul Ehrlich's "magic bullet" does not have enough technological sophistication for the post-sputnik readership.) This kind of predictable hyperbole by the media about scientific discoveries can easily be dismissed—except, of course, by cancer patients and their families who, on reading such articles, ask the oncologist to use this latest "breakthrough" in the treatment of their own intractable disease.

No scientific justification could be offered then, or now, for many of these extravagant claims. Certain examples of liposome targeting, such as within the vascular and lymphatic systems, may still become reality, but others—particularly ambitious proposals for targeting liposomes to tumor or normal organ parenchymal cells in the extravascular compartment—must be viewed as having an extremely low probability of success. Even though a more critical perspective about the feasibility of liposome targeting *in vivo* is emerging, the legacy of earlier speculation about liposome targeting still survives in portions of current literature. Even in 1983, uncritical generalizations and proposals for liposome targeting continue to be published that have little rationale when examined in terms of current knowledge of anatomy, physiology, and pathology. The myriad problems that must be overcome if liposome targeting is to achieve routine clinical use have received scant attention from proponents of the concept. These merit critical review, together with discussion of other conceptual and technical issues that raise serious doubts about many of the proposed uses of liposomes in cancer therapy.

In the majority of studies listed in Table II, the antitumor activity of liposome-associated drugs has been tested under conditions conducive to effective therapy. These include the use of very small tumor burdens and initiation of treatment within only a few hours of tumor cell inoculation (usually less than 24 hr). In certain studies tumor cells were even pretreated *in vitro* before being transplanted *in vivo*.

The use of localized ascites tumors and well-vascularized, rapidly growing nonmetastasizing tumors implanted subcutaneously (sc) or intramuscularly (im) also favors successful therapy. Although these tumor models allow simple monitoring of the cytotoxic effects of liposome-associated drugs, they do not approximate the therapeutic challenge posed by established metastatic disease.

TABLE II

Therapy of Experimental Animal Tumors with Liposome-Associated Antineoplastic Drugs

Tumor	Host	Drug	Dose and regimen	Liposome[a]	Results	Reference
L1210 ip (10^5 cells)	DBA/2 mice	Methotrexate	2.5–50 mg/kg iv or ip on day 1	SUV (PC:C:SA = 3.25:2.25:1)	No increase in therapeutic efficacy of liposome-treated groups as compared to control groups	Kimelberg and Atchison, 1978
L1210 ip (10^5 cells)	CD2/F1 mice	Ara-C	50 mg/kg ip on day 1, multiple doses; single dose on day 5	MLV (SM:SA:C = 20:2:15)	Single dose ip on day 1 very effective; multiple doses ip allow use of lower individual doses; single dose ip on day 5 (advanced disease) less effective than treatment on day 1; iv route less effective than sc or ip dosing	Kobayashi et al., 1977
Ehrlich ascites ip (2 × 10^5 cells)	DDY mice	Illudin S	150–350 µg/kg ip on day 1	SUV (PC:C:SA = 3.2:2.2:1)	Increased MST and number of long-term survivors	Shinozowa et al., 1979
L1210 ip (1 × 10^5 cells)	CD2/F1 mice	Ara-C	3.1–100 mg/kg ip on day 1	SUV (SM:C:SA = 2:1.5:0.22)	Increased MST and number of long-term survivors	Kobayashi et al., 1975
Sarcoma 180 sc (5 × 10^5 cells)	NMRI mice	cis-Dichlorodi-amine platinum II	0.7–1.2 mg/kg iv on day 7 followed by 1 hr hyperthermia	(DSPC:DPPC = 7:1)	Liposome–drug followed by hyperthermia more effective than controls in slowing tumor growth; no evidence presented for tumor regression	Yatvin et al., 1981
Ehrlich ascites ip (1 × 10^6 cells)	ICR Swiss albino mice	Nitrogen mustard (BCNU)	2.5 mg/kg ip on day 2	MLV (DPPC)	Increased number of long-term survivors compared with free drugs; drug need not be encapsulated but must be given within 10 min of liposome preparation	Ritter et al., 1981
1210 ip (1 × 10^5 cells)	CD/F1 mice	Nitrogen mustard (BCNU)	2.5 mg/kg ip on day 2	MLV (DPPC)		Ritter et al., 1981
Ehrlich ascites ip (1 × 10^5 cells)	Swiss albino mice	Trimethylamine carboxyborane	2.5 mg/kg ip on days 1–10	MLV (PC:C:SA = 10:3:2)	Increase in MST and number of long-term survivors at lower dose than free drug	Sur et al., 1981
P-388 ip (1 × 10^5 cells)	BD/F1 mice	Adriamycin	4 mg/kg ip on day 1	(PC:PS:C = 10:4:1)	As effective as free drug but less cardiotoxicity	Rahman et al., 1980

Tumor model	Host	Drug	Dose/schedule	Liposome composition	Result	Reference
Lewis lung sc (1 × 10^5 cells)	CD/F1 mice	Adriamycin	4 mg/kg iv on days 8, 10, and 12	(PC:C:SA = 10:4:3)	As effective as free drug but less toxicity; no dose titration to demonstrate enhancement	Rhaman et al., 1980
Ridgeway osteosarcoma sc (200-mg implant)	AKR mice	Methotrexate	0.125–8.0 mg/kg iv on day 1	SUV (PC:C:SA = 18:4:5)	Ineffective when administered in liposomes	Kaye, 1981
Ridgeway osteosarcoma (no cell number)	AKR mice	Actinomycin D Actinomycin D	5–40 mg/kg iv on day 1 0.8 mg/kg iv on day 1	MLV (PC:C:SA = 18:4:5)	Effective but no increase over free actinomycin D Less effective than free drug on mg/kg basis	Kaye, 1981 Kaye and Ryman, 1980
Ehrlich ascites ip	MRI mice	Methotrexate	7.5 mg/kg iv on days 1–5	SUV (PC:C:DCP = 5:5:1)	Reduction in tumor burden	Freise et al., 1979
Nitrosamine-induced hepatoma	Wistar rats	Methotrexate	7.5 mg/kg iv on days 1–5	SUV (PC:C:DCP = 5:5:1)	Minimal uptake of liposome–MTX by primary hepatoma compared with nontumor tissue from same organ	Freise et al., 1979
L1210 ip (10^6 cells)	DBA/2J mice	Ara-C	10 mg/kg iv on day 1	REV (DPPC:C = 1:1)	Single injection of liposome–Ara-C as effective as an iv infusion of free drug and significantly increases long-term survivors	Mayhew et al., 1980
L1210 iv (10^5–10^6 cells)	DBA/2J mice	Ara-C	10 mg/kg iv on day 1	MLV or SUV (PS:PC:C = 1:4:5)	Increased MST; few long-term survivors	Rustum et al., 1979
L1210 ip (10^5–10^6 cells)	DBA/2 mice	Ara-C	12–50 mg/kg ip on day 1	MLV or SUV (PC:C:SA = 3:3:1)	Increase in MST and number of long-term survivors compared with free drug	Rustum et al., 1979
L1210 ip (no cell number)	DBA/2 mice	8-Azaguanine	1.6 mg/kg drug ip on days 1–8	MLV, SUV (DPPC:C:SA = 6:2:1.4)	No difference in survival times of liposome-treated or free drug groups	Fendler and Romero, 1976
L1210 ip (5 × 10^5 cells)	B6D/F1 mice	RFCNU (water-insoluble nitrosurea)	5–200 mg/kg ip on days 1, 5, and 9	MLV (PC)	Increase in MST with liposome-encapsulated RFCNU in the higher doses (60–100 mg/kg) as compared with free drug	Mathe and Bothorel, 1981
Ehrlich ascites tumor cells ip (5 × 10^6 cells)	DDY mice	Neocarzinostatin	(1) 10–350 μg/kg ip on day 1 (2) 600–700 μg/kg iv on days 1, 3, and 5,	SUV (PC:C = 7:2) (PC:C:DCP = 7:2:1) (PC:C:SA = 7:2:1)	Increase in MST compared with free drug; few long-term survivors	Shinozawa et al., 1980
L1210 iv (1 × 10^5 cells)	B6D/F1 mice	Daunoblastin	5–80 mg/kg iv on day 1	MLV or SUV (PC:C:PA = 7:2:1)	Increase in MST at high doses compared with free drug; no significant difference at lower doses	Fitchner et al., 1981

(continued)

TABLE II (*Continued*)

Tumor	Host	Drug	Dose and regimen	Liposome[a]	Results	Reference
Renal adenocarcinoma (5×10^5 cells intrarenally)	BALB/c mice	Actinomycin D	300 mg/kg ip, no dosage schedule	Composition not reported	Free drug more effective than liposome-associated actinomycin D in increasing survival time; no difference in metastatic tumor burden in lung	Kedar et al., 1980
ADJ/PC6A 1 mm³ trocar implant (no site) (no cell number)	BALB/c mice	cis-Dichlorocyclo-pentylamine platinum II	13.6 mg/kg iv on day 26 after implant	SUV (PC:C:PA = 7:2:1) (DPPC:C:PA = 7:2:1)	Increased retention of liposome–drug compared with free drug in tumor; no information on cytotoxic activity	Deliconstantinos et al., 1977
Ehrlich ascites ip (no cell number)	Swiss albino mice	5-Fluorouracil	1 mg/kg iv or ip on days 2–8	SUV (DPPC:C:PA = 7:2:1)	Increase in MST compared with free drug	Mazumder, 1981
L1210 ip (1×10^5 cells)	CD2/F1 mice	Ara-C	5–40 mg/kg ip on day 1 as single and multiple doses	SUV (PC:C:ICP = 1:1:0.14; 1:0.5:0.14; 1:0.1:0.14)	Increase in MST with P:C ratio 1:1; acts as slow-release formulation	Ganapathi et al., 1980
Hepatoma A sc footpad (0.05 ml of a 10% ascites suspension); pulmonary adenocarcinoma sc footpad (4 × 10⁵ cells)	A/He mice	cis-Diamino-dichloro-platinum II	0.01 mg/kg every 48 hr (four doses) sc in ipsilateral footpad prior to tumor resection	SUV (PC)	50% reduction in number of mice with lymph node metastases; no effect on distant metastases when administered iv or sc	Kaledin et al., 1981
Lewis lung carcinoma iv or sc (10^5 cells)	C57BL/6 mice	Methyl CCNU	20–40 mg/kg iv or ip on day 7	(PC:C:SA = 5:5:1)	Decreased number of metastatic colonies in the lung; no difference between liposome-encapsulated and free drug on sc tumors after iv or ip treatment	Inaba et al., 1981

Tumor model	Host	Drug	Dose/schedule	Liposome	Result	Reference
Mammary adenocarcinoma 13762 (sc) (no cell number)	Fischer 344 rats	Melphalan	0.125 mg/kg sc 3 days after resection of sc tumor in calf	SUV (PC:C = 2:1)	Significant reduction of regional lymph node weight	Khato et al., 1982
Ehrlich ascites tumor cells sc (2 × 10⁶ cells)	ICR mice	Adriamycin	1.25 mg/kg ip on days 7, 8, and 9	SUV (PC:C:DCP = 7:2:1) (PC:C:SA = 7:2:1)	Significant reduction in tumor weight	Shinozawa et al., 1981
L1210 sc (0.5–20 × 10⁶ cells)	B6D2/F1 mice	Methotrexate	3 mg/kg iv on days 1, 2, and 3	SUV (DPPC:DSPC = 7:3)	Significant delay in tumor growth; effect not significant at lower MTX doses	Weinstein et al., 1980
P1798 lymphosarcoma sc (no cell number)	CD/F1 mice	Methotrexate	1 mg/kg ip on days 10–13	SUV (PC:C:SA = 4:3:1)	Significant reduction in tumor weights and diameters	Koslowski et al., 1978
Murphy–Sturman lymphosarcoma sc (no cell number)	Sprague–Dawley rats	Methotrexate	0.5 mg/kg ip on days 11–14			
Ehrlich ascites ip (1 × 10⁶ cells)	ICR mice	Carboquone	1.25 mg/kg ip on day 1 after tumor inoculation	MLV (DSPC)	Significant increase in MST; few long-term survivors	Hisaoka et al., 1982
J-6456 lymphoma iv (10⁶ cells)	BALB/c mice	Adriamycin	6 mg/kg iv on days 3, 10, 17, and 24 after tumor inoculation	SUV (PS:PC:C = 3:7:10)	Increase in MST	Gabezon et al., 1982
Hepatoma 129 ip (10⁶ cells)	C3H mice	Methotrexate	2–3 mg/kg iv or ip on day 1 after tumor inoculation	MLV or SUV (DPPC:C:SA = 34:23:10)	Treatment iv was ineffective: ip treatment increased MST	Patel et al., 1982

[a] Abbreviations used: C, cholesterol; DCP, dicetylphosphate; DPPC, dipalmitoylphosphatidylcholine; DSPC, disteroylphosphatidylcholine; MST, mean survival time; PA, phosphatidic acid; PC, phosphatidylcholine; PS, phosphatidylserine; SA, steroylamine; SM, sphingomyelin.

Successful eradication of metastases demands that therapeutic drug concentrations be achieved in the vicinity of multiple lesions that are often located in different organs.

Intravenous (iv) drug administration presently offers the only practical route of administration for most agents used in treating metastatic disease. In any situation in which a cytotoxic drug is introduced into the circulation, effective therapy requires that the drug reach therapeutic levels in the vicinity of tumor cells. In the case of solid tumors and their metastases growing in extravascular sites, this means that drugs must exist from the circulation and penetrate into the organ parenchyma. In the case of targeted drug delivery in which a drug is associated with a carrier that recognizes the target cell, the intact drug–carrier complex must thus extravasate. As we will see, in the case of particulate drug carriers such as liposomes this is far from guaranteed. Valuable improvements in therapy using particulate drug carriers could still be obtained, however, if ways could be found to achieve selective localization of these vehicles in the vascular bed of tumor-bearing tissues. In this sense they would be used in a fashion analogous to drug delivery via organ catheterization. Although the carrier would remain within the bloodstream, release of entrapped drug would produce high local concentration of drugs. With the exception of organ catheterization, exclusive drug delivery to tumor-bearing organs has yet to be demonstrated.

Drug delivery to metastases disseminated in different organs, including the brain, represents a considerably greater technical challenge than the therapy of most localized tumors. The animal tumor(s) selected for evaluating new antitumor agents should thus attempt to address the problem of metastasis.

Intraperitoneal therapy of a minimal ascites tumor burden localized in the peritoneal cavity does not meet this requirement, since the drug or the drug carrier can gain immediate access to tumor cells without interference from anatomical barriers. Similarly, well-vascularized, transplanted tumors growing sc or im, though more difficult to eradicate than ip tumors, also fail to provide a sufficiently demanding model for evaluating the effectiveness of agents in treating metastases. Implantation of tumor cells into host tissues by injection disrupts the local tissue microvasculature and enhances vascular permeability at the injection site. This effect, which persists until vascular repair is achieved within 2 to 3 days, will affect the efficiency with which materials injected iv localize in the tumor. Administration of drug within 24 to 48 hr of tumor implantation can therefore result in unusually high concentrations of drugs within the tumor. Furthermore, the blood supply of transplanted tumors is established by emigration of new capillary sprouts into the tumor from surrounding host vessels (review in Folkman and Haudenschild, 1981). During this initial angiogenic response, the newly forming capillary sprouts are highly permeable because of gaps between adjacent endothelial cells and open terminal ends. The sprouts allow virtually unlimited passage of materials, including erythrocytes, into the surrounding extravascular tissue (see Folkman and Haudenschild, 1981). Penetration of transplanted tumors by liposomes, antibodies, or other circulating materials may thus be artificially high and provide little or no insight into the behavior of these materials in the vascular bed of human tumors or spontaneous animal tumors, in which the vascular supply will evolve in an entirely different fashion in concert with progressive enlargement of the tumor cell population. In this regard it is of interest to note that circulating liposomes have been reported to localize in a number of transplanted animal tumors, but liposome uptake into a series of histologically diverse human neoplasms was not detected following iv administration (Ryman *et al.*, 1978; Richardson *et al.*, 1979).

In the formation of hematogenous metastases, circulating tumor cells arrest in capillaries, extravasate, and grow initially as pericapillary colonies in the extravascular parenchyma (micrometastases) before the angiogenic response needed to support the additional cell growth and formation of clinically significant metastases occurs (review in Poste and Fidler, 1980). There is no evidence that capillary permeability is drastically altered by tumor cell extravasation in micrometastasis formation. Thus, if liposomes—or any particulate drug carrier—are to gain access to micrometastases, they must cross structurally intact microvessels. As discussed later, there is no evidence to suggest that this can occur on any significant scale.

All animal tumors are flawed in some regard as models for human neoplasms (reviews in Fidler and White, 1982; Poste, 1982). However, this does not mean that an effort should not be made to use models that share as many features as possible with human malignancies. We consider that at a minimum this requires that experimental chemotherapy regimens be evaluated for their activity against established metastases in an adjuvant therapy protocol comparable to that undertaken routinely in the clinic following removal or reduction of the primary tumor.

Our rationale in proposing that experimental therapies be tested for activity against established metastases is not based on the premise that the therapeutic responses of cells in metastases may differ from tumor cells in the primary lesion. The fact that tumors are heterogeneous and contain subpopulations of cells with differing metastatic abilities and responses to therapeutic agents is well documented (reviews in Poste and Fidler, 1980; Owens *et al.*, 1982; Poste, 1982; and Section V,A). However, it is not established that metastatic tumor cell subpopulations exhibit unique responses to therapeutic agents that are not seen in nonmetastatic cells. Both nonmetastatic and metastatic cells appear to display an extraordinary level of diversity in their responses to anticancer drugs, but no correlation with metastatic ability is evident. Consequently, there is no reason to assume that the chemosensitivity of metastatic tumor cell subpopulations could not be determined by merely assaying the response of a heterogeneous tumor cell population containing both metastatic and nonmetastatic cell subpopulations implanted sc or im.

The more compelling rationale for using metastatic tumor models is to establish that the disposition and pharmacokinetics of a drug or a delivery system are consistent with achieving therapeutic drug concentrations in the organs typically affected by metastases in the neoplasm of interest. Since metastases in the same host vary significantly in their size, growth rates, cell growth fraction, and vascular supply, the use of metastatic models also yields useful secondary information about the efficacy of a drug delivery system in circumventing these factors.

Numerous metastatic animal tumors are available that could be used for this purpose (review in Poste, 1982; Poste and Nicolson, 1983). In addition, methods have been described recently that permit reproducible metastasis of human tumor xenografts in nude mice (review in Hanna, 1982), and this approach will probably find increasing use in the testing of new antineoplastic agents.

Most of the concepts just discussed are relevant to the search for new anticancer agents at large and do not apply solely to studies with liposomes. There are, however, features peculiar to liposomes and related particulate drug carriers that affect their usefulness as drug delivery systems. As discussed later, the use of liposomes in drug delivery to cells *within* the bloodstream (Section IV) and in treating lymph node metastases by sc administration (Section IX) appears to offer realistic opportunities for the therapy of certain aspects of neoplastic disease. However, the rationale for the much more widely publicized proposals to use liposomes administered iv to target drugs to tumor cells growing in the extravascular tissues does not withstand critical examination in terms of either current knowledge about the influence of anatomical and physiological factors on liposome disposition *in vivo* or our understanding of the cell biology of malignant tumors. Specifically, proposals to employ targeted liposomes in the therapy of solid tumors growing in extravascular locations have largely failed to ask the basic question whether liposomes administered iv can escape from the bloodstream. A major portion of this chapter will be devoted to this issue (Section IV). Similarly, inadequate attention has been given to the possibility of novel toxicity problems that might result from the altered disposition of liposome-encapsulated antitumor drugs in which high concentrations of cytotoxic drugs are delivered to mononuclear phagocytes in the reticuloendothelial system (RES) and the bone marrow (Section X). In addition to toxicities produced by the direct action of drugs on mononuclear cells involved in clearing liposomes from the bloodstream, the risk of impaired RES and bone marrow function arising from saturation of their clearance capacities induced by multiple dosing also warrants careful attention (Section X). Finally, in common with many other current approaches to drug delivery in cancer therapy, most of the proposed uses of liposomes in cancer therapy do not offer a realistic strategy for dealing with the widely differing responses to therapy displayed by different subpopulations of tumor cells within the same tumor (Section V,A). In a related vein, proposals for targeting liposomes to tumor cells using monoclonal antibodies directed against tumor-associated antigens make little or no mention of how this would be achieved in the face of the extensive antigenic heterogeneity displayed by different tumor cell subpopulations (Section V,B). Many of these problems apply equally, however, to other drug delivery systems. This is particularly true for the so-called particulate drug delivery systems (nanoparticles, microspheres, microbeads), which share many of the advantages and disadvantages of liposomes. However, if particulate drug systems do prove sufficiently effective to stimulate commercial development, liposomes may be at a disadvantage to other particulate systems, which offer tangible advantages with respect to formulation homogeneity, storage stability, and lower production cost (Section XI).

IV. LIPOSOME TARGETING

The clinical appeal and the therapeutic advantage of targeting drugs to different cell types in the body do not need to be stated. Cancer probably represents the most obvious, and is certainly the most quoted, example of a disease in which targeted drug delivery and selective destruction of tumor cells would produce truly dramatic therapeutic gains. It thus comes as no surprise that this goal is a common focal point for most current experimental approaches to drug delivery *in vivo*, whether via liposomes and other particulate carriers or via antibody–drug conjugates or immunotoxins.

We will confine our remarks to the issue of targeting *in vivo*. Development of methods for targeting liposomes to cultured cell populations *in vitro* is considered to be of less value, since in most cases the convenience of working with well-characterized cells in culture enables liposomes to be added directly to the desired target cell. *In vitro* experiments will, of course, be useful in developing methods that might eventually be used *in vivo*. Liposomes bearing cell-specific ligands and liposomes without ligands may interact with cells in entirely different fashions, and it is important to understand how such differences may affect drug uptake and activity. Analysis of such questions is logically undertaken using cultured cells *in vitro*.

Targeting of liposomes (or any carrier) to a specific cell type *in vivo* requires successful completion of several independent steps: (1) access to the appropriate target cell, (2) recognition and selective interaction with the target cell, and (3) selective uptake by the target cell with little or no uptake by nontarget cells. In addition, the liposome–drug combination must not produce unacceptable levels of toxicity, and the drug must remain associated with the liposome for sufficient time to enable therapeutically effective drug concentrations to be delivered to the target cells. Finally, if widespread clinical use and commercial development are ever to occur, the carrier system must be pharmaceutically and clinically acceptable with respect to formulation homogeneity, stability on storage, sterilization, cost of manufacture, and ease of administration.

A distinction will be made in this chapter between passive and active targeting. Both can be exploited therapeutically, but the technical demands of the two approaches are considerably different. The term "passive targeting" refers to the natural localization patterns of liposomes prepared from phospholipids (alone or in combination with cholesterol) when introduced into the body. As discussed in detail later, liposomes injected iv localize predominantly in mononuclear phagocytes of the RES in the liver, spleen, and bone marrow, and in circulating macrophages (monocytes). This distribution pattern can be exploited to target liposomes to these cells, albeit in a passive manner (see Section VII). Similarly, sc or im injection of liposomes results in uptake into lymphatics and significant retention of liposomes within lymph nodes. This offers a way of passively targeting liposomes to lymph nodes for the therapy of lymph node metastases or imaging changes in lymph node architecture (see Section IX). Other examples of passive targeting include instillation into anatomically isolated compartments such as the lung via aerosolization, injection into joint cavities, and introduction into different regions of the urogenital tract. Injection of liposomes into major body cavities could also be viewed as examples of passive mechanical targeting, but liposomes instilled into the peritoneum or the pleural cavity can enter serosal lymphatics and return to the circulation (see Section IX).

The term "active targeting" refers to the experimental strategy of attempting to alter the natural (passive) tissue disposition pattern(s) of liposomes administered by different routes to engineer interaction with specific cells, tissues, or organs that ordinarily have little or no interaction with liposomes. The principal strategy presently advocated for active targeting is to construct liposomes bearing ligands that "recognize" and bind to specific molecular or macromolecular determinants on the surface of the target cell(s). Antibodies have been by far the most popular ligands adopted for this purpose to date (see Section V,B), but attempts to achieve cell-specific targeting *in vivo* using synthetic glycopeptides and glycolipids, glycosylated cholesterol derivatives, asialoglycoproteins, lectins, and virus envelope glycoproteins have also been evaluated (for references, see reviews by Poste, 1980; Gregoriadis *et al.,* 1982a; Widder *et al.,* 1982; Yatvin and Lelkes, 1982; Poste, 1983).

A third strategy for liposome targeting can be classified as "physical targeting." This approach involves construction of liposomes with physicochemical properties that result in breakdown of the liposomal membrane(s) and release of encapsulated drug when exposed to specific environmental conditions such as changes in temperature or pH (review in Yatvin and Lelkes, 1982; and Section VIII).

**Behavior of Liposomes Administered Intravenously:
Implications for Drug Targeting**

1. Localization in Mononuclear Phagocytes

Numerous studies have shown that the majority of liposomes injected iv are
retained in the liver and spleen, irrespective of liposome size, structural class
(unilamellar or multilamellar), or composition (review in Poste, 1983). Tissue
fractionation studies have established that retention of liposomes injected iv in
these organs is due primarily to their uptake by phagocytic reticuloendothelial
(RE) cells that line microvasculature sinusoids in these organs (see Poste, 1983).
In addition to uptake by fixed phagocytes of the RES, liposomes injected iv are
also phagocytized by circulating blood monocytes (Poste *et al.,* 1982).

The rapid clearance of iv-injected liposomes from the bloodstream and their
uptake by RE phagocytes and blood monocytes is analogous to the behavior of
other inert particulate materials when injected iv, including colloidal carbon,
latex beads, erythrocytes, immune complexes, microorganisms, and particulate
drug carriers such as nanoparticles and microspheres (reviews in Altura, 1980;
Donald, 1980; Juliano, 1982; Poste, 1983).

Although liposome composition exerts a significant effect on the rate of
liposome clearance from the circulation (for references, see Gregoriadis *et al.,*
1982b), liposomes with markedly different half-lives within the circulation share
common tissue disposition patterns, localizing primarily in the liver and spleen
(see Poste, 1983). The kinetics of liposome retention in these organs varies
substantially, however, as a result of the different liposome clearance times
(Gregoriadis *et al.,* 1982b).

In discussing the clearance and tissue disposition of liposomes *in vivo,* it is
important to note that a number of seemingly minor technical issues can affect
these two features of liposome behavior *in vivo* and thus represent a potential
source of experimental variation in studies reported by different laboratories.
These factors include (1) purity of phospholipids, (2) size heterogeneity within
liposome preparations, (3) storage conditions, (4) liposome permeability and rate
of leakage of encapsulated material, (5) dose (amount of phospholipid per kilogram of body weight, particles per kilogram of body weight, total surface area of
particles administered), (6) the age, weight, and sex of inoculated animals, and
(7) the exact site of injection. Also, in the case of liposomes injected iv, the
volume of the inoculum, the diluent, and the rate of administration may also
affect the kinetics of liposome clearance from the circulation and their tissue
disposition (see Poste, 1983; Abra and Hunt, 1981, 1982).

Although phagocytic Kupffer cells lining hepatic sinusoids represent the major
site of liposome accumulation *in vivo,* liposomes can also interact with liver

parenchymal cells (hepatocytes). Small sonicated unilamellar liposomes can be taken up by hepatocytes as intact particles (see Poste *et al.*, 1982; Scherphof, 1982; loc cit). In contrast, uptake of intact liposomes of larger size by hepatocytes, if it occurs, is more limited (see Poste *et al.*, 1982; Scherphof, 1982). This is presumed to result from the inability of larger particles to penetrate the gaps in the endothelium lining hepatic sinusoids (see later). Exchange of phospholipids between large MLV liposomes and hepatocytes has been described (see Scherphof, 1982). This can occur either via direct phospholipid exchange or via indirect transfer of liposomal lipids to high-density lipoproteins (HDL), which, in turn, transfer lipid to hepatocytes (Scherphof, 1982). Scherphof and his colleagues have also obtained evidence that suggests that lipids from liposomes taken up by phagocytic Kupffer cells in the liver can be transferred subsequently to hepatocytes (see Scherphof, 1982).

The other major sites of liposome retention after iv injection are the spleen and the bone marrow (Poste, 1983). As discussed later, liposome accumulation in the spleen is enhanced under conditions where hepatic uptake of liposomes is eliminated. Splenic retention thus represents "spillover" of liposomes from the liver. Saturation of the ability of the spleen to retain liposomes results, in turn, in increased "spillover" of liposomes to the bone marrow. Multiple injections of liposomes can eventually "exhaust" the particle retention capacities of liver, spleen, and bone marrow (Poste, 1983; and Section X).

Apart from the reports of uptake of intact small sonicated SUV liposomes by hepatocytes described earlier, there is no evidence of uptake of iv-administered liposomes as intact structures by cells other than mononuclear phagocytes of the RES and circulating blood monocytes.

2. Redistribution of Circulating Liposomes Away from the Mononuclear Phagocyte System

The retention and uptake of criculating liposomes by RE cells and blood monocytes is a major obstacle to experimental efforts to target liposomes to other cell types. This problem has stimulated efforts to devise methods to reduce the localization of liposomes in the RES and blood monocytes with the aim of increasing liposome uptake by other cell types. Two different strategies have been adopted. The first involves efforts to manipulate liposome composition to create liposomes that are cleared less rapidly from the circulation. The second approach has been to attempt to reduce the clearance capacity of the mononuclear phagocyte system by "blockading" the phagocytic uptake mechanisms of these cells by predosing with saturation doses of liposomes or other inert particles.

Small SUV liposomes (<700-Å diameter) are cleared from the circulation more slowly than larger MLV, REV, and LUV liposomes (reviews in Juliano *et al.*, 1983; Poste, 1983). This has led to proposals that SUV liposomes, or perhaps all classes of liposomes that are cleared slowly from the circulation, might be a more effective vehicle for the delivery of therapeutic agents to sites other than the mononuclear phagocyte system (see Gregoriadis *et al.*, 1982b). However, apart from the uptake of SUV liposomes by hepatocytes mentioned earlier, there is no evidence that SUV liposomes, or liposomes with prolonged half-lives in the circulation, accumulate to any significant degree in sites other than the liver, spleen, and bone marrow (Poste, 1983). Although the kinetics of accumulation of such liposomes in the RES is slower, their final tissue disposition is identical to that of large liposomes, which are cleared rapidly from the circulation (Poste, 1983). This, together with the limited internal volume and low encapsulation efficiency of SUV, dictates that there is no compelling reason to accept the view that SUV or liposomes with prolonged circulating half-lives represent the optimal carrier vehicle for drug delivery to sites outside of the RES.

Liposomes with extended half-lives in the circulation as a result of delayed clearance by the RES may still be useful, however, as vehicles for maintaining therapeutic drug levels in cancer therapy and a variety of other drug treatments. By serving as a controlled-release depot for drugs, such liposomes might avoid major fluctuations in drug levels in the blood and the accompanying risks of lack of therapeutic benefit (low drug levels) or toxic side effects (high drug levels).

Liposomal encapsulation of drugs that are rapidly inactivated or degraded by blood components could also provide an effective method for prolonging the biological half-life of labile drugs. The merits of this approach are illustrated by studies with cytosine arabinoside (Ara-C). This drug has a very short half-life in the circulation and must be administered by infusion. Mayhew *et al.* (1982) have shown that iv administration of Ara-C incorporated in liposomes is as effective as a 5-day iv infusion of free Ara-C in treating L1210 tumor cells implanted ip. These results were interpreted by Mayhew *et al.* as indicating that liposomes act by slowly releasing Ara-C in the circulation.

Therapeutic exploitation of liposomes as controlled-release vehicles for antineoplastic agents demands, of course, that liposomes can be constructed with highly reproducible permeability characteristics to ensure that the rate of drug release is consistent with sustaining therapeutic levels of drug in the blood. Ironically, the search for highly stable liposomes with very low permeability characteristics and long circulating half-lives may be of limited value if the rate of drug release is so slow that therapeutic drug levels are never achieved. (See Hunt, 1982, for a fuller discussion of this issue and other aspects of the pharmacokinetics of liposome-associated drugs.)

The second approach that has been explored as a possible way of limiting uptake of iv-injected liposomes by the RES has been to predose animals with liposomes or other inert particles that localize in the RES and thus "blockade" the ability of the RES to take up a second (therapeutic) dose of liposomes given during the period of the RE blockage (Abra *et al.*, 1980; Kao and Juliano, 1981;

Ellens *et al.*, 1982; Proffitt *et al.*, 1983). However, the value of this method in the context of liposome-mediated drug delivery remains equivocal.

Even though a reversible RE blockade can be imposed with relative ease, it is not accompanied by any significant increase in liposome uptake by tissues outside of the mononuclear phagocyte system (Poste, 1983). Also, repeated iv injections of liposomes at regular intervals are accompanied by long-term paralysis of RE function (Poste, 1983; and Section X). Since many of the proposed clinical applications of liposomes would require multiple dosing, this problem represents a potentially serious drawback.

To date, none of the approaches described earlier have been successful in achieving their stated aim of producing major alterations in liposome disposition *in vivo*. Even if the goal of limiting liposome retention in the RES and blood monocytes were to be achieved, the issue of whether liposomes can exit from the circulation to reach target cells in extravascular tissues must still be addressed (see next section).

3. Can Circulating Liposomes Escape from the Microcirculation?

Many of the more ambitious uses proposed for liposomes in drug delivery, and targeted drug delivery in particular, are based on the assumption that after iv injection they can traverse blood vessels to gain access to cells located in extravascular tissues. In view of the crucial importance of this issue in establishing the feasibility of the most frequently cited advantage of liposomes as a drug carrier, it is remarkable that so little attention has been given to this fundamental question. This deficiency probably reflects the considerable technical difficulties involved in answering this question.

a. Liposome–Capillary Interactions in Normal Tissues. The anatomy of the microcirculation in different tissues and organs can reasonably be expected to be of crucial importance in determining whether liposomes can escape into the surrounding extravascular tissue (review in Poste, 1983). The present discussion will be limited to a discussion of possible events in the microcirculation, since it is considered more likely that liposomes injected iv will arrest in capillaries and postcapillary venules rather than in larger vessels. The extensive adventitial elements of venules, arterioles, and larger vessels also probably present too large a mechanical barrier to be breached. Liposome extravasation, in common with the extravasation of circulating blood cells, might thus be expected to be restricted to capillaries and small-diameter postcapillary venules that possess minimal adventitial elements.

Blood capillaries are classified according to the architecture of the lining endothelium and the underlying subendothelial basement membrane (basal lami-

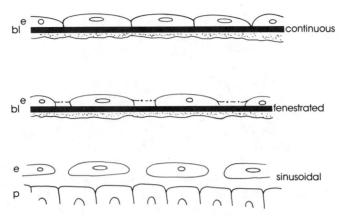

Fig. 1. Schematic illustration of the structure of different classes of blood capillaries. *Continuous capillary:* The endothelium is continuous with tight junctions between adjacent endothelial cells. The subendothelial basement membrane is also continuous. *Fenestrated capillary:* The endothelial cells exhibit a series of fenestrae that are sealed by a membranous diaphragm. The subendothelial basement membrane is continuous. *Discontinuous (sinusoidal) capillary:* The overlying endothelium contains numerous gaps of varying size, enabling materials in the circulation to gain access to the underlying parenchymal cells. The subendothelial basement is either absent (liver) or present as a fragmented interrupted structure (spleen, bone marrow).

na) into three different groups (Fig. 1): continuous capillaries, fenestrated capillaries, and discontinuous or so-called sinusoidal capillaries (reviews in Weiss and Greep, 1977; Wolff, 1977).

In continuous capillaries adjacent endothelial cells adhere via tight junctions to form a ''continuous'' lining. In addition, continuous capillaries typically possess an uninterrupted subendothelial basement membrane. In fenestrated capillaries, the endothelium is interrupted by fenestrae that vary from 300 to 800 Å in diameter. However, with the exception of fenestrated endothelial cells in the renal glomeruli, the fenestrae do not represent simple openings and the fenestrae are spanned by a thin membranous diaphragm (40–60 Å thick) (see Wolff, 1977). As in continuous capillaries, the subendothelial basal lamina in fenestrated capillaries is continuous. The final class of capillaries, the discontinuous (sinusoidal) capillaries, are thin-walled vessels found only in the liver, spleen, and bone marrow. The endothelium in these vessels has large gaps, which may be as large as several thousand angstroms in diameter. In most species the sinusoidal capillaries of the liver lack a basement membrane, but an interrupted basement membrane is present in these vessel in the spleen and the bone marrow (see Weiss and Greep, 1977).

Viewed simply from a mechanical standpoint, it is clear that continuous and fenestrated capillaries represent a major barrier to the escape of liposomes from the circulation. In contrast, liposomes might be expected to penetrate the relatively large gaps in the endothelium in sinusoidal capillaries and thus come into immediate contact with the underlying organ parenchymal cells.

Extravasation of liposomes in organs lined by sinusoidal capillaries would therefore appear to be limited only by the diameter of the gaps in the endothelium. Typically, these gaps in hepatic sinusoids are less than 0.1 μm in diameter (see Morta and Makable, 1980). Small sonicated SUV liposomes should thus be able to pass through such openings, whereas larger liposomes would be retained within the sinusoid. This is supported by the data discussed earlier (Section IV,1). The endothelium of hepatic sinusoids also contains openings larger than 0.1 μm in diameter and which are large enough to allow penetration of MLV, REV, or LUV liposomes. However, the lower frequency of these openings and their irregular distribution within sinusoids dictate that extravasation of large liposomes will probably be less efficient than with SUV liposomes.

Extravasation of materials from the bloodstream in continuous and fenestrated capillaries is more complicated and typically occurs by one of two pathways. The so-called small-pore pathway is limited to materials of <90 Å diameter and thus does not represent an obvious pathway for liposome extravasation, since the smallest SUV are 250–300 Å in diameter.

The so-called large-pore system is permeable to materials up to 700 Å in diameter. In fenestrated capillaries this system is believed to be represented by the fenestrated openings within endothelial cells, but, as emphasized earlier, the presence of a membranous diaphragm in the fenestrations dictates that permeability is not defined simply by the diameter of the fenestration. The permeability of diaphragmed fenestrae appears to vary significantly in different tissues (review in Simionescu and Palade, 1982). Fenestrated capillaries in tissues such as submaxillary gland, renal medulla, pancreas, and intestine are permeable to molecules such as ferritin [Eistein–Stokes radius (ESR) 61 Å]. However, the proportion of intestinal capillaries that are permeable to dextrans of differing sizes (ESR 62.5–100 Å) and glycogens (ESR 110–150 Å) can vary between 20 and 70% (see Simionescu and Palade, 1982). On the other hand, some fenestrated capillaries, such as those in the choriocapillaris, are not permeable to tracers with ESR of >32 Å (Pino and Essner, 1982).

In continuous capillaries, the large-pore permeability pathway is provided by the endothelial vesicle system. Until recently, the predominant view was that vesicles formed at the lumenal surface of endothelial cells and then passed across to the cell to fuse with the ablumenal plasma membrane and discharge their contents. Since endothelial vesicles do not exceed 700 Å diameter, they would not accommodate large MLV or REV liposomes. It is by no means certain, however, that SUV liposomes of less than 700 Å diameter could be transported across capillaries in this system. There is no evidence that the lumenal plasma membrane of endothelial cells is able to "flow" around a liposome (or other particle) bound to the cell surface in the way that actively phagocytic cells such

as macrophages and PMN engulf particles by surrounding them with pseudopo-
dial extensions. Endothelial cells in the liver, spleen, and newly formed capillaries exhibit significant phagocytic activities, but most endothelial cells do not
(review in Weiss and Greep, 1977). Consequently, uptake and transport of
materials via the endothelial vesicle system may be limited to materials whose
diameter does not exceed the width of the "neck" (diameter 60–100 Å) at the
opening of a vesicle at the lumenal surface. If this is correct then even the
smallest SUV liposomes would be too large to be transported by this pathway.

Additional doubts about the size of materials that can enter endothelial vesicles
have been raised as a result of recent studies suggesting that endothelial vesicles
may not be a dynamic system as proposed originally, in which new vesicles are
formed constantly at the lumenal surface, internalized, and translocated to the
ablumenal surface to undergo exocytotic fusion. Careful three-dimensional mor-
phometric studies using serial sections suggest that vesicles are static structures
(review in Bungaard, 1983). Additional evidence suggesting that lumenal vesicles are static and open to the vessel lumen via a constricted channel comes from
studies showing that tracers are taken up by vesicles under conditions where
membrane internalization should not occur. For example, vesicles in fixed
tissues take up tracers, as do vesicles in tissues exposed to anoxia, metabolic
poisons, or low temperature (for references, see Bungaard, 1983).

While these new findings do not exclude the contribution of endothelial vesicles as a pathway for macromolecular transport, the possibility of particles such
as liposomes being transported in this system seems remote, since access to such
vesicles will be limited by the size of the channel (diameter, 60–100 Å) by which
the vesicles open to the vessel lumen.

From this brief review of capillary structure, it is evident that at least for
continuous and fenestrated capillaries, it might be predicted on the basis of
theoretical considerations alone, that there are major anatomical barriers that can
hinder the escape of circulating liposomes into the surrounding extravascular
tissues. Experimental evidence to support this interpretation has been obtained in
our laboratory (Poste, 1983; Poste et al., 1982, 1983b).

The capacity of liposomes to cross continuous capillaries has been studied by
analyzing extravasation of small sonicated SUV liposomes (mean diameter of
600 Å) and MLV liposomes (diameter 0.4 μm) containing encapsulated [125]I-
labeled bovine serum albumin (^{125}I-BSA) in the microcirculation of the mouse
lung (Poste et al., 1982). Extravasation of MLV liposomes injected iv was
assayed by their presence within pulmonary macrophages recovered from pulmonary alveoli by bronchial lavage. However, studies in which the blood monocyte
populations of mice were depleted experimentally demonstrated that liposomes
were unable to exit from pulmonary capillaries but were instead engulfed within
the bloodstream by blood monocytes that subsequently migrated into the alveoli
(Poste et al., 1982). Similar passive translocation of MLV within macrophages

could presumably provide a mechanism for liposome extravasation in other tissues where the anatomy of the microcirculation impedes extravasation of free liposomes.

Further evidence for the inability of liposomes to cross continuous capillaries in the lung has been obtained using classical methods of monitoring capillary permeability. Extravasation of materials from circulating blood in the lung can be measured by recovery and analysis of lung lymph (review in Dawson *et al.*, 1982). By measuring the concentration of a marker molecule in the blood and in pulmonary lymph, it is possible to measure capillary permeability, to identify dynamic changes in capillary permeability, and to distinguish whether the increase in permeability is due to enhanced hydrostatic pressure (filtration) or leakage. Using a heart–lung perfusion preparation, we have examined the ability of SUV and MLV liposomes containing ^{125}I-BSA to cross pulmonary capillaries and be recovered in the lymph (Poste, 1983; Poste *et al.*, 1983b). In this system no extravasation of liposome-associated ^{125}I-BSA was detected even under conditions in which significant extravasation of unencapsulated (free) ^{125}I-BSA occurred as a result of elevated hydrostatic pressure induced by increasing left atrial pressure via an indwelling balloon catheter (or by administration of vasoactive drugs that increase capillary leakage).

Continuous capillaries in other tissues are equally impermeable to liposomes. Using isolated perfused preparations of cat gastrocnemius muscle, we have failed to detect extravasation of either SUV or MLV liposomes (see Poste *et al.*, 1983a).

Analogous organ perfusion techniques have also been used to evaluate the permeability of fenestrated capillaries in dog colon and cat submandibular gland to SUV or MLV liposomes containing ^{125}I-BSA. Liposome extravasation was not detected in either tissue (see Poste, 1983; Poste *et al.*, 1983b).

These observations indicate that liposomes are probably unable to exist from the microcirculation in organs lined with either continuous capillaries (skeletal, smooth, and cardiac muscles, connective tissue, central nervous system, exocrine pancreas, gonads, lung) or fenestrated capillaries (most exocrine and endocrine glands, gastrointestinal tract, renal glomeruli and peritubular capillaries, choroid plexus). Although permeability measurements have not been made on capillaries in all of these tissues, the data described earlier from studies on capillaries in lung, skeletal muscle, gut, and salivary gland at least confirm experimentally what might reasonably be predicted on mechanical considerations, namely that the endothelial lining and/or the continuous basal lamina found in these classes of capillaries represent major anatomical barriers to liposome extravasation.

Hwang *et al.* (1982) have claimed that SUV (diameter 200 Å; sphingomyelin:cholesterol ratio 2:1) can pass across capillaries in the stomach, intestine, and skin. This claim was advanced on the basis of evidence showing gradual accumulation of liposome-derived ^{111}In in the intestine, stomach, and skin over a period of several days. However, this study did not establish whether the radioactivity in these tissues was associated with intact liposomes, and the question whether intact liposomes had entered the extravascular compartment cannot therefore be answered. Furthermore, the increase in liposome-derived radioactivity in the gut is as likely to represent biliary excretion of encapsulated material from liposomes taken up and broken down within the liver. In agreement with our previous findings (Poste *et al.*, 1982), these investigators found no evidence of liposome extravasation in the lung or in skeletal muscle.

The most zealous protagonists of liposome targeting will probably continue to argue that until similar capillary permeability measurements are made on *all* tissues using liposomes of the smallest size and of endlessly variable composition, the feasibility of targeting liposomes to extravascular tissues cannot be totally discounted. This is undoubtedly true, but the evidence available to date argues against this possibility. Until experimental data are obtained showing that liposomes can successfully cross continuous or fenestrated capillaries in a particular tissue, we consider that proposals for targeting liposomes to parenchymal cells in the extravascular compartment of tissues lined by these two classes of capillaries should be viewed with considerable skepticism. Extravasation of liposomes from continuous or fenestrated capillaries may be occurring on a limited scale below the detection limits of the assay methods used in the foregoing experiments. Even if this is the case, the more important issue is whether such low levels of extravasation could be exploited therapeutically.

The preceding discussion refers only to situations in which the endothelial lining retains its structural integrity. In inflammation and ischemia this is not guaranteed, and such conditions may alter endothelial cell architecture and, in turn, affect vessel permeability (see Section IV,3,b). Arrest of very large liposomes or large aggregates of liposomes within a capillary could conceivably impair blood flow downstream. The resulting hypoxia could evoke reversible retraction of endothelial cells downstream (see Nicolson and Poste, 1983) and allow particles comparable in size to liposomes to extravasate.

That liposomes can occasionally pass through the junctional spaces between organized endothelial cells and reach the underlying basement membrane is demonstrated by the work of Lubec *et al.* (1981). These investigators presented electron microscopic evidence showing penetration of positively charged MLV (PC:SA:C) between adjacent glomerular endothelial cells in the rat kidney. However, the frequency of this phenomenon was not quantified, and occurrence of the same phenomenon in capillaries of other organs was not examined. Once again, however, the issue is not so much whether penetration of the endothelium may occur in particular tissues and/or certain conditions, but rather whether it occurs with sufficient frequency to be useful therapeutically.

Even if penetration of endothelial cells by liposomes were taking place on a significant scale, the question then arises whether liposomes can penetrate the subendothelial basement membrane. In the study by Lubec *et al.* (1981) cited earlier, liposomes were observed between and beneath endothelial cells, but no examples were seen of liposomes that had penetrated the basement membrane or the surrounding adventitial elements to reach the extravascular compartment.

Ultrastructural studies using electron-dense tracers of differing molecular weights and known Einstein–Stokes radii have shown convincingly that the subendothelial basement membrane in continuous and fenestrated capillaries provides a highly efficient barrier to the penetration of materials whose ESR are considerably lower than the diameter of the smallest SUV liposomes (reviews in Weiss and Greep, 1977; Fishman, 1982). Clearly, blood-borne materials, including cells and motile parasitical larvae, can cross subendothelial basement membranes. Current concepts of basement membranes interpret these structures as representing fully hydrated gels with thixotropic properties that undergo gel–sol transformations in response to localized deforming pressures to create "sol" channels that allow materials to pass (review in Simpson, 1981). As fully hydrated gels, thixotropic basement membranes would be freely permeable to water, small solutes, and low molecular weight drugs, which can pass through the lattice in its fully hydrated "gel" state. In contrast, passage of larger molecules and cells requires that they induce localized deformation of the lattice to cause transformation to the "sol" phase. In the case of cells, this would be induced by the cell's own motile activity. However, for macromolecules and inert particles such as liposomes that lack active, energy-dependent motility systems, passage would be possible only if pulsatile intracapillary pressure was adequate to initiate local deformation of the basement membrane (see Simpson, 1981).

The energy of deformation needed to induce a gel–sol transformation in a local area of sufficient size to permit entry of even the smallest liposomes would be greater than that needed to create similar "sol" zones for smaller plasma proteins. Consequently, it seems likely that the intracapillary pressure conditions necessary to induce successful transit of liposomes across the basement membrane would simultaneously render the vessel highly permeable to a variety of blood macromolecules. The experiments described earlier using the heart–lung preparation indicates that leakage of this kind does not occur, since the lymph:plasma protein ratio remains stable after iv infusion of liposomes (Poste, 1983). This suggests that normal vascular hemodynamics are not sufficient to serve as a "driving force" to induce thixotropic deformation of endothelial basement membrane on the scale needed to permit extravasation of liposomes.

b. Liposome–Capillary Interaction at Sites of Inflammation and Ischemia.
It is well known that capillary permeability increases significantly during inflammation (review in Gabbiani and Majno, 1980). However, studies in our laborato-

ry using the granuloma pouch assay to monitor the permeability of vessels in an inflammatory lesion have revealed that liposomes do not extravasate even under conditions in which extensive macromolecular leakage occurs (Poste, 1983; Poste et al., 1983b).

There is evidence, however, that capillaries at sites of tissue ischemia become permeable to liposomes. Occlusion of the coronary arteries in dogs or guinea pigs for various intervals has been shown to cause preferential accumulation of iv-injected liposomes in the resulting areas of ischemic myocardium (Caride and Zaret, 1977; Wikman-Coffelt et al., 1980; Mueller et al., 1981). Similar accumulation of circulating liposomes at sites of ischemia has been reported in the rat intestine following experimental ligation of the mesenteric artery (Palmer et al., 1981). Electron microscopic studies of ischemic myocardium reveal liposomes in both intravascular and extravascular locations (Mueller et al., 1981). Damage to capillaries was evident as shown by swelling, distortion, and retraction of endothelial cells and structural abnormalities in the underlying basement membrane. These changes, albeit of a nonspecific nature, would be expected to enhance capillary permeability to liposomes and many other circulating materials. This is consistent with previous studies showing that a wide range of low and high molecular weight solutes, drugs, and particulate materials such as colloidal carbon will accumulate in the ischemic myocardium (for references, see Mueller et al., 1981).

c. Liposome–Capillary Interactions in Tumors. Even though extravasation of circulating liposomes from the microcirculation may prove to be a major limitation in targeting liposomes in tissues with a normal vascular supply, proponents of liposome-mediated drug delivery in cancer therapy have speculated that targeted drug delivery to tumors may still be possible because of the enhanced vascular permeability found in tumors. This argument is not confined to advocates of liposome targeting and is voiced with equal conviction by proponents of other targeted drug delivery systems such as immunotoxins and drug–antibody conjugates.

The factors affecting the localization and retention of circulating materials in tumors are complex, variable, unpredictable, and poorly understood (reviews in Peterson, 1979; Anghileri, 1982). Most of the available information on this topic has come from studies of the localization of radiopharmaceuticals and antitumor antibodies employed in tumor imaging, and from studies with labeled cells and particulates used in estimating the volume of the vascular bed in tumors (review in Anghileri, 1982). The following are among the more important factors in determining the efficiency with which materials introduced into the circulation localize in tumors: total blood flow, tissue perfusion rates and pressure, the properties of the circulating material(s), microvascular architecture and permeability, and the properties of the tumor cells.

The only safe conclusion that can be drawn from the large body of experimental data accumulated over the last 20 years is that any generalization about the role of these factors is likely to be overly simplistic and that predictions about vascular hemodynamics in any given tumor are highly imprecise. Total blood flow, rates of perfusion, and the efficiency with which circulating materials localize in tumors can vary considerably in tumors of similar histological origin and clinical staging in different patients, in different regions of the same tumor, and in different metastases in the same host. Also, as emphasized earlier, the structure and function of the vascular supply in tumors transplanted sc or im may be completely different from spontaneous tumors and metastases. Furthermore, the vascular system in these different types of lesions is not static and will change during progressive tumor growth and after therapeutic assault.

In common with other tissues, tumors have an arterial supply, a capillary network to distribute blood, and a venous drainage system. Except where they are invaded by neoplastic cells or compressed by expanding masses of tumor cells, the arteries of tumors show minimal or no structural changes from their normal counterparts (Willis, 1973). Structural changes in venous structures of tumors are more common. Invasion of veins is an almost universal finding in malignant tumors (review in Willis, 1973), and foci of necrotic endothelial cells are not uncommon in tumor venules (see Dvorak *et al.*, 1980).

It is in the structure of capillaries that tumors show the most dramatic departure from the vascular anatomy of normal tissues. The microvessels found in tumors fall into four general classes: continuous, discontinuous, sinusoidal blood channels, and giant capillaries (Fig. 2). Continuous capillaries of tumors are the most like normal microvessels. They are lined by an uninterrupted sheet of endothelial cells joined by typical tight junctions and resting on a well-formed basement membrane that is sometimes reduplicated (Papadimitriou and Woods,

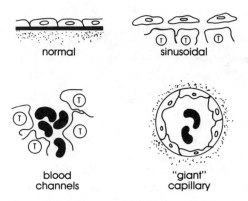

Fig. 2. Schematic illustration of the structure of different types of capillaries and other microvessels commonly found in neoplastic tissue (see text for description).

1975; Dvorak *et al.*, 1980). Continuous capillaries in tumors are usually supported by incomplete layers of pericytes and bundles of collagen fibers. An increased frequency of fenestrated endothelial cells has also been reported in certain tumor microvessels (see Ward *et al.*, 1974; loc. cit.), but such vessels usually possess a continuous subendothelial basement membrane that will present a substantial mechanical barrier to extravasation of liposomes and other particulate materials.

Discontinuous capillaries have an incomplete endothelial lining with the endothelial cells lying on a continuous or fragmented basement membrane (Cavallo *et al.*, 1973; Warren, 1979), reminiscent of capillaries in areas of inflammation (Majno and Palade, 1961). Alternatively, the lumen can be lined almost exclusively by tumor cells, with only scattered endothelial cells (see Warren, 1979). Newly forming capillaries may also be grouped in this category, because they commonly have large gaps between adjacent endothelial cells (see Cavallo *et al.*, 1973). Blood can also circulate within tumors through vascular channels lined exclusively by tumor cells (T, Fig. 2) rather than endothelial cells. The circulation pattern in this type of vessel is such that blood simply percolates around solid cords of tumor cells (see Warren, 1979).

The so-called giant capillaries are common at the growing edge of tumors, and their lumen may exceed 50 μm in diameter. Although such vessels may easily be confused with venules on histological analysis, ulstrastructural studies have shown that they are composed only of a single layer of endothelial cells with little or no supporting connective tissue and thus warrant classifcation as capillaries.

On mechanical grounds alone, the discontinuous capillaries and blood channels found in tumors represent sites at which circulating materials have ample opportunity to penetrate into the extravascular space. What is not known, and cannot be predicted with any measure of accuracy for any given tumor, is what fraction of the total tumor vasculature is composed of these highly permeable vessels. Even within the same tumor, structurally normal capillaries can be observed in close proximity to abnormal vessels (review in Warren, 1979). Although structural defects in a proportion of vessels might be useful in allowing liposomes containing antitumor agents to gain access to tumor cells, the presence of many normal vessels in other portions of the same tumor will probably ensure that a significant number of tumor cells will remain inaccessible to liposomes injected iv.

In discussing the feasibility of targeting any drug carrier to tumors, it is important that changes in the vascular permeability within tumors not be overstated, since the alterations are relative, and unlimited permeability is found only in a minor group of microvessels with marked structural changes.

Success in using imaging agents for tumor angiography and measurements of the vascular volume of tumors using radiolabeled erythrocytes and microspheres both rely on the fact that these materials will not escape from tumor vessels into the extravascular compartment. This is well illustrated by the behavior of sodium diatrizoate (M_r 600), an X-ray contrast medium commonly used in angiography, which circulates unbound to plasma proteins yet does not rapidly extravasate into tumor tissue (Abrams, 1961).

The kinetics of partition of molecules between the intra- and extravascular compartments are also relevant to the present discussion. Once again, great variability is the rule, as illustrated by the following examples. Goldacre and Sylvén (1962) found that the dye Lissamine green extravasated within as little as 30 sec in both normal and tumor tissues following iv injection. However, certain areas were commonly seen in tumors that were found to contain large numbers of viable tumor cells but failed to stain at any time after dye infusion. Gullino and Grantham (1964) found that high molecular weight (500,000) dextran took between 1 and 5 hr to appear in the interstitial fluid of a series of rat tumors. Underwood and Carr (1977) observed that while extensive leakage of Evans blue into the extravascular compartment of a transplanted rat sarcoma occurred within 1 hr after iv injection, extravasation of particles of colloidal carbon (diameter 30 nm) or saccharated iron (diameter 3–10 nm) did not occur. Extravasation of the latter, but not the former, could be elicited by intratumoral injection of histamine.

The most definitive and comprehensive analysis of the permeability of tumor blood vessels completed to date is provided by the work of Peterson and his colleagues (review in Peterson, 1979). Their elegant studies on the partition between blood and tumor tissue of radiolabeled molecules of differing molecular weights indicate that although tumors in general may display a higher permeability to plasma proteins than normal tissues, considerable barriers to free permeation exist in a significant fraction of the tumor vasculature.

Even tumor microvessels that lack an endothelial cell lining do not necessarily represent sites of unrestricted permeability. Martinez-Palomo (1970) examined the permeability of junctions between adjacent tumor cells in the blood channels within several rat and mouse tumors. Using colloidal lanthanum as an ultrastructural probe of junctional permeability, he found that while many junctions allowed greater penetration of lanthanum than endothelial junctions in normal vessels, others were identified that completely excluded lanthanum. Although termed colloidal lanthanum, the probe used by Martinez-Palomo has been found by others to be largely ionic in nature (Schatzki and Newsome, 1975). That some junctional areas are able to exclude an ionic probe also argues against the likelihood of free passage of particulates. Penetration of circulating particulate materials into the extravascular compartment of tumors can occur, however, as shown by Long et al. (1978) for fluorocarbon emulsions and by Bugelski et al. (1983a) for aggregates formed between ionic lanthanum and serum proteins.

Detailed information on the permeability of tumor vessels to liposomes is lacking. Several studies have reported significant localization of iv-administered liposomes in tumors implanted sc or im (Gregoriadis and Neerunjun, 1975; Gregoriadis *et al.*, 1977; Yatvin *et al.*, 1982; Proffitt *et al.*, 1983; loc cit), but a systematic analysis of the effect of liposome size, composition, dose, and tumor characteristics on liposome localization and retention in solid tumors has still to be undertaken.

The data just reviewed indicate that the permeability of the microcirculation in tumors is often greater than that found in normal tissues, but this is a highly variable and unpredictable element of tumor physiology. Enhanced vascular permeability in tumors is still relative, however, and free access of circulating materials to the extravascular interstitium is not found, even for serum proteins. Inorganic colloids and proteins that have effective diameters of the order of 30 nm (e.g., colloidal carbon and IgM) have only limited access to the extracellular space of tumors and localize rapidly within the RES (Dobson and Jones, 1982). Since the smallest SUV liposomes have typical diameters of 25 to 35 nm, it seems likely that only a small fraction of such liposomes would have the opportunity to extravasate in tumors before being cleared by the RES. Larger liposomes are cleared even more rapidly by the RES and will thus have an even lower probability of extravasation. Blockade of the RES by predosing with liposomes or other particulate materials can increase the opportunities for the localization of SUV liposomes in tumors (see Proffitt *et al.*, 1983). However, as discussed in more detail in Section X, this strategy is clinically unacceptable for two reasons. First, effective therapy of tumors will almost certainly involve a multiple dosing protocol, whether liposome-encapsulated drug or some other treatment is employed. If RES blockade must be imposed before each liposome treatment, this introduces additional risk in that repeated blockade can impair both RES function and bone marrow hematopoiesis (Section X). Second, even under conditions of RES blockade, a higher concentration of liposome-associated drug may still accumulate in macrophages of the RES than in unblockaded animals treated with free drug (for example, see Table 1 in Proffitt *et al.*, 1983). This altered drug disposition may be of little consequence for many classes of drugs, but for the highly cytotoxic agents used in cancer therapy this can cause destruction of the RES (see Section X).

In debating the fading prospects for successful targeting of circulating liposomes to extravascular sites, advocates of the concept argue that ways might still be found to render vessels permeable to liposomes. Such methods could probably be devised, but for what purpose and at what risk? It is difficult to envisage how any selectivity could be imposed on this process and how it could be localized to the microcirculation of interest. Vessels "permeabilized" for this purpose may instead become highly leaky for a wide array of macromolecules that do not ordinarily penetrate into the extravascular space (and should not). In our opinion such proposals are naive and pose the risk of significant toxicity. Even if this questionable strategy were pursued and methods developed to allow safe "permeabilization'' of limited regions of the microvasculature in specific tissues and organs,.this remarkable achievement would virtually eliminate the need for using liposomes as drug carriers, since free drug would also be able to extravasate in larger amounts.

V. TUMOR CELL HETEROGENEITY AND CANCER THERAPY

A. Variation in the Responsiveness of Tumor Cells to Antineoplastic Drugs

The phenotypic heterogeneity of tumor cell subpopulations coexisting within the same tumor is probably the single most important factor contributing to the current lack of success in treating many solid malignancies. Malignant tumors are not uniform entities populated by cells with identical properties but instead contain multiple subpopulations of cells with diverse phenotypes, including metastatic properties and responses to antineoplastic agents (reviews in Owens *et al.,* 1982; Poste, 1982; Poste and Greig, 1982). Liposome-mediated drug delivery presently offers no tangible advantage over other approaches in addressing this vexing problem. Even if liposomes containing a single drug or several antitumor drugs do prove to be more effective than the free drug(s) in treating certain tumors, the probability is still high that drug-resistant tumor cell subpopulations will be present in the tumor and will survive to produce recurrent disease.

Consequently, whether liposomes or any other delivery systems are adopted, the only successful therapeutic strategy will be one that can circumvent the diverse chemosensitivities of different tumor cell subpopulations present in any given tumor. Current strategies to achieve this goal fall into two nonexclusive categories.

The first involves the use of multiple antineoplastic agents in an effort to address the presence of multiple subpopulations of cells with widely differing sensitivities to drugs and other therapeutic modalities coexisting in the same lesion. Logically, the trend is toward the use of increasingly large combinations of drugs.

The second strategy attempts to limit the emergence of drug-resistant subpopulations by reducing the rate at which new subpopulations of cells with variant phenotypes are generated. Among the concepts being explored in this context are accelerated staging of multiagent therapy (see Poste and Greig, 1982; Nicolson and Poste, 1983) and the use of short cycles of alternating multiagent therapy instead of administering the same agents in nonalternating, sequential fashion (see Goldie, 1983).

Neither of these strategies precludes the use of liposome-associated drugs.

However, given the trend toward multiagent therapy, the effectiveness of liposomes as a drug delivery vehicle must be compatible with this type of protocol, whether liposomes are used to deliver one, some, or all of the drugs in the protocol.

B. Antigenic Heterogeneity of Tumor Cells and Antibody-Mediated Drug Targeting

The appeal of antibodies as a means of targeting drugs to specific cell types *in vivo* has long been recognized (Ehrlich, 1906). The feasibility of this approach could not be explored fully before because of the highly variable properties of polyclonal antisera obtained from immunized animals. However, with the advent of hybridoma technology, this situation has changed dramatically. Highly purified monoclonal antibodies of defined class and antigen specificity can now be produced in virtually unlimited quantities, and the range of antigens to which monoclonal antibodes are commercially available is growing rapidly. Antibodies to tumor cell surface antigens have attracted considerable interest because of their possible value in cancer diagnosis and in targeting drugs, toxins, and other therapeutic agents to tumor cells (reviews in McMichael and Fabre, 1982; Baldwin and Pimm, 1983; Levy and Miller, 1983). Antibody-mediated targeting of liposomes is a logical extension of this concept, and several methods have been described for covalent coupling of intact antibody molecules or antibody fragments to the outer bilayer of liposomes (review in Leserman *et al.*, 1983).

Despite its theoretical simplicity, major practical problems have still to be solved before antibody-mediated targeting of drugs and drug carriers can fulfill its therapeutic promise. Few of these problems are unique to antibody-mediated targeting of liposomes and apply equally to any situation in which antibodies are used therapeutically, either as cytotoxic molecules in their own right or as targeting ligands for covalently bound drugs or toxins.

The first, and obvious, requirement is for antibodies that recognize tumor-associated antigens and that display little or no cross-reactivity with normal cells. With the exception of idiotypes on B-cell tumors, such antigens have not yet been found. A large panel of antibodies to tumor-associated antigens have now been described that have a high affinity for tumor cells in histologically diverse neoplasms but that also show varying reactivity with the normal tissues from which the tumors arose (see Levy and Miller, 1983). This lack of absolute specificity may prove to be only a temporary technical difficulty, and by expanding the number of hybridoma clones examined, it might be possible to identify antibodies with the desired selectivity for tumor cells.

Less optimism can be expressed, however, about how antibody-mediated targeting will overcome the problem of antigenic heterogeneity among tumor cells within the same tumor. Studies in many laboratories have revealed quantiative and qualitative differences in the tumor-associated antigens expressed by different tumor cell subpopulations both within the primary tumor and in different metastases (reviews in Poste and Fidler, 1980; Poste, 1982; Baldwin and Pimm, 1983). Also, neoplasms of seemingly similar histological origin in different patients can exhibit different patterns of antigen expression (see Mazauric *et al.*, 1982). The available evidence thus suggests that for monoclonal antibodies to be effective in directing drugs to tumor cells, whether bound to liposomes or as drug–antibody conjugates, it will be necessary to use a large panel of antibodies, and that different antibody panels would be required in treating different patients. Whether a single antibody or multiple antibodies are chosen, antigenic modulation and immunoselection of tumor cell variants that lack the antigen(s) in question represent real risks. (See Olsson, 1983, for a critical discussion of these problems and their implications for the use of monoclonal antibodies in cancer therapy.) Observations reported by Webb *et al.* (1983) also raise the troubling possibility that the risk of antigenic modulation may be greater in cells exposed to a panel of antibodies rather than to a single antibody. They found that two antigens (Pro 3 and Pro 5) expressed by human prostate carcinoma cells were not modulated by exposure to monoclonal antibodies directed against either antigen alone, but both antigens modulated rapidly following treatment with a mixture of the two antibodies.

Intravenous infusion of monoclonal antibodies has been reported to eliminate leukemia cells from the bloodstream in both humans and animals (review in Levy and Miller, 1983), but access of antibodies to solid tumors and their metastases situated in extravascular locations may be far less efficient. The efficiency of tissue penetration will be even lower in antibody-mediated targeting of particles such as liposomes that are too large to extravasate.

Free-antigen blockade poses another potential drawback to antibody-mediated drug targeting *in vivo* (see Levy and Miller, 1983). Preliminary evidence suggests that antibody molecules covalently bound to liposomes are less susceptible than free antibody to inhibition by blocking antigens (Bragman *et al.*, 1983), but further studies using a variety of antibodies are needed to establish whether this is a general feature of antibodies bound to liposomes.

Repeated infusion of antibodies also carries the risk of eliciting anti-idiotypic antibodies, which may not only block the interaction of the original antibody with its target cell but also increase the risk of adverse hypersensitivity reactions during subsequent antibody treatments (see Levy and Miller, 1983).

The shortcomings listed earlier are common to all efforts to use antibodies as therapeutic agents, either as cytotoxic molecules in their own right or as ligands conjugated to drugs, toxins, or particulate drug carriers such as liposomes. However, antibody-mediated targeting of liposomes and other particulate carriers poses additional problems. Covalent addition of a targeting antibody to liposomes will not enhance their ability to escape from the circulation, and this issue thus remains a major limitation in the targeting of liposomes to solid tumors or to organ parenchymal cells by iv administration. In fact, coupling of antibodies to liposomes may result in even more rapid clearance by the RES and circulating monocytes if antibodies are coupled in a way that leaves the Fc region exposed and available to bind to Fc receptors on these cells. In the case of liposomes containing cytotoxic drugs, inadvertent targeting to Fc receptor-bearing cells can result in destruction of important host defense functions (Section X).

Another unexpected complication in the use of antibodies to target liposomes containing drugs to tumor cells has been revealed in the elegant studies of Leserman and his colleagues (Machy *et al.*, 1982, 1983). These investigators examined the targeting of liposomes containing methotrexate (MTX) to mouse T and B lymphocytes using a series of monoclonal antibodies directed against three different cell surface antigens. Binding and uptake of liposomes by the same cell type was found to differ significantly depending on the target cell antigen selected. Liposomes directed against the same target antigen on B and T cells also exhibited significantly different binding and internalization patterns. Of most interest, however, was the finding that liposome uptake by the same cell type was significantly different when monoclonal antibodies directed against different epitopes on the same target cell antigen were used as targeting ligands. Although these experiments were undertaken with liposomes, there is no a priori reason to conclude that similar phenomena may not be operating in other examples of antibody-mediated drug targeting such as drug–antibody conjugates and immunotoxins.

Other studies by the same investigators have shown that small SUV liposomes of 800 Å diameter are more effective in delivering MTX to mouse spleen cells when targeted via monoclonal antibodies to H-2K^k surface antigens than larger liposomes (diameter 2000–4000 Å) targeted to the same antigen (Machy and Leserman, 1983). Since the total volume of encapsulated drug bound to cells is greater for the larger liposomes, and the therapeutic action of the drug is proportional to the amount internalized, these data suggest that small liposomes may be a more suitable vehicle for drug delivery. However, further studies will be needed to establish if similar relationships are valid for drug delivery by liposomes targeted to different surface antigens or when different antibodies directed against the same target antigen are used.

These findings introduce an additional level of technical complexity to the task of antibody-mediated targeting. It now becomes necessary to establish not only that the targeting antibody has the desired target cell specificity but also that on binding to the target antigen it can stimulate cellular uptake of the antibody–drug/toxin or antibody–carrier complex.

The issues reviewed in this section, together with the low extravasation efficiency of liposomes injected iv, suggest that the prospects for antibody-mediated targeting of liposomes to solid tumors in extravascular sites are extremely poor. Antibody-mediated targeting of liposomes to cells within the bloodstream (Section VI) or lympth nodes (Section IX) remains feasible, but it is clear that substantial technical problems must still be overcome before this approach would be suitable for routine clinical use.

VI. LIGAND-DIRECTED TARGETING OF LIPOSOMES
WITHIN THE VASCULAR COMPARTMENT

Even though the anatomy of the microcirculation seems likely to frustrate targeting of liposomes to cells outside of the vasculature in most tissues and organs, significant opportunities may nonetheless exist for targeting liposomes to cell types within the vasculature. These opportunities fall into four different groups: (1) passive targeting to the RES, (2) active targeting to circulating tumor cells and tumor cells in the bone marrow, (3) active targeting to specific subsets of circulating blood cells, and (4) active targeting to vascular endothelial cells.

Passive targeting of liposomes injected iv to the RES and to blood monocytes will be discussed in the next section.

The key issue in *active* targeting of liposomes to cells other than mononuclear phagocytes within the vascular system is whether uptake of liposomes by the RES and circulating monocytes can be avoided. By comparison, the availability of appropriate recognition ligands for such cells may prove less of a problem. As our knowledge of the surface properties of specific cell expands, a panel of cell-specific surface determinants will almost certainly become available. As outlined in the following, this process has already begun.

The more critical issue, at least for the immediate future, is how liposomes bearing such ligands could be prevented from localizing in mononuclear phagocytes. It is possible, of course, that equipping liposomes with ligands that have a high affinity for cells other than the RES or blood monocytes may be sufficient to achieve this goal. As emphasized in the last section, this is by no means certain. Any exposure of Fc regions in antibody molecules used as targeting ligands will result in rapid clearance of liposomes via their binding to Fc receptors on circulating monocytes and RE cells.

Remarkable progress has been made over the last few years using monoclonal antibodies and other immunological probes to classify the major classes of circulating blood cells into subsets bearing defined differentiation antigens (reviews in Greaves *et al.* 1981; Olsson, 1983). The rapid pace of discovery in this subject area continues, and further subdivision of current subsets of cells into even more detailed classification schemes will almost certainly occur. These cell surface markers represent potential target molecules for ligand-directed targeting of liposomes (and also other drug carriers). Monoclonal antibodies currently repre-

sent the major class of ligand available for this purpose. However, as biochemical characterization of the surface properties of defined subsets of blood
cells progresses, additional ligands such as drugs and hormones will probably be
identified.

The ability to direct liposomes containing therapeutic agents to specific subsets of circulating blood cells in the bloodstream and in the bone marrow has
many potential clinical applications. One obvious example would be to exploit
the abnormal expression of lymphocyte differentiation antigens on leukemia cells
as target molecules for ligand-directed targeting of liposomes containing anticancer drugs. The feasibility of using these molecules for selective drug targeting
has already been demonstrated in studies using immunotoxins (Youhle and Neville, 1980; Raso *et al.* 1982; loc cit). Even if liposomes can be targeted successfully to specific subsets of lymphocytes, or other circulating blood cells, subsets
may differ significantly in their capacity to internalize liposomes bound to the
cell surface (see Machy *et al.,* 1982; and Section V,B).

Ligand-directed targeting of liposomes to vascular endothelial cells also merits
investigation. The antigens and drug receptors expressed by endothelial cells
may vary quantitatively and qualitatively in different regions of the vascular tree
(see Poste, 1983). These observations raise the possibility that these molecules
could serve as targets in ligand-directed localization of liposomes to specific
regions of the vasculature. As in the case of circulating blood cells, new information on the expression of differentiation antigens and other cell surface molecules
on endothelial cells will emerge in the next few years. This knowledge could
create fascinating opportunities for site-specific targeting of drugs within the
vascular system.

VII. PASSIVE TARGETING OF LIPOSOME-
ENCAPSULATED DRUGS TO MONONUCLEAR
PHAGOCYTES AND AUGMENTATION OF HOST
RESISTANCE TO TUMORS AND
MICROORGANISMS

The localization of liposomes injected iv in cells of the mononuclear phagocyte system, though frustrating to investigators who wish to direct liposomes
to other cells, offers a potentially powerful method for targeting therapeutic
agents to these cells. This type of targeting will be referred to as passive targeting, since it simply exploits the natural fate of liposomes in being taken up by
mononuclear phagocytes.

The central importance of the RES and blood monocytes in myriad host
defense functions is well documented. In addition to its role in removing "foreign" particulate materials, microorganisms, immune complexes, effete cells,

dead cells, and cell debris from the circulation, the functional state of the RES is also important in determining host responses to hemorrhage, circulatory shock, septic shock, trauma, burns, surgery, X irradiation, prolonged tissue ischemia, and responses to drugs. Impaired RES function also occurs secondarily to the development of other common disease states such as diabetes, liver disease, chronic heart failure, and malnutrition, and also as a general consequence of the aging process (review in Altura, 1980). Many of the host defense functions performed by the RES are also discharged by blood monocytes and tissue macrophages, most notably host defense against pathogenic microorganisms, parasites, and tumor cells.

The diverse repertoire of host defense functions performed by mononuclear phagocytes means that an efficient method for delivery of therapeutic agents to these cells to augment host defense reactions might have many potential clinical applications. Liposomes represent such a system, although there is presently no reason to assume that liposomes offer any tangible advantage for this purpose over other particulate drug carriers, such as nanoparticles and other synthetic microparticle systems that also localize in the RES and blood monocytes following iv injection.

A. Liposome-Encapsulated Immunomodulators and Macrophage-Mediated Destruction of Tumor Cells

The discouraging results that have been obtained in both experimental and clinical efforts to develop specific active immunotherapeutic regimens for the treatment of neoplastic diseases has stimulated a renaissance in studying non-specific host defense mechanisms. The increasing evidence that cells of the mononuclear phagocyte series play a significant role in host defense against both microbial and neoplastic diseases has led to a reevaluation of the potential therapeutic value of augmenting host defenses by the selective activation of macrophages *in vivo*. Once activated by a variety of synthetic or naturally occurring agents, macrophages appear capable of selectively recognizing tumor cells irrespective of their degree of phenotypic diversity, and in addition, macrophage-mediated tumoricidal activity appears devoid of the problem of generation of resistance that is often observed in therapy with cytotoxic drugs (review in Poste and Fidler, 1982). For these reasons, a significant effort is now being undertaken in many laboratories to identify novel agents (biological response modifiers, BRM) that can selectively enhance macrophage-mediated tumoricidal activity *in vivo* (review in Poste and Kirsh, 1982).

The localization of liposomes injected iv within fixed macrophages of the RES and circulating blood monocytes, discussed at length in this chapter, provides a highly efficient means of targeting BRM agents to these cells.

There is increasing evidence that the activated macrophage is an important effector cell in host defense against tumors and against metastases in particular. Studies in our laboratory, in collaboration with Dr. I. J. Fidler and his colleagues at the Frederick Cancer Research Facility of the National Cancer Institute in Maryland, have shown that systemic administration of liposomes containing immunomodulators that activate macrophages to render them cytotoxic for tumor cells is highly effective in augmenting macrophage-mediated destruction of tumor cells *in vitro* and established lung metastases *in vivo* (reviews in Fidler and Poste, 1981b; Fidler *et al.*, 1980a,b, 1982; Poste and Fidler, 1981, 1982; Poste and Kirsh, 1980; Poste *et al.*, 1979, 1980, 1982). A full description of the use of liposomes containing immunomodulators in the treatment of experimental animal tumors is provided in several review articles (Fidler and Poste, 1981; Poste and Fidler, 1981, 1982; Poste *et al.*, 1982).

The optimal conditions for therapy with liposome-encapsulated immunomodulators and the efficacy of this modality in treating metastatic tumor burdens of increasing size have still to be defined. It is considered unlikely that liposome-encapsulated immunomodulators could serve as a single modality in treating advanced metastatic disease. In common with many other antitumor therapies, optimal application will probably involve its use in combination with other antitumor agents. For example, if the ratio of macrophages to tumor cells required for optimal macrophage-mediated tumoricidal activity *in vivo* is similar to that operating *in vitro,* then, even allowing for maximum recruitment of monocytes from the blood, there are insufficient macrophages in the lung to permit effective destruction of pulmonary metastatic tumor burdens exceeding 10^8 tumor cells per lung (Poste and Fidler, 1980). Since tumor burdens of this size are easily attained, it is clear that therapeutic stimulation of macrophage-mediated antitumor activity will be unsuccessful in treating large metastatic foci, no matter how effective this modality at activating macrophages. Thus, potential therapeutic regimens designed to stimulate the antitumor properties of macrophages will thus almost certainly have to be used in combination with other treatments such as chemotherapy, which would be used to reduce the "bulk" tumor burden to a level sufficient to allow activated macrophages to kill the surviving tumor cells. Studies to evaluate the efficacy of liposome-encapsulated immunodulators in combination with chemotherapeutic regimens in treating metastatic disease of differing severity in experimental animals are currently in progress.

Evaluation of the efficacy of therapeutic agents in augmenting macrophage-mediated reactions to tumors has been hindered by the lack of methods for quantifying the macrophage content of metastases. We have described a new double-label histochemical method that not only enables macrophages to be identified reliably in histological sections of metastases but also allows macrophages that have entered lesions during therapy to be distinguished from those present at the onset of therapy (Bugelski *et al.*, 1983a). In evaluating macrophage responses to tumors, it is also necessary to quantify changes in macrophage content that can occur at different stages in tumor growth. Morphological analysis of several hundred lung metastases produced by the B16 melanoma using serial sections of each metastasis has revealed marked heterogeneity in the macrophage content of individual metastases present in the same animal (Bugelski *et al.,* 1983b). This study also revealed that the macrophage density falls rapidly as metastases increase in size, reaching a uniform low level in metastases with median cross-sectional areas of 0.01 mm^2 or greater (Fig. 3). Lesions of this size typically contain between 400 and 1000 tumor cells. Assuming exponential cell growth within metastases, tumor cells with a doubling time of 24 hr would take only 1 week to generate a metastasis of this size from a single cell.

These findings provide a possible explanation for the failure of nonspecific immunotherapy in treating large metastatic burdens. These data further reinforce the view that successful therapy of established metastatic disease will require multiagent and/or multimodality treatment regimens.

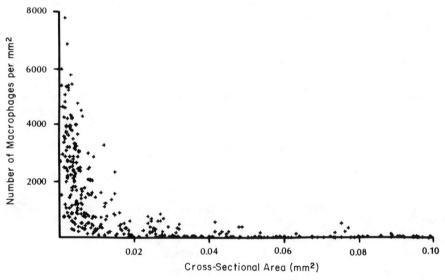

Fig. 3. Scatter diagram of macrophage density versus cross-sectional area of lung micrometastases. C57BL/6J mice were injected with 1×10^5 B16F$_1$ cells (tail vein) and subsequently injected with colloidal iron–dextran, iv (tail vein) 8, 14, or 22 days after injection of tumor cells, to label tumor-associated macrophages. Mice were sacrificed 24 hr after injection of colloidal iron and their lungs fixed in Formalin. Paraffin sections were first treated with potassium ferrocyanide to convert colloid iron to Prussian blue and then stained for pseudoperoxidase activity with diaminobenzidine. Staining cells were counted and the cross-sectional area of individual metastases determined and macrophages per unit area calculated using a Zeiss Videoplan. Each point represents an individual metastasis. Data from 335 separate metastasis sections are shown. Metastases with cross-sectional areas up to 3 mm^2 have been examined and show uniformly low macrophage density.

B. Liposomes and Antimicrobial Chemotherapy

Liposomes containing biological response modifier agents are also highly effective in stimulating macrophage-mediated host resistance to microbial infections. Systemic administration of MLV liposomes containing muramyl dipeptide (MDP) produces a significant increase in the ability of experimental animals to resist acute infections by both bacteria (*Listeria* sp., *Salmonella* sp., *Klebsiella* sp., *Pseudomonas aeruginosa*) and fungi (*Candida albicans*). Evidence has also been obtained demonstrating synergy in the action of liposome-encapsulated MDP and antibiotics in the therapy of experimental infections produced by these classes of microorganisms (G. Poste, unpublished observations).

In addition to their role in destroying invading microorganisms, mononuclear phagocytes also serve as sites of infection. A number of viruses, bacteria, fungi, and pathogenic protozoa replicate within macrophages. Intracellular infections of this kind are difficult to treat and are often refractory to conventional antimicrobial–antiparasitic agents because of poor drug penetration into cells. Administration of the same agents in association with liposomes offers a potential solution to this problem. Assuming that infected macrophages retain their phagocytic capacity, systemic administration of liposomes containing a drug active against the invading microorganisms or parasite provides a method for effective drug delivery directly to the site of infection. By so doing, the drug concentration used can often be reduced in relation to the amount of free drug ordinarily given and thus reduce potential toxic side effects. The merits of liposomes as drug carriers in the chemotherapy of infectious agents and parasites that reside in the RES and/or blood monocytes has been demonstrated by several investigators (Alving and Steck, 1979; New *et al.*, 1981; Fountain *et al.*, 1981; Graybill *et al.*, 1982; Taylor *et al.*, 1982; Lopez-Berestein *et al.*, 1983).

The success of this approach in treating disseminated fungal infections produced by *C. albicans* (Lopez-Berenstein *et al.*, 1983), *Cryptococcus neoformans* (Graybill *et al.*, 1982), and *Histoplasma capsulatum* (Taylor *et al.*, 1982) is particularly encouraging.

Opportunistic fungal infections caused by *C. albicans, Aspergillus* sp., and *Mucor* sp. are a major problem in oncology, particularly in patients with leukemia and lymphomas (Bodey, 1966; Wright *et al.*, 1981; Degregorio *et al.*, 1982; Louria and Sen, 1982). The prospect of improved therapy of systemic mycoses using liposome-encapsulated drugs is exciting. Of particular note is the marked improvement in the therapeutic index of amphotericin B when encapsulated in liposomes (Graybill *et al.*, 1982; Taylor *et al.*, 1982; Lopez-Berenstein *et al.*, 1983). This agent and many other systemic antifungal agents are highly toxic, and the ability to reduce their toxic side effects with no loss in efficacy is an important therapeutic gain. If this proves to be a general feature of other antifungal agents when administered in liposomes, it may become possible to undertake clinical trials with other agents that display potent antifungal properties but whose development was previously curtailed on the grounds of unacceptable host toxicity.

The success of liposome-encapsulated antifungal agents in treating disseminated fungal infections might reasonably be expected to be limited to infections in which the organism resides within macrophages and becomes exposed to high drug concentrations following uptake of liposomes by infected macrophages. Since growth of the more common opportunistic fungal pathogens such as *C. albicans* and *Aspergillus* sp. is not confined to tissue cells but also involves extensive extracellular growth, particularly in advanced infections, the value of liposome-mediated drug delivery to macrophages may be less effective in treating extracellular infections. However, selective delivery of antifungal drugs to macrophages may still be useful even in extracellular infections. Phagocytic uptake of fungi by macrophages that also contain drug would be expected to enhance the killing of the phagocytosed organisms. In addition, macrophages could also conceivably act as a mobile slow-release vehicle for drug delivery. For example, macrophages could engulf liposomes within the bloodstream, migrate to the sites of infection, and release drug over a period of several hours or even days.

C. Liposomes and Chemotherapy of Malignancies of the Mononuclear Phagocyte System

Theoretically, passive uptake of systemically administered liposomes containing cytotoxic drugs by macrophages in the liver, spleen, or bone marrow offers a potential method for selective ablation of these cells. This strategy could thus be useful in treating neoplasms arising in cells of the mononuclear phagocyte system such as histiocytic medullary reticulosis, monocytic leukemia, hairy cell leukemia, and certain forms of Hodgkin's disease.

VIII. PHYSICOCHEMICAL TARGETING OF LIPOSOMES IN CANCER CHEMOTHERAPY

Yatvin *et al.* (1982) and Magin and Weinstein (1982) have explored the intriguing concept of constructing liposomes from phospholipids or phospholipid mixtures that have a transition temperature (T_c) slightly above normal physiological temperature. Such liposomes should only become permeable and release their contents in tissues warmed to the T_c by local hyperthermia. By localized heating of a tumor, it might be possible to confine drug release to the tumor. This strategy assumes, of course, that liposomes retain their temperature-sensitive properties after interaction with various blood components and that they remain in the circulation for a sufficient time to allow maximum drug release by hyperthermia before being cleared by the RES. Initial experiments using "physical" targeting of this kind to enhance release of methotrexate from temperature-sensitive liposomes in L1210 tumors implanted sc were successful in achieving tumor-associated drug ratios in heated versus unheated tumors of between 4:1 and 14:1. However, in reviewing a more extensive series of experiments using this strategy, Yatvin and Lelkes (1982) indicate that this approach may be less effective with other drugs and different tumor models.

A further major drawback is that this method is not applicable to the therapy of metastatic disease. Whole-body hyperthermia cannot be used, since uniform elevation of the body "core" temperature will induce generalized drug release throughout the body. Enthusiasm for the use of hyperthermia is also dampened by reports showing that local and whole-body hyperthermia significantly enhance metastasis of experimental animal tumors (Walker et al., 1978; Urano et al., 1983).

In an effort to apply the concept of "physical" targeting of liposomes to the treatment of established metastases, Yatvin and his colleagues have constructed "pH-sensitive" liposomes that release their contents only when exposed to tissue environments of low pH (see Yatvin and Lelkes, 1982). The rationale for this approach comes from reports showing that the pH of interstitial fluids in a variety of human and animal tumors is lower (pH 6.0–6.5) than in normal tissues (pH > 6.5). Yatvin has succeeded in developing liposomes that release encapsulated material five to six times faster at pH 6.0 than at pH 7.4, but their effectiveness in achieving site-specific drug delivery to metastases has still to be determined.

It is unclear to what extent the assumption on which this strategy is based reflects a general feature of neoplastic tissue. For example, Jahde et al. (1982) were unable to detect any significant difference in the pH of interstitial fluids sampled from normal and neoplastic tissues. In their study, tissue fluid was sampled using pH microelectrodes with a diameter of <10 μm. In contrast, the earlier measurements reporting lowered pH values in neoplastic tissues were done with sampling electrodes with tip diameters of >0.1 mm. The tissue compression and trauma accompanying insertion of the larger electrodes may have produced significant cell death and release of lysosomal enzymes with resulting artifactual lowering of tissue pH values.

Physical targeting of liposomes using external magnets to direct liposomes containing ferromagnetic particles to specific organs has also been suggested (Gordon et al., 1979), in a fashion analogous to earlier reports of magnetic targeting of microspheres (Widder et al., 1979) and microcapsules (Kato, 1982). Small particles such as liposomes and microspheres are suitable for drug delivery to capillary beds in specific organs. However, the much larger microcapsules (>20 μm) arrest in larger vessels and are unable to return to the venous circulation. The smaller size of liposomes may be a disadvantage in controlling liposomes that are circulating within major supply vessels. For example, a magnetic field of 8000 Oe was required to achieve localization of 50% of an injected dose of small microspheres within the rat tail artery with a flow rate of only 0.6 ml/min (Widder *et al.*, 1979). In contrast, a similar 50% level of magnetic control efficiency could be achieved for large microcapsules at magnetic fields of only 250 Oe/cm in the dog abdominal aorta in which the blood flow rates are as high as 240 ml/min (Kato, 1982). These data suggest that magnetic control and targeting of liposomes containing ferromagnetic particles may be feasible only if combined with arterial catherterization techniques to achieve initial delivery to the organ of interest.

IX. LIPOSOMES AND DRUG DELIVERY TO LYMPH NODES

Liposomes injected sc or im are cleared slowly from the injection site by absorption into lymphatics, after which they localize in the draining regional lymph node(s) (Jackson, 1981; Kaledin *et al.*, 1981, 1982; Khato *et al.*, 1982). The ability of liposomes to enter tissue lymphatics as intact structures from the surrounding tissue is not at variance with the apparent inability of liposomes to traverse continuous and fenestrated capillaries mentioned earlier.

The terminal lymphatics (synonyms: lymphatic capillaries, small lymphatics, lymphatic rootlets, and initial lymphatics) offer a far less formidable mechanical barrier than these two classes of capillaries. Continuous and fenestrated capillaries possess a continuous, uninterrupted subendothelial basement membrane. These supporting structures are minimal in terminal lymphatics, and when they are present, their thickness is highly variable. In many terminal lymphatics, a basal lamina and other supporting structures are completely absent and only the lining endothelium is present (review in Casley-Smith, 1977). The cellular junctions between endothelial cells in terminal lymphatics also differ significantly from those in blood capillaries. Zonula adherens are common features, and adjacent endothelial cells are separated at these sites by 20 nm. However, it is equally common to find sites in which large gaps measuring 0.1 μm or larger, are present between adjacent endothelial cells (Fig. 4). These gaps enlarge dramatically at sites of inflammation and are also very common in tissues where there is constant motion or frequent variation in tissue pressure (see Casley-Smith, 1977). These gaps are believed to be dynamic structures that are ''opened'' by active movement of the endothelial cells produced by cytoskeletal elements resembling microfilaments that are attached to ablumenal surface of the endothelial cells (Fig. 4). In the ''open'' configuration the gaps in the lymphatic endothelium are of sufficient size to accommodate SUV liposomes without difficulty and would also be expected to allow penetration of larger liposomes (MLV, REV) of up to 0.5 to 1.0 μm in

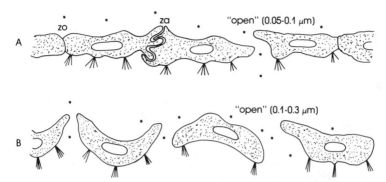

Fig. 4.   Schematic illustration of the structural relationships between adjacent endothelial cells in terminal lymphatics. (A) Zona occludens (zo) and zona adherens (za) junctions between adjacent endothelial cells limit permeability, but at other sites large gaps may be present that are freely permeable to materials of the indicated size. In contrast to the structure of blood capillaries shown in Fig. 1, these vessels lack a subendothelial basement membrane and extensive adventitial elements. (B) At sites of inflammation, edema, constant tissue motion, or frequent variation in the tissue pressure, all endothelial cells may be in the "open" configuration, allowing penetration of materials of relatively large size. The size of the gap between adjacent endothelial cells is believed to be regulated by cytoskeletal elements that are associated with the ablumenal side of the cells and are believed to alter endothelial cell morphology by their contraction and relaxation.

diameter. The terminal lymphatics drain into increasingly larger lymphatics (the so-called collecting lymphatics). The endothelial junctions in these vessels are typically closed. The larger collecting lymphatics also possess an extensive basement membrane are impermeable to molecules of $M_r >6000$ (see Casley-Smith, 1977). It is thus considered unlikely that any class of liposomes would be able to penetrate these vessels.

Lymphatic uptake of liposomes and their localization within regional lymph nodes provides a potentially useful system for the delivery of cytotoxic anti-cancer drugs for treatment of lymph node metastases (Kaledin *et al.*, 1981, 1982; Khato *et al.*, 1982) and the delivery of radioimaging agents in diagnostic monitoring of lymph node architecture and infiltration of nodes by metastatic tumor cells (see Ryman and Barratt, 1982). This approach might also be valuable in delivering BRM agents to lymph node macrophages to augment destruction of small nodal tumor burdens.

Lymphatic uptake of liposomes containing cytotoxic drugs avoids the potential toxicity to the RES seen with iv injection (Section X). In addition, lymphatic uptake can achieve more efficient drug localization and higher ratios of drug retention in nodal metastases compared with iv administration.

Active targeting of liposomes to specific cell types within lymph nodes may also be feasible. Liposomes carried in the lymph will have direct access to the various cell types that reside on the reticulum cell meshwork within the nodes.

Anatomical barriers such as basement membranes that frustrate active ligand-directed targeting from the bloodstream are not present. Nonetheless, macrophages will probably still play a major role in liposome uptake in lymph nodes because of their phagocytic capacity, their presence in large numbers, and their anatomical location within the node that permits them to "filter" particulate material from lymph immediately after its entry into the node. However, growth of metastatic tumor cells within the node can radically alter lymph circulation patterns and thus induce changes in intranodal liposome disposition.

X. LIPOSOME TOXICITY AND ADVERSE COMPLICATIONS OF LIPOSOME UPTAKE BY MONONUCLEAR PHAGOCYTES

A. Toxicity of the Liposomal Carrier

Liposomes prepared from most phospholipids and/or cholesterol are biodegradable, and single doses are apparently well tolerated by rodents and dogs over a wide dose range (review in Poste, 1983). Less is known, however, about the effect of repeated iv administration of liposomes on RE activity or other body functions. Many of the proposed clinical applications of liposomes will require repeated dosing extending over periods of several weeks or even months.

We have begun to evaluate the effects of single and multiple liposome doses on RE clearance capability with respect to the onset, extent, and duration of RE depression (Poste, 1983; Poste et al., 1983b). These experiments demonstrated that after a single dose of MLV liposomes, the ability to retain a subsequent liposome dose in the liver, spleen, and bone marrow recovers fully within 24 hr. In contrast, dextran sulfate, which is relatively nonbiodegradable by macrophages, induces a more prolonged period of RES hyporesponsiveness that requires at least 96 hr for complete recovery. Additional studies comparing liposome clearance in normal hosts and in X-irradiated, monocytopenic experimental animals indicate that recovery of RES clearance functions after exposure to liposomes involves both recovery of particle uptake capabilities by existing RE cells and recruitment of new phagocytic cells from the circulation (Poste et al., 1983a).

To evaluate the influence of repeated doses of liposomes on the clearance of a subsequent test dose, mice were injected iv with up to 20 injections of MLV liposomes (PS:PC:C = 3:3:4; 5 μM/mouse) at 3-day intervals prior to injection of a radiolabeled test dose of homologous liposomes. Animals that received more than 10 doses of MLV liposomes displayed a significantly decreased capacity to retain the subsequent test dose. This depression in RE phagocytic capability was not accompanied by a compensatory increase in liposome retention by non-RE organs (Poste, 1983). The impaired RE phagocytic capability induced by multiple liposome injections is not limited to liposome clearance. Mice given multiple frequent injections of liposomes (10 injections; 3- or 7-day intervals) also display an impaired ability to clear erythrocytes and other particulate materials from the bloodstream (Poste *et al.*, 1983b).

The onset, extent, and duration of impaired RES function is dependent on liposome size, dose, dosage frequency, and lipid composition (Abra and Hunt, 1981; Poste, 1983). Mice given multiple doses of liposomes (5 μM phospholipid/mouse) at either 3-, 7-, or 30-day intervals all display significant differences in their ability to clear a subsequent particle dose, with the extent of suppression being more pronounced with the more aggressive dosing schedules. Liposomal lipid composition also influences the retentive capability of the RES (see Poste *et al.*, 1983b). Liposomes containing dicetyl phosphate or sterylamine induced a more rapid onset and a more severe RE suppression than liposomes prepared from phospatidylserine (PS) and phosphatidylcholine (PC) or disteroylphosphatidylcholine (DSPC) and cholesterol. In addition to direct functional suppression of RE particle clearance pathways, multiple doses of multilamellar liposomes induce bone marrow hypoplasia with resulting decreases in the numbers of circulating monocytes and granulocytes (Poste *et al.*, 1983b).

Reports of the formation of antibodies to a wide range of phospholipids following iv injection of liposomes (review in Alving and Richards, 1983) also emphasize the need for caution before a decision is taken to use a multidose liposome regimen in humans.

Reference is often made, during formal discussion periods at scientific meetings on liposomes, to the clinical use of intravenous fat emulsions such as Intralipid and Liposyn in total parenteral nutrition (TPN), as a clinical precedent for the "safety" of lipid emulsions. The analogy between these products and liposomes is simplistic, and statements that these lipid emulsions are "without deleterious effects" (Yatvin and Lelkes, 1982, p. 160) are misleading and incorrect.

The literature is replete with reports of adverse reactions associated with intravenous fat emulsions. In reviewing these, care must be exercised in determining which product is being implicated. Most of the toxic reactions described before 1970 related to Lipomul, which was prepared from cottonseed oil and was withdrawn in the United States in 1965 following reports of a "fat overloading syndrome." The introduction of Intralipid and Liposyn in the 1970s provided clinicians with valuable products for TPN; however, in common with other pharmaceutical products, a broad spectrum of toxic reactions of varying severity have now been reported with these newer agents (review in Pelham, 1981). Notwithstanding the poor clinical status of many patients receiving TPN, most of the reported complications occur with prolonged use of intravenous fat emulsions and are associated with abnormal hepatic function, thrombophlebitis, lipid accumulation in the RES and other organs, impaired RES clearance function, and increased susceptibility to infection (review Pelham, 1981, for references).

B. Toxicity Resulting from Altered Disposition of Liposome-Encapsulated Drugs

Little attention has been given to the potential toxicities that might arise from the localization of liposome-associated materials within macrophage populations in the liver, spleen, bone marrow, and blood. The disposition of drugs administered in association with liposomes will, in most cases, differ substantially from that observed with conventional unencapsulated formulations of the same drugs. As discussed in Section VII, this can be advantageous if the therapeutic goal is to "concentrate" drugs in mononuclear phagocytes. In other situations, however, the altered pharmacodistribution of liposome-associated drugs may be less desirable, and in certain instances may be harmful. Perhaps the most obvious example of a potential problem concerns the proposed use of liposome-encapsulated cytotoxic drugs in cancer treatment. By delivering large amounts of such drugs to the RES and circulating blood monocytes, the use of liposomes may cause toxic ablation of a vital element of host defense function. The risk of toxic destruction of mononuclear phagocytes will differ depending on the mechanism of action of the cytotoxic drug being used. Inhibitors of DNA synthesis might be expected to have little toxic effect on nondividing macrophage populations, but cytotoxic drugs that impair RNA and protein synthesis may well produce toxic destruction of macrophages. Studies in our laboratory have confirmed that this fear is justified. Systemic administration of bleomycin and several other antitumor drugs encapsulated within both SUV and MLV liposomes was found to enhance the metastatic spread of several malignant animal tumors (Poste, 1983; Poste *et al.,* 1983b). This effect was not seen when liposomes were injected sc or im. The increased metastasis in mice treated with liposomes containing bleomycin could be reversed by transfusion of syngeneic macrophages 12 hr after each treatment cycle. This indicates that the iatrogenic enhancement of metastases produced by liposome therapy is probably caused by toxic destruction of mononuclear phagocytes. These data indicate that the rationale for using liposomes as a carrier vehicle for drug delivery in cancer treatment may be seriously flawed if the class of drug being used is able to destroy host macrophages.

That this complication was not reported earlier, despite the large number of published studies on the use of liposome-encapsulated cytotoxic drugs in treating experimental animal tumors (Table II), once again emphasizes the importance of working with tumor models that are more representative of the clinical setting in which a drug will be used. With the exception of studies on the effect of sc injection of liposome-encapsulated drugs on lymph node metastases (see Section IX), none of the publications in Table II examined the effect of treatment on metastatic burden. Nonmetastasizing tumors transplanted ip or sc were used in the majority of studies, and even in studies in which metastatic tumors were used, no data were provided on metastatic burden. Instead, the effectiveness of the therapy was assayed as either a reduction in the size of the primary tumor or increased survival time. Neither of these end points excludes the possibility that the metastatic burden may be enhanced. Many of the tumors listed in Table II are highly aggressive and kill the host within 10 to 20 days. Significant therapeutic effects on survival time in these tumors are measured in days rather than weeks or months. Although statistically significant, such small increases in host survival times are not of sufficient duration to allow detection of new metastases. The risk of iatrogenic metastases caused by toxic ablation of the RES will be greater after several treatments and will thus tend to occur in the relatively later stages of growth of these highly aggressive tumors, and metastatic lesions may not reach macroscopic size by the time of death. The probability of detecting iatrogenic metastases induced by liposome-mediated chemotherapy will thus be greater in more slowly growing metastasizing tumors that allow the host to survive for a minimum of 6 weeks and that produce a low yet reproducible metastatic burden that facilitates reliable identification of any change in metastatic burden. The B16 melanoma cell line used in the studies of Poste (1983), as well as several other metastatic rodent tumors, fulfills these criteria.

The ability of certain cytotoxic antitumor drugs to produce toxic destruction of the RES when administered in association with liposomes was perhaps predictable in the light of existing knowledge identifying the RES as the major site of liposome localization *in vivo*. This phenomenon is not unique to liposomes, and similar impairment of RES function has been reported in mice injected iv with erythrocyte ghosts containing encapsulated bleomycin (Lynch *et al.*, 1980).

It is less easy, however, to predict whether systemic administration of liposomes containing drugs that are not known to be toxic for macrophages will produce toxic alterations in macrophages that similarly limit the value of liposomes as a drug delivery system.

Collectively, the observations reviewed in this section emphasize the need for caution in using liposomes as a drug delivery system, particularly for cytotoxic drugs. It is important to ensure that neither the liposomal carrier nor the encapsulated agent suppresses the mononuclear phagocyte system, since impaired RES function may predispose a host to infections, endotoxemia, hepatocellular injury, and suppression of both primary and secondary immune responses (review in Altura, 1980).

XI. CLINICAL TRIALS AND COMMERCIAL DEVELOPMENT OF LIPOSOMES AS DRUG CARRIERS

Parenteral administration of liposomes to human patients and volunteers has been described in a few reports. Liposomes have been injected iv into cancer patients to study their disposition (Richardson *et al.*, 1979) and to assess their value in detecting tumor foci in diagnostic imaging (Ryman and Barratt, 1982). Efforts have also been made to treat lysosomal storage diseases in two patients by iv administration of liposomes containing th missing enzyme(s) (review in Gregoriadis, 1981). Liposomes containing dipalmitoylphosphatidylcholine (DPPC) and dipalmitoylphosphatidylglycerol administered as aerosols into the airways have been reported to enhance survival of human neonates suffering from severe respiratory distress syndrome (Ivey *et al.*, 1980). A small clinical trial in which liposomes containing cortisol palmitate were injected intraarticularly to determine possible efficacy in treating rheumatoid arthritis has also been reported (DeSilva *et al.*, 1979). With the exception of the last study, which was done in collaboration with a pharmaceutical company, these studies were conducted with liposomes prepared in the investigators' own laboratories and used within hours of preparation.

Widespread clinical use of liposomes in cancer and other diseases will depend, however, on the routine availability of commercial preparations. For this to become a reality, a lengthy series of complex and costly preclinical and clinical studies must first be undertaken to demonstrate the safety and efficacy of these products to fulfill the stringent requirements set by international agencies responsible for regulating the production and marketing of pharmaceuticals.

In an earlier review of the prospects for commercial development of liposomes, Fildes (1981) stated that "the realistic chance of industrial development of a medicine based on the liposome in the near future is not high." Little has changed in the intervening 2 years. Current studies on passive targeting of liposomes to macrophages to augment macrophage-mediated host defense functions and to treat parasites and microorganisms residing in these cells undoubtedly present exciting clinical opportunities. However, from the industrial standpoint clinical trials to evaluate these opportunities could be pursued more easily using other particulate carrier systems (see later).

The pharmaceutical industry operates in a highly competitive environment, and its research and development activities must achieve adequate financial return. This requirement becomes even more crucial in an era when the development costs and time needed to bring a product to the marketplace are increasing dramatically. As with any drug delivery system, industrial development of liposomes requires a clear definition of the medical need and its technical feasibility. The former is determined by the frequency of the disease, its seriousness, and the adequacy of current therapies. In the case of cancer therapy, the medical need is self-evident. However, assessment of the technical feasibility of developing liposomes as a drug delivery system involves many more uncertainties.

To achieve success it will be necessary to develop preparative methods suitable for commercial scale and to acquire a safe product with stable, reproducible characteristics that can be manufactured in sterile fashion under conditions acceptable to regulatory authorities, have a minimum shelf life of 12 mo under adverse storage conditions, offer the physician and patient maximum convenience, and also meet the increasing demand for cost effectiveness being set by both government-sponsored and private health care systems. In discussing the technical difficulties involved in meeting these criteria, emphasis has been given to events needed to fulfill regulatory requirements in the United States set by the Food and Drug Administration (FDA).

The response of regulatory authorities to liposomes is itself uncertain. Precedent from other drug delivery systems suggests that liposome-associated drug formulations would be treated as totally new drug substances and be required to meet the full range of tests demanded of any new chemical entity. It is unclear, however, whether this classification would apply to lymphokines and other natural mediators that are presently classified as "biologicals" by the FDA. Will such molecules retain their traditional classification if administered in association with liposomes? Commercially this is not a trivial question, since the complexity, time, and cost of developing a product as a "biological" for review by the Office of Biologics are considerably less than for a "new chemical entity" reviewed by the Office of Drug Evaluation.

The situation becomes even more confused as a result of a proposal published in the *Federal Register* (1983) by the FDA, which states that products involving "coupled antibodies, i.e., products that consist of an antibody component coupled with a drug or radionuclide in which both components provide a pharmacological effect but the biological component determines the site of action" should be submitted to the Office of Biologics for review.

Whether the FDA would in reality allow drugs encapsulated in liposomes bearing antibodies to be treated as "biologicals" rather than as "chemical entities" is far from certain. Further ambiguity is also introduced by the FDA's delay in publishing requirements for monoclonal antibody preparations injected iv.

To develop a suitable liposome preparation for clinical trial and eventual commercial development, the biopharmaceutical and metabolic characteristics of the liposome–drug complex tabulated here must be defined:

> Liposome size and tolerance limits
> Properties of membrane-associated ligands
> Sterility
> Stability of liposome ($\pm$ cell recognition ligand):
> >   Chemical stability at different storage temperatures
> >   In diluent
> >   Lyophilized and after reconstitution
> >   Retention of encapsulated drug
> >   Size changes, aggregation, or sedimentation
> Metabolism studies
> >   Dose–response relationships
> >   Pharmacodistribution

Metabolite identification
Routes and rates of excretion
Initial toxicity studies (two species)
Acute
Subacute

For water-insoluble drugs that partition into the liposome membrane, storage as freeze-dried aqueous solutions or as freeze-hydrated solids reconstituted with sterile diluent presents few problems. These are compatible with dosage form production facilities available in most pharmaceutical companies. Substantial problems remain, however, in achieving stable liposome preparations containing low molecular weight, water-soluble drugs. The low encapsulation efficiency of hydrophilic drugs means that reconstitution of lyophilized lipid–drug mixtures will also involve subsequent separation of free drug. The high rate of leakage of molecules from fully formed liposomes also introduces the need for separation techniques unless the levels of free drug can be tolerated. In either case, few clinical centers would have the facilities or the motivation to adopt complex separation methods as routine clinical practice. Several techniques are being studied to reduce drug loss from liposome storage. These include chemical modification of drugs to render them more hydrophobic and the use of higher molecular weight absorbent molecules that would interact with water-soluble drugs and retain them within the liposome. To date, however, a satisfactory solution has not been found.

Even with the availability of stable, homogeneous liposome formulations, additional development studies to evaluate the toxicology and clinical efficacy of a liposome–drug complex will be both costly and time consuming. Foremost among the problems involved is the need to produce several hundred kilograms of phospholipid. This enormous quantity of material is required to fulfill the extensive metabolic and toxicological studies mandated by the FDA and to undertake extensive clinical trials to demonstrate clinical efficacy. (Typically between 1000 and 3000 patients are studied in clinical trials of most drugs in the United States.)

The problems that must be solved before liposomes can become a commercially viable dosage form are substantial. In many respects liposomes behave in a fashion similar to multiphase emulsions and biodegradable microparticles (nanoparticles, microspheres, and microparticles). The feasibility of preparing several of these carriers as homogeneous stable, cost-effective formulations on an industrial scale has already been demonstrated, and they must therefore be viewed as logical alternatives to liposomes.

The comments in this section may seem unduly pessimistic, certainly to those who own or invest in new companies that have been formed in the last few years to develop liposomes as a commercial drug delivery system. In our opinion, liposomes have been and will continue to be a valuable experimental tool for manipulation of cells *in vitro* and for demonstrating the feasibility of using particulate carriers for drug delivery *in vivo*. Exciting therapeutic opportunities for drug delivery to macrophages and lymph nodes have already emerged from such studies. However, the commercial factors needed to translate these applications into routine clinical practice presently favor the use of alternative particulate carriers. Biodegradable microspheres are able to mimic most of the desired features of liposomes and can be produced as pharmaceutically acceptable uniform formulations at far less cost than liposomes using methods and manufacturing equipment already available within the pharmaceutical industry.

XII. CONCLUSIONS

Sufficient experimental observations on liposome behavior *in vivo* have been made over the last decade to enable several general conclusions to be made regarding the value of liposomes as a drug delivery system in cancer therapy.

Much of the interest in liposomes as a potential drug delivery system has stemmed from widely publicized speculations that liposomes could be "targeted" to tumor cells by incorporating ligands into the liposomal membrane that could recognize and bind to surface determinants on tumor cells. Unfortunately, it is now clear that many of the more ambitious proposals for targeting liposomes to tumor cells *in vivo* do not withstand critical scrutiny in the light of newer knowledge. To be effective in treating solid tumors, liposomes must have access to tumor cells residing in the extravascular tissues. Two problems dictate that the probability of achieving this objective is very low. First, the problem of liposome localization in macrophages must be overcome. Second, to gain access to target cells in extravascular tissues, circulating liposomes within the bloodstream must cross blood vessel walls.

The evidence reviewed here indicates that extravasation of liposomes from the blood to extravascular sites in normal tissues is limited to organs lined by sinusoidal capillaries. Extravasation of liposomes does not apparently occur on any significant scale in tissues lined by continuous or fenestrated capillaries. Little information is available concerning liposome extravasation in the microcirculation of tumors. Data on the permeability of tumor microvessels to other materials suggest that vascular permeability may often be higher than in normal tissues, but this property is extremely variable and cannot be predicted with any certainty for any given tumor. Even if liposome extravasation occurs in hyperpermeable regions of tumors, it remains to be shown whether it occurs on a sufficient scale to achieve therapeutic drug concentrations within the tumor. The kinetics of liposome localization within a tumor will be crucial in this regard. To be of therapeutic value, liposome extravasation would need to occur more rapidly than the rate of liposome clearance from the blood by the RES and circulating macrophages.

Notwithstanding the major problem of liposome extravasation, current proposals to use monoclonal antibodies directed against tumor cells to target liposomes to tumor cells fail to address the problem of antigenic heterogeneity in tumor cell subpopulations coexisting within the same tumor.

Experimental efforts to induce significant redistribution of liposomes administered iv away from the mononuclear phagocytes to other sites by "blockading" the ability of these cells to take up circulating liposomes have not been successful to date. Similarly, efforts to reduce liposome uptake into mononuclear phagocytes by modification of liposome composition, though effective in prolonging liposome lifetimes within the circulation, merely delay the process of uptake by macrophages and have failed to produce the desired redistribution of liposomes to cells other than macrophages. It thus seems unlikely that either of these strategies will be of value in targeting liposomes to tumor cells.

The predominant localization of liposomes in circulating and fixed macrophages after iv injection offers a convenient method for "passive targeting" of drugs to those cells. Experimental evidence has been obtained in several laboratories describing the value of this approach in the delivery of biological response modifiers to stimulate macrophage-mediated destruction of tumor cells and invading microorganisms. The same strategy has also been used to deliver antimicrobial and antiprotozoal drugs to macrophages to destroy microorganisms and parasites residing inside these cells.

Paradoxically, the dominant role of the mononuclear phagocyte system in determining the disposition of liposomes injected iv, may also be the greatest liability in the use of liposomes as a drug carrier, and in cancer chemotherapy in particular.

New evidence suggests that repeated uptake of liposomes by the RES may exhaust the capacity of the RES to clear particulate materials from the circulation. Consequently, until conditions are defined in which this risk can be excluded, treatment regimens that require multiple liposome treatments (>10) with short intervals between treatments may lead to unacceptable toxicity.

Passive localization of liposomes containing cytotoxic antineoplastic drugs within the RES may pose an even greater hazard. Liposome-mediated delivery of cytotoxic drugs that impair macrophage function can cause iatrogenic destruction of the RES. In tumor-bearing hosts this can enhance metastasis. The risk of iatrogenic destruction of the RES has received scant mention by proponents of liposome targeting. This, together with the fading prospects for ligand-directed targeting of liposomes to tumor cells located in extravascular sites, suggests that liposomes offer little promise as a drug delivery system in the chemotherapy of metastatic disease.

Even though opportunities for ligand-directed targeting of liposomes to extravascular tumor cells seem remote, the use of cell recognition ligands to target liposomes to specific cell types or subsets of cells within the vascular system remains a viable option. This approach could be particularly valuable in directing drugs to specific subsets of circulating blood cells, hematopoietic stem cells, and vascular endothelial cells, although in each of these examples it will again be necessary to guard against complications that could result from untoward drug localization within the RES.

The potential value of liposomes as a drug delivery system is not limited to intravenous administration. A variety of therapeutic opportunities can be envisaged for utilizing liposomes in slow-release formulations for drugs injected into anatomically isolated compartments such as joints and the urogenital tract. When implanted subcutaneously or intramuscularly, liposomes may provide an effective carrier system for enhancing lymphatic absorption of drugs and retention within lymph nodes. This application offers particularly exciting prospects for the therapy of lymph node metastases and in the diagnosis of nodal metastases.

Several important issues remain to be addressed before liposomes can be used clinically on any significant scale. Foremost among these is the need to develop cost-effective methods for large-scale preparation of homogeneous formulations that are stable for relatively long periods. Additional information is also needed to examine the safety of liposomes when administered repeatedly at frequent intervals over periods of several weeks or months. Resolution of these questions will be crucial in determining whether liposomes become a commercially viable dosage form. At the present time alternative particulate carriers are available that can duplicate the positive attributes of liposomes and have the additional advantage that they can be produced as stable, homogeneous preparations in a cost-effective manner using existing formulation techniques and manufacturing equipment. However, many of the unanswered questions regarding the toxicity of liposomes apply to particulate drug delivery systems at large.

The next few years will be decisive in determining whether liposomes can be developed as a commercially viable dosage form or will join the ranks of other drug carriers that have failed to attain their initial promise.

REFERENCES

Abra, R. M., and Hunt, C. A. (1981). Liposomes disposition in vivo. III. Dose and vesicle-size effects. *Biochim. Biophys. Acta* **666,** 493–503.

Abra, R. M., and Hunt, C. A. (1982). Liposome disposition in vivo. IV. The interaction of sequential doses of liposomes having different diameters. *Res. Commun. Chem. Pathol. Pharmacol.* **36,** 17–31.

Abra, R. M., Bosworth, M. E., and Hunt, C. A. (1980). Liposome disposition in vivo: Effects of pre-dosing with liposomes. *Res. Commun. Chem. Pathol. Pharmacol.* **29,** 346–360.

Abrams, H. (1961). "Angiography." Little Brown, Boston, Massachusetts.

Altura, B. M. (1980). Reticuloendothelial cells and host defence. *Adv. Microcirc.* **9,** 252–294.

Alving, C. R., and Richards, R. L. (1983). Immunological aspects of liposomes. *In* "The Liposomes" (M. Ostro, ed.), pp. 209–287. Dekker, New York.

Alving, C. R., and Steck, E. A. (1979). The use of liposome-encapsulated drugs in leishmaniasis. *Trends Biochem. Sci.* **4,** N175–177.

Anghileri, L. J., ed. (1982). "General Processes of Radiotracer Localization," Vols. I and II. CRC Press, Boca Raton, Florida.

Baldwin, R. W., and Pimm, M. V. (1983). Antitumor monoclonal antibodies for radioimmunodetection of tumors and drug targeting. *Cancer Metastasis Rev.* **2,** 89–106.

Bodey, G. P. (1966). Fungal infections complicating acute leukemia. *J. Chron. Dis.* **19,** 667.

Bragman, K. S., Heath, T. D., and Papahadjopoulos, D. (1983). Simultaneous interaction of monoclonal antibody-targeted liposomes with two receptors on K562 cells. *Biochim. Biophys. Acta* **730,** 187–195.

Bruck, S. D., ed. (1982). "Controlled Drug Delivery." CRC Press, Boca Raton, Florida.

Bugelski, P., and Poste, G. (1982). Recruitment of macrophages in experimental metastases. *Proc. Am. Assoc. Cancer Res.* **23,** 1004.

Bugelski, P., Kirsh, R., and Poste, G. (1983a). A new histochemical method for measuring intratumoral macrophages and macrophage recruitment into experimental metastases. *Cancer Res.* **43,** 5493–5501.

Bugelski, P., Kirsh, R., Sowinski, J., and Poste, G. (1983b). Changes in the macrophage content of lung metastases at different stages in tumor growth (submitted for publication).

Bundgaard, M. (1983). Vesicular transport in capillary endothelium. Does it occur? *Fed. Proc., Fed. Am. Soc. Exp. Biol.* **42,** 2425–2430.

Caride, V. J., and Zaret, B. L. (1977). Liposome accumulation in regions of experimental myocardial infarction. *Science* **198,** 735–737.

Casley-Smith, J. R. (1977). Lymph and lymphatics. *In* "Microcirculation" (G. Kaley and B. M. Altura, eds.), Vol. I, pp. 423–502. Univ. Park Press, Baltimore, Maryland.

Cavallo, T., Sade, R., Folkman, J., and Cotran, R. S. (1973). Ultrastructural autoradiographic studies of the early vasoproliferative responses in tumor angiogenesis. *Am. J. Pathol.* **70,** 345–362.

Chien, Y. W., ed. (1982). "Novel Drug Delivery Systems." Dekker, New York.

Counsell, R. E., and Ponland, R. C. (1982). Lipoproteins as potential site-specific delivery systems for diagnostic and therapeutic agents. *J. Med. Chem.* **25,** 1115–1120.

Dawson, C. A., Linehan, J. H., and Rickaby, D. A. (1982). Pulmonary microcirculatory dynamics. *Ann. N. Y. Acad. Sci.* **384,** 90–106.

Degregorio, M. W., Lee, W. M. F., Linker, C. A., Jacobs, R. A., and Ries, C. A. (1982). Fungal infections in patients with acute leukemia. *Am. J. Med.* **73,** 543–548.

Deliconstantinos, G., Gregoriadis, G., Abel, G., Jones, M., and Robertson, D. (1977). Incorporation of *cis*-dichloro-bis-cyclopentylamine platinumII into liposomes enhances its uptake by ADJ/PC6A tumors implanted subcutaneous into mice. *Biochem Soc. Trans.* **5,** 1326–1328.

DeSilva, M., Hazleman, B. L., Page-Thomas, D. P., and Wraight, P. (1979). Liposomes in arthritis: A new approach. *Lancet* **1,** 1320–1322.

Dobson, E. L., and Jones, H. B. (1982). The behavior of intravenously injected particulate material. Its rate of disappearance from the blood stream as a measure of liver blood flow. *Acta Med. Scand.* **273,** 1–71.

Donald, K. (1980). Ultrastructure of reticuloendothelial clearance. *In* "The Reticuloendothelial System: A Comprehensive Treatise" (I. Carr and W. T. Daems, eds.), Vol. 1, pp. 525–554. Plenum, New York.

Dvorak, A. M., Mihm, M. C., Osage, J. E., and Dvorak, H. F. (1980). Melanoma: An ultrastructural study of the host inflammatory and vascular responses. *J. Invest. Dermatol.* **75,** 388–393.

Ehrlich, P. (1906). "Collected Studies on Immunity," Vol. 2, pp. 442–447. Wiley, New York. (Reprinted.)

Ellens, H., Mayhew, E., and Rustum, Y. M. (1982). Reversible depression of the reticuloendothelial system by liposomes. *Biochim. Biophys. Acta* **714,** 479–485.

Federal Register (1983). Food and Drug Administration. Proposed new drug, antibiotic and biologic drug product regulations. *Fed. Regist.* **48,** 26720–26749 (June 9, 1983).

Fendler, J. H., and Romero, A. (1976). Encapsulation of 8-azaguanine in single multiple compartment liposomes. *Life Sci.* **18,** 1453–1458.

Fidler, I. J., and Poste, G. (1981a). Functional activity of macrophages in vivo: destruction of micrometastases. *In* "Manual of Macrophage Methodology" (H. B. Herscowitz, H. T. Holden, J. A. Bellanti, and A. Ghaffer, eds.), pp. 431–438. Dekker, New York.

Fidler, I. J., and Poste, G. (1981b). Treatment of spontaneous murine metastases by the systemic administration of liposomes containing macrophage-activating agents. *In* "Cancer: Achievements, Challenges and Prospects for the 1980's" (J. H. Burchenall and H. F. Oettgen, eds.), Vol. 2, pp. 77–89. Grune and Stratton, New York.

Fidler, I. J., and White, R. W., eds. (1982). "Design of Models for Testing Cancer Chemotherapeutic Agents." Van Nostrand-Reinhold, Princeton, New Jersey.

Fidler, I. J., Raz, A., Fogler, W. E., Kirsh, R., Bugelski, P., and Poste, G. (1980a). Design of liposomes to improve delivery of macrophage-augmenting agents to alveolar macrophages. *Cancer Res.* **40,** 4460–4466.

Fidler, I. J., Raz, A., Fogler, W. E., Hoyer, L. C., and Poste, G. (1980b). The role of plasma membrane receptors and the kinetics of macrophage activation by lymphokines encapsulated in liposomes. *Cancer Res.* **41,** 495–504.

Fidler, I. J., Barnes, Z., Fogler, W. E., Kirsh, R., Bugelski, P., and Poste, G. (1982). Involvement of macrophages in the eradication of established metastases following intravenous injection of liposomes containing macrophage activators. *Cancer Res.* **42,** 496–501.

Fildes, F. J. T. (1981). Liposomes: The industrial viewpoints. *In* "Liposomes: From Physical Structure to Therapeutic Applications" (C. G. Knight, ed.), pp. 464–485. Elsevier, Amsterdam.

Fishman, A. P., ed. (1982). "Endothelium." N. Y. Acad. Sci., New York.

Fitchner, I., Reszka, R., Elbe, B., and Arndt, D. (1981). Therapeutic evaluation of liposome encapsulated daunoblastin in murine tumor models. *Neoplasma* **28,** 141–149.

Folkman, J., and Haudenschild, C. (1981). Induction of capillary growth *in vitro*. *In* "Cellular Interactions" (J. T. Dingle and J. L. Gordon, eds.), pp. 119–136. Elsevier, Amsterdam.

Forssen, E. A., and Tokes, Z. A. (1981). Use of anionic liposomes for the reduction of chronic doxorubicin-induced cardiotoxicity. *Proc. Natl. Acad. Sci. U.S.A.* **78,** 1873–1877.

Forssen, E. A., and Tokes, Z. A. (1983). Improved therapeutic benefits of doxorubicin by entrapment in anionic liposomes. *Cancer Res.* **43,** 546–550.

Fountain, M. W., Dees, C., and Schultz, R. D. (1981). Enhanced intracellular killing of *Staphylococcus aureus* by canine monocytes treated with liposomes containing amikacin, gentamicin, kanamycin, and tobramycin. *Curr. Microbiol.* **6,** 737–376.

Freise, J., Schmidt, F. W., and Magerstedt, P. (1979). Effect of liposome entrapped methotrexate on Ehrlich ascites tumor cells and uptake into primary liver cell tumor. *J. Can. Res. Clin. Oncol.* **94,** 21–27.

Gabbiani, G., and Majno, G. (1980). Pathophysiology of small vessel permeability. *In* "Microcirculation" (G. Kaley and B. M. Altura, eds.), Vol. III, pp. 143–163. Univ. Park Press, Baltimore, Maryland.

Gabizon, A., Dagan, A., Goren, D., Barenholz, Y., and Fuks, Z. (1982). Liposomes as in vivo carriers of adriamycin: Reduced cardiac uptake and preserved antitumor activity in mice. *Cancer Res.* **42**, 4734–4739.

Ganapathi, K., Krishan, A., Wodinsky, I., Zubrod, C. G., and Lesko, L. J. (1980). Effect of cholesterol content on antitumor activity and toxicity of liposome encapsulated 1-β-D-arabino furanosylcytosine in vivo. *Cancer Res.* **40**, 630–633.

Goldacre, R. J., and Sylvén, B. (1962). On the access of blood-borne dyes to various tumor regions. *Br. J. Cancer* **16**, 306–322.

Goldie, J. H. (1983). New thoughts on resistance to chemotherapy. *Hosp. Practice* **18**, 165–177.

Gordon, R. T., Hines, J. R., and Gordon, D. (1979). Intracellular hyperthermia. A biophysical approach to cancer treatment via intracellular temperature and biophysical alterations. *Med. Hypothesis* **5**, 83–102.

Graybill, J. R., Craven, P. C., Taylor, R. L., Williams, D. M., and Magee, W. E. (1982). Treatment of murine cryptococcosis with liposome associated amphotericin B. *J. Infect. Dis.* **145**, 748–751.

Greaves, M., Delia, D., Sutherland, R., Rao, J., Verbi, W., Kemshead, J., Hariri, G., Goldstein, G., and Kung, P. (1981). Expression of the OKT monoclonal antibody defined antigenic determinants in malignancy. *Int. J. Immunopharmacol.* **3**, 283–300.

Gregoriadis, G. (1981). Targeting of drugs: Implications in medicine. *Lancet* **2**, 241–244.

Gregoriadis, G., and Neerunjun, E. D. (1975). Homing of liposomes to target cells. *Biochem. Biophys. Res. Commun.* **65**, 537–540.

Gregoriadis, G., Neerunjun, E. D., and Hunt, R. (1977). Fate of liposome-associated agents injected into normal and tumor-bearing rodents. Attempts to improve localization in tumor tissues. *Life Sci.* **21**, 357–361.

Gregoriadis, G., Senior, J., and Trouet, A., eds. (1982a). "Targeting of Drugs." Plenum, New York.

Gregoriadis, G., Kirby, C., Large, P., Meehan, A., and Senior, J. (1982b). Targeting of liposomes: Study of influencing factors. *In* "Targeting of Drugs" (G. Gregoriadis, J. Senior, and A. Trouet, eds.), pp. 155–184. Plenum, New York.

Gullino, P., and Grantham, F. H. (1984). The vasculature of growing tumors. *Cancer Res.* **24**, 1727–1732.

Hanna, N. (1982). Role of natural killer cells in control of cancer metastasis. *Cancer Met. Rev.* **1**, 45–64.

Hauser, H. (1982). Methods of preparation of lipid vesicles: Assessment of their suitability for drug encapsulation. *Trends Pharm. Sci.* **3**, 274–277.

Hisaoka, M., Tsukada, K., Mouoka, T., Inomata, T., and Arakawa, M. (1982). Studies on liposome encapsulated carboquone. IV. Enhancement of antitumor activity of carboquone against Ehrlich ascites carcinoma by encapsulation. *T. Pharm. Dyn.* **42**, 4734–4739.

Hunt, C. A. (1982). Liposomes disposition in vivo. V. Liposome stability in plasma and implications for drug carrier function. *Biochim. Biophys. Acta* **719**, 450–463.

Hwang, K. J., Luk, K.-F. S., and Beaumier, P. L. (1982). Volume of distribution and transcapillary passage of small unilamellar vesicles. *Life Sci.* **31**, 949–955.

Inaba, M., Yoshida, N., and Tsukagoshi, S. (1981). Preferential action of liposome entrapped 1-(2-chloroethyl)-3-(4-methylcyclohexyl)-1-nitrosourea on lung metastasis of Lewis lung carcinoma as compared with free drug. *Gann* **72**, 341–345.

Ivey, H. H., Kattwinkel, J., and Roth, S. (1980). Nebulization of sonicated phospholipids for treatment of respiratory distress syndrome of infancy. *In* "Liposomes and Immunobiology" (B. H. Tom and H. R. Six, eds.), pp. 301–314. Elsevier, Amsterdam.

Jackson, A. J. (1981). Intramuscular absorption and regional lymphatic uptake of liposome-entrapped inulin. *Drug Metab. Dispos.* **9**, 535–540.

Jahde, E., Rajewsky, M. F., and Baumgartl, H. (1982). pH distributions in transplanted neural tumors and normal tissues of BDIX rats as measured with pH microelectrodes. *Cancer Res.* **42**, 1498–1504.

Juliano, R. L. (1982). Liposomes and the reticuloendothelial system: Interactions of liposomes with macrophages and behavior of liposomes *in vivo. In* "Targeting of Drugs" (G. Gregoriadis, J. Senior, and A. Trouet, eds.), pp. 285–300. Plenum, New York.

Juliano, R. L., Lopez-Berenstein, G., Mehta, R., Hopfer, R., Mehta, K., and Kasi, L. (1983). Pharmacokinetic and therapeutic consequences of liposomal drug delivery: Fluorodeoxyuridine and amphotericin B as examples. *Biol. Cell* **47**, 39–46.

Kaledin, V. I., Matienko, N. A., Nikolin, V. P., Gruntenko, Y. V., and Budker, V. G. (1981). Intralymphatic administration of liposome-encapsulated drugs to mice: Possibility for suppression of the growth of tumor metastases in the lymph nodes. *JNCI, J. Natl. Cancer Inst.* **66**, 881–887.

Kaledin, V. I., Matienko, N. A., Nikolin, V. P., Gruntenko, Y. V., Budker, V. G., and Vakhrusheva, T. E. (1982). Subcutaneously injected radiolabeled liposomes: Transport to the lymph nodes in mice. *JNCI, J. Natl. Cancer Inst.* **69**, 67–71.

Kao, Y. J., and Juliano, R. L. (1981). Interactions of liposomes with the reticuloendothelial system. Effects of reticuloendothelial blockade on the clearance of large unilamellar vesicles. *Biochim. Biophys. Acta* **677**, 453–461.

Kato, T. (1)82). Encapsulated drugs in targeted cancer therapy. *In* "Controlled Drug Delivery" (S. D. Bruck, ed.), Vol. 11, pp. 189–240. CRC Press, Boca Raton, Florida.

Kaye, S. B. (1981). Liposomes—problems and promise as selective drug carriers. *Cancer Treat. Rep.* **8**, 27–50.

Kaye, S. B., and Ryman, B. E. (1980). The fate of liposome entrapped-actinomycin D *in vivo* and its therapeutic effect in a solid murine tumor. *Biochem. Soc. Trans.* **8**, 107–108.

Kedar, A., Mayhew, E., Moore, R. H., Williams, P., and Murphy, G. P. (1980). Effect of actinomycin D–containing lipid vesicles on murine renal adenocarcinoma. *J. Surg. Oncol.* **15**, 363–365.

Khato, J., Priester, E. R., and Sieber, S. M. (1982). Enhanced lymph node uptake of melphalan following liposomal entrapment and effects on lymph node metastasis in rats. *Cancer Treat. Rep.* **66**, 517–527.

Kimelberg, H. K., and Atchison, M. A. (1978). Effects of entrapment in liposomes on the distribution, degradation and effectiveness of methotrexate in vivo. *Ann. N. Y. Acad. Sci.* **308**, 395–409.

Kobayashi, T., Tsukagoshi, S., and Sakurai, Y. (1975). Enhancement of the cancer chemotherapeutic effect of cytosine arabinoside entrapped in liposomes on mouse leukemia L-1210. *Gann* **66**, 719–720.

Kobayashi, T., Kataoka, T., Tsukagoshi, S., and Sakurai, Y. (1977). Enhancement of antitumor effect of β-D-arabinofuranosylcytosine by encapsulation in liposomes. *Int. J. Cancer* **20**, 581–587.

Koskowski, M. J., Rosen, F., Millholland, R. J., and Papahadjopoulos, D. (1978). Effect of lipid vesicle (liposome) encapsulation of methotrexate on its chemotherapeutic efficacy in solid rodent tumors. *Cancer Res.* **38**, 2848–2853.

Leserman, L. D., Machy, P., Devaux, C., and Barbet, J. (1983). Antibody-bearing liposomes: Targeting in vivo. *Biol. Cell* **47**, 111–116.

Levy, R., and Miller, R. A. (1983). Tumor therapy with monoclonal antibodies. *Fed. Proc., Fed. Am. Soc. Exp. Biol.* **42**, 2650–2656.

Long, D. M., Multer, F. K., Greenberg, A. G., Peskin, G. W., Lasser, E. C., Wickham, W. G., and Sharts, C. M. (1978). Tumor imaging with X-rays using macrophage uptake of radio-opaque fluorocarbon emulsions. *Surgery* **84**, 104–112.

Lopez-Berenstein, G., Mehta, R., Hopfer, R. L., Mills, K., Kasi, L., Mehta, K., Fainstein, V., Luna, M., Hersh, E. M., and Juliano, R. (1983). Treatment and prophylaxis of disseminated infection due to *Candida albicans* in mice with liposome-encapsulated amphotericin B. *J. Infect. Dis.* **5,** 939–945.

Louria, D. B., and Sen, P. (1982). Fungal infections with a particular focus on the compromised host. *Del. Med. J.* **54,** 11–19.

Lubec, G., Kuhn, K., Latzka, U., and Reale, E. (1981). Glomerular permeability for proteins of high molecular weight entrapped in liposomes. *Renal Physiol.* **4,** 131–136.

Lynch, W. E., Sartiano, G. P., and Ghaffar, A. (1980). Erythrocytes as carriers of chemotherapeutic agents for targeting to the reticuloendothelial system. *Am. J. Hematol.* **9,** 249–259.

Machy, P., and Leserman, L. D. (1983). Small liposomes are better than large liposomes for specific drug delivery in vitro. *Biochim. Biophys. Acta* **730,** 313–320.

Machy, P., Barbet, J., and Leserman, L. D. (1982). Differential endocytosis of T and B lymphocyte surface molecules evaluated with antibody-bearing fluorescent liposomes containing methotrexate. *Proc. Natl. Acad. Sci. U.S.A.* **79,** 4148–4152.

McMichael, A. J., and Fabre, J. W., eds. (1982). "Monoclonal Antibodies in Medicine." Academic Press, New York.

Magin, R. L., and Weinstein, J. (1982). Delivery of drugs in temperature-sensitive liposomes. *In* "Targeting of Drugs" (G. Gregoriadis, J. Senior, and A. Trouet, eds.), pp. 202–221. Plenum, New York.

Majno, G., and Palade, G. E. (1961). Studies on inflammation. The effect of histamine and serotonin on vascular permeability: An electron microscopic study. *J. Biophys. Biochem. Cytol.* **11,** 571–605.

Martinez-Palomo, A. (1970). Ultrastructural modifications of intercellular junctions in some epithelial tumors. *Lab. Invest.* **22,** 605–614.

Mathe, G., and Bothorel, P. (1981). In vivo enhancement of the experimental oncostatic effects of RSCNU by its encapsulation in liposomes. *Biomedicine* **35,** 201–202.

Mayhew, E., Rustum, Y., and Szoka, F. (1980). Efficacy of liposome-entrapped cytosine arabinoside (ARA-C) compared with infused "free" ARA-C against L1210 tumor. *Proc. Am. Assoc. Can. Res.* **21,** 293.

Mayhew, E., Rustum, Y. M., and Szoka, F. (1982). Therapeutic efficacy of cytosine arabinoside trapped in liposomes. *In* "Targeting of Drugs" (G. Gregoriadis, J. Senior, and A. Trouet, eds.), pp. 249–260. Plenum, New York.

Mazauric T., Mitchell, K. F., Letchworth, G. J., III, Koprowski, H., and Steplewski, Z. (1982). Monoclonal antibody-defined human lung cell surface protein antigens. *Cancer Res.* **42,** 150–154.

Mazunder, A. (1981). Effect of liposome entrapped 5-fluorouracil on Ehrlich ascites tumor bearing mice. *Ind. J. Biochem. Biophys.* **18,** 120–123.

Motta, P., and Makable, S. (1980). Foetal and adult liver sinusoids and Kupffer cells as revealed by scanning electron microscopy. *In* "The Reticuloendothelial System and the Pathogenesis of Liver Disease" (H. Liehr and M. Grun, eds.), pp. 11–16. Elsevier, Amsterdam.

Mueller, T. M., Marcus, M. L., Mayer, H. E., Williams, J. K., and Hermsmeyer, K. (1981). Liposome concentration in canine ischemic myocardium and depolarized myocardial cells. *Cir. Res.* **49,** 405–415.

New, R. R. C., Chance, M. L., and Heath, S. (1981). The treatment of experimental cutaneous leishmaniasis with liposome-entrapped Pentostam. *Parasitology* **83,** 519–527.

Newmark, P. (1983). Priority by press release. *Nature (London)* **304,** 108.

Nicolau, C., and Poste, G., eds. (1983). Liposomes in vivo. *Biol. Cell.* (Special Issue) **47,** 1–133.

Nicolson, G. L., and Poste, G. (1983). Tumor cell diversity and host responses in cancer metastasis. Host immune responses and therapy of metastases. *Curr. Concepts Cancer* **7,** 3–42.

Olson, F., Mayhew, E., Maslow, D., Rustum, Y., and Szoka, F. (1982). Characterization, toxicity and therapeutic efficacy of adriamycin encapsulated in liposomes. *Eur. J. Cancer Clin. Oncol.* **18,** 167–176.

Olsson, L. (1983). Phenotypic diversity in leukemia cell populations. *Cancer Met. Rev.* **2,** 153–164.

Owens, A. H., Coffey, D. S., and Baylin, S. B., eds. (1982). "Tumor Cell Heterogeneity: Origins and Implications." Academic Press, New York.

Palmer, T. N., Caride, V. J., Fernandez, L. A., and Twickler, J. (1981). Liposome accumulation in ischaemic intestine following experimental mesenteric occlusion. *BioScience Rep.* **1,** 337–344.

Papadimitriou, J. M., and Woods, A. E. (1975). Structural and functional characteristics of the microcirculation in neoplasms. *J. Pathol.* **116,** 65–72.

Patel, K. R., Jonah, M. M., and Rahman, Y. R. (1982). In vitro uptake and therapeutic application of liposome-encapsulated methotrexate in mouse hepatoma 129. *Eur. J. Cancer Clin. Oncol.* **18,** 833–843.

Pelham, L. D. (1981). Rational use of intravenous fat emulsions. *Am. J. Hosp. Pharm.* **38,** 198–208.

Peterson, H.-I., ed. (1979). "Tumor Blood Circulation: Angiogenesis, Vascular Morphology and Blood Flow of Experimental and Human Tumors." CRC Press, Boca Raton, Florida.

Pino, R. M., and Essner, E. (1981). Permeability of rat choriocapillaris to hemeproteins. Restriction of tracers by a fenestrated endothelium. *J. Histochem. Cytobiochem.* **29,** 281–290.

Poste, G. (1980). The interaction of lipid vesicles (liposomes) with cultured cells and their use as carriers for drugs and macromolecules. *In* "Liposomes in Biological Systems" (G. Gregoriadis and A. C. Allison, eds.), pp. 101–151. Wiley, New York.

Poste, G. (1982). Experimental systems for analysis of the malignant phenotype. *Cancer Met. Rev.* **1,** 141–199.

Poste, G. (1983). Liposome targeting *in vivo:* Problems and opportunities. *Biol. Cell.* **47,** 19–39.

Poste, G., and Fidler, I. J. (1980). The pathogenesis of cancer metastasis. *Nature (London)* **283,** 139–146.

Poste, G., and Fidler, I. J. (1981). Stimulation of macrophage-mediated destruction of lung metastases by administration of immunomodulators encapsulated in liposomes. *In* "Liposomes, Drugs and Immunocompetent Cell Functions" (C. Nicolau and A. Paraf, eds.), pp. 147–162. Academic Press, New York.

Poste, G., and Fidler, I. J. (1982). Active non-specific immunotherapy of lung metastases by macrophage activating agents encapsulated in liposomes. *Alfred Benzon Symp.* No. 17, pp. 418–429.

Poste, G., and Greig, R. (1982). On the genesis and regulation of cellular heterogeneity in malignant tumors. *Invas. Metast.* **2,** 137–176.

Poste, G., and Kirsh, R. (1979). Rapid decay of tumoricidal activity and loss of responsiveness to lymphokines in inflammatory macrophages. *Cancer Res.* **39,** 2582–2590.

Poste, G., and Kirsh, R. (1982). Liposome-encapsulated macrophage activation agents and active non-specific immunotherapy of neoplastic disease. *In* "Cell Function and Differentiation" (G. A. Koyunoglou, A. E. Evangelopoulos, J. Georgatsos, G. Palarologos, A. Trakatellis, and C. P. Tsiganos, eds.), Part A, pp. 309–319. Alan R. Liss, New York.

Poste, G., and Nicolson, G. L. (1983). Experimental systems for analysis of the surface properties of metastatic tumor cells. *In* "Biomembranes" (A. Nowotny, ed.), Vol. II, pp. 341–364. Plenum, New York.

Poste, G., Kirsh, R., Fogler, W., and Fidler, I. J. (1979). Activation of tumoricidal properties in mouse macrophages by lymphokines encapsulated in liposomes. *Cancer Res.* **39,** 881–892.

Poste, G., Kirsh, R., Raz, A., Sone, S., Bucana, C., Fogler, W. E., and Fidler, I. J. (1980). Activation of tumoricidal properties in macrophages by liposome-encapsulated lymphokines:

In vitro studies. *In* "Liposomes in Immunobiology" (B. Tom and H. Six, eds.), pp. 93–108. Elsevier, Amsterdam.

Poste, G., Bucana, C., Raz, A., Bugelski, P., Kirsh, R., and Fidler, I. J. (1982). Analysis of the fate of systemically administered liposomes and implications for their use in drug delivery. *Cancer Res.* **42**, 1412–1422.

Poste, G., Kirsh, R., Koestler, T., Bugelski, P., and Lewis, H. (1983a). Analysis of the interaction of liposomes with mononuclear phagocytes in the liver, spleen and bone marrow (submitted for publication).

Poste, G., Kirsh, R., and Koestler, T. (1983b). The challenge of liposome targeting in vivo. *In* "Liposome Technology" (G. Gregoriadis, ed.), Vol. III, pp. 1–28. CRC Press, Boca Raton, Florida.

Proffitt, R. T., Williams, L. E., Presant, C. A., Tin, G. W., Uliana, J. A., Gamble, R. C., and Baldeschwieler, J. D. (1983). Liposomal blockade of the reticuloendothelial system: Improved tumor imaging with small unilamellar vesicles. *Science* **220**, 502–505.

Rahman, A., Kessler, A. More, N., Sikic, B., Rowden, G., Woolley, P., and Schein, P. S. (1980). Liposomal protection of adriamycin-induced cardiotoxicity in mice. *Cancer Res.* **40**, 1532–1537.

Rahman, A., More, N., and Schein, P. S. (1982). Doxorubicin-induced chronic cardiotoxicity and its protection by liposomal administration. *Cancer Res.* **42**, 1817–1825.

Raso, V., Ritz, J., Basala, M., and Schlossman, S. T. (1982). Monoclonal antibody-ricin A chain conjugate selectively cytotoxic for cells bearing the common acute lymphoblastic leukemia antigen. *Cancer Res.* **42**, 457–464.

Richardson, V. J., Ryman, B. E., Jewkes, R. F., Jeyasingh, K., Tattersall, M. N. H., Newlands, E. S., and Kaye, S. B. (1979). Tissue distribution and tumour localization of 99m-technetium-labelled liposomes in cancer patients. *Br. J. Cancer* **40**, 35–43.

Ritter, C., Iyengar, C. L., Rutman, R. J. (1981). Differential enhancement of antitumor effectiveness by phospholipid vesicles (Liposomes). *Cancer Res.* **41**, 2366–2371.

Rustum, Y., Dave, C., Mayhew, E., and Papahadjopoulos, D. (1979). Role of liposome type and route of administration in the antitumor activity of 1-β-D arabinofuranosylcytosine against mouse L1210 leukemia. *Cancer Res.* **33**, 1390–1395.

Ryman, B. G., and Barratt, G. M. (1982). Liposomes—further considerations of their possible role as carriers of therapeutic agents. *In* "Targeting of Drugs" (G. Gregoriadis, J. Senior, and A. Trouet, eds.), pp. 235–248. Plenum, New York.

Ryman, B. G., Jewkes, R. F., Jeyasingh, K., Osborne, M. P., Patel, H. M., Richardson, V. J., Tattersall, N. H. N., and Tyrell, D. A. (1978). Potential applications of liposomes in therapy. *Ann. N. Y. Acad. Sci.* **308**, 281–296.

Schatski, P. F., and Newsome, A. (1975). Neutralized lanthanum solution: A largely noncolloidal ultrastructural tracer. *Stain Technol.* **50**, 171–178.

Scherphof, G. L. (1982). Interaction of liposomes with biological fluids and fate of liposomes in vivo. *In* "Liposome Methodology" (L. D. Leserman and J. Barbet, eds.), pp. 79–92. Inserm, Paris.

Shinozawa, S., Tsutsui, K., and Oda, T. (1979). Enhancement of the antitumor effect of illudin S by including it in liposomes. *Experentia* **35**, 1102–1103.

Shinozawa, S., Araki, Y., and Oda, T. (1980). Antitumor effects of neocarzinostatin entrapped in liposomes. *Gann* **71**, 107–111.

Shinozawa, S., Anaki, Y., and Oda, T. (1981). Tissue distribution and antitumor effect of liposome-entrapped doxorubicin (adriamycin) in Ehrlich ascites solid tumor bearing mice. *Acta Med. Okayama* **35**, 395–405.

Simionescu, M., Simionescu, N., and Palade, G. E. (1982). Biochemically differentiated microdomains of the cell surface of capillary endothelium. *Ann. N.Y. Acad. Sci.* **401**, 9–24.

Simpson, L. O. (1981). *In* "Biological Thixotropy of Basement Membranes: the Key to the Understanding of Capillary Permeability" (D. Garlick, ed.), pp. 55–66. Committee in Postgraduate Medical Education, Univ. of New South Wales.

Sur, P., Roy, D. K., and Das, M. K. (1981). The efficacy of trimethylamine carboxyborane by liposomal encapsulation in the treatment of EAC in mice. *ICRS Med. Sci.* **9**, 1066–1067.

Szoka, F., and Papahadjopoulos, D. (1981). Liposomes. Preparation and characterization. *In* "Liposomes: From Physical Structure to Therapeutic Applications" (C. G. Knight, ed.), pp. 51–82. Elsevier, Amsterdam.

Taylor, R. L., Williams, D. M., Craven, P. C., Graybill, J. R., Drutz, D. J., and Magee, W. E. (1982). Amphotericin B in liposomes: A novel therapy for histoplasmosis. *Am. Rev. Respir. Dis.* **125**, 610–611.

Tomlinson, G. (1983). Microsphere delivery systems for drug targeting and controlled release. *Int. J. Pharm. Technol. Prod. Mgmt.* (in press).

Underwood, J. C. E., and Carr, I. (1972). The ultrastructure and permeability characteristics of the blood vessels of a transplanted rat sarcoma. *J. Pathol.* **107**, 157–166.

Urano, M., Rice, L., Epstein, R., Suit, H. D., and Chu, A. M. (1983). Effect of whole-body hyperthermia on cell survival, metastasis frequency, and host immunity in moderately and weakly immunogenic murine tumors. *Cancer Res.* **43**, 1039–1043.

Walker, A., McCallum, H. M., Wheldon, T. E., Nias, A. H., and Abdelaal, A. S. (1978). Promotion of metastasis of C3H mouse mammary carcinoma by local hyperthermia. *Br. J. Cancer* **38**, 561–563.

Ward, J. D., Hadfield, M. G., Becker, D. P., and Lovings, E. T. (1974). Endothelial fenestrations and other vascular alterations in primary melanoma of the central nervous system. *Cancer* **34**, 1982–1991.

Warren, B. A. (1979). The vascular morphology of tumors. *In* "Tumor Blood Circulation: Angiogenesis, Vascular Morphology and Blood Flow of Experimental and Human Tumors" (H.-I. Peterson, ed.), pp. 1–48. CRC Press, Boca Raton, Florida.

Webb, K. S., Ware, J. L., Parks, S. F., Briner, W. H., and Paulson, D. F. (1983). Monoclonal antibodies of different epitopes on a prostate tumor-associated antigen: Implications for immunotherapy. *Cancer Immunol. Immunother.* **14**, 155–166.

Weinstein, J. N., Majin, R. L., Cysyk, R. L., and Zeharko, D. S. (1980). Treatment of solid L1210 murine tumors with local hyperthermia and temperature-sensitive liposomes containing methotrexate. *Cancer Res.* **40**, 1388–1395.

Weiss, L., and Greep, R. O. (1977). "Histology," 4th ed. McGraw-Hill, New York.

Widder, K. J., Senyei, A. G., and Ranney, D. F. (1979). Magnetically responsive microspheres and other carriers for the biophysical targeting of antitumor agents. *Adv. Pharmacol. Chemother.* **16**, 213–267.

Widder, K. J., Senyei, A. E., and Sears, B. (1982). Experimental methods in cancer therapeutics. *J. Pharm. Sci.* **71**, 379–387.

Wikman-Coffelt, J., Leung, J., and Mason, D. T. (1980). In vivo localization of liposomes in skeletal and cardiac muscle following experimental coronary ligation in guinea pigs. *Biochem. Med.* **23**, 87–93.

Willis, R. A. (1973). "Pathology of Tumors," 4th ed., p. 157. Butterworth, London.

Wolff, J. R. (1977). Ultrastructure of the terminal vascular bed as related to function. *In* "Microcirculation" (G. Kaley and B. M. Altura, eds.), Vol. I, pp. 95–130. Univ. Park Press, Baltimore, Maryland.

Wright, D. G., Dale, D. C., Fauci, A. S., and Wolff, E. M. (1981). Human cyclic neutropenia: clinical review and long-term follow-up of patients. *Medicine* **60**, 1–13.

Yatvin, M. B., and Lelkes, P. I. (1982). Clinical prospects for liposomes. *Med. Phys.* **9**, 149–175.

Yatvin, M. B., Muhlensiepen, H., Porschen, W., Weinstein, J. N., and Feinendegen, L. E. (1981).

Selective delivery of liposome associated *cis*-dichloro-diamine platinumII by heat and its influence on tumor drug uptake and growth. *Cancer Res.* **41**, 1602–1607.

Yatvin, M. B., Cree, T. C., and Gipp, J. I. (1982). Hyperthermia-mediated targeting of liposome-associated anti-neoplastic drugs. *In* "Targeting of Drugs" (G. Gregoriadis, J. Senior, and A. Trouet, eds.), pp. 223–248. Plenum, New York.

Youhle, R. J., and Neville, D. M. (1980). Anti-thy 1.2 monoclonal antibody linked to ricin is a potent cell-type-specific toxin. *Proc. Natl. Acad. Sci. U.S.A.* **77**, 5483–5486.

6

Macrophage Activation by Lymphokines: Usefulness as Antimetastatic Agents

EUGENIE S. KLEINERMAN*
Laboratory of Molecular Immunoregulation
Biological Response Modifiers Program
Frederick Cancer Research Facility
National Cancer Institute
Frederick, Maryland

ISAIAH J. FIDLER*
Cancer Metastasis and Treatment Laboratory
Litton Biomedics, Inc.—Basic Research Program
Frederick Cancer Research Facility
National Cancer Institute
Frederick, Maryland

I.	Introduction	232
II.	Interaction of Macrophages with Heterogeneous Neoplasms	233
III.	Manipulations of Macrophages for Treatment of Metastases	235
IV.	Activation of Tumoricidal Properties of Human Monocytes *in Vitro* by Liposome-Encapsulated Human Lymphokines	237
V.	Selective Destruction of Tumor Cells by Human Monocytes Activated with Liposome-Encapsulated MAF	241
VI.	Conclusions	243
	References	244

*Present address: Department of Cell Biology, M. D. Anderson Hospital and Tumor Institute, The University of Texas System Cancer Center, P.O. Box HMB-173, Houston, Texas 77030.

231

Novel Approaches to Cancer Chemotherapy
Copyright © 1984 by Academic Press, Inc.
All rights of reproduction in any form reserved.
ISBN 0-12-676980-X

I. INTRODUCTION

The most devastating aspect of cancer is the propensity of malignant neoplasms to spread from their primary site of growth to distant organs where secondary tumors, metastases, can develop. Despite remarkable advances in aggressive adjuvant therapy and improvements in general patient care, most deaths of patients with solid cancers are caused by progressive growth of metastatic lesions that are resistant to conventional therapies. There are several reasons for the current failure to treat cancer metastasis successfully. First, because early disseminated lesions are microscopic, they often are undetected when the primary tumor is diagnosed and excised, only to be detected later after substantial growth has taken place. Second, even when metastases are diagnosed, their location and number may not permit complete and total surgical resection. Likewise the location and number of lesions may limit the effective dose of therapeutic agents (i.e., radiation and/or cytotoxic drugs) that can be delivered to the lesion without being toxic to the normal tissues. Third, the most formidable obstacle to successful treatment of metastasis is the heterogeneous nature of malignant neoplasms and the rapid emergence of metastases that are resistant to conventional therapeutic regimens (Fidler, 1978a; Poste and Fidler, 1979; Fidler and Kripke, 1980).

There is now a large body of data to indicate that at the time of diagnosis, malignant neoplasms are heterogeneous and contain cells with diverse characteristics such as antigenicity and/or immunogenicity (Prehn, 1965, 1970; Sugarbaker and Cohen, 1972; Faraci, 1974; Goldman *et al.*, 1974; Killion and Kollmorgen, 1976; Fidler *et al.*, 1976; Byers and Johnston, 1977; Biddison and Palmer, 1977; Fidler and Bucana, 1977; Fugi *et al.*, 1977; Killion, 1978; Kripke *et al.*, 1978; Miller and Heppner, 1979; Kolb and Muller, 1979; Kerbel, 1979; Schirrmacher *et al.*, 1979; Olsson and Ebbesen, 1979), growth rate (DeWys, 1972; Schabel, 1975; Cifone *et al.*, 1979; Cifone and Fidler, 1980; Miller *et al.*, 1980), protein production (Gray and Pierce, 1964; Niles and Makarski, 1978; Fidler *et al.*, 1981), karyotypes (Ito and Moore, 1967; Mittleman, 1971; Ohno, 1971; Bohm and Sondritter, 1975; Vindelov, 1977; Siracky, 1979; Vindelov *et al.*, 1980), cell surface receptors (Tao and Burger, 1977; Brunson and Nicolson, 1978; Raz *et al.*, 1980; Reading *et al.*, 1980), hormone receptors (Franks, 1960; Sluyser and Van Nie, 1974; Baylin *et al.*, 1975, 1978; Sluyser *et al.*, 1976), response to a variety of cytotoxic drugs (Barranco *et al.*, 1972, 1973; Hakansson and Trope, 1974a,b; Trope, 1975; Trope *et al.*, 1975, 1979; Fugmann *et al.*, 1977; Heppner *et al.*, 1978; Barranco *et al.*, 1978; Lotan, 1979; Lotan and Nicolson, 1979; Calabresi *et al.*, 1979; Tsuruo and Fidler, 1981), and metastatic potential (Fidler and Kripke, 1977; Nicolson and Brunson, 1977; Nicolson *et al.*, 1978; Fidler and Cifone, 1979; Liotta *et al.*, 1980; Fidler and Hart, 1981). The recognition that malignant neoplasms are composed of cells with diverse biological behaviors has initiated studies into the nature of this heterogeneity and its implications for therapy.

Heterogeneity in sensitivity to cytotoxic drugs exists among tumor cells populating primary neoplasms. For example, cells isolated from a rat hepatocellular carcinoma (Barranco et al., 1978), a methylcholanthrene-induced murine sarcoma (Hakansson and Trope, 1974b), and a murine mammary tumor (Heppner et al., 1978), have been shown in vitro and in vivo to have different sensitivities to a variety of chemotherapeutic agents. These observations are not restricted to experimental tumor systems. Various human neoplasms such as melanoma (Lotan, 1979), lymphoma (Baylin, 1981), and adenocarcinomas isolated from the colon (Trope, 1981), stomach (Trope et al., 1979), breast (Lotan, 1979), and ovary (Trope et al., 1979) also have been shown to be heterogeneous for drug response. Moreover, even within the same patient, different metastases can exhibit different susceptibilities to chemotherapeutic agents (Tsuruo and Fidler, 1981). The emergence of drug-resistant tumor cell variants in clinical oncology is well documented. For example, small-cell carcinoma of the lung usually is initially sensitive to chemotherapy with or without radiotherapy. In contrast, recurrences, which are a common feature of this neoplasm, are resistant to chemotherapy regardless of the magnitude of the initial response to therapy (Abelff et al., 1979; Livinston, 1979). These tumor cells that are resistant to chemotherapy can proliferate unchecked following the destruction of the sensitive populations. Thus, to treat successfully tumors that are difficult to reach or resect completely, and particularly tumors that have already metastasized, agents that can circumvent both the cellular heterogeneity and drug resistance of tumors must be developed and incorporated into cancer therapeutic regimens.

Although specific immunotherapy has been disappointing in the treatment of cancer, "nonspecific" or "natural" host antitumor defense mechanisms such as macrophage-mediated tumoricidal activity may offer a different and more successful approach to the problem of eradicating metastases.

II. INTERACTION OF MACROPHAGES WITH HETEROGENEOUS NEOPLASMS

The macrophage is recognized as an important component of host defense against bacterial, fungal, and parasitic infections. In addition, the role of macrophages in host defense against neoplasms has attracted increasing attention (Fidler and Poste, 1982). The macrophage may provide surveillance in the detection and destruction of neoplastic cells (Hibbs et al., 1972; Evans and Alexander, 1976). Lurie (1964) noticed that in rabbit tumor systems the incidence of uterine cancer, dependent on age and strain, was parallel to the natural resistance to tuberculosis (the most resistant strain having the lowest incidence of cancer). In addition, the resistance of the rabbits to tuberculosis was directly related to the bactericidal capacity of their macrophages. These studies suggested a correlation between the activity of the macrophages and the observed resistance to neoplasia. Studies by Droller and Remington (1975) supported this concept. In their investigations, mice infected with the intracellular protozoan *Toxoplasma gondii* were more resistant to viral induction of neoplasms and to tumors resulting from the transplantation of syngeneic tumor cells. The macrophages harvested from the protozoan-infected mice were cytotoxic *in vitro* to the transplanted tumor cells.

The importance of macrophages in carcinogenesis was revealed from studies by Norbury and Kripke (1979), who investigated whether treatment of mice with either a macrophage stimulant (pyran copolymer) or macrophage toxins (trypan blue or silica) would influence the latency and/or incidence of skin carcinogenesis induced by ultraviolet radiation. Treatment of mice with pyran copolymer lengthened the latent period of tumor development and reduced the incidence and number of the skin tumors that resulted from suboptimal exposures to ultraviolet radiation. Conversely, treatment of mice with macrophage toxins shortened the latent period for induction of skin cancer by ultraviolet radiation. Similarly, in transplantable tumor systems, the impairment of macrophage function by agents such as carrageenan or silica was found to be associated with an increase in the incidence of spontaneous (Jones and Castro, 1977; Sadler *et al.*, 1979) and experimental metastases (Mantovani *et al.*, 1980).

Evidence of the effectiveness of activated macrophages in controlling cancer metastasis *in vivo* comes from adoptive transfer studies. Intravenous injections of syngeneic murine macrophages that had been rendered tumoricidal by *in vivo* or *in vitro* manipulations reduced the incidence of experimental metastases (Fidler, 1974; Liotta *et al.*, 1977; Fidler *et al.*, 1979). Similarly, macrophages activated *in vitro* have been shown to inhibit the growth of tumors at primary sites (Den Otter *et al.*, 1977).

Although tumor cell populations are heterogeneous with regard to many characteristics, they appear to be susceptible to destruction by activated (tumoricidal) macrophages. The term macrophage activation is quite vague. In some studies, activation is taken to represent a change in the behavior of macrophages, such as increased adherence to glass, increased mobility, increased phagocytic capability, or increased enzymatic activity (Fidler and Raz, 1981). In this chapter, however, the term macrophage activation is reserved for the process whereby noncytotoxic macrophages acquire tumor-cytotoxic or tumoricidal properties.

Activated macrophages have the ability to recognize and destroy neoplastic cells (Hibbs, 1974a; Piessens and Churchill, 1975; Fidler, 1978b), regardless of the *in vivo* biological behavior of the tumor cell. Melanoma variant cell lines that have a low or high metastatic potential, that have invasive or noninvasive characteristics, and that are either susceptible or resistant to lysis mediated by syngeneic T cells are lysed *in vitro* by activated macrophages (Fidler, 1978b; Fidler and Poste, 1982). Similarly, several cloned cell lines that were isolated from a murine fibrosarcoma induced by ultraviolet radiation and that vary in their degree of immunogenicity and/or invasive and metastatic potential *in vivo* (Kripke *et al.*, 1978) are all susceptible to destruction *in vitro* by tumoricidal macrophages (Fidler and Cifone, 1979). The nature of target cell susceptibility to destruction by activated macrophages has also been examined with virus-transformed cell lines in which various characteristics of the transformed phenotype are temperature dependent (Fidler *et al.*, 1978). These studies demonstrated that the tumor cells were lysed by macrophages regardless of whether they expressed cell surface LETS protein or Forssman antigens, displayed surface charges that permitted agglutination by low doses of plant lectins, expressed Simian virus 40 (SV40) T antigen, had a low saturation density, or exhibited density-dependent inhibition of DNA synthesis (Fidler *et al.*, 1978). Moreover, attempts to select *in vitro* tumor cell variant lines that are resistant to macrophage-mediated lysis have proved unsuccessful (Fidler and Poste, 1982); the techniques were similar to those used previously to select successfully tumor cell lines that are resistant to lysis by syngeneic T lymphocytes (Fidler *et al.*, 1976) or natural killer cells (Hanna and Fidler, 1980). We have attempted to select for macrophage-resistant tumor variants using 11 mouse tumors of different histological classification, etiology, and histocompatibility. Despite rigorous selection pressures, we were unable to isolate macrophage-resistant tumor cell populations.

Because activated macrophages are able to kill phenotypically diverse tumor cells, including cells that are resistant to killing by other components of the host defense system and various anticancer drugs (Fidler and Poste, 1982), the activation of these cells to the tumoricidal state is an intriguing possibility for the treatment of individuals with metastatic disease.

III. MANIPULATIONS OF MACROPHAGES
FOR TREATMENT OF METASTASES

As discussed in the previous section, the intravenous injection of nonspecifically activated macrophages into mice bearing metastases has been shown to inhibit tumor growth both in the primary site (Den Otter *et al.*, 1977) and in metastases (Fidler, 1974; Liotta *et al.*, 1977; Fidler *et al.*, 1979); therefore, intravenous administration of activated macrophages might be useful in augmenting host resistance to disseminated neoplastic disease. For clinical use, however, this strategy has two serious shortcomings: the transfusion of a large number of histocompatible or autologous macrophages is required, and most intravenously injected macrophages are likely to become arrested in the capillary bed of the lung and not reach other relevant sites. A more promising approach is to develop methods whereby autologous macrophages can be activated *in situ*.

One of the major pathways for macrophage activation *in vivo* is believed to result from the action of the lymphokine component [macrophage-activating factor (MAF)], which is released from sensitized lymphocytes. MAF can be produced by incubating lymphocytes *in vitro* with an antigen to which the donor of the lymphocytes has been previously sensitized. MAF specifically interacts with macrophages bearing appropriate receptors (Fidler and Raz, 1981; Poste *et al.*, 1979a). Subsequently, MAF-treated macrophages can recognize and destroy neoplastic cells both *in vitro* and *in vivo* (Cameron and Churchill, 1979; Churchill *et al.*, 1975; Fidler, 1978b; Fidler and Raz, 1981; Poste *et al.*, 1979b; Kleinerman and Fidler, 1983; Kleinerman *et al.*, 1983) by a nonimmunological mechanism that requires cell-to-cell contact (Hibbs, 1974b; Bucana *et al.*, 1976; Marino and Adams, 1982; Key *et al.*, 1982). Lymphokines are also released spontaneously from lymphoid cell cultures (McDaniel *et al.*, 1976; Papermaster *et al.*, 1976) or from normal lymphocytes in suspension following their interaction with nonspecific mitogens such as phytohemagglutinin and concanavalin A (Fidler and Raz, 1981).

To date, an exact chemical definition for MAF is lacking. Direct measurement of the amount of MAF required to activate macrophages cannot be made because the only assay for its activity now available involves biological assay of its action on macrophages. Thus, for convenience and brevity in this chapter, lymphocyte culture supernatant fluids rich in MAF activity will be referred to as MAF.

Therapeutic use of MAF is hindered by the lack of purified preparations of this mediator, and efforts to activate the tumoricidal properties of macrophages *in vivo* by parenteral injection of crude preparations of lymphokines have proved unsuccessful. Injection of lymphokines into skin (Yoshida and Cohen, 1972) or skin tumors (Papermaster *et al.*, 1974; Salvin *et al.*, 1975) provoked local inflammatory reactions and histological changes suggestive of macrophage activation that resulted in the regression of small cutaneous tumors; however, systemic activation of macrophages is more difficult for several reasons: (1) Lymphokines injected into venous circulation have a short half-life, probably because of rapid dilution, undesirable clearance, and binding to plasma proteins (Poste and Kirsh, 1979). (2) Only a small fraction of the macrophages may be capable of responding to MAF. (3) Macrophages can be activated by lymphokines only within a relatively short period following their emigration into tissues from the circulation (Poste and Kirsh, 1979). (4) The tumoricidal properties of macrophages are short-lived (2–3 days), and macrophages are refractory to reactivation by lymphokines (Poste and Kirsh, 1979). Even under ideal conditions, at least an 8-hr interaction between human monocytes and free MAF is required for successful activation (Cameron and Churchill, 1979; Kleinerman *et al.*, 1983); therefore, the systemic administration of soluble lymphokines will not result in monocyte/macrophage activation because of the short half-life of the lymphokines. In addition, the systemic administration of crude unfractionated preparations of lymphokines may cause undesirable side effects and thus may not be feasible.

Consequently, efficient therapeutic activation of macrophages *in vivo* requires an agent that is stable, nontoxic, and nonimmunogenic, and that can provide sufficient interaction time with the target cells. The concept of devising a carrier vehicle to transport the activating agent to the macrophages *in situ* would seem to fulfill these requirements.

IV. ACTIVATION OF TUMORICIDAL PROPERTIES OF HUMAN MONOCYTES *IN VITRO* BY LIPOSOME-ENCAPSULATED HUMAN LYMPHOKINES

To overcome the shortcomings of using free MAF as an activating agent *in situ,* our laboratory has focused on the use of multilamellar liposomes as vehicles for delivering substances such as MAF directly to the phagocytic cell. Most investigations of macrophage activation *in vitro* and *in vivo* have used rodent systems; however, we have begun to investigate the use of liposome-encapsulated lymphokines to activate human blood monocytes to the tumoricidal state. To serve as vehicles for the delivery of compounds to monocytes and macrophages, liposomes must avidly bind to and become endocytosed by the cells. Similar to the phagocytosis by rodent alveolar and peritoneal macrophages, the phagocytosis of liposomes by human blood monocytes is influenced by the chemical composition and surface charge of the liposomes (Kleinerman *et al.,* 1983; Kleinerman and Fidler, 1983). Neutral liposomes made up exclusively of phosphatidylcholine (PC) were inefficiently internalized by monocytes, whereas the uptake of multilamellar liposomes consisting of PC and phosphatidylserine (PS) admixed in a 7:3 mole ratio was greater than 10-fold (Kleinerman *et al.,* 1983). When the PC/PS liposomes were injected iv into mice, 80–90% were taken up by the reticuloendothelial system in the liver and spleen, and 8–10% were localized in the pulmonary microcirculation, where they were able to interact with blood monocytes in the lung (Fidler *et al.,* 1980; Fidler and Poste, 1982). No local or systemic toxicity was observed following multiple intravenous injections of PC/PS multilamellar liposomes.

The human MAF used in our studies was prepared by incubating human mononuclear leukocytes (MNL) with Sepharose-bound concanavalin A (S-Con A) for 48 hr and then harvesting the cell-free supernatant. All MAF activity was attributed to a soluble mediator released by the stimulated lymphocytes. The MAF activity could not be attributed to the direct effects of S-Con A on the monocytes (Kleinerman *et al.,* 1983; Table I). Furthermore, unlike S-Con A, our

TABLE I

Effect of Various Control Supernatants on Monocyte-Mediated Cytotoxicity

Treatment of monocytes with culture supernatants from[a]	Generated cytotoxicity[b] (%)
Medium + S-Con A	−0.09
MNL + medium	−0.014
MNL + S-Con A for 2 hr	−0.018
MNL + S-Con A for 48 hr	43.0
MNL + S-Con A for 48 hr, then heat treatment (100°C for 2 min)	44.0
Control: lipopolysaccharide (1 μg)	71.0

[a] 1×10^5 human monocytes were plated and incubated for 24 hr with the indicated agents. The cells were washed, and 1×10^4 ^{125}I-IUdR-labeled A375 cells were added. Cytotoxicity was assessed after 3 days of cocultivation.

[b] Cytotoxicity as compared to monocytes treated with medium.

preparations were heat stable (100°C × 2 min, Table I). They were also free of endotoxins (<0.125 ng/ml as determined by the *Limulus* amebocyte lysate assay). In addition, the MAF preparations were found negative for α- and β-interferons by the virus neutralization test (<5 U/ml). Although our MAF preparations did contain 100–1000 U of γ-interferon/ml, the direct addition of 1–10,000 U of γ-interferon to our human monocyte preparations did not, in and of itself, activate the monocyte tumoricidal properties (Table II). Furthermore, the heat treatment of our MAF preparation stated previously (100°C × 2 min) removed detectable levels of γ-interferon as determined by the virus neutralization test, yet it had no effect on the activation of cytotoxic activity (Table I, Fig. 1). Finally, when our MAF preparations were treated with antibody to γ-interferon (kindly donated by Dr. Erwin Braude), there was no detectable decrease in activity (Fig. 1). Therefore, we believe that the effects of MAF described here cannot be attributed to Con A, endotoxin, or interferon.

MAF can be encapsulated within the liposomes between the concentric phospholipid bilayers. When these liposomes containing MAF are injected into mice, they are cleared from the circulation by phagocytic cells of the reticuloendothelial system as well as by free monocytes (Fidler *et al.*, 1980; Fidler and Poste, 1982). Thus, preferential delivery of the encapsulated substance can be achieved *in vivo*, because only the cells that phagocytize the liposomes are exposed to the liposome-entrapped agent. Once phagocytized, the biologically active material can be released into the cytoplasm of the phagocyte. This "targeting" therefore circumvents the problems of lymphokine dilution, serum protein binding, rapid undesirable clearance, and the elicitation of undesirable side effects.

TABLE II

Effect of γ-Interferon (γ-INF) on Monocyte-Mediated Tumoricidal Activity

Treatment of monocytes[a]	Generated cytotoxicity[b] (%)
MAF	58
γ-INF 10^4 U	2
γ-INF 10^3 U	−2
γ-INF 10^2 U	1
γ-INF 10^1 U	−17
γ-INF 10^0 U	−23

[a] 1×10^5 human monocytes were plated and incubated for 24 hr with the indicated agents. The cells were washed, and 1×10^4 ^{125}I-IUdR-labeled A375 cells were added. Cytotoxicity was assessed after 3 days of cocultivation.

[b] Cytotoxicity as compared to monocytes treated with medium.

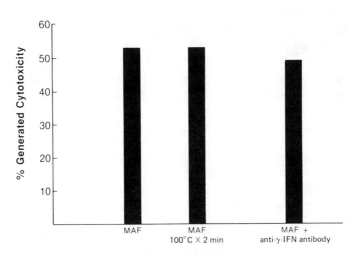

Treatment of Monocytes

Fig. 1. Removal of γ-interferon activity from MAF supernatants by heat treatment or treatment with specific antibody does not affect activation of monocyte-mediated tumoricidal properties. Human monocytes were incubated for 24 hr with MAF, MAF treated at 100°C for 2 min, or MAF treated with anti-γ-interferon antibody for 30 min at 37°C. Tumoricidal activity was subsequently assayed against ^{125}I-IUdR-labeled A375 human melanoma cells at a 10:1 ratio of effector cells to target cells. Cytotoxicity is expressed as compared to monocytes treated with medium.

In rodent systems, MAF encapsulated within liposomes activated macrophages both *in vitro* (Fidler and Raz, 1981; Poste *et al.*, 1979b; Fogler *et al.*, 1980; Sone *et al.*, 1980) and when injected *in vivo* (Fidler, 1980; Fidler *et al.*, 1980, 1982). Similarly, we have shown that human monocytes can be efficiently activated by liposome-encapsulated human MAF (Kleinerman *et al.*, 1983). Dose–response measurements indicate that the liposome-encapsulated preparations induce maximum levels of tumoricidal activity at significantly lower doses than do nonencapsulated "free" preparations (Kleinerman *et al.*, 1983).

Activation of human monocytes to the tumoricidal state by liposome-encapsulated MAF requires a period of 1 to 2 hr for phagocytic uptake of the liposomes and a subsequent lag period of 2 to 4 hr before tumoricidal activity is expressed (Kleinerman *et al.*, 1983). This 1- to 2-hr uptake period is much more feasible than the 8-hr interaction that is required for activation by free MAF (Cameron and Churchill, 1979; Kleinerman *et al.*, 1983). Even under conditions of rapid clearance from the circulation, complete clearance usually requires 1–2 hr after injection. Therefore, in addition to the benefits previously mentioned, liposome-encapsulated MAF has the advantage of giving a sufficient interaction time following injection.

Participation of monocyte/macrophage surface receptors is not required, suggesting that activation results from the interaction of MAF with an intracellular target(s). Unlike activation by free MAF, which requires binding of MAF to a fucoglycolipid receptor on the macrophage surface (Poste *et al.*, 1979a), liposome-encapsulated MAF can activate macrophages that lack functional receptors for MAF (Poste *et al.*, 1979b). Moreover, liposome-encapsulated MAF can induce activation of subpopulations of tissue macrophages and intratumoral macrophages (Poste and Kirsh, 1979; Poste *et al.*, 1979b) that are completely refractory to activation by free MAF.

These findings raised the possibility that macrophage-activating agents encapsulated within liposomes could be similarly efficient in activating mononuclear phagocytes *in vivo* and provide a therapeutic modality for enhancing host resistance against metastases. To test this possibility, we gave mice bearing spontaneous pulmonary metastases intravenous injections of liposome-encapsulated MAF. Multiple intravenous injections of liposome-encapsulated MAF, but not free MAF or control liposome preparations, eradicated spontaneous visceral metastases in C57BL/6NCr mice from which a syngeneic melanoma had been surgically removed. Of the mice treated with liposome-encapsulated MAF, 70% survived at least 200 days. Thus, the intravenous injection of liposome-encapsulated MAF brought about the complete regression of established pulmonary and lymph node metastases.

The mechanism(s) responsible for the regression of established metastases after the systemic administration of liposomes containing MAF probably involved the activation of macrophages to become tumoricidal. Several lines of evidence tend to support this conclusion. First, administration of macrophage-activating agents encapsulated within liposomes that are not retained in the lung fails to activate lung macrophages, and there is no regression of lung metastases (Fidler *et al.*, 1982). Second, the pretreatment of tumor-bearing animals with agents that are toxic for macrophages (silica, carrageenan, hyperchlorinated drinking water) before systemic therapy with liposome-encapsulated lymphokines or other agents abrogates the response to liposome therapy, and such animals rapidly die of metastatic disease (Fidler *et al.*, 1982). Third, intravenous injection of macrophages activated *in vitro* by incubation with liposomes containing MAF produced a reduction in metastatic burden comparable to that achieved by systemic administration of liposome-encapsulated activators (Fidler *et al.*, 1982). In addition, neither functional T lymphocytes nor natural killer cells were found to be necessary for stimulation of host antitumor responses by liposome-encapsulated lymphokines.

It is encouraging that findings from our *in vitro* studies with human monocytes and liposome-encapsulated MAF are similar to findings from studies with various rodent systems. We feel, therefore, that augmentation of human macrophage tumoricidal activity *in situ* can also be achieved by the intravenous injection of liposomes containing MAF.

V. SELECTIVE DESTRUCTION OF TUMOR CELLS BY HUMAN MONOCYTES ACTIVATED WITH LIPOSOME-ENCAPSULATED MAF

A successful approach to the therapy of neoplasms and their metastases may involve the activation of tumoricidal properties of the host's own macrophages. A severe limitation of many cancer therapies is their lack of selectivity and the resultant toxicity to the patient. Therefore, in addition to circumventing both tumor heterogeneity and cell resistance, macrophages must also be able to distinguish between normal and tumorigenic targets so as to avoid nonspecific destruction of the normal tissue.

We have begun to investigate the interaction of activated human monocytes with tumorigenic and nontumorigenic target cells and to determine whether nontumorigenic cells could be lysed as "innocent bystanders." In these experiments tumorigenic and nontumorigenic human cell lines were cocultivated alone, with monocytes preincubated with control liposomes, and with monocytes preincubated with liposomes containing MAF. To determine whether lysed cells were nontumorigenic or tumorigenic cells, the target cells were prelabeled *in vitro* with either [^{3}H]thymidine ([^{3}H]TdR) or [^{14}C]thymidine ([^{14}C]TdR). The human target cells used were A375 melanoma cells, HT-29 colon carcinoma cells, NATUSCH glioblastoma cells, nontumorigenic embryonic lung fibroblasts, and

TABLE III

Monocyte-Mediated Cytotoxicity against
Tumorigenic and Nontumorigenic Targets:
Cocultivation Experiments[a]

Target cells labeled with	
[³H]TdR	[¹⁴C]TdR
A375 mel. (47)	A375 mel. (54)
A375 mel. (45)	HT-29 carc. (37)
A375 mel. (48)	NAT-glio. (47)
A375 mel. (41)	Lung cells (0)
A375 mel. (40)	Kidney cells (0)
Lung cells (0)	A375 mel. (36)
Lung cells (0)	HT-29 carc. (35)
Lung cells (−1)	NAT-glio. (41)
Lung cells (0)	Lung cells (0)
Lung cells (0)	Kidney cells (0)
HT-29 carc. (36)	Lung cells (0)
HT-29 carc. (45)	Kidney cells (−3)
NAT-glio. (38)	Lung cells (0)
NAT-glio. (45)	Kidney cells (1)
Kidney cells (1)	A375 mel. (49)
Kidney cells (0)	HT-29 carc. (45)
Kidney cells (1)	NAT-glio. (35)
Kidney cells (−2)	Lung cells (0)
Kidney cells (−3)	Kidney cells (1)

[a]In these experiments target cells were cultured alone, with monocytes preincubated with liposomes containing medium, or with liposomes containing MAF. Control monocytes were not cytotoxic to any of the targets. The numbers in parentheses are percentages of target cell lysis as compared with control monocytes and target cells ($p < .001$). Abbreviations used: A375 mel., A375 melanoma; HT-29 carc., H-29 colon carcinoma; NAT-glio., NATUSCH glioblastoma.

nontumorigenic kidney cells. Upon injection into nude mice, A375, HT-29, and NATUSCH cells produced progressively growing tumors, whereas cells from the two nontumorigenic lines did not.

Control monocytes did not demonstrate detectable levels of spontaneous cytotoxicity against either tumorigenic or nontumorigenic target cells. However, as shown in Table III, human monocytes activated *in vitro* with liposomes containing MAF were cytolytic to A375, HT-29, and NATUSCH cells but left the lung or kidney cells unharmed, even under conditions of cocultivation.

Furthermore, when two different tumorigenic target cell lines were cocultivated with tumoricidal monocytes, release of both isotopes was observed. In contrast, neither radiolabel was released from cocultivated nontumorigenic target cell lines. This selective lysis was not due merely to an inherent resistance of normal cells to lysis mediated by immune cells, but was associated with activated monocytes. We base the conclusion on the findings that both tumorigenic and nontumorigenic cells were equally susceptible to *in vitro* lysis mediated by normal phytohemagglutinin-stimulated peripheral blood mononuclear leukocytes. The ability of activated monocytes/macrophages to destroy tumorigenic cells selectively while leaving normal cells unharmed is another reason that activation of macrophages may be a beneficial addition to cancer therapeutic regimens.

VI. CONCLUSIONS

The successful approach to eradication of metastases must fulfill the following criteria: (1) It must circumvent the problem of tumor heterogeneity, (2) it must circumvent the problem of cell resistance, and (3) it must be selective (i.e., destroy tumor but not normal cells). Since tumoricidal macrophages fulfill all these criteria, the activation and/or augmentation of the host's natural macrophage-mediated immune processes may be a significant adjuvant to the treatment of solid tumors and their metastases. Activated macrophages, by virtue of their ability to destroy tumor cells regardless of phenotypic diversity, offer a particularly attractive approach to the elimination of micrometastases that are not detected when the primary tumor is diagnosed as well as the residual tumor cells that are not killed by chemotherapy or are not fully excised during surgery.

The destruction of large tumor burdens may not be feasible because the number of macrophages is too low. We therefore see liposome-encapsulated macrophage-activating agents like MAF being used as an addition to existing chemotherapeutic and surgical regimens rather than as the sole treatment for massive tumor burdens. Once the major tumor burden is eliminated by surgery, radiation, and/or chemotherapy, the activated macrophage can perhaps destroy the residual tumor cells. Because activated macrophages appear able to lyse the tumor cells selectively while leaving the normal cells unharmed, this therapy may become a powerful weapon for the oncologist.

The *in situ* activation of tumoricidal macrophages may thus provide an attractive approach for the treatment of disseminated cancer. Our *in vitro* human studies are very encouraging and have demonstrated that human monocytes respond well to activation by MAF entrapped within liposomes. These findings, coupled with the successful treatment of mice bearing metastases using systemic administration of liposomes containing MAF, suggest that further clinical trials are warranted.

REFERENCES

Abeloff, M. D., Ettinger, D. S., Khouri, N. F., and Lenhard, R. E. (1979). Intensive induction therapy for small cell carcinoma of the lung. *Cancer Treat. Rep.* **63,** 519–524.

Barranco, S. C., Ho, D., Derwinko, B., Romsdahl, M. M., and Humphrey, R. M. (1972). Differential sensitivities of human melanoma cells grown *in vitro* to arabinosylcytosine. *Cancer Res.* **32,** 2733–2736.

Barranco, S. C., Derwinko, B., and Humphrey, R. M. (1973). Differential response by human melanoma cells to 1,3-bis-(2-chloroethyl)-1-nitrosourea and bleomycin. *Mutat. Res.* **19,** 277–280.

Barranco, S. C., Hanenelt, B. R., and Gea E. L. (1978). Differential sensitivities of five rate hepatoma cell lines to anticancer drugs. *Cancer Res.* **38,** 656–660.

Baylin, S. B. (1981). Clonal selection and heterogeneity of human solid neoplasms. *In* "Design of Models for Testing Cancer Therapeutic Agents" (I. J. Fidler and R. J. White, eds.), pp. 50–63. Van Nostrand-Reinhold, Princeton, New Jersey.

Baylin, S. B., Abeloff, M. D., Wieman, K. C., Tomford, J. W., and Ettinger, D. S. (1975). Elevated histaminase (diamine oxidase) activity in small-cell carcinoma of the lung. *N. Engl. J. Med.* **293,** 1286–1290.

Baylin, S. B., Weisburger, W. R., Eggleston, J. C., Mendelsohn, G., Bearnen, M. A., Abeloff, M. D., and Ettinger, D. S. (1978). Variable content of histaminase, L-dopa decarboxylase and calcitonin in small-cell carcinoma of the lung: Biological and clinical implications. *N. Engl. J. Med.* **299,** 105–110.

Biddison, W. E., and Palmer, J. C. (1977). Development of tumor cell resistance to syngeneic cell-mediated cytotoxicity during growth of ascitic mastocytoma P815Y. *Proc. Natl. Acad. Sci. U.S.A.* **74,** 329–333.

Bohm, N., and Sondritter, W. (1975). DNA in human tumors: A cytophotometric study. *Curr. Top. Pathol.* **60,** 152–219.

Brunson, K. W., and Nicolson, G. L. (1978). Selection and biologic properties of malignant variants of a murine lymphosarcoma. *JNCI, J. Natl. Cancer Inst.* **61,** 1499–1503.

Bucana, C., Hoyer, L. C., Hobbs, B., Breesman, S., McDaniel, M., and Hanna, M. G., Jr. (1976). Morphological evidence for translocation of lysosomal organelles from cytotoxic macrophages into the cytoplasm of tumor target cells. *Cancer Res.* **36,** 4444–4458.

Byers, W. S., and Johnston, J. O. (1977). Antigenic differences among osteogenic sarcoma tumor cells taken from different locations in human tumors. *Cancer Res.* **37,** 3173–3183.

Calabresi, P., Dexter, D. L., and Heppner, G. H. (1979). Clinical and pharmacological implications of cancer cell differentiation and heterogeneity. *Biochem. Pharmacol.* **28,** 1933–1941.

Cameron, D. J., and Churchill, W. H. (1979). Cytotoxicity of human macrophage for tumor cells: Enhancement by human lymphocyte mediators. *J. Clin. Invest.* **63,** 977–984.

Churchill, W. H., Jr., Piessens, W. F., Sulis, C. A., and David, J. R. (1975). Macrophages activated as suspension cultures with lymphocyte mediators devoid of antigen become cytotoxic for tumor cells. *J. Immunol.* **115,** 781–786.

Cifone, M. A., and I. J. Fidler. (1980). Correlation of patterns of anchorage-independent growth with *in vivo* behavior of cells from a murine fibrosarcoma. *Proc. Natl. Acad. Sci. U.S.A.* **77,** 1039–1043.

Cifone, M. A., Kripke, M. L., and Fidler, I. J. (1979). Growth rate and chromosome number of tumor cell lines with different metastatic potential. *J. Supramol. Struct.* **11,** 467–476.

Den Otter, W., Dullens Hub, J. J., Can Lovern, H., and Pels, E. (1977). Anti-tumor effects of macrophages injected into animals: A review. *In* "The Macrophage and Cancer" (K. James, B. McBride, and A. Stuart, eds.), pp. 119–141. Econoprint, Edinburgh.

Droller, M. J., and Remington, J. S. (1975). A role for the macrophage in *in vivo* and *in vitro* resistance to murine bladder tumor cell growth. *Cancer Res.* **35,** 49–53.

DeWys, W. D. (1972). Studies correlating the growth rate of a tumor and its metastases and providing evidence for tumor-related systemic growth-retarding factors. *Cancer Res.* **32,** 374–379.

Evans, R., and Alexander, P. (1976). Mechanisms of extracellular killing of nucleated mammalian cells by macrophages. *In* "The Immunobiology of the Macrophage" (D. S. Nelson, ed.), pp. 562–576. Academic Press, New York.

Faraci, R. P. (1974). *In vitro* demonstration of altered antigenicity of metastases from a primary methycholanthrene-induced sarcoma. *Surgery (St. Louis)* **76,** 469–473.

Fidler, I. J. (1974). Inhibition of pulmonary metastasis by intravenous injection of specifically activated macrophages. *Cancer Res.* **34,** 1074–1078.

Fidler, I. J. (1978a). Tumor heterogeneity and the biology of cancer invasion and metastasis. *Cancer Res.* **37,** 2481–2486.

Fidler, I. J. (1978b). Recognition and destruction of target cells by tumoricidal macrophages. *Isr. J. Med.* **14,** 177–191.

Fidler, I. J. (1980). Therapy of spontaneous metastases by intravenous injection of liposomes containing lymphokines. *Science* **208,** 1469–1471.

Fidler, I. J., and Bucana, C. (1977). Mechanism of tumor cell resistance to lysis by syngeneic lymphocytes. *Cancer Res.* **37,** 3945–3956.

Fidler, I. J., and Cifone, M. A. (1979). Properties of metastatic and nonmetastatic cloned subpopulations of an ultraviolet-light-induced murine fibrosarcoma of recent origin. *Am. J. Pathol.* **97,** 633–648.

Fidler, I. J., and Hart, I. R. (1981). The origin of metastatic heterogeneity in tumors. *Eur. J. Cancer* **17,** 487–494.

Fidler, I. J., and Kripke, M. L. (1977). Metastasis results from preexisting variant cells within a malignant tumor. *Science* **197,** 893–895.

Fidler, I. J., and Kripke, M. L. (1980). Biological variability within murine neoplasms. *Antibiot. Chemother. (Basel)* **28,** 123–129.

Fidler, I. J., and Poste, G. (1982). Macrophage-mediated destruction of malignant tumor cells and new strategies for the therapy of metastatic disease. *Springer Semin. Immunopathol.* **5,** 161–174.

Fidler, I. J., and Raz, A. (1981). The induction of tumoricidal capacities in mouse and rat macrophages by lymphokines. *In* "Lymphokines" (E. Pick, ed.), pp. 345–363. Academic Press, New York.

Fidler, I. J., Gersten, D. M., and Budman, M. B. (1976). Characterization *in vivo* and *in vitro* of tumor cells selected for resistance to syngeneic lymphocyte-mediated cytotoxicity. *Cancer Res.* **36,** 3160–3165.

Fidler, I. J., Roblin, R. O., and Poste, G. (1978). *In vitro* tumoricidal activity of macrophages against virus-transformed lines with temperature-dependent transformed phenotypic characteristics. *Cell. Immunol.* **38,** 131–146.

Fidler, I. J., Fogler, W. E., and Connor, J. (1979). The rationale for the treatment of established experimental micrometastases with the injection of tumoricidal macrophages. *In* "Immunobiology and Immunotherapy of Cancer" (W. D. Terry and Y. Yamamura, eds.), pp. 361–375. Elsevier, New York.

Fidler, I. J., Raz, A., Fogler, W. E., Kirsh, R., Bugelski, P., and Poste, G. (1980). Design of liposomes to improve delivery of macrophage-augmenting agents to alveolar macrophages. *Cancer Res.* **40,** 4460–4466.

Fidler, I. J., Gruys, E., Cifone, M. A., Barnes, Z., and Bucana, C. (1981). Demonstration of multiple phenotypic diversity in a murine melanoma of recent origin. *JNCI, J. Natl. Cancer Inst.* **67**, 947–956.

Fidler, I. J., Barnes, Z., Fogler, W. E., Kirsh, R., Bugelski, P., and Poste, G. (1982). Involvement of macrophages in the eradication of established metastases following intravenous injection of liposomes containing macrophage activators. *Cancer Res.* **42**, 496–501.

Fogler, W. E., Raz, A., and Fidler, I. J. (1980). *In situ* activation of murine macrophages by liposomes containing lymphokines. *Cell. Immunol.* **53**, 214–219.

Franks, L. M. (1960). Estrogen-treated prostatic cancer. *Cancer* **13**, 490–501.

Fugi, H., Mihich, E., and Pressman, D. (1977). Differential tumor immunogenicity of L1210 and its sublines. *J. Immunol.* **119**, 983–986.

Fugmann, R. A., Anderson, J. C., Stoli, R., and Martin, D. S. (1977). Comparison of adjuvant chemotherapeutic activity against primary and metastatic spontaneous murine tumors. *Cancer Res.* **37**, 496–500.

Goldman, L. I., Flaxman, B. A., Wernick, G., and Zabriski, J. B. (1974). Immune surveillance and tumor dissemination: *In vitro* comparison of the B16 melanoma in primary and metastatic form. *Surgery (St. Louis)* **76**, 50–56.

Gray, J. M., and Pierce, G. B. (1964). Relationship between growth rate and differentiation of melanoma *in vivo. JNCI, J. Natl. Cancer Inst.* **32**, 1201–1211.

Hakansson, L., and Trope, C. (1974a). On the presence within tumors of clones that differ in sensitivity to cytostatic drugs. *Acta Pathol. Microbiol. Scand. Sect. A* **82**, 35–40.

Hakansson, L., and Trope, C. (1974b). Cell clones with different sensitivity to cytostatic drugs in methylcholanthrene-induced mouse sarcomas. *Acta Pathol. Microbiol. Scand. Sect. A* **82**, 41–47.

Hanna, N., and Fidler, I. J. (1980). Role of natural killer cells in the destruction of circulating tumor emboli. *JNCI, J. Natl. Cancer Inst.* **65**, 801–809.

Heppner, G. H., Dexter, D. L., DeNucci, T., Miller, F. R., and Calabresi, P. (1978). Heterogeneity in drug sensitivity among tumor cell subpopulations of a single mammary tumor. *Cancer Res.* **38**, 3758–3763.

Hibbs, J. B., Jr. (1974a). Discrimination between neoplastic and nonneoplastic cells *in vitro* by activated macrophages. *JNCI, J. Natl. Cancer Inst.* **53**, 1487–1492.

Hibbs, J. B., Jr. (1974b). Heterocytolysis by macrophages activated by bacillus Calmette-Guérin: Lysosome exocytosis into tumor cells. *Science* **184**, 468–471.

Hibbs, J. B., Lambert, L. H., and Remington, J. S. (1972). Control of carcinogenesis: A possible role for the activated macrophage. *Science* **177**, 998–1000.

Ito, E., and Moore, G. E. (1967). Characteristic differences in clones isolated from an S37 ascites tumor *in vitro. Exp. Cell Res.* **48**, 440–447.

Jones, P. D. E., and Castro, J. E. (1977). Immunological mechanisms in metastatic spread and the antimetastatic effects of *C. parvum. Br. J. Cancer* **35**, 519–527.

Kerbel, R. S. (1979). Implications of immunological heterogeneity of tumors. *Nature (London)* **280**, 358–360.

Key, M. E., Hoyer, L., Bucana, C., and Hanna, M. G., Jr. (1982). Mechanisms of macrophage-mediated tumor cytolysis. *Adv. Exp. Med. Biol.* **146**, 265–310.

Killion, J. J. (1978). Immunotherapy with tumor subpopulations: I. Active, specific immunotherapy of L1210 leukemia. *Cancer Immunol. Immunother.* **4**, 115–119.

Killion, J. J., and Kollmorgen, G. M. (1976). Isolation of immunogenic tumor cells by cell-affinity chromatography. *Nature (London)* **259**, 674–676.

Kleinerman, E. S., and Fidler, I. J. (1983). Production and utilization of human lymphokines containing macrophage-activating factor (MAF) activity. *Lymphokine Res.* **2**, 7–12.

Kleinerman, E. S., Schroit, A. J., Fogler, W. E., and Fidler, I. J. (1983). Tumoricidal activity of human monocytes activated *in vitro* by free and liposome-encapsulated human lymphokines. *J. Clin. Invest.* **72,** 1–12.

Kolb, E., and Muller, E. (1979). Local responses in primary and secondary human lung cancers: II. Clinical conclusions. *Br. J. Cancer* **40,** 410–416.

Kripke, M. L., Gruys, E., and Fidler, I. J. (1978). Metastatic heterogeneity of cells from an ultraviolet light-induced murine fibrosarcoma of recent origin. *Cancer Res.* **38,** 2962–2967.

Liotta, L. A., Gattozzi, C., Kleinerman, J., and Saidel, G. (1977). Reduction of tumor cell entry into vessels by BCG-activated macrophages. *Br. J. Cancer* **36,** 639–641.

Liotta, L. A., Tryggvason, K., Gabrisa, A., Hart, I. R., and Foltz, C. M. (1980). Metastatic potential correlates with enzymatic degradation of basement membrane collagen. *Nature (London)* **284,** 67–68.

Livinston, R. B. (1979). Treatment of small cell carcinoma: Evaluation and future directions. *Semin. Oncol.* **5,** 299–308.

Lotan, R. (1979). Different susceptibilities of human melanoma and breast carcinoma cell lines to retinoic acid-induced growth inhibition. *Cancer Res.* **39,** 1014–1019.

Lotan, R., and Nicolson, G. L. (1979). Heterogeneity in growth inhibition by β-transretinoic acid of metastatic B16 melanoma clones and in vivo-selected cell variant lines. *Cancer Res.* **39,** 4767–4771.

Lurie, H. (1964). "Resistance to Tuberculosis: Experimental Studies in Native and Acquired Defense Mechanisms." Harvard Univ. Press, Cambridge, Massachusetts.

McDaniel, M. C., Laudico, R., and Papermaster, B. W. (1976). Association of macrophage-activation factor from a human cultured lymphoid cell line with albumin and α_2 macroglobulin. *Clin. Immunol. Immunopathol.* **5,** 91–104.

Mantovani, A., Giavazzi, R., Polentanitti, N., Spreafico, F., and Garattini, S. (1980). Divergent effects of macrophage toxins on growth of primary tumors and lung metastases in mice. *Int. J. Cancer* **25,** 617–624.

Marino, P. A., and Adams, D. O. (1982). The capacity of activated murine macrophages for augmented binding of neoplastic cells: Analysis of induction by lymphokine containing MAF and kinetics of the reaction. *J. Immunol.* **128,** 2816–2823.

Miller, F. R., and Heppner, G. H. (1979). Immunologic heterogeneity of tumor cell subpopulations from a single mouse mammary tumor. *JNCI, J. Natl. Cancer Inst.* **63,** 1457–1463.

Miller, B. E., Miller, F. R., Leith, J., and Heppner, G. H. (1980). Growth interaction in vivo between tumor subpopulations derived from a single mouse mammary tumor. *Cancer Res.* **40,** 3977–3981.

Mittleman, F. (1971). The chromosomes of fifty primary Rous rat sarcomas. *Hereditas* **69,** 155–186.

Nicolson, G. L., and Brunson, K. W. (1977). Organ specificity of malignant B16 melanoma: *In vivo* selection for organ preference of blood-borne metastasis. *Cancer Res.* **20,** 15–24.

Nicolson, G. L., Brunson, K. W., and Fidler, I. J. (1978). Specificity of arrest, survival, and growth of selected metastatic variant cell lines. *Cancer Res.* **38,** 4105–4111.

Niles, R. M., and Makarski, J. S. (1978). Hormonal activation of adenylate cyclase in mouse melanoma metastatic variants. *J. Cell Physiol.* **96,** 35–359.

Norbury, K., and Kripke, M. L. (1979). Ultraviolet-induced carcinogenesis in mice treated with silica, trypan blue or pyran copolymer. *J. Reticuloendothel. Soc.* **26,** 827–837.

Ohno, S. (1971). Genetic implication of karyological instability of malignant somatic cells. *Physiol. Rev.* **51,** 496–526.

Olsson, L., and Ebbesen, P. (1979). Natural polyclonality of spontaneous AKR leukemia and its consequence for so-called specific immunotherapy. *JNCI, J. Natl. Cancer Inst.* **62,** 623–627.

Papermaster, B. W., Holtermann, O. A., Rosner, D., Klein, E., Dao, T., and Djerassi, I. (1974). Regressions produced in breast cancer lesions by a lymphokine fraction from a human lymphoid cell line. *Res. Commun. Chem. Pathol. Pharmacol.* **8,** 413–428.

248   Eugenie S. Kleinerman and Isaiah J. Fidler

Papermaster, B. W., Holtermann, O. A., Klein, E., Parmett, S., Dobkin, D., Laudico, R., and Djerassi, I., (1976). Lymphokine properties of a lymphoid cultured cell supernatant fraction active in promoting tumor regression. *Clin. Immunol. Immunopathol.* **5,** 48–59.
Piessens, W. F., and Churchill, W. H., Jr. (1975). Macrophages activated *in vitro* with lymphocyte mediators kill neoplastic but not normal cells. *J. Immunol.* **114,** 293–299.
Poste, G., and Fidler, I. J. (1979). The pathogenesis of cancer metastasis. *Nature (London)* **283,** 139–146.
Poste, G., and Kirsh, R. (1979). Rapid decay of tumoricidal activity and loss of responsiveness to lymphokines in inflammatory macrophage. *Cancer Res.* **39,** 2582–2590.
Poste, G., Kirsh, R., and Fidler, I. J. (1979a). Cell surface receptors for lymphokines. *Cell. Immunol.* **44,** 71]71–87.
Poste, G., Kirsh, R., Fogler, W. E., and Fidler, I. J. (1979b). Activation of tumoricidal properties in mouse macrophages by lymphokines encapsulated in liposomes. *Cancer Res.* **39,** 881–891.
Prehn, R. T. (1965). Cancer antigens in tumors induced by chemicals. *Fed. Proc., Fed. Am. Soc. Exp. Biol.* **24,** 1018–1028.
Prehn, R. T. (1970). Analysis of antigenic heterogeneity within individual 3-methylcholanthrene–induced mouse sarcomas. *JNCI, J. Natl. Cancer Inst.* **45,** 1039–1044.
Raz, A., McLellan, W. E., Hart, I. R., Bucana, C. D., Hoyer, L. C., Sela, B. A., Dragsten, P., and Fidler, I. J. (1980). Cell surface properties of B16 melanoma variants with differing metastatic potential. *Cancer Res.* **40,** 1645–1651.
Reading, C. L., Belloni, D. N., and Nicolson, G. L. (1980). Selection and *in vivo* properties of lectin-attachment variants of malignant murine lymphosarcoma cell lines. *JNCI, J. Natl. Cancer Inst.* **64,** 1241–1249.
Sadler, T. E., Jones, D. D. E., and Castro, J. E. (1979). The effects of altered phagocytic activity on growth of primary and metastatic tumors. *In* "The Macrophage and Cancer" (J. F. McBride and A. Stuart, eds.), pp. 115–163. Econoprint, Edinburgh.
Salvin, S. B., Youngner, J. S., Nishio, J., and Neta, R. (1975). Tumor suppression by a lymphokine released into the circulation of mice with delayed hypersensitivity. *JNCI, J. Natl. Cancer Inst.* **55,** 1233–1236.
Schabel, F. M. (1975). Concepts for systemic treatment of micrometastases. *Cancer* **35,** 15–24.
Schirrmacher, V., Bosslet, K., Shantz, G., Claver, K., and Hubsch, D. (1979). Tumor metastases and cell-mediated immunity in a model system in DBA/2 mice. IV. Antigenic differences between a metastasizing variant and the parental tumor line revealed by cytotoxic T lymphocytes. *Int. J. Cancer* **23,** 245–252.
Siracky, J. (1979). An approach to the problem of heterogeneity of human tumor cell populations. *Br. J. Cancer* **39,** 570–577.
Sluyser, M., and Van Nie, R. (1974). Estrogen receptor content and hormone-responsive growth of mouse mammary tumors. *Cancer Res.* **34,** 3252–3257.
Sluyser, M., Evers, S. G., and DeGoey, C. C. (1976). Sex hormone receptors in mammary tumours of GR mice. *Nature (London)* **263,** 386–389.
Sone, S., Poste, G., and Fidler, I. J. (1980). Rat alveolar macrophages are susceptible to activation by free and liposome-encapsulated lymphokines. *J. Immunol.* **124,** 2197–2201.
Sugarbaker, E. V., and Cohen, A. M. (1972). Altered antigenicity in spontaneous pulmonary metastases from an antigenic murine sarcoma. *Surgery (St. Louis)* **72,** 155–166.
Tao, T. W., and Burger, M. M. (1977). Nonmetastasizing variants selected from metastasizing melanoma cells. *Nature (London)* **270,** 437–438.
Trope, C. (1975). Different sensitivity to cytostatic drugs of primary tumor and metastasis of the Lewis carcinoma. *Neoplasma* **22,** 171–180.
Trope, C. (1981). Different susceptibilities of tumor cell subpopulations to cytotoxic agents. *In*

"Design of Models for Testing Cancer Therapeutic Agents" (I. J. Fidler and R. J. White, eds.), pp. 64–79. Van Nostrant–Reinhold, Princeton, New Jersey.

Trope, C., Hakansson, L., and Dencker, H. (1975). Heterogeneity of human adenocarcinomas of the colon and the stomach as regards sensitivity to cytostatic drugs. *Neoplasma* **22**, 423–430.

Trope, C., Aspergen, K., Kullander, S., and Astredt, B. (1979). Heterogeneous response of disseminated human ovarian cancers to cytostasis in vitro. *Acta Obstet. Gynecol. Scand.* **58**, 543–546.

Tsuruo, T., and Fidler, I. J. (1981). Differences in drug sensitivity among tumor cells from parental tumors, selected variants, and spontaneous metastases. *Cancer Res.* **41**, 3058–3064.

Vindelov, L. V. (1977). Flow microfluoremetric analysis of nuclear DNA in cells from solid tumors and cell suspensions. *Virchows Arch. B.* **24**, 227–242.

Vindelov, L. V., Hansen, H. H., Christensen, I. J., Spange-Thomsen, M., Hirsch, F. R., Hansen, M., and Nissen, N. I. (1980). Clonal heterogeneity of small-cell anaplastic carcinoma of the lung demonstrated by flow cytometric DNA analysis. *Cancer Res.* **40**, 4295–4300.

Yoshida, T., and Cohen, S. (1972). Lymphokine activity *in vivo* in relation to circulating monocyte levels and delayed skin reactivity. *J. Immunol.* **122**, 1540–1546.

7

Tuftsin: A Naturally Occurring Immunomodulating Antitumor Tetrapeptide

KENJI NISHIOKA

Department of General Surgery/Surgical Research Laboratory, and
Department of Biochemistry and Molecular Biology
M.D. Anderson Hospital and Tumor Institute
The University of Texas System Cancer Center
Houston, Texas

I.	Introduction	251
II.	Biology and Chemistry of Tuftsin	252
	A. Generation of Tuftsin	252
	B. Abnormality and Deficiency of Tuftsin	253
	C. Tuftsin Receptor	254
	D. Measurement of Tuftsin	256
	E. Biological Activities of Tuftsin	256
	F. Mechanism of Action of Tuftsin	257
	G. Chemical Synthesis and Purification of Tuftsin	257
III.	Antitumor Activity of Tuftsin	258
IV.	Antimicrobial Activity of Tuftsin	262
V.	Concluding Remarks	263
	References	264

I. INTRODUCTION

The host immunological system plays crucial roles in combating occurrence of neoplasms and in protecting against infections. Although much emphasis in tumor immunology had been placed on studies on lymphocyte functions, sub-

251

Novel Approaches to Cancer Chemotherapy
ISBN 0-12-676980-X

stantial data have been accumulated that indicate that macrophages, natural killer (NK) cells, and polymorphonuclear leukocyte neutrophils (PMN) are also likely to perform equally important roles *in vivo*. Moreover, it has been suggested that macrophages and NK cells impose the predominant lethal effect on tumor cells (James *et al.*, 1977; Herberman, 1980). PMN have also been shown to exert a cytotoxic effect on neoplastic cells (Klebanoff and Clark, 1978). Additionally, macrophages, PMN, and possibly NK cells are capable of manifesting anti-neoplastic effects through antibody-dependent cellular cytotoxicity (ADCC). A great deal of interest has been centered around various agents that have been shown to activate macrophages and NK cells in a nonspecific or specific manner. These include endotoxins, lipid A, double-stranded RNA, bacillus Calmette-Guérin (BCG), *Corynebacterium parvum,* levamisole, glucan, polyanions, muramyl dipeptides, and interferons (Chirigos, 1978; Hersh *et al.*, 1981).

Although tuftsin belongs to the category of immunomodulator and/or immuno-stimulating agents within the broad definition of biological response modifiers (Oldham, 1982), it should be considered as a peptide hormone considering its physiological origin and mechanism of action (Nishioka *et al.*, 1981a). An enormous number of factors or mediators are undoubtedly involved in the regulation of the immunological system. Yet very few of these immunological mediators are chemically well defined. Tuftsin is one of a very few factors whose chemical identification has been convincingly established.

II. BIOLOGY AND CHEMISTRY OF TUFTSIN

A. Generation of Tuftsin

The presence of this mediator was first reported by Najjar and Nishioka (1970) in the sera of dogs and humans as a phagocytosis-stimulating factor of PMN. In the phagocytosis system, a specific fraction of the immunoglobulin G (leuko-philic IgG) binds to the circulating blood PMN and stimulates their phagocytic activity. Since splenectomized animals failed to show the phagocytosis stimulation activity (Najjar *et al.*, 1968), it became clear that the spleen plays an essential role in the generation of this factor. The presence of the phagocytosis-enhancing activity was then chemically localized on the heavy chain of the IgG. Furthermore, early studies on the kinetics of phagocytosis stimulation by the leukophilic IgG clearly demonstrated that a specific factor (tuftsin) was released from the IgG fraction. In view of this, the partially purified leukophilic IgG fraction was then treated by crude PMN membrane preparation and the phagocytosis-stimulatory activity recovered in 80% ethanol fraction. Treatment of this fraction by a variety of enzymes indicated that tuftsin was a peptide. Therefore, this peptide was isolated, sequenced as L-Thr-L-Lys-L-Pro-L-Arg (Nishioka *et*

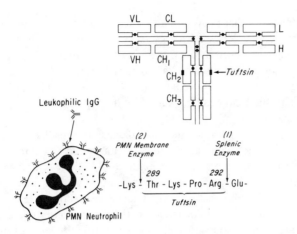

Fig. 1. Two-step enzymatic release of tuftsin.

al., 1972, 1973a), and chemically synthesized to confirm the structure (Nishioka *et al.*, 1972, 1973b). The presence of the tuftsin sequence was actually shown to exist in the CH_2 domain of human IgG (Edelman *et al.*, 1969). On the basis of these accumulated studies, we currently envision the mechanism of enzymatic release of tuftsin from the leukophilic IgG as depicted in Fig. 1. First, the specific splenic enzyme (tuftsin-endocarboxypeptidase) cleaves the carboxy-terminus of tuftsin, the Arg-Glu bond. The leukophilic IgG travels via the blood circulation in this form with the free tuftsin carboxy-terminus. Upon binding of the IgG to the Fc receptors of PMN, the second enzyme (leukokininase) sets tuftsin free by cleaving the amino-terminus of tuftsin, the Lys-Thr bond. Thus released, tuftsin then binds to its specific receptors on the surface of PMN and initiates its biological functions. Our study indicates that tuftsin receptors are entirely separate molecules from those of Fc receptors (Amoscato *et al.*, 1983a).

B. Abnormality and Deficiency of Tuftsin

Demonstration of a genetic disorder of tuftsin brought about a critical insight in considering physiological significance of this agent. Among pediatric patients who suffered from repeated staphylococcal infections, several patients with a tuftsin abnormality have been documented. Detailed studies of these patients showed the presence of abnormal tuftsin that could effectively compete with normal tuftsin molecules. Further studies indicated that this abnormality was a gene-linked condition with undetectable tuftsin activity occurring in one of the parents and sometimes in other siblings (Najjar and Constantopoulos, 1972; Constantopoulos and Najjar, 1973a; Inada *et al.*, 1979). This finding, combined with the observation that many tuftsin analogs are also inhibitors, suggests that patients with a congenital abnormality carry a tuftsin inhibitor in which one of the amino acids is replaced by another amino acid, a typical feature of molecular disease. One patient was shown to have abnormal tuftsin with a sequence of Thr-Glu-Pro-Arg with Lys $\rightarrow$ Glu replacement (Najjar et al., 1980; Konopinska et al., 1981). This alteration can be caused by the replacement of a single base in the DNA sequence.

As mentioned in the previous section, splenectomy results in tuftsin deficiency. Likhite (1975), however, successfully demonstrated that chronically splenectomized rats were able to restore leukophilic IgG in their sera upon heterotropic autotransplantation of splenic tissue. In human studies (Najjar and Constantopoulos, 1972), while patients who underwent elective splenectomy showed undetectable tuftsin activity in their sera, patients who were subjected to splenectomy after traumatic incidents usually showed normal levels of tuftsin activity. This observation was supported by a study of Spirer et al. (1977), who established a radioimmunoassay for tuftsin. Patients with elective splenectomy showed serum tuftsin levels roughly one-third of normal subjects, whereas patients who underwent traumatic splenectomy exhibited close to normal levels of tuftsin. This phenomenon can be well explained on the basis of splenosis, in which recurrent splenic tissue is detectable by a spleen scan as reported by Pearson et al., (1978). This probably also corresponds to the reduced frequency of overwhelming sepsis observed in pediatric patients with traumatic splenectomy (Singer, 1973; Balfanz et al., 1976). On the basis of this finding, Aigner et al. (1980), Patel et al. (1981), and Millikan et al. (1982) have reported on the potential importance of reimplantation of splenic tissue in humans.

Patients with acute myelocytic leukemia or myelofibrosis are also known to have low serum levels of tuftsin. In addition, their PMN responded poorly to tuftsin in vitro as examined by phagocytosis assay (Constantopoulos et al., 1973). Having found reduced levels of tuftsin in the sera of patients with idiopathic thrombocytopenic purpura and sickle cell disease, Spirer et al. (1977, 1980) suggested that these low levels of tuftsin without splenectomy were indicators of splenic hypofunction.

C. Tuftsin Receptor

The presence of specific tuftsin receptors on the surface of PMN was originally demonstrated by abolishing the responsiveness of PMN to tuftsin by neuraminidase treatment (Constantopoulos and Najjar, 1973b). Stabinsky et al. (1978) then reported a systematic study of these receptors employing [^{3}H]tuftsin. This study indicated that the specific receptors for tuftsin existed on human PMN and monocytes with K_D 130 and 125 nM, respectively. The numbers of binding sites were approximately 50,000 and 10,000 per cell, respectively. Lymphocytes showed only a threshold binding capacity (5% relative to PMN). This partially purified lymphocyte fraction, however, appeared to contain NK cells, suggesting to us the possible presence of tuftsin receptors on NK cells. This implication thus led us to perform studies on NK cells. The erythrocyte fraction exhibited no detectable binding. However, Nair *et al.* (1978) demonstrated the binding of tuftsin to lymphocytes in addition to PMN and monocytes employing [^{14}C]tuftsin and ^{125}I-labeled tuftsin. Bar-Shavit *et al.* (1979) studied the binding of tuftsin to murine peritoneal macrophages and found that the macrophage possessed 72,000 tuftsin receptors per cell with K_D 53 nM, which was lower than that of the human monocyte. The finding of tuftsin receptors on macrophages corresponds to the observation that tuftsin was capable of stimulating phagocytosis of macrophages (Constantopoulos and Najjar, 1972). Tuftsin is now also known to bind other murine cells such as mononuclear phagocytes differentiated *in vitro* from bone marrow cells and P-388D$_1$ cells (Bar-Shavit *et al.*, 1980a).

Substance P and neurotensin possess a similar primary sequence in their structure: Arg-Pro-Lys-Pro at the N-terminal of substance P and Lys-Pro-Arg in neurotensin. These neuropeptides stimulate phagocytosis and compete with tuftsin for its binding sites (Bar-Shavit *et al.*, 1980b; Bar-Shavit and Goldman, 1982). This observation may be related to the central effect of tuftsin including an analgesic effect (Herman *et al.*, 1980; Kamenskii *et al.*, 1980; Val'dman *et al.*, 1981).

In order to study further the binding of tuftsin to the receptor and the subsequent fate of the tuftsin molecule upon binding, we labeled the molecule with fluorescein specifically at its N-terminal amino group. This fluorescein-labeled tuftsin was purified by high-performance liquid chromatography (HPLC). The compound was shown to retain full biological activity of the native molecule as evidenced by phagocytosis and bactericidal assays. Binding of this agent to living human PMN was then studied by means of video intensification fluorescence microscopy. At 37°C, diffuse membrane fluorescence was seen initially, followed by rapid aggregation and internalization. These processes are temperature dependent and rely on specific binding to the tuftsin receptor. The labeled tuftsin was also shown to bind to macrophages and NK cells but not to T or B lymphocytes or erythrocytes. The fluorescein-labeled agent did not compete with IgG aggregates, indicating that tuftsin receptors are entirely independent from Fc receptors (Amoscato *et al.*, 1983a,b).

Conformation studies of tuftsin have been controversial (Fridkin and Gottlieb, 1981). It appears to us now that tuftsin does not take on a definite structure (Blumenstein *et al.*, 1979) until it binds to the receptor. In addition to tuftsin receptors, an ectoenzyme, leucine aminopeptidase, is also localized on the surface of PMN. This enzyme may cleave threonine from tuftsin, thus producing Lys-Pro-Arg, which is an inhibitor of tuftsin (Nagaoka and Yamashita, 1981). This may then lead to inhibition of tuftsin activity at high concentrations.

D. Measurement of Tuftsin

At the beginning of tuftsin research, the factor was primarily assayed employing a phagocytosis procedure. This assay lacked precision and reproducibility, and was also quite tedious. Spirer et al. (1977) subsequently introduced the radioimmunoassay procedure for tuftsin. They raised antituftsin antibodies in rabbits, employing antigen that was produced by chemically coupling tuftsin to bovine serum albumin (BSA). Antituftsin antibodies were also successfully raised in chickens (Nair et al., 1978) by using BSA–tuftsin and IgG–tuftsin conjugates. Currently we are attempting to produce specific antituftsin monoclonal antibodies to develop an enzyme-linked immunosorbent assay for tuftsin. A sensitive procedure for tuftsin quantification is also being developed employing HPLC in our laboratory. To examine the biological activity of tuftsin, we also developed cytotoxicity and bactericidal assays (Phillips et al., 1981; Amoscato et al., 1981).

E. Biological Activities of Tuftsin

In addition to antitumor and antimicrobial activities, tuftsin possesses a variety of other biological properties. These properties may contribute to antitumor and/or antimicrobial activities of tuftsin either directly or indirectly. Tuftsin is chemotactic and also enhances migration of leukocytes as well as their phagocytic and pinocytic activities. We observed an increase in the peritoneal leukocyte count of mice upon intraperitoneal (ip) injection of tuftsin (Nishioka, 1979a). This observation led us to in vitro examination of tuftsin. Subsequently, chemotactic and migration-enhancing activities of tuftsin were confirmed in vitro, employing human PMN and monocytes (Nishioka et al., 1972, 1973b; Nishioka, 1978; Babcock et al., 1983). Among the reports published by other investigators (Goetzl, 1975, 1976; Horsmanheimo et al., 1978; Giroud et al., 1980; Yamanaka et al., 1979; Kavai et al., 1981), the results obtained by Goetzl (1975, 1976) and Horsmanheimo et al. (1978) are somewhat at variance with the others. This discrepancy appears to be due to the relative purities of the tuftsin preparations used for their experiments. Using our migration inhibition factor assay system, the ability of tuftsin to enhance migration of human mononuclear cells could not be inhibited (Nishioka, 1978). We have also examined by video microscopy the morphological alterations of human monocytes upon introduction of tuftsin (Babcock et al., 1983). Initially the monocyte became extended, exhibited active membrane ruffling, and began to migrate. With time the monocytes became round again.

In our laboratory, we have observed mitogenic and differentiation-inducing activities of tuftsin (Nishioka et al., 1981a; Babcock et al., 1983). Tuftsin showed relatively weak mitogenic activity toward murine spleen cells and human monocytes as examined by the incorporation of [^{3}H]thymidine into these cells.

The potential of tuftsin to induce differentiation in murine monocytes was studied by employing P-388D$_1$ cells. This cell line consisted of immature monocytes, which are not cytotoxic unless they are induced to differentiate. In the presence of tuftsin, the P-388D$_1$ cells incorporated [^{3}H]thymidine and elicited cytotoxicity against L1210 leukemia cells. In addition, tuftsin promoted bone marrow colony formation, indicating the ability of tuftsin to enhance the differentiation of committed progenitor cells in murine bone marrow. The colonies contained either mononuclear or granulocytic cells. Tuftsin also shows effect on antibody formation. Florentin *et al.* (1978) demonstrated that tuftsin-treated mice possessed a potentiated antibody response to a thymus-dependent antigen. Tzehoval *et al.* (1978) showed that tuftsin enhanced the antigen-specific macrophage-dependent education of T cells in mice.

It has been reported by Luftig *et al.* (1977) that addition of tuftsin to the murine leukemia virus-infected cell resulted in an increase of virion-associated reverse transcriptase. This could be due to the presence of a sequence of tuftsin in the structural protein p12, which is coded by the *gag* gene of Rauscher murine luekemia virus (Oroszlan *et al.*, 1978).

F. Mechanism of Action of Tuftsin

The molecular mechanism of action of tuftsin is not precisely known at present. However, it appears certain that tuftsin binds to its specific receptor and manifests its biological activities. Spirer *et al.* (1975) reported that tuftsin enhanced reduction of nitro blue tetrazolium by human leukocytes. This suggests that tuftsin activates the hexose monophosphate shunt and in turn increases production of superoxide, hydroxyl radical, and hydrogen peroxide. Tritsch and Niswander (1982), and Hartung and Toyka (1983) have demonstrated that tuftsin stimulates release of superoxide and hydrogen peroxide. The latter group, in addition, showed the enhanced release of thromboxane from macrophages by tuftsin. Stabinsky *et al.* (1980) reported that tuftsin caused PMN and macrophages to increase intracellular cyclic GMP and concomitantly to decrease cyclic AMP with enhanced release of calcium ions.

G. Chemical Synthesis and Purification of Tuftsin

We have reported the chemical synthesis of tuftsin using the solid-phase procedure (Nishioka *et al.*, 1972). Since then, this peptide was synthesized by various investigators using a number of procedures (Fridkin and Gottlieb, 1981; Siemion and Konopinska, 1981). Since we obtained extremely variable results in our biological experiments depending on the sources of tuftsin used for those experiments, we decided to concentrate on analysis of various tuftsin preparations and subsequently on development of a purification procedure for tuftsin. A commercial preparation of tuftsin was then carefully analyzed employing our established reverse-phase HPLC procedure (Amoscato *et al.*, 1981). This preparation gave roughly 12 separate peaks with the purity of 85%. A further detailed study suggested that the majority of contaminating peaks were diastereomers. This inactive commercial preparation became fully active in stimulating phagocytosis and the bactericidal activity of PMN upon the HPLC purification. This purification procedure is now routinely used to purify tuftsin preparations synthesized in our laboratory using both solid- and solution-phase procedures. This finding regarding impurities in tuftsin preparations may explain the various discrepancies among the studies published on biological effects of tuftsin, and suggests an essential need for extensve purification of tuftsin preparations.

While a variety of tuftsin analogs and derivatives have been synthesized by various investigators (reviews in Fridkin and Gottlieb, 1981; Siemion and Konopinska, 1981), there has been no tuftsin analog that exhibits clearly higher biological activities than those of tuftsin. This type of study has served to emphasize the structural requirements and specificities for expression of tuftsin activities, since some tuftsin analogs turned out to be effective tuftsin inhibitors. The known important tuftsin inhibitors are Thr-Lys-Pro-Pro-Arg, Ser-Lys-Pro-Arg, Ala-Lys-Pro-Arg, Thr-Glu-Pro-Arg, and Lys-Pro-Arg.

III. ANTITUMOR ACTIVITY OF TUFTSIN

By 1972 it had become apparent that tuftsin augmented the phagocytic activity of both PMN and macrophages. In view of this, we began to wonder if tuftsin could also stimulate tumor cytotoxicity by these effector cells. If that is the case, a definite role of tuftsin in the immunotherapy of tumor is indicated. To examine this possibility, we initiated our animal studies using the L1210 leukemia model in 1976. Although tuftsin showed significant antitumor activity in this model, we encountered two critical problems as we repeated this experiment.

1. Apparently because of the difference in antigenicity in different cell lines, L1210 cell lines obtained from different sources gave very different survival curves.
2. Tuftsin preparations from different sources also produced vastly different effects indicating the importance of the purity of tuftsin employed.

To examine the cellular mechanism behind the ability of tuftsin to inhibit the growth of L1210 leukemia cells, we also performed *in vitro* experiments. To rule out the possibility that tuftsin exerts direct antitumor activity or is cytotoxic to tumor cells, the effect of tuftsin on the incorporation of [³H]thymidine by tumor target cells, such as L1210 leukemia cells and Cloudman S91 melanoma cells, was examined. No direct cytotoxicity of tuftsin was found. Therefore, the antitumor effect of tuftsin was considered to be exerted through the stimulation of immune effector cells. We then examined the effect of tuftsin on the cytotoxicity of peritoneal macrophages obtained from DBA/2 mice against cultured L1210 leukemia cells. Monolayered macrophages were treated with tuftsin for 18 hr in microtiter plates. After washing, L1210 target cells labeled with [^{3}H]proline were introduced to each well at an effector:target cell ratio of 50:1. After 48 to 72 hr of incubation, the cytotoxicity of the macrophages was determined by examining the released [^{3}H]proline. In this system the tuftsin treatment gave significantly elevated macrophage cytotoxicity (Nishioka, 1979a; Nishioka *et al.*, 1981b).

To examine further the antitumor activity of this peptide, the Cloudman S91 murine melanoma system was utilized. DBA/2 mice were injected subcutaneously (sc) with 2.5×10^5 tissue culture S91 melanoma cells and 10 μg tuftsin in the hind leg. The growth of melanoma was monitored for 48 days. The tumors in the tuftsin-treated group grew slower than those in the control group (Nishioka *et al.*, 1981b). To evaluate this antitumor effect of tuftsin in a more quantitative fashion, melanoma colonies were established in the lung by injecting the Cloudman S91 murine melanoma cells into the tall vein of DBA/2 mice. The pigmented melanoma colonies thus formed were counted upon pneumonectomy 30 days after the inoculation of the tumor cells (Takami and Nishioka, 1981; Nishioka *et al.*, 1981c). The experimental mice received 1×10^5 melanoma cells on day 0, and were then treated with ip injections of tuftsin three times per week. The tuftsin-treated mice clearly showed significant reductions in the melanoma lung colonies formed. Mice treated with tuftsin 2 weeks after the inoculation of melanoma cells still displayed the antitumor activity (Noyes *et al.*, 1981). In order to examine this phenomenon *in vitro*, the cytotoxic activity of alveolar macrophages was studied, because they represent the major class of effector cells in the lungs. The alveolar macrophages, collected from DBA/2 mice by endobronchial lavage by the aid of lidocaine, were treated with tuftsin and ^{51}Cr-labeled Cloudman S91 melanoma cells introduced. The standard 18-hr ^{51}Cr-release assay clearly exhibited the augmented cytotoxicity by tuftsin treatment, whereas the untreated effector cells conspicuously displayed no significant cytotoxicity. We also observed the stimulation of alveolar macrophages *in vivo* by administering tuftsin to DBA/2 mice. Upon a single injection of various doses of tuftsin, alveolar macrophages were collected at different time points and examined by using the *in vitro* cytotoxicity assay. Although the kinetics differ somewhat between ip and intravenous (iv) administrations, the peak cytotoxicity of alveolar macrophages was attained in several days with gradual decline of the cytotoxicity with time (Babcock *et al.*, 1981; Nishioka *et al.*, 1983).

In order to confirm this antitumor effect of the peptide, we introduced two primary tumor models. In the Rous sarcoma system, upon injection of the oncogen preparation in the thigh within 24 hr of birth, C57BL/10Sn mice gave a

65% incidence of Rous sarcoma. Tuftsin treatment of these mice significantly reduced the tumor incidence. In the 3-methylcholanthrene-induced primary fibrosarcoma, C57BL/10 mice were treated with tuftsin following the injection of the carcinogen in the thigh. The mean tumor latent period for the tuftsin-treated group was significantly longer than that for mice in the control group (Nishioka et al., 1983; Banks et al., 1983).

We have also attempted to examine the antimetastatic activity of tuftsin in addition to its antitumor activity. Thus, we selected another murine tumor model. In the CH1 B-cell lymphoma system, 1×10^6 CH1 cells were injected iv to syngeneic mice, followed 1 day later by different dosages of tuftsin given iv every other day. The majority of mice receiving 10 or 100 μg of tuftsin per dose exhibited no tumor growth at 150 days after tumor inoculation. In this model we also examined the antimetastatic effect of tuftsin by observing the appearance of sc nodules. Mice receiving 1 μg of tuftsin per dose showed a reduced number of sc tumors, whereas no metastatic tumors were observed in mice receiving 10 or 100 μg of tuftsin (Babcock et al., 1982). To determine the cellular mechanism by which tuftsin exerts its antitumor activity, we introduced the carrageenan treatment, which is known to suppress mostly macrophages (Catanzaro et al., 1971) and NK cells (Quan et al., 1980). Carrageenan given in combination with tuftsin reduced the survival of mice to control level. This suggests that one or both of these effector cells are probably responsible for the antitumor activity. This interpretation was further supported by the observation that the carrageenan treatment by itself reduced the survival time of the mice compared with the control animals.

In collaboration with Dr. Sunkara, the combination therapy of tuftsin with α-difluoromethyl ornithine (DFMO) was evaluated employing the B16 murine melanoma system (Sunkara et al., 1983). DFMO is an inhibitor of the biosynthesis of polyamines and inhibits specifically ornithine decarboxylase irreversibly (Metcalf et al., 1978). DFMO by itself inhibited 80% of the tumor growth, and addition of tuftsin to this model blocked the tumor growth almost completely.

A number of studies by other investigators have been published demonstrating the antitumor activity of this naturally occurring peptide. Bruley-Rossett et al. (1981a) examined the effect of tuftsin on the occurrence of spontaneous tumors by treating 12-month-old C57BL/6 mice with 10 μg tuftsin every week for 6 months. An untreated control group showed 22% incidence of spontaneous tumors, while no tumor was detected in the tuftsin-treated group upon careful pathological examination. They also observed that these repeated administrations of tuftsin restored the aging-related impaired cytotoxic capabilities of macrophages and cytolytic T cells to the levels of those effector cells obtained from younger mice (Bruley-Rosset et al., 1981a,b). Since we failed to demonstrate the direct binding of fluorescein-labeled tuftsin to T cells, it appears that the activation of T cells was brought about indirectly through the activation of macrophages. Najjar *et al.* (1980, 1981) reported *in vivo* antitumor effect of tuftinyltuftsin in the L1210 leukemia model. Catane *et al.* (1983) demonstrated the antitumor effect of tuftsin in a transplantable fibrosarcoma model in C3H mice. Florentin *et al.* (1978) treated mice with tuftsin *in vivo,* collected macrophages and spleen cells from these mice, and examined these effector cells *in vitro.* The macrophages showed enhanced cytostatic effect, and the spleen cells exhibited the stimulation of ADCC activity. In this experiment, tuftsin did not appear to induce nonspecific splenic suppressor cells, because the response of normal spleen cells to mitogens *in vitro* was not depressed when cultivated in the presence of spleen cells from tuftsin-treated mice. We observed the direct *in vitro* activation of spleen cells by tuftsin in ADCC assay. We also became interested in possible activation of PMN cytotoxicity. Purified human PMN were treated with tuftsin and tested against established human melanoma cell lines and a normal human embryonic lung cell line WI-38. The PMN showed significant cytotoxicity against human melanoma cell lines, but not against the WI-38 line (Nishioka, 1979b). Although untreated murine peritoneal macrophages always showed substantial natural cytotoxicity against tumor cells, human PMN, like murine alveolar macrophages, did not display detectable cytotoxicity without tuftsin treatment.

As mentioned previously, we observed the direct binding of tuftsin to human NK cells. In order to examine the significance of this observation, experiments were performed in a murine system. *In vitro* treatment of mouse splenic cells with tuftsin induced a pronounced enhancement of NK cell cytotoxicity against ^{51}Cr-labeled Yac-1 lymphoma cells. The elimination of macrophages, monocytes, T cells, and Ig-bearing cells did not alter this activation (Phillips *et al.,* 1981). In a similar manner, human peripheral leukocytes were examined using K562 human leukemia cells and 39.5 human melanoma cells as tumor target cells. Since similar results were obtained, an attempt was made to purify NK cells from human peripheral blood employing discontinuous density gradients of Percoll. This purified preparation of NK cells displayed the cytotoxicity of 40% against K562 cells after 6 hr incubation using a 3:1 (effector cell:target cell) ratio. In the presence of tuftsin, 100% cytotoxicity was obtained.

To examine the effect of tuftsin from the viewpoint of natural cell-mediated cytotoxicity, various murine leukocyte fractions from CBA/J mice were tested for cell-mediated cytotoxicity against tumor cells without apparent presensitization. In the presence of tuftsin, all of the leukocyte fractions used, splenic macrophages, peripheral blood PMN, and splenic NK cells, exhibited enhanced cytotoxicity against the Yac-1 cells in 18-hr ^{51}Cr-release assay. Subsequently, the *in vivo* effect of tuftsin was also examined. Following a single iv injection of different doses of tuftsin, unfractionated spleen cells and bone marrow cells were collected from mice at various time points, and the cytotoxicities of these cell fractions were measured as described earlier. The clear augmentation of cytotoxicity by tuftsin was observed in both cell fractions. The same *in vitro* procedure already described was then applied to human peripheral blood leukocytes. All cell fractions applied—monocytes, PMN, and NK cells—clearly manifested tuftsin-enhanced cytotoxicities against the K562 human leukemia cells (Phillips *et al.*, 1983).

On the basis of experimental results obtained by us and others, we envision that the following properties of tuftsin contribute to the *in vivo* antitumor activity of tuftsin:

1. Monocyte-macrophages, PMN, and NK cells have direct cytotoxic action.
2. Other effector cells are indirectly stimulated through release of factors by tuftsin-activated cells. As mentioned previously, the activation of cytolytic T cells may be achieved in this manner.
3. The augmentation of antibody production may lead to effective killings of tumor cells through ADCC.
4. The mitogenic activity of tuftsin may result in increased numbers of effector cells, and the induction of differentiation by tuftsin may lead to maturation of young effector cells to cytotoxic cells.
5. The chemotaxis and migration-enhancing properties of tuftsin may help mobilize effector cells to the sites of tumors.

IV. ANTIMICROBIAL ACTIVITY OF TUFTSIN

After its discovery, the biological activity of tuftsin was measured by phagocytosis assay. In 1977, however, Martinez *et al.* reported that mice treated with tuftsin showed drastic increase in the clearance of different bacteria and also observed that the peritoneal macrophages from these tuftsin-treated mice manifested enhanced bactericidal activity, thus indicating that tuftsin administration brought about both increased phagocytosis and killing of bacteria.

As previously mentioned, splenectomized patients possess reduced levels of tuftsin in their sera. The mortality rate of postsplenectomy sepsis is more than 50% (Franke and Neu, 1981). It is also known that patients with tumors tend to have much more frequent infections than the normal population and that the major cause of death among these patients is infection. In view of this, a splenectomy performed on a cancer patient requires special attention. A typical example of this complication can be found among splenectomized pediatric patients with Hodgkin's disease (Chilcote *et al.*, 1976). To combat fulminant infection in this particular group of patients, Mikulski *et al.* (1977) suggested a clinical trial of tuftsin.

It is also well known that candidiasis is a life-threatening infection in the management of terminal cancer patients. Hisatsune *et al.* (1983) have observed beneficial effects of tuftsin using an animal model. We have also observed a similar effect in our murine candidiasis system.

V. CONCLUDING REMARKS

As mentioned earlier, tuftsin possesses a wide range of activities on various populations of leukocytes. Tuftsin therefore appears to be a promising peptide hormone in the treatment of cancer and infections. The toxicity of tuftsin has been shown to be very low (mouse LD_{50} by iv administration: 2.4 g/kg body weight) (Catane *et al.*, 1983). The toxicity of tuftsin has been also examined in the dog (Catane *et al.*, 1983) and monkey (Mathe *et al.*, 1983) models. As expected from our study on mitogenicity of tuftsin, leukocytosis was observed in these animal studies upon the administration of tuftsin. A human study was then initiated using tuftsin as a single agent (Catane *et al.*, 1983). The preliminary phase 1 study with 15 terminal cancer patients showed no toxicity up to 0.96 mg tuftsin per kilogram of body weight. One patient with nasopharyngeal carcinoma showed a definite response with shrinkage of the tumor. Their phase 2 study had only three patients. Tuftsin treatment induced remission in one patient with chronic myelocytic leukemia who had a blast crisis. Many of these tuftsin-treated patients manifested leukocytosis and increases in mononuclear cell cytotoxicity.

Since various traumas including surgery and burns are known to impair the natural immunological system, we are currently attempting to improve this impaired system by employing tuftsin, with some promising results. Tuftsin may also be effective in repairing a variety of suppressed immune conditions, including acquired immune deficiency syndrome and congenital immune diseases, in addition to congenital tuftsin abnormalities and tuftsin deficiencies. As exemplified by the combination treatment employing tuftsin and DFMO, effective combination regimens of tuftsin with other agents should be exploited. Considering the apparent advantages of this peptide as a natural biological response modifier—(1) its physiological origin, (2) enhancement of antitumor and antimicrobial activities of the hosts, (3) low toxicity, and (4) availability of an immunoassay to measure serum tuftsin levels at any given time—wider clinical applications of tuftsin are anticipated in the future.

Acknowledgments

The author wishes to acknowledge Dr. M. Romsdahl for his encouragement, Dr. G. Babcock, Dr. J. Phillips, Mr. A. Amoscato, Dr. R. Banks, Mr. T. Elhagin, Ms L. Yoshimura, Dr. D. Chu, and Dr. S. Schantz for their scientific contributions, and Ms. L. Lerma for her assistance in preparing the manuscript. Work in our laboratory was supported in parts by Grants CA-27330, CA-32666, and CA-30115 awarded by the National Cancer Institute, Department of Health and Human Services.

REFERENCES

Aigner, K., Dobroschke, J., Weber, E. G., Schwemmle, K., Bauer, M., Teuber, J., and Helmke, K. (1980). Successful reimplantation of splenic tissue after neonatal abdominal trauma. *Lancet* **1**, 360–361.

Amoscato, A. A., Babcock, G. F., and Nishioka, K. (1981). Analysis of contaminants in commercial preparations of the tetrapeptide tuftsin by high-performance liquid chromatography. *J. Chromatogr.* **205**, 179–184.

Amoscato, A. A., Davies, P. J. A., Babcock, G. F., and Nishioka, K. (1983a). Receptor-mediated internalization of tuftsin. *Ann. N.Y. Acad. Sci.* **419**, 114–134.

Amoscato, A. A., Davies, P. J. A., Babcock, G. F., and Nishioka, K. (1983b). Receptor-mediated internalization of tuftsin by human polymorphonuclear leukocytes. *J. Reticuloendothel. Soc.* **34**, 53–67.

Babcock, G. F., Noyes, R. D., and Nishioka, K. (1981). The effect of tuftsin, an immunopotentiating peptide, on Cloudman S-91 melanoma *in vivo*. *In* "Pigment Cell 1981: Phenotypic Expression in Pigment Cell" (M. Seiji, ed.), pp. 623–628. Univ. Tokyo Press, Tokyo.

Babcock, G. F., Phillips, J. H., and Nishioka, K. (1982). The immunotherapeutic effect of the peptide tuftsin on the B cell lymphoma, CH1. *In* "B and T Cell Tumors" (E. S. Vitetta, ed.), pp. 481–485. Academic Press, New York.

Babcock, G. F., Amoscato, A. A., and Nishioka, K. (1983). Effect of tuftsin on the migration, chemotaxis and differentiation of macrophages and granulocytes. *Ann. N.Y. Acad. Sci.* **419**, 64–74.

Balfanz, J. R., Nesbit, M. E., Jr., Jarvis, C., and Krivit, W. (1976). Overwhelming sepsis following splenectomy for trauma. *J. Pediatr. (St. Louis)* **88**, 458–460.

Banks, R. A., Babcock, G. F., and Nishioka, K. (1983). Effect of tuftsin on *in vivo* murine oncogenesis. *Proc. Am. Assoc. Cancer Res.* **24**, 194.

Bar-Shavit, Z., and Goldman, R. (1982). Tuftsin and substance P as modulators of phagocyte functions. *Adv. Exp. Med. Biol.* **141**, 549–558.

Bar-Shavit, Z., Stabinsky, Y., Fridkin, M., and Goldman, R. (1979). Tuftsin–macrophage interaction: Specific binding and augmentation of phagocytosis. *J. Cell. Physiol.* **100**, 55–62.

Bar-Shavit, Z., Bursuker, I., and Goldman, R. (1980a). Functional tuftsin binding sites on macrophage-like tumor line P388D1 and on bone marrow cells differentiated *in vivo* into mononuclear phagocytes. *Mol. Cell. Biochem.* **30**, 151–155.

Bar-Shavit, Z., Goldman, R., Stabinsky, Y., Gottlieb, P., Fridkin, M., Teichberg, V. I., and Blumberg, S. (1980b). Enhancement of phagocytosis—A newly found activity of substance P residing in its N-terminal tetrapeptide sequence. *Biochem. Biophy. Res. Commun.* **94**, 1445–1451.

Blumenstein, M., Layne, P. P., and Najjar, V. A. (1979). Nuclear magnetic resonance studies on the structure of the tetrapeptide tuftsin, L-threonyl-L-lysyl-L-prolyl-L-arginine, and its pentapeptide analogue L-threonyl-L-lysyl-L-prolyl-L-prolyl-L-arginine. *Biochemistry* **18**, 5247–5253.

Bruley-Rosset, M., Hercend, T., Martinez, J., Rappaport, H., and Mathe, G. (1981a). Prevention of spontaneous tumors of aged mice by immunopharmacologic manipulation: Study of immune antitumor mechanisms. *JNCI, J. Natl. Cancer Inst.* **66**, 1113–1119.

Bruley-Rosset, M., Florentin, I., and Mathe, G. (1981b). Macrophage activation by tuftsin and muramyl-dipeptide. *Mol. Cell. Biochem.* **41**, 113–118.

Catane, R., Schlanger, S., Weiss, L., Penchas, S., Fuks, Z., Treves, A. J., and Fridkin, M. (1983). Toxicology and antitumor activity of tuftsin. *Ann. N.Y. Acad. Sci.* **419**, 251–260.

Catanzaro, P. J., Schwartz, H. J., and Graham, R. C. (1971). Spectrum and possible mechanism of carrageenan cytotoxicity. *Am. J. Pathol.* **64**, 387–404.

Chilcote, R. R., Baehner, R. L., and Hammond, D. (1976). Septicemia and meningitis in children splenectomized for Hodgkin's disease. *N. Engl. J. Med.* **295,** 798–800.

Chirigos, M. A. (1978). "Immune Modulation and Control of Neoplasia by Adjuvant Therapy." Raven, New York.

Constantopoulos, A., and Najjar, V. A. (1972). Tuftsin, a natural and general phagocytosis stimulating peptide affecting macrophages and polymorphonuclear granulocytes. *Cytobios* **6,** 97–100.

Constantopoulos, A., and Najjar, V. A. (1973a). Tuftsin deficiency syndrome. *Acta Paediatr. Scand.* **62,** 645–648.

Constantopoulos, A., and Najjar, V. A. (1973b). The requirement for membrane sialic acid in the stimulation of phagocytosis by the natural tetrapeptide, tuftsin. *J. Biol. Chem.* **248,** 3819–3822.

Constantopoulos, A., Likhite, V., Crosby, W. H., and Najjar, V. A. (1973). Phagocytic activity of the leukemic cell and its response to the phagocytosis-stimulating tetrapeptide, tuftsin. *Cancer Res.* **33,** 1230–1234.

Edelman, G. M., Cunningham, B. A., Gall, W. E., Gottlieb, P. D., Rutishauser, U., and Waxdal, M. J. (1969). The covalent structure of an entire γG immunoglobulin molecule. *Proc. Natl. Acad. Sci. U.S.A.* **63,** 78–85.

Florentin, I., Bruley-Rosset, M., Kiger, N., Imbach, J. L., Winternitz, F., and Mathe, G. (1978). In vivo immunostimulation by tuftsin. *Cancer Immunol. Immunother.* **5,** 211–216.

Franke, E. L., and Neu, H. C. (1981). Postsplenectomy infection. *Surg. Clin. North Am.* **61,** 135–155.

Fridkin, M., and Gottlieb, P. (1981). Tuftsin, Thr-Lys-Pro-Arg: Anatomy of an immunologically active peptide. *Mol. Cell. Biochem.* **41,** 73–97.

Giroud, J. P., Roch-Arveiller, M., Muntaner, O., and Bradshaw, D. (1980). Action comparée et de la tuftsine sur le chimiotactisme des polynucléaires de rat. *Nouv. Rev. Fr. Hematol.* **22,** 69–76.

Goetzl, E. J. (1975). Plasma and cell-derived inhibitors of human neutrophil chemotaxis. *Ann. N.Y. Acad. Sci.* **256,** 210–221.

Goetzl, E. J. (1976). Modulation of human eosinophil polymorphonuclear leukocyte migration and function. *Am. J. Pathol.* **85,** 419–435.

Hartung, H. P., and Toyka, K. V. (1983). Tuftsin stimulates the release of oxygen radicals and thromboxane from macrophages. *Immunol. Lett.* **6,** 1–6.

Herberman, R. B. (1980). "Natural Cell-Mediated Immunity against Tumors." Academic Press, New York.

Herman, Z. S., Stachura, Z., Siemion, I. Z., and Nawrocka, E. (1980). Analgesic activity of tuftsin analogs. *Naturwissenschaften* **67,** 613–614.

Hersh, E. M., Chirigos, M. A., and Mastrangelo, M. J. (1981). "Augmenting Agents in Cancer Therapy." Raven, New York.

Hisatsune, K., Nozaki, S., Ishikawa, T., Hayashi, M., Nagaki, K., and Ogawa, H. (1983). Biochemical study of phagocytic activities of tuftsin and its analogues. *Ann. N.Y. Acad. Sci.* **419,** 205–213.

Horsmanheimo, A., Horsmanheimo, M., and Fudenberg, H. H. (1978). Effect of tuftsin on migration of polymorphonuclear and mononuclear human leukocytes in leukocyte migration agarose test. *Clin. Immunol. Immunopathol.* **11,** 251–255.

Inada, K., Nemoto, N., Nishijima, A., Wada, S., Hirata, M., and Yoshida, M. (1979). A suspected case of tuftsin deficiency. *In* "Phagocytosis: Its Physiology and Pathology" (Y. Kokubun and N. Kobayashi, eds.), pp. 101–108. Univ. Park Press, Baltimore, Maryland.

James, K., McBride, B., and Stuart, A. (1977). "The Macrophage and Cancer." Univ. of Edinburgh, Edinburgh.

Kamenskii, A. A., Antonova, L. V., Samoilova, N. A., Galkin, O. M., Andreev, S. M., and

Ashmarin, I. P. (1980). Excitatory action of the tetrapeptide tuftsin on activity of albino rats. *Bull. Exp. Biol. Med.* **89**, 911–914.

Kavai, M., Lukacs, K., Szegedi, G., Szeherke, M., and Erchegyi, J. (1981). Chemotactic and stimulating effect of tuftsin and its analogues on human monocytes. *Immunol. Lett.* **2**, 219–224.

Klebanoff, S. J., and Clark, R. A. (1978). "The Neutrophil: Function and Clinical Disorders." North-Holland Publ., New York.

Konopinska, D., Najjar, V. A., and Callery, M. (1981). Solid phase synthesis of L-threonyl-L-glutamyl-L-prolyl-L-arginine, as the mutant analog of tuftsin. *Arch. Immunol. Ther. Exp.* **29**, 851–856.

Likhite, V. V. (1975). Opsonin and leucophilicγ-globulin in chronically splenectomized rat with and without heterotropic autotransplanted splenic tissue. *Nature (London)* **253**, 742–744.

Luftig, R. B., Yoshinaka, Y., and Oroszlan, S. (1977). Sequence relationship between Rauscher leukemia virus (RLV) p 65-70 (*gag* gene product) and tuftsin as monitored by the p 65-70 proteolytic factor. *J. Cell Biol.* **25**, 397a.

Martinez, J., Winternitz, F., and Videl, J. (1977). Nouvelles syntheses et propriétés de la tuftsine. *Eur. J. Med. Chem.-Chim. Ther.* **12**, 511–516.

Mathe, G., Bruley-Rosset, M., and Rappaport, H. (1983). Spontaneous development of tumors in C57BL/6 mice associated with aging: Pharmacoprevention by tuftsin. Conference on Anti-neoplastic, Immunogenic and Other Effects of the Tetrapeptide Tuftsin: A Natural Macrophage Activator, p. 22.

Metcalf, B. W., Bey, P., Danzin, C., Jung, M. J., Casara, P., and Vevert, J. P. (1978). Catalytic irreversible inhibition of mammalian ornithine decarboxylase (E.C.4.1.1.17) by substrate and product analogues. *J. Am. Chem. Soc.* **100**, 2551–2553.

Mikulski, S. M., Von Hoff, D. D., Rozencweig, M., and Muggia, F. M. (1977). Tuftsin—Unimportant or forgotten? *N. Engl. J. Med.* **296**, 454.

Millikan, J. S., Moore, E. E., Moore, G. E., and Stevens, R. E. (1982). Alternative to splenectomy in adults after trauma, repair, partial resection, and reimplantation of splenic tissue. *Am. J. Surg.* **144**, 711–716.

Nagaoka, I., and Yamashita, T. (1981). Inactivation of phagocytosis-stimulating activity of tuftsin by polymorphonuclear neutrophils: A possible role of leucine aminopeptidase as an ecto-enzyme. *Biochim. Biophy Acta* **675**, 85–93.

Nair, R. M. G., Ponce, B., and Fudenberg, H. H. (1978). Interactions of radiolabeled tuftsin with human neturophils. *Immunochemistry* **15**, 901–907.

Najjar, V. A., and Constantopoulos, A. (1972). A new phagocytosis-stimulating tetrapeptide hormone, tuftsin, and its role in disease. *J. Reticuloendothe. Soc.* **12**, 197–215.

Najjar, V. A., and Nishioka, K. (1970). 'Tuftsin': A physiological phagocytosis stimulating peptide. *Nature (London)* **288**, 672–673.

Najjar, V. A., Fidalgo, B. V., and Stitt, E. (1968). The physiological role of the lymphoid system. VII. The disappearance of leucokinin activity following splenectomy. *Biochemistry* **7**, 2376–2379.

Najjar, V. A., Chaudhuri, M. K., Konopinska, D., Beck, B. D., Layne, P. P., and Linehan, L. (1980). Tuftsin (Thr-Lys-Pro-Arg) a physiological activator of phagocytic cells: A possible role in cancer suppression and therapy. *In* "Augmenting Agents of Cancer Therapy" (E. M. Hersh, A. Chirigos, and M. Mastrangelo eds.), pp. 459–478. Raven, New York.

Najjar, V. A., Konopinska, D., Chaudhuri, M. K., Schmidt, D. E., and Linehan, L. (1981). Tuftsin, a natural activator of phagocytic functions including tumoricidal activity. *Mol. Cell. Biochem.* **41**, 3–12.

Nishioka, K. (1978). Migration enhancement by tuftsin of human mononuclear cells and its effect on the migration inhibition factor test with tumor antigens. *Gann* **69**, 569–572.

Nishioka, K. (1979a). Anti-tumor effect of the physiological tetrapeptide, tuftsin. *Br. J. Cancer* **39**, 342–345.

Nishioka, K. (1979b). *In vitro* induction of human granulocyte cytotoxicity by tuftsin. *Gann* **70**, 845–846.

Nishioka, K., Constantopoulos, A., Satoh, P. S., and Najjar, V. A. (1972). The characteristics, isolation and synthesis of the phagocytosis stimulating peptide tuftsin. *Biochem. Biophys. Res. Commun.* **47**, 172–179.

Nishioka, K., Constantopoulos, A., Satoh, P. S., Mitchell, W. M., and Najjar, V. A. (1973a). Characteristics and isolation of the phagocytosis-stimulating peptide, tuftsin. *Biochim. Biophys. Acta* **310**, 217–229.

Nishioka, K., Satoh, P. S., Constantopoulos, A., and Najjar, V. A. (1973b). The chemical synthesis of the phagocytosis-stimulating tetrapeptide tuftsin (Thr-Lys-Pro-Arg) and its biological properties. *Biochim. Biophys. Acta* **310**, 230–237.

Nishioka, K., Amoscato, A. A., and Babcock, G. F. (1981a). Tuftsin: A hormone-like tetrapeptide with antimicrobial and antitumor activities. *Life Sci.* **28**, 1081–1090.

Nishioka, K., Babcock, G. F., Phillips, J. H., and Noyes, R. D. (1981b). Antitumor effect of tuftsin. *Mol. Cell. Biochem.* **41**, 13–18.

Nishioka, K., Takami, H., Noyes, R. D., and Babcock, G. F. (1981c). Cloudman S-91 melanoma colony assay in the lungs of mice and profiles of the biochemical tumor markers, tyrosinase and polyamines. *In* "Pigment Cell 1981: Phenotypic Expression in Pigment Cell" (M. Seiji, ed.), pp. 617–621. Univ. Tokyo Press, Tokyo.

Nishioka, K., Babcock, G. F., Phillips, J. H., Banks, R. A., and Amoscato, A. A. (1983). *In vivo* and *in vitro* antitumor activities of tuftsin. *Ann. N.Y. Acad.* **419**, 234–241.

Noyes, R. D., Babcock, G. F., and Nishioka, K. (1981). Antitumor activity of tuftsin on murine melanoma *in vivo*. *Cancer Treat. Rep.* **65**, 673–675.

Oldham, R. K. (1982). Biological response modifiers program. *J. Biol. Resp. Modif.* **1**, 81–100.

Oroszlan, S., Henderson, L. W., Stephenson, J. R., Copeland, T. D., Long, C. W., Ihle, J. N., and Gilden, R. V. (1978). Amino- and carboxy-terminal amino acid sequences of proteins coded by *gag* gene of murine leukemia virus. *Proc. Natl. Acad. Sci. U.S.A.* **75**, 1404–1408.

Patel, J., Williams, J. S., Shmigel, B., and Hinshaw, R. (1981). Preservation of splenic function by autotransplantation of traumatized spleen in man. *Surgery (St. Louis)* **90**, 683–688.

Pearson, H. A., Johnston, D., Smith, K. A., and Touloukin, R. J. (1978). The born-again spleen: Return of splenic function after splenectomy for trauma. *N. Engl. J. Med.* **298**, 1389–1392.

Phillips, J. H., Babcock, G. F., and Nishioka, K. (1981). Tuftsin: A naturally occurring immunopotentiating factor I. *In vitro* enhancement of murine natural cell-mediated cytotoxicity. *J. Immunol.* **126**, 915–921.

Phillips, J. H., Nishioka, K., and Babcock, G. F. (1983). Tuftsin-induced enhancement of murine and human natural cellmediated cytotoxicity. *Ann. N.Y. Acad. Sci.* **419**, 192–204.

Quan, P.-C., Kolb, J.-P., and Lespinats, G. (1980). NK activity in carrageenan-treated mice. *Immunology* **40**, 495–503.

Siemion, I. Z. (1981). Tuftsin analogs and their biological activity. *Mol. Cell. Biochem.* **41**, 99–112.

Singer, D. B. (1973). Postsplenectomy sepsis. *Perspect. Pediatr. Pathol.* **1**, 285–305.

Spirer, Z., Zakuth, V., Golander, A., Bogair, N., and Fridkin, M. (1975). The effect of tuftsin on the nitrous blue tetrazolium reduction of normal human polymorphonuclear leukocytes. *J. Clin. Invest.* **55**, 198–200.

Spirer, A., Zakuth, V., Bogair, N., and Fridkin, M. (1977). Radioimmunoassay of the phagocytosis-stimulating peptide tuftsin in normal and splenectomized subjects. *Eur. J. Immunol.* **7**, 69–74.

Spirer, A., Weisman, Y., Zakuth, V., Fridkin, M., and Bogair, N. (1980). Decreased serum tuftsin concentrations in sickle cell disease. *Arch. Dis. Child.* **55**, 566–567.

Stabinsky, Y., Gottlieb, P., Zakuth, V., Spirer, Z., and Fridkin, M. (1978). Specific binding sites for the phagocytosis stimulating peptide tuftsin on human polymorphonuclear leukocytes and monocytes. *Biochem. Biophys. Res. Commun.* **83,** 599–606.

Stabinsky, Y., Bar-Shavit, Z., Fridkin, M., and Goldman, R. (1980). On the mechanism of action of the phagocytosis-stimulating peptide tuftsin. *Mol. Cell Biochem.* **30,** 71–77.

Sunkara, P. S., Prakash, N. J., and Nishioka, K. (1983). Potentiation of antitumor activity of α-difluoromethyl ornithine by immunomodulating peptide tuftsin. *Ann. N.Y. Acad. Sci.* **419,** 268–272.

Takami, H., and Nishioka, K. (1980). Raised polyamines in erythrocytes from melanoma-bearing mice and patients with solid tumors. *Br. J. Cancer* **41,** 751–756.

Tritsch, G. L., and Niswander, P. W. (1982). Positive correlation between superoxide release and intracellular adenosine deaminase activity during macrophage membrane perturbuation regardless of nature or magnitude of stimulus. *Mol. Cell. Biochem.* **49,** 49–51.

Tzehoval, E., Segal, S., Stabinsky, Y., Fridkin, M., Spirer, Z., and Feldman, M. (1978). Tuftsin (an Ig-associated tetrapeptide) triggers the immunogenic function of macrophages: Implications for activation of programmed cells. *Proc. Natl. Acad. Sci. U.S.A.* **75,** 3400–3404.

Val'dman A. V., Kozlovskaya, M. M., Ashmarin, I. P., Mineeva, M. F., and Anokhin, K. V. (1981). Central effects of the tetrapeptide tuftsin. *Bull. Exp. Biol. Med.* **92,** 890–892.

Yamanaka, N., Fukushima, M., Matsuoka, H., Nishida, K., and Ota, K. (1979). Effect of tuftsin on polymorphonuclear leukocyte metabolism. *In* "Phagocytosis: Its Physiology and Pathology" (Y. Kokubun and N. Kobayashi, eds.), pp. 93–100. Univ. Park Press, Baltimore, Maryland.

8

5α-Reductase: A Target Enzyme for Prostatic Cancer

VLADIMIR PETROW
Department of Pharmacology
Duke University Medical Center
Durham, North Carolina

GEORGE M. PADILLA
Department of Physiology
Duke University Medical Center
Durham, North Carolina

	I. Introduction	270
II.	Historical Background	271
	A. 5α-Reductase	274
	B. Mechanism of Action of 5α-Reductase	276
III.	The Androgen Receptor and the Mechanism of Action of Androgens within the Prostatic Cell	276
IV.	5α-Reductase, Dihydrotestosterone, and the Human Prostate	277
V.	Dihydrotestosterone and Prostatic Cancer	280
	A. Rat Studies	280
	B. Human Studies	281
	C. Elimination of Testosterone from the Prostate	281
VI.	Steroid Biochemistry of the Normal Prostatic Cell	282
	A. Receptors	282
	B. Steroid-Metabolizing Enzymes Identified in the Human Prostate	283
VII.	Hormone Sensitivity of the Neoplastic Prostatic Cell	286
	A. Latent Lesions	286
	B. Androgen-Responsive Lesions	286
	C. Androgen-Insensitive Lesions	287
	D. Endocrine Correlates of Autonomous Cellular Change	287
VIII.	A New Approach to Palliative Treatment of Prostate Cancer	288

Novel Approaches to Cancer Chemotherapy
Copyright © 1984 by Academic Press, Inc.
All rights of reproduction in any form reserved.
ISBN 0-12-676980-X

    A. Proposition I 288
    B. Proposition II... 288
    C. Proposition III.. 289
    D. Proposition IV.. 289
  IX. 5α-Reductase as a Target Enzyme for Prostatic Cancer 289
   X. 5α-Reductase Inhibitors Active *in Vivo* 291
    A. Competitive Reversible Inhibitors 292
    B. Active-Site-Directed Inhibitors (k_{cat} Inhibitors) 294
  XI. Summary 297
    Addendum 298
    References 298

The etiology of prostatic cancer is not known at the present time so that discussion of treatment must be based on the pragmatism of experiment. In addition, the paucity of information on the human disease enforces reliance upon animal data with all its attendant pitfalls. There must consequently be considerable speculation and oversimplification in a contribution of this type. It is nevertheless hoped that the concepts presented herein will receive sympathetic consideration and will help stimulate interest in a hitherto untried approach to palliative therapy.

"Start New Opinions of an Old Disease"
George Crabbe
Letter VII Professions—Physic
The Borough, 1810

I. INTRODUCTION

It was known as long ago as 1786 that castration leads to atrophy of the prostate gland. By 1865 prostatic cancer had been recognized as a clinical entity and its metastatic character established by 1891. In the early 1940s the pioneering studies of Huggins and Hodges (1941) had delineated the regulatory role of the testes and testicular androgens in prostatic cancer, studies that had led them to introduce castration and estrogens for treatment of the disease. Though representing a major therapeutic breakthrough—which has remained virtually unchallenged for the last 40 years—the theoretical concepts behind the use of castration and estrogens were based on early biochemical data that are now in need of major revision (see Section V). It is now clear that 5α-dihydrotestosterone (DHT) (**III**) and not testosterone (T) (**I**) is the pivotal androgen of the prostate (see Fig. 1). *Elimination of dihydrotestosterone and not testosterone from the economy of the prostate gland must consequently represent the primary goal of palliative therapy.* Such elimination of dihydrotestosterone can theoretically be achieved by inhibiting the enzyme 5α-reductase. If this is indeed the case, then the way is open to a new and improved form of palliative therapy that avoids the trauma of immolative surgery.

II. HISTORICAL BACKGROUND

Following isolation of the testicular hormone T (**I**) in crystalline form (David *et al.*, 1935), two groups (Butenandt *et al.*, 1935; Ruzicka and Goldberg, 1935) simultaneously converted it into 17β-hydroxy-5α-androstan-3-one (DHT) (**III**) by catalytic hydrogenation. DHT proved to be inferior to the parent T in androgenic activity as measured by Tschopp's chick comb-growth assay (1935) and so aroused little contemporary interest. In the same year, Callow and Deansley (1935) reported data on the response of the prostate and seminal vesicles to an androgen (androsterone) in the prepubertally castrated rat. Two years later Kochakian (1937) demonstrated the anabolic effect of T in the castrated dog as measured by nitrogen retention. In 1950 Kochakian followed up this early observation by showing that DHT was equipotent with T in this assay. Because nitrogen retention studies were so time consuming, Eisenberg and Gordon (1950) suggested that comparison of the effects of steroids on the levator ani muscle and on the ventral prostate and seminal vesicles of the castrated rat formed a reasonable indicator of protein-anabolic potency. Introduction of this assay and modifications thereof led to a major effort, mostly by pharmaceutical companies, to identify an anabolic steroid with minimal androgenic activity. It also led to the recognition that DHT was about twice as active as T in stimulating the growth of the prostate (Dorfman and Kincl, 1963; Dorfman, 1969; Saunders, 1963).

While these purely endocrine studies were in progress, important advances were being made in the metabolism of the steroid hormones. It was found that αβ-unsaturated ketones such as **I** were metabolized in the body primarily by reductive reactions involving ring A to give 5α (**III**) and/or 5β (**IV**) dihydroderivatives (see Dorfman and Ungar, 1965). Rat liver preparations, in particular, contained enzymes that catalyzed both these processes in the presence of reduced pyridine nucleotide as cofactor (Tomkins and Isselbacher, 1954; Tomkins, 1957; Schneider, 1952). Further study by Forchielli and Dorfman (1956) and Forchielli *et al.* (1958) showed that fractions prepared from livers of adult male rats contained both a soluble Δ^4,5β-hydrogenase and a microsomal Δ^4,5α-hydrogenase, which, in the presence of NADPH, readily reduced T (**I**) to the dihydro derivatives (**III** and **IV**) (Fig. 1).

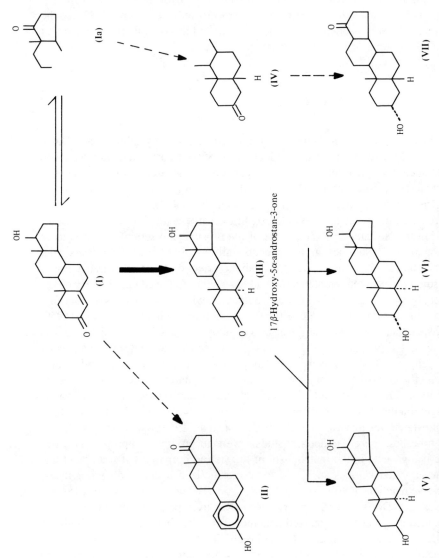

Fig. 1. Metabolism of testosterone. **I** = Testosterone; **Ia** = androstenedione; **II** = estrone; **III** = 5α-dihydrotestosterone; **IV** = 5β-dihydrotestosterone; **V** = 5α-androstane-3β,17β-diol; **VI** = 5α-androstane-3α,17β-diol; **VII** = 3α-hydroxy-5β-androstan-17-one.

That the prostate contained similar reductases was unequivocally established a few years later. In 1963 Farnsworth and Brown incubated radiotestosterone with minces of rat prostate and with slices of human benign hypertrophic prostate and obtained in both cases DHT (**III**) and 5α-androstane-3α,17β-diol (**VI**) as major metabolites. The same metabolites resulted from perfusion of [1,2-^{3}H]-testosterone through the prostate of the anesthetized rat. Simultaneously, Pearlman (1963) infused intact adult male rats with [7-^{3}H]4-androstene-3,17-dione (cf. **Ia**) and identified 3α-hydroxy-5α-androstan-17-one, 3α-hydroxy-5β-androstan-17-one (**VII**), and 5α-androstane-3,17-dione as metabolic products of the ventral prostate. This organ, he observed, retained androgens to a somewhat greater extent than does blood. It is not clear if liver 5α- and 5β-reductases are indeed identical with those found in prostate. Present evidence is equivocal (see McGuire and Tomkins, 1959).*

It had been realized as early as 1958 (Butler and Schade, 1958) that the synthesis of proteins and nucleic acids in prostatic tissue of castrated rats was rapidly and markedly increased by administration of T. With recognition that T itself undergoes rapid metabolism in the prostate to the more potent androgen DHT, attention was directed by three groups, working independently, on the role DHT might play in this biochemical sequence.

By injecting [1,2-^{3}H]testosterone into rats, Bruchovsky and Wilson (1968a) found that within 1 min T was taken up by the prostate. At least 90% was converted into DHT (**III**) + androstanediols + androsterone. From prostatic nuclei, however, only [^{3}H]testosterone (25–50%) and [^{3}H]DHT (50–75%) could be recovered up to 2 hr following injection. Moreover, formation of the less androgenic androstanediols and androsterone occurred only in the cytoplasm. Bruchovsky and Wilson (1968b) concluded that the prostatic cell and its nucleus possessed an NADPH-dependent enzymatic mechanism that converted T into DHT. Binding of DHT to prostatic nucleic, moreover, markedly exceeded that of T itself (in a ratio of 4:1 to 13:1 in different experiments) (Bruchovsky and Wilson, 1968a), leading to the conclusion that DHT might indeed be the biologically active form of the hormone in this and other sex accessory tissues.

The appearance of the 1968 paper by Bruchovsky and Wilson triggered publications by Anderson and Liao (1968) and by Baulieu et al. (1968) expanding and further delineating these fundamental concepts. Anderson and Liao pointed out that prostate nuclear chromatin, but not other tissues that are insensitive to androgen, contains an androgen receptor that can selectively retain DHT and that is specific for DHT. The soluble fraction of the cytoplasm from prostatic tissue

*McGuire and colleagues (1959, 1960, 1960) have provided evidence supporting the view that there is a multiplicity of 5α-reductase enzymes in the body. Leshin and Wilson (1982), in contrast, take the opposite view that there is only one 5α-reductase enzyme. We believe that further work is required to establish this point.

contained a spectrum of androstane-3,17-diols and other metabolites with less than 5% of total radioactivity as DHT. In contrast, liver cells, which can convert T to DHT, do not retain DHT in the nuclei, presumably through lack of the appropriate receptor. They believed DHT was the active form of androgen in the prostate. Baulieu *et al.* (1968) studied the effects of T and its metabolites on prostatic epithelium to determine if the biological effects of T were caused by the hormone per se, or by its metabolites. Their results suggested that the action of T on the prostate may be related to local metabolism and that DHT was implicated in the control of cell division.

The following year Fang *et al.* (1969) described studies on the retention of DHT by prostatic cell nuclei and cytoplasm *in vivo* and *in vitro*. They made the key observation that whereas DHT was selectively retained by prostatic nuclei following incubation of minced rat prostate with radiolabeled T, DHT did not bind to isolated nuclei unless a cytosolic fraction was added. A cytosolic 3.5 S protein was isolated that spontaneously and selectively bound DHT at 0°C. DHT-binding capacity was enhanced over the temperature range 15–50°C. Testosterone significantly had only some 20% of the binding affinity of DHT. Fang *et al.* (1969) concluded that prostatic cell nuclei had specific sites for retaining the DHT–protein complex but not the protein moiety alone. The nuclear localization of radiolabeled androgen in the prostate was elegantly illustrated the following year by Sar *et al.* (1970), employing dry-mount autoradiography. Surprisingly, they used T and not its dihydro derivative for this purpose. The stage was set for characterization of both the androgen receptor and of the enzyme Δ^4,3-ketosteroid 5α-reductase (5α-reductase) and for elucidation of their respective roles in molecular terms in the integrated biochemistry of the prostatic cell.

A. 5α-Reductase

The metabolism of androstenedione to a 5α-dihydro derivative by rat prostate was first reported by Lemon *et al.* (1953). This was followed in the late 1950s by metabolic studies on T employing rat liver 5α- and 5β-reductases (cf. Dorfman and Ungar, 1965). Prostatic 5α-reductase came into its own, however, only after the clear demonstration by Farnsworth and Brown in 1963 that incubation of T with rat or human prostate preparations led to formation of DHT as major metabolite (cf. Pearlman, 1963; Goldzieher and Acevedo, 1962). Two years later Shimazaki *et al.* (1965) successfully prepared concentrates of 5α-reductase from microsomal and mitochondrial fractions of rat ventral prostate. Activity of the enzyme fractions was determined by incubating them with labeled T in the presence of NADPH as cofactor, followed by isolation of the steroids and quantitation of DHT after chromatography. This method of assay, with modifications, remains in use to the present day.

The impetus of research on 5α-reductase now passed to the United States, where scientists such as J. D. Wilson, N. Bruchovsky, and others took up the challenge of discovery of an enzyme that plays so important a role in the differentiation of the male genotype.

Gloyna and Wilson (1969a) carried out comparative studies on the conversion of T to DHT in a number of animal species. They reached the conclusion that DHT may mediate the cellular proliferative effects of T but was not an obligatory feature of androgen-induced secretion by the prostate (cf. Baulieu *et al.*, 1968). They observed that DHT formation was high in adult prostates in those species that develop benign prostatic hypertrophy (man, dog, lion). Studies on the human enzyme were greatly simplified by the observation of Voigt *et al.* (1970) that human foreskin readily provided a microsomal fraction rich in enzyme. The nuclear fraction, however, proved to be relatively poor in enzyme content. In rat prostate, in contrast, distribution of enzyme was about equally divided between nuclear membrane and the endoplasmic reticulum (Frederiksen and Wilson, 1971; Moore and Wilson, 1972). Enzyme levels in the rat prostate fell upon castration (Shimazaki *et al.*, 1969), but increased some sevenfold above normal levels on treatment with testosterone propionate (TP) for 8 days, when enzyme activity correlated with growth response of the prostate to androgen (Moore and Wilson, 1973).

5α-Reductase is a membrane-bound enzyme requiring NADPH as cofactor. It is tightly bound to cell membranes, including the nuclear membrane and the endoplasmic reticulum, and has not been purified or solubilized. It is unstable *in vitro* at 25°C even in intact membrane preparations, but can be stored at −20°C for prolonged periods. From study of nuclear and microsomal extracts, it has an apparent molecular weight of the order of 250,000 to 350,000 as estimated by gel filtration, a sedimentation coefficient of 13.5 to 15 S as determined by density gradient centrifugation, and a pH optimum of 6.6 ± 0.3 (Moore and Wilson, 1974, 1975). 5α-Reductase is widely distributed in bacteria (Davidson and Talalay, 1966), and in many animals as evidenced by their excretion of 5α-reduced metabolites. In animals such as rat and in man, 5α-reductase plays a necessary role in providing DHT for the accessory sex tissues. Its presence in certain regions of the brain (Verhoeven *et al.*, 1974) reflects the need of such neuroendocrine tissues for 5α-reduced metabolites (see, for example, Nuti and Karavolas, 1977). It is also found in such organs as the liver (cf. Dorfman and Ungar, 1965; Graef *et al.*, 1981) and lungs (rat, Hartiala *et al.*, 1976; Verhoeven *et al.*, 1974; human, Milewich *et al.*, 1978). These contain relatively large amounts of enzyme. Thus, Moore and Wilson (1975) point out that, in toto, rat liver contains about 500 times as much 5α-reductase activity as does the prostate. Such efficient metabolic capacity toward androgens does not seem to be linked to the androgen responsiveness of these tissues and may represent a mechanism for androgen inactivation.

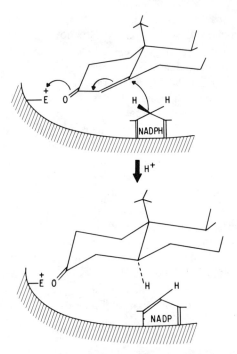

Fig. 2.   Interaction of testosterone and NADPH at the active site of 5α-reductase. (From Petrow and Lack, 1981. Reproduced by permission of Alan R. Liss, Inc.)

B. Mechanism of Action of 5α-Reductase

The mechanism of action of 5α-reductase is illustrated in Fig. 2. Saturation of the Δ^4 double bond is accomplished by incorporation of a hydrogen ion at C-4 from a water molecule (McGuire and Tomkins, 1960) and stereospecific introduction of the H_S-hydride provided by NADPH into position C-5 of the steroid with creation of a new chiral center (Abul-Hajj, 1972; Lemm and Wenzel, 1977).

III. THE ANDROGEN RECEPTOR AND THE MECHANISM OF ACTION OF ANDROGENS WITHIN THE PROSTATIC CELL

It is a basic tenet of this chapter that DHT and not T plays a pivotal role in prostatic cancer. To express its oncogenic potential and to modulate growth, DHT must enter the nucleus and bind to the genome. Incubation of isolated nuclei with DHT, however, does not lead to entry of the steroid into the nucleus. For this to happen, a high-affinity androgen-binding receptor protein is required

(Fang *et al.*, 1969), a protein, moreover, that is present in both cytosol and nucleus (see the review by Tymoczko *et al.*, 1978).

The isolation of a cytosolic androgen receptor protein (rat) with high binding affinity for DHT was described by Baulieu and Jung in 1970. Subsequent studies have shown that T has less binding affinity for this protein. Estradiol shows some binding affinity, whereas the androstanediols **V** and **VI** do not bind. Studies (Tymoczko *et al.*, 1978) have shown that T has only 20% of the binding affinity of DHT for this receptor protein (rat).

Baulieu and Jung (1970) had pointed out that both nuclei and the endoplasmic reticulum network contain receptor proteins and enzymatic 5α-reductase, and suggested that a close relationship existed between them. That they are separate entities was proved by Mainwaring (1970), who pointed out that metabolism of T to DHT *in vivo* probably precedes binding to receptor proteins, because (1) T has low binding affinity for the receptor compared to DHT and (2) protein-bound steroids are generally considered to be protected from enzymatic action (Westphal, 1969). The following year Mainwaring and Peterken (1971), using a reconstituted cell-free system, demonstrated the need for DHT–receptor binding to ensure entry of DHT into the nucleus and its binding to specific acceptor sites on the nuclear chromatin. As a result of these and other findings (reviewed by King and Mainwaring, 1974), Mainwaring (1975, 1977) put forward a schematic model for the mechanism of action of androgens, which has been incorporated into Fig. 3.

In simplistic terms, T, derived almost entirely from the testes, is transported in blood as the stable complex with sex steroid-binding β-globulin (man) or corticosteroid-binding α_2-globulin (rat). On reaching the prostatic cell, it enters by a process that has not yet been fully elucidated. Once inside the cell it is subjected to extensive metabolism with formation of DHT as a principal metabolite (>90%). This metabolite binds with high affinity to a cytoplasmic receptor protein to form a DHT–receptor complex. The latter then undergoes a change in structure and configuration, resulting in an activated complex that now undergoes translocation to the nucleus where it binds to a specific acceptor site(s) on the nuclear chromatin, thereby initiating biochemical events that are manifested as the androgenic DHT response. The DHT–receptor complex finally breaks down, with release of steroid. All interactions between DHT, cytoplasmic receptor protein, and genome are reversible, so that the steroid may be extracted with organic solvents throughout the entire process.

IV. 5α-REDUCTASE, DIHYDROTESTOSTERONE, AND THE HUMAN PROSTATE

The foregoing review of the molecular mechanisms governing androgen action is based almost entirely on studies using the rat prostate. They show conclusively

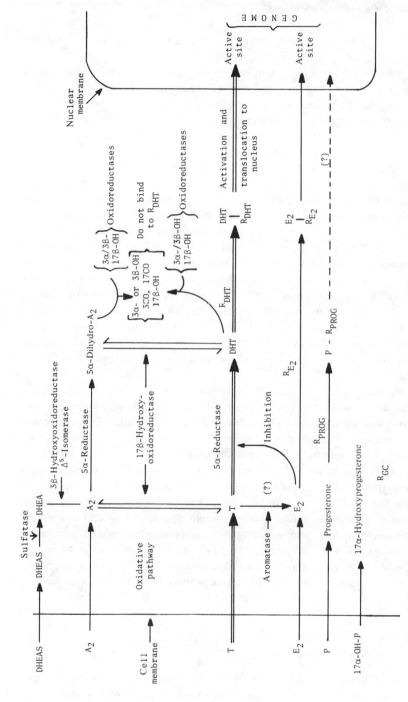

Fig. 3. Steroid biochemistry of the prostatic cell. A_2 = androstenedione; E_2 = estradiol; R = cytoplasmic receptors for individual steroids as indicated in subscripts. Other abbreviations as indicated in text.

that in this animal species DHT is the key androgen governing normal growth. In other species, however, DHT does not play so unique a role (cf., for example, Walsh and Wilson, 1976; Siiteri and Wilson, 1970). There is consequently a need to establish that DHT is likewise the pivotal androgen in the human prostate, thereby opening the way to a discussion of the role of this androgen in prostatic cancer, both in the rat and in man.

It is not possible to distinguish histologically between the male and female fetal gonads in humans up to the seventh week of development. At this point the "indifferent gonad" begins the typical morphological changes that lead to its differentiation into the testes or ovaries. At this critical juncture in embryogenesis, T secretion by the testes begins and stimulates differentiation of the Wolffian anlage into the epididymis, vas deferens, and seminal vesicles. 5α-Reductase is absent from these structures until after differentiation is complete, so that T is undoubtedly the hormone involved. 5α-Reductase, in contrast, is present in the urogenital sinus, urogenital tubercle, and urogenital swellings, where it converts T into DHT, with resulting differentiation of these structures into male genitalia and prostate (Josso, 1973; Siiteri and Wilson, 1974). It follows that DHT and not T is the critical androgen responsible for prostatic growth in man. That this is indeed the case is elegantly illustrated by studies on male human pseudohermaphrodites with 5α-reductase deficiency. This small group of affected subjects at birth have a clitoris-like phallus, bifid scrotum, and urogenital sinus. Masculinization of the internal structures, however, is normal. At puberty the subjects develop a muscular male habitus with growth of phallus and scrotum and change of voice. They have erections, ejaculations, complete spermatogenesis, a small or absent prostate, and a libido directed toward females. Plasma T levels fall within the normal range. The conversion ratio of T to DHT is less than 1% (Imperato-McGinley et al., 1974; Peterson et al., 1977; Fisher et al., 1978). Decreased 5α-reductase activity is present (Walsh et al., 1974), coupled with normal cytosolic binding of [³H]DHT in fibroblasts derived from genital and nongenital skin (Saenger et al., 1978). The syndrome consequently stems from an enzyme deficiency and not from an androgen receptor defect.

In these subjects it is difficult to reconcile the association of a small or vestigial prostate with normal circulating levels of T and normal populations of androgen receptors without drawing the obvious conclusion that in man, as in the rat, DHT is the key androgen modulating prostatic growth. That this is indeed the case is further supported by the key observation of Peterson et al. (1977) that administration of DHT to hermaphrodite subjects with 5α-reductase deficiency results in prostatic growth.

With this background, the way is open to consideration of the putative role of DHT in prostatic cancer, both in the rat and in man.

V. DIHYDROTESTOSTERONE AND PROSTATIC CANCER

A. Rat Studies

There has been inadequate recognition among biologists that, insofar as prostatic growth is concerned, T functions almost entirely as a precursor of DHT, which is de facto the active agent (see Shain *et al.*, 1977b). This detracts in some degree from the significance of studies otherwise characterized by an enviable professionalism. For the purpose of this section, the biological effects resulting from T administration will be equated with those of DHT.

The induction of prostatic tumors by androgens has been reported by several groups. Noble (1977a) described the spontaneous occurrence of prostatic adenocarcinoma in the Nb rat strain. Incidence was relatively low at 0.45%, but was increased to 20% by prolonged administration of T. The parameters of the Nb tumor, moreover, closely resemble those of human prostatic adenocarcinoma, including response to chemotherapy and castration (Drago *et al.*, 1980). A further example of an androgen-induced prostatic tumor has been reported by Shain *et al.* (1977a, 1979). These workers first observed the occurrence of spontaneous prostatic adenocarcinoma in 7 of 41 senescent virgin A × C rats kept in a germ-free environment for 34 to 37 mo. Of a second group of 33 rats (30–46 mo old), 12 were treated with exogenous T for 6 weeks before sacrifice, when the detected incidence of spontaneous prostatic adenocarcinoma rose to 70%. Although DHT was invariably the principal metabolite of T in the young A × C rat, with increasing age 5α-reductase and DHT levels very slowly declined, with some increase in the oxidative pathway leading to androstenedione (Fig. 3). Shain *et al.* (1977a) concluded that this biochemical alteration may be an early manifestation of neoplastic transformation. Androstenedione does not bind significantly to the androgen receptor (Mainwaring, 1969; Shain *et al.*, 1979) and so will not translocate to the (DHT–receptor) acceptor site in the genome. It is a preferred substrate for the enzyme aromatase, which converts it to estrone (*Ia* in Fig. 5), itself a 5α-reductase inhibitor, so that the enzymatic shift to an oxidative pathway may also represent a defense mechanism. Finally, Pollard *et al.* (1982) have successfully induced prostatic adenocarcinomas in Lobund Wistar rats by implanting silastic chambers containing testosterone propionate (TP). After 8 to 14 months, microscopic tumors, of which 18% were large and grossly visible, were detected in 40% of the rats. One of these adenocarcinomas had metastasized to the lungs.

The clear-cut experimental induction of prostatic adenocarcinomas in these genetically susceptible animals unequivocally links the appearance of such prostatic neoplasms to DHT stimulation, which must be regarded as a causative agent. For obvious reasons, parallel experimental evidence is not available for man. Nevertheless, the data outlined in the following paragraphs provide, we believe, compelling reasons for the conclusion that in man, too, DHT is a pivotal component in the genetic changes that commit normal prostatic cells to proliferation and altered control of cellular differentiation.

B. Human Studies

Prostatic cancer (and benign prostatic hypertrophy, BPH) has not been detected in males over the age of 45 who have undergone castration before the age of 40 (Moore, 1944). The presence of a functioning testis is thus a prerequisite for appearance of the disease. As discussed earlier, the testicular hormone T undergoes reduction to DHT within the prostatic cell. The DHT thus formed is then translocated by the androgen receptor to its acceptor site on the genome, where it sets in motion the molecular events that lead to prostatic growth. Unless DHT is present, prostatic growth does not occur. Thus, in the absence of DHT but in the presence of T, prostatic growth is vestigial (cf. Imperato-McGinley *et al.*, 1974). Moreover, androgen concentration (as DHT) within the prostate is nearly fourfold that in blood and increases to still higher levels on development of cancer. While, therefore, the etiology of prostatic cancer is unknown, the conclusion that DHT plays a pivotal role in its induction and progression is unavoidable. The demonstration that malignant tissue possesses an enriched androgen environment, moreover, vindicates the 40 years of effort to control the disease by androgen depletion (Farnsworth and Brown, 1976).

C. Elimination of Testosterone from the Prostate

Elimination of testosterone from the economy of the prostate presently forms the main therapeutic approach to the palliative treatment of endocrine-responsive prostatic cancer. Such T elimination is achieved by castration and/or estrogen therapy.

The testes produce approximately 95% of circulating testosterone in man. Bilateral orchidectomy results in a reduction of approximately 93% in plasma T levels (normal, 611 ng/100 ml; castrate 43 ng/100 ml). The adrenal cortex, however, continues to elaborate androgens and in particular dehydroepiandrosterone (DHEA, **IX**) and its sulfate (DHEAS, **VIII**). These two steroids are present in high concentrations in the plasma (DHEA, 0.46–0.54 μg/100 ml; DHEAS, 48–217 μg/100 ml). The prostate is rich in sulfatase, which is inhibited by T and its metabolites. Following castration there is consequently a compensatory increase in DHEAS hydrolysis with conversion of formed DHEA to T and thence DHT (Farnsworth, 1975). It is therefore not surprising that patients who respond poorly to castration and/or estrogen therapy may show rapid temporary clinical improvement following bilateral adrenalectomy if done within 3 mo of immolative surgery (Schoonees *et al.*, 1972). Elimination of T by castration, however, is followed by undesirable side effects. These include psychotropic effects and in particular a depressive symptomatology and decrease in mental performance (see Hermann and Beach, 1976). Libido is diminished (cf., for example, Davidson *et al.*, 1979), and there is significant loss of muscle (cf. Kochakian, 1976). In addition, because testosterone and androstenedione form the main substrates for estrogen biosynthesis in man (cf. the review by Siiteri, 1982), there is disruption of estrogen production. Estrogen biosynthesis occurs selectively in tissues containing the enzyme aromatase. Such tissues usually possess estrogen receptor, so that estrogen is utilized immediately on biosynthesis and only an overspill enters the general circulation (see Marks and Petrow, 1983). Circulating levels of estrogen consequently fail to reflect the contribution of this hormone at the tissue level to well-being and homeostasis. Its endocrine synergism with T requires no comment. Elimination of T by castration must consequently be accompanied by loss of tissue and circulating estrogen, with unfavorable effects on psyche, muscle, bone, reticuloendothelial system, and so on.

Administration of estrogen, with or without orchidectomy, likewise results in virtual loss of circulating T through decreases in luteinizing hormonal (LH) and follicle-stimulating hormone (FSH) levels. The unfavorable side effects that follow estrogen therapy include those mentioned earlier in association with loss of T, together with impotence and a significant incidence of gynecomastia and cardiovascular death (cf., for example, Blackard *et al.*, 1970; Bailar and Byar, 1970; Blackard, 1975; Murphy *et al.*, 1975; Smith *et al.*, 1976) due to induced antithrombin III deficiency (Buller *et al.*, 1982). A further undesirable side effect of estrogen therapy lies in its suppression of immunity to tumor-associated antigens in patients with prostatic cancer. Such reduced efficiency of immunosurveillance of tumors may contribute to exacerbation of the disease (Ablin *et al.*, 1979a), and is only produced by therapeutic and not by physiological levels of the hormone (see Ablin *et al.*, 1979b).

VI. STEROID BIOCHEMISTRY OF THE NORMAL PROSTATIC CELL

The normal prostatic cell is well endowed with biochemical mechanisms for the utilization and metabolism of steroid hormones (cf. Fig. 3).

A. Receptors

Steroid receptor proteins identified in the human prostate include those discussed in the following paragraphs.

1. Androgen Receptor

An androgen receptor in human prostate was first reported by Mainwaring and Milroy (1973), and has since been confirmed, inter alia, by Geller et al. (1975) and also by Wiebert et al. (1983).

2. Estrogen Receptor

The presence of estrogen receptor protein in prostatic tissue was shown by Wagner et al. (1975) and subsequently confirmed by Pontes et al. (1982) and others.

3. An Atypical Androgen–Progesterone Receptor

[3H]Methyltrienolone (R1881, 17β-hydroxy-17α-methyl-4,9,11-estratrien-3-one), a highly potent anabolic steroid (Azadian-Boulanger et al., 1975), is widely used as a tracer for study of the androgen receptor in tissues. On applying it to rat prostatic cytosol, a high-affinity binding protein was isolated with ligand specificity characteristic of androgen receptor. Thus, the probe was displaced by DHT and not by progesterone. With human prostatic cytosol, in contrast, a different picture emerged. Progesterone proved to be a more effective ligand than 19-nor-testosterone (Asselin et al., 1976). Similar results were obtained by Menon et al. (1978). It should be noted that for progestagens to affect the genome there must be an acceptor site on the latter for the progesterone–receptor complex, and this has not yet been established. Progesterone and 17α-hydroxyprogesterone, however, are present in the prostate (Hammond, 1978).

4. Glucocorticoid Receptor

Some evidence exists that glucocorticoid (GC) receptors are present in human prostate with localization in stromal tissue (Hawkins et al., 1976; Cowan et al., 1976). Again, their role is not clear.

B. Steroid-Metabolizing Enzymes Identified in the Human Prostate (cf. Fig. 3)

1. 5α-Reductase

This NADPH-dependent enzyme not only converts T to DHT (as discussed in Section II) but also reduces 4-androstene-3,17-dione to 5α-androstane-3,17-dione. It has the capacity to reduce most 3-oxo-Δ^4-steroidal components of the prostatic cell to 5α-dihydro derivatives including progesterone (cf. Leshin and Wilson, 1982).

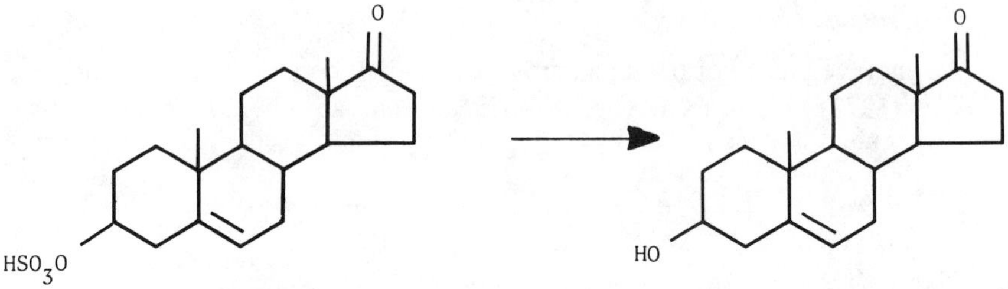

(VIII)

DHEAS

(IX)

DHEA

Fig. 4. Conversion of dehydroepiandrosterone sulfate (DHEAS, **VIII**) to dehydroepiandrosterone (DHEA, **IX**) by sulfatase.

2. Sulfatase

The prostate is rich in sulfatase with an average hydrolytic capacity of 200 pmol DHEAS/mg prostatic protein/hr. This is calculated to be sufficient to hydrolyze a total day's production of DHEAS (**VIII**) to DHEA (**IX**) by the adrenals in a few hours (Farnsworth, 1975) (cf. Fig. 4).

3. 3β-Hydroxy-5-ene Steroid Oxidoreductase/5 → 4-ene,3-Ketosteroid Isomerase

This enzyme complex converts DHEA (**IX**) into A_2 (**Ia**) (cf. Fig. 5) and pregnenolone/17α-hydroxypregnenolone into progesterone/17α-hydroxyprogesterone (cf. Yates and Deshpande, 1975). That the prostate converts adrenal DHEA into T has been reported by Boyns *et al.* (1972). Both progesterone and 17α-hydroxyprogesterone are present in normal prostate (Hammond, 1978), but it is not yet known if these typically adrenal steroids are synthesized within the prostate

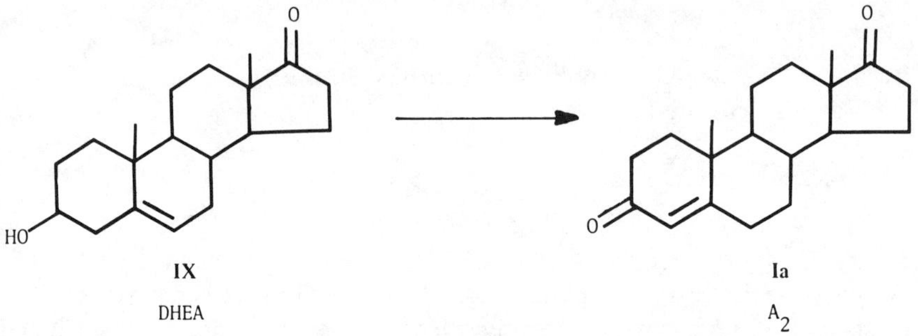

IX

DHEA

Ia

A_2

Fig. 5. Conversion of dehydroepiandrosterone (DHEA) to androstenedione (A_2, **Ia**).

from pregnenolone. It seems likely that they originate in the adrenals and testes, respectively (Vermulen and Verdonck, 1976). It may be mentioned that testicular homogenates from patients with prostatic cancer, in the presence of NADPH, readily convert progesterone into its 17α-hydroxy derivative and hence into A_2 and T (Murota et al., 1965).

4. 3α/3β-Hydroxy- and 17β-Hydroxyoxidoreductases

These enzymes maintain a reversible equilibrium between keto and hydroxyl residues at C-3 and C-17, respectively, giving rise to isomeric 5α-dihydrodiols, dione, and ketols [see Fig. 6(i)]. These structures have only weak affinity for the DHT receptor.

17β-Hydroxyoxidoreductase reversibly converts A_2 into T [Fig. 6 (ii)].

5. Aromatase

The NADPH-dependent enzyme aromatase converts androstenedione (**Ia**) into estrone (**II**) (see Siiteri, 1982). Its presence in human BPH tissue was reported by Farnsworth (1966). Smith et al. (1982), however, failed to establish aromatization of androgen by BPH tissue under their experimental conditions. Marks and Petrow (1983) found low levels of aromatase in rat prostate using the assay method of Thompson and Siiteri (1974). It seems likely that the enzyme is present in small amounts in the human gland.

Estrogen plays an important role in the biochemistry of the prostate. Thus, estrogen is able to increase cytosolic and nuclear androgen receptor populations in experimental prostatic carcinoma of the rat with no change in estrogen receptor levels and to increase prostatic androgen receptor concentrations in patients with BPH compared to untreated controls (Kliman et al., 1980; see also Bouton et al., 1981). It inhibits 5α-reductase (Shimazaki et al., 1965) and decreases the

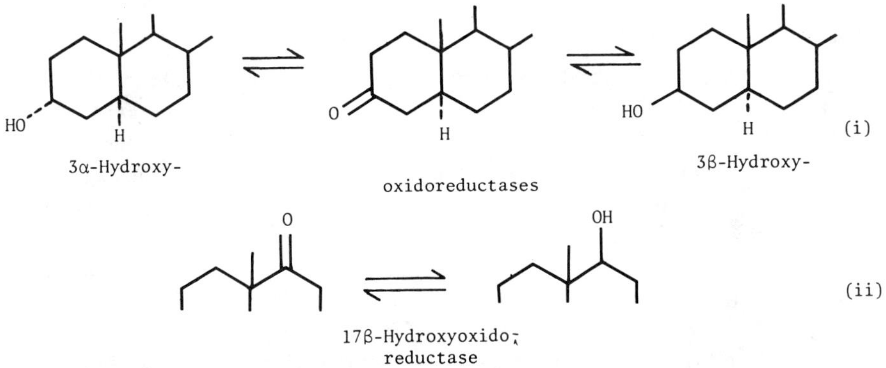

Fig. 6. Reversible equilibria maintained by 3α/3β-hydroxy- and 17β-hydroxyoxidoreductases.

production of DHT from T and A_2 (Bard and Lasnitzki, 1977). It accumulates in the stroma (see Ruberg $et\ al.$, 1982). It binds to the nuclear fraction (Fang and Liao, 1969), thereby revealing an acceptor site on the genome. At physiological dose levels, it modulates immunological defense mechanisms (see Ablin $et\ al.$, 1979a,b) and stimulates the reticuloendothelial system (Nicol $et\ al.$, 1952).

VII. HORMONE SENSITIVITY OF THE NEOPLASTIC PROSTATIC CELL

Because of the many difficulties attending human experimentation, there is a paucity of data on steroid biochemistry in prostatic cancer. In seeking to develop a rationale for the use of a 5α-reductase inhibitor for this intractable disease, we have been forced to draw freely on animal data, fully recognizing the pitfalls inherent in this approach.

The prostate tumor in its early hormone-responsive phase is characterized by a heterogeneity of neoplastic cells that coexist side by side in a competitive but mutually associated growth pattern. This mixed population of clones in simplest terms may be divided into the four types described in the following paragraphs.

A. Latent Lesions

Latent lesions occur frequently in the aging male and often remain stationary, particularly in certain ethnic populations such as the Japanese (see Rotkin, 1979; Hutchison, 1981). Bruchovsky and his colleagues (Van Doorn $et\ al.$, 1976) have pointed out that the synthesis of R_{DHT} is tightly coupled to cell proliferation in the growing rat prostate and that, in resting cells and presumably in latent lesions, there is no further synthesis of nuclear receptor.

B. Androgen-Responsive Lesions

The premalignant stage of prostatic cancer is characterized by the persistence into old age of cells histologically similar to those of the young adult. Persistence of youthful activity is presumably correlated with high R_{DHT} and androgen levels coupled with a deficiency in normal feedback and constraint mechanisms. Such maintenance of epithelial activity must stem from alteration of the genome and be the harbinger of that inexorable neoplastic epithelial autonomy that kills the patient. Further development of the premalignant lesion leads to frank carcinoma, which is normally well differentiated at this stage and contains a majority of hormone-responsive cells. This is followed by progressive loss of differentiation, increase of malignant potential with metastasis, loss of hormone dependence, and finally, death of the patient (see McNeal, 1979).

The evolutionary sequence from the "youthful" premalignant phase to the undifferentiated metastatic malignant phase is accompanied by changes in cellular steroid biochemistry. Drawing on the work of Hammond (1978), the premalignant phase is characterized by high T, DHT, and R_{DHT} levels with low A_2 levels. Gradual loss of differentiation and loss of endocrine dependence appear to be accompanied by loss of androgen receptor (Kliman *et al.*, 1978; see also Shain *et al.*, 1975), diminished DHT-synthetic capacity (Shain *et al.*, 1977a), and a shift in metabolism to the oxidative pathway leading to A_2 (cf. Habib *et al.*, 1976). It should be noted that with aging there is a gradual reduction in R_{DHT} content (Shain *et al.*, 1975), coupled with a statistically significant increase in the efficiency with which circulating androstenedione is converted to estrone (Hemsell *et al.*, 1974).

C. Androgen-Insensitive Lesions

Androgen-insensitive lesions are believed to be present from the beginning of the neoplastic process and are the pivotal problem in prostatic cancer therapy. Whereas cells of type B may be controlled by endocrine manipulation, androgen-insensitive cells are extremely resistant to all forms of therapy. Although initially they are believed to represent only a small fraction of the malignant growth, they ultimately outgrow the endocrine-responsive cells and kill the patient.

D. Endocrine Correlates of Autonomous Cellular Change

As early as 1969, Foulds had drawn attention to the disturbing possibility that therapeutic measures designed to retard or suppress the growth of endocrine-dependent tumors might in themselves lead to progression from the responsive to the autonomous state with devastating results to the host. That this may indeed be the case was established in the experimental animal by Noble (1977c, 1979).

By treating the Nb rat with testosterone propionate (TP), plus estrogen (E), or E alone, Noble produced a number of hormone-dependent tumors. Employing an estrogen-dependent mammary tumor in male Nb rats, Noble studied the effects of endocrine manipulation on it and made the following observations:

1. Withdrawal of hormone therapy (90–100%) was accompanied by regression followed by regrowth of tumors that were now autonomous.
2. Partial withdrawal of hormone therapy (75–80%) led to marked reduction in tumor progression and autonomy (14–40%).
3. *Production of a stationary growth pattern appeared to inhibit the appearance of autonomous cells.* Similar results were obtained with an

adenocarcinoma of the dorsal prostate that grew only in the estrogen-treated host (Noble, 1977a). He concluded that

a reduction in hormone levels sufficient to prevent advancing tumor growth, but adequate to reduce the extent of regression, also reduced the frequency or prevented the development of autonomous change. Although regression per se was not a prerequisite for autonomous change, the paradox was evident that progression towards autonomous growth was accelerated with procedures expected to check tumor growth and was minimal with procedures that accelerated it [p. 82].

From an analysis of these data, Bruchovsky and Rennie (1979) concluded that a revised approach to therapy might involve ablative surgery followed by fractional hormone replacement.

VIII. A NEW APPROACH TO PALLIATIVE TREATMENT OF PROSTATE CANCER

On the assumption that animal models of prostatic cancer yield information on the human disease, many of the foregoing experimental data can be rationalized into the following four propositions, which are directed toward the cellular kinetics of neoplastic growth under hormonal stimulation.

A. Proposition I

During the early endocrine-dependent phase of growth, the cell types that make up a tumor do not proliferate in an independent and haphazard manner but have an overall growth pattern modulated by the rapidly growing *endocrine-responsive* cells. The latter appear to have the capacity to control or influence their proliferation and/or conversion to autonomy by unknown negative feedback mechanisms and constraints, thereby stabilizing the relative proportions of the various clones that make up the tumor.

In this connection it will be remembered that even a short serial passage of individual clones isolated from a tumor leads to rapid emergence of variant subclones with different metastatic properties and that, if several such clones are mixed and cocultivated, this instability is not expressed (cf. the work of Fidler and associates, for example, in Poste *et al.*, 1981; see also Miller *et al.*, 1981).

B. Proposition II

Removal of endocrine support leads to regression and/or autophagy of endocrine-responsive cells, with resulting loss of the negative feedback mechanisms and constraints that inhibit growth of latent and autonomous cells. This results in unrestrained autonomous growth.

C. Proposition III

Maintenance of cellular mechanism patterns characteristic of hormone responsiveness, and in particular maintenance of some R_{DHT} levels, or the mechanism for production of R_{DHT}, by endocrine manipulation may be expected to protect against and/or delay autonomous change.

D. Proposition IV

Endocrine manipulations that shift cell biochemistry away from that characteristic of hormone dependence and toward autonomy by inter alia lowering of R_{DHT} levels accelerate autonomous change.

If these propositions do indeed reflect the growth characteristics of human as well as animal prostatic cancer, then the following conclusion may be drawn:

The aim of palliative therapy should be directed toward attenuation or inhibition of neoplastic growth by endocrine manipulation and not toward enforced regression and/or autophagy by trophic hormone elimination through castration. In this way, optimal conditions may be created for a shift in cellular kinetics toward latency or pseudolatency and away from autonomy. Furthermore, such endocrine manipulation should also act as a prophylactic against prostatic cancer in genetically susceptible individuals.

How this can best be done forms the subject of the next section.

IX. 5α-REDUCTASE AS A TARGET ENZYME FOR PROSTATIC CANCER

As mentioned earlier, castration, with or without supplemental estrogen therapy, was introduced for palliative treatment of prostatic cancer some 40 years ago (Huggins and Hodges, 1944; Huggins et al., 1941). It was based on the incorrect premise that it was the testicular hormone T that was responsible for prostatic growth. Elimination of T by castration thus formed the logical cornerstone of therapy, and it was supported by a wealth of impressive clinical data. That such therapy had little impact on overall survival of patients with advanced prostatic cancer was accepted at the time as an inevitable consequence of the disease (cf. Lepor et al., 1982; Blackard et al., 1970). Castration, however, is often refused for reasons that require no comment. It behooves the scientist, in these circumstances, to develop palliative therapies that avoid the trauma of castration, if only to help those patients who are unwilling to undergo immolative surgery.

The newer knowledge of prostate biochemistry shows the following:

1. DHT and not T is the main trophic hormone of the prostate.
2. DHT is formed from circulating T by reduction within the prostate by the NADPH-dependent enzyme 5α-reductase.

3. 5α-Reductase deficiency in the adult male does not produce any apparent psychological or physiological stigmata and is unlikely even to be recognized. Thus, adult male pseudohermaphrodites with 5α-reductase deficiency and approximately $1/2.8\times$ normal levels of circulating DHT have a normal male habitus, psyche, and libido. They do not develop male pattern alopecia or prostatic cancer. They possess vestigial prostates that nevertheless respond to DHT stimulation (Peterson *et al.*, 1977, quoted in Imperato-McGinley, 1974). These observations unequivocally establish that the human prostate requires DHT and not T for normal growth and development. It provides clear-cut evidence that the androgen acceptor site on the genome of the prostate cell is activated by the DHT:R_{DHT} complex and cannot be activated by the T:R_{DHT} complex.

It follows that regression and/or autophagy of the prostate can be enforced by (partial) elimination of DHT from the economy of the prostate cell *in the presence of circulating levels of T*. If, therefore, the prime objective of castration is the removal of androgen support from the prostate, then theoretically this objective can be reached equally well by inhibiting prostatic 5α-reductase or by castration. As this has now been done in the experimental animal (see later), the way is open to a new therapy that no longer relies on ablative surgery that has dominated the field for the past two generations.

The endocrine insult of castration leads to elimination of some 95% of circulating T. The subsequent natural history of the lesion follows the behavioral pattern defined in propositions I and II (given earlier), with dramatic regression of the tumor followed by burgeoning growth of autonomous cells. In the experimental animal, as described earlier, *partial withdrawal of trophic support* leads to an attenuated or static growth pattern with concomitant delay in conversion to autonomy. Such a static growth pattern is highly characteristic of the human disease and occurs naturally in man. Thus, epidemiological studies of prostate cancer among the Japanese, who seldom die from the disease, have shown a "Western" incidence of latent lesions (Rotkin, 1979; Hutchison, 1981). Nearer home, liver cirrhotics with lowered androgen and raised estrogen levels have lower rates of prostate cancer than do controls (see Henderson *et al.*, 1982). That reversion of proliferating cells to attenuated growth or latency is theoretically possible, moreover, is rendered likely by experimental reversal of the premalignant hyperplasia induced by methycholanthrene in mouse prostate preparations in organ culture (Chopra and Wilkoff, 1976). In addition, prolonged remissions of prostatic cancer occasionally occur following estrogen therapy (Johansson and Ljunggren, 1981). If it is accepted as a working hypothesis that partial withdrawal of trophic support from the prostatic neoplasm by means of a 5α-reductase inhibitor can lead to an attenuated or static growth pattern, then the question must be asked what effect this would have on the steroid biochemistry of the cell in the light of propositions III and IV. Castration, it will be noted, leads to virtual disappearance of R_{DHT} with production of prostatic cells that are now identical—in this respect at least—with their autonomous counterparts. Therapy with a 5α-reductase inhibitor, in contrast, is expected to maintain R_{DHT} levels (see Van Doorn and Bruchovsky, 1978), thereby ideally providing some defense against autonomous change.

At the risk of repetition, it must be stressed that castration and treatment with a 5α-reductase inhibitor are not equivalent forms of palliative therapy, nor are they interchangeable procedures. Unless this is clearly understood, the biochemical differences that characterize them can become lost in a welter of arguments on the pros and cons of castration. Castration is irreversible and absolute. No partial form of castration is possible, nor is there any flexibility in this approach. It results in virtual elimination of T, DHT, R_{DHT}, 5α-reductase (+ E), with rapid regression of the tumor followed later by a rebound of devastating autonomous growth. Treatment with a 5α-reductase inhibitor is reversible and has no anticipated side effects. Significant changes in T and R_{DHT} are not expected. DHT and 5α-reductase levels, theoretically at least, can be varied at will, providing a unique flexibility of endocrine support that, it is hoped, can be profiled to induce tumor reversion to pseudolatency or an attenuated growth pattern conducive to increased expectation of life. A comparison between the two approaches is summarized in Table I.

X. 5α-REDUCTASE INHIBITORS ACTIVE *IN VIVO*

Although a number of steroids have been shown to inhibit prostatic 5α-reductase *in vitro,* nearly all of them are virtually inactive *in vivo* (Lotz, 1980). The reasons for this are threefold: (1) administered steroidal inhibitors run the risk of metabolism before reaching the prostate, (2) the enzyme 5α-reductase is widely distributed within the body with greater quantities found in the liver and lungs than are present within prostate (Verhoeven *et al.,* 1974), and (3) only a tiny fraction of an administered steroid (such as T) finds its way to, and is localized within, the prostate (Tveter and Attranmandal, 1968). The problem of finding a prostatic 5α-reductase inhibitor is thus basically a problem in logistics that is rendered more difficult by an almost complete lack of knowledge of the structural requirements governing prostate selectivity. Despite these handicaps, several steroidal inhibitors of 5α-reductase have now been discovered with sufficient antiprostate activity *in vivo* to warrant study in a tumor-bearing animal.

Enzyme inhibitors fall into three main classes: (1) competitive reversible inhibitors, (2) nonspecific irreversible inhibitors, which are basically alkylating agents with structural resemblance to the normal substrate, and (3) specific

TABLE I

Comparison of Some Effects of Castration and Castration plus Estrogen with 5α-Reductase Deficiency in Human Males and 5α-Reductase Inhibition in Rats

Parameter	Castration	Castration + estrogen	5α-Reductase inhibition
Human			
T levels	95%	95%	Normal
DHT levels	Very low	Very low	Low
R_{DHT}	Very low	Very low	No change expected
Prostatic 5α-reductase	Very low	Very low	Present
Psychotropic effect	Negative	Negative	None observed
Muscle	Loss	Loss	Normal
Prostate	Decreased	Decreased	Decreased
Gynecomastia	—	Significant	Not observed
Reversibility	No	No	Yes
Immunity to tumor antigens	—	Suppressed	Not anticipated
Sexual potency	Very low	Very low	Normal
Sperm production	None	None	Normal
Mental performance	Decreased	Decreased	Normal
Cardiovascular death	—	Increased	Not observed
Estrogen biosynthesis	Decreased	—	No effect anticipated
Alopecia	—	—	Possible slowing down
Rats			
DHT levels	Very low	Very low	Varies with dose of inhibitor
Prostatic 5α-reductase	Very low	Very low	Varies with dose of inhibitor
Reversibility	No	No	Yes

irreversible inhibitors, also known as active-site-directed inhibitors or k_{cat} inhibitors. The latter are believed to be of particular interest in the present context, because irreversible inactivation of the enzyme is widely regarded as a means of achieving enzyme selectivity and of combating the effects of physiological dilution (cf., for example, Shaw, 1980).

A. Competitive Reversible Inhibitors (Fig. 7)

1. 17β-Carboxy-4-androsten-3-one (X)

In 1969, Nayfeh and Baggett pointed out that utilization of [^{14}C]progesterone by rat testicular homogenates was inhibited by the methyl ester of 17β-carboxy-4-androsten-3-one. Extension of this early study by Voigt and Hsia (1975) led to the discovery that 17β-carboxy-4-androsten-3-one (X) was an inhibitor of

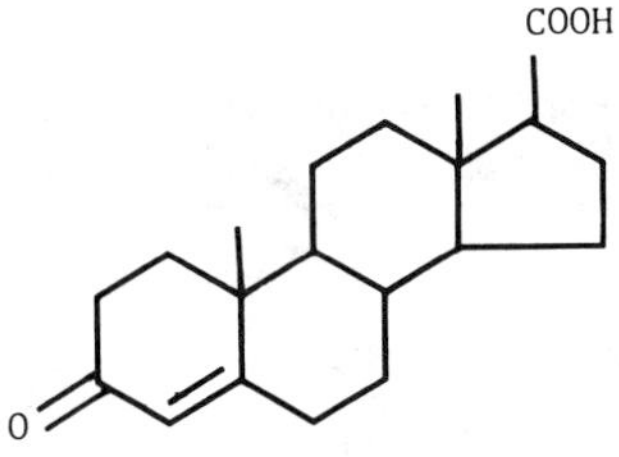

Fig. 7.   5α-Reductase inhibitors. See text for details.

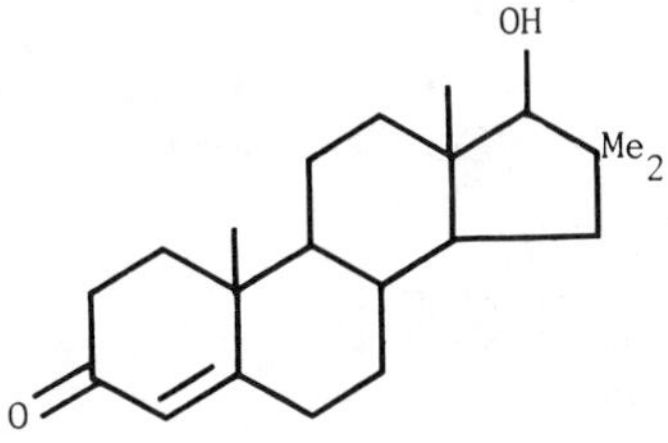

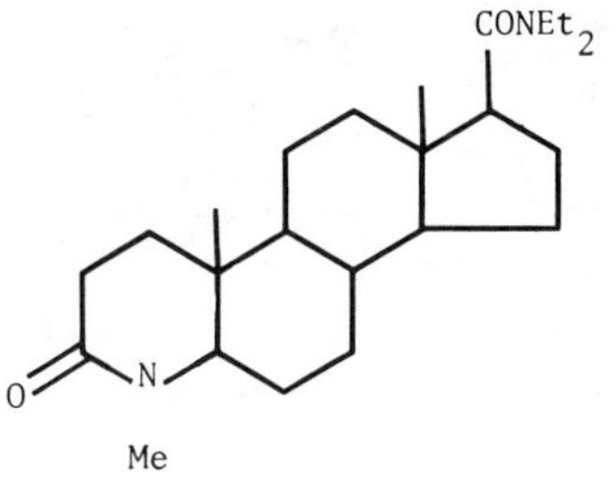

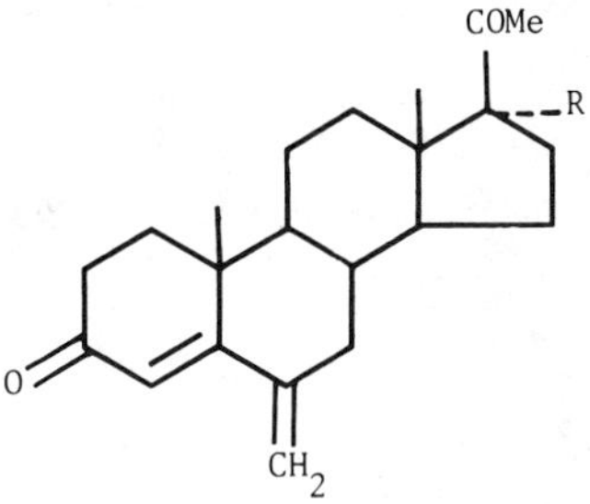

5α-reductase that, moreover, was without overt hormonal activity. Antiprostatic effect was established using the 4-week-old Sprague–Dawley rat. After castration, the rats were treated sc for 7 days with 0.08 mg TP in sesame oil with and without the inhibitor. The results obtained are shown in Table II.

A similar study but lasting only 4–5 days in mature castrated rats has been reported by Kao and Weisz (1979). The hormone and inhibitor were separately incorporated into silastic sheets that were cut to appropriate size and implanted. An antiprostatic effect was observed, but quantitative evaluation requires more data than reported.

2. *16,16-Dimethyl-17β-hydroxy-4-androsten-3-one* (XI)

The antiprostatic activity of structures of this type was reported by the Beecham group (1976), who found that they possess both antiandrogenic and 5α-reductase-inhibiting activity. In our hands, **XI** was virtually inactive as an enzyme inhibitor (Petrow *et al.*, 1983), so that its antiprostatic action derives from its antiandrogenicity.

TABLE II

Effect of 17β-Carboxy-4-androsten-3-one (X) on the Ventral Prostate of 4-Week-Old Sprague–
Dawley Rats following 7 Days' Treatment

Treatment (mg/rat/day)	Ventral prostate (mg)	Body weight gain (g)
Castrate	24	46.7
+ 0.08 mg TP	96	57.4
+ 0.08 mg TP + 8 mg (X)	52	43.1
+ 0.08 mg TP + 0.8 mg (X)	45	55.0
Intact	50	49.2

3. 17β-N,N-Diethylcarbamoyl-4-methyl-4-aza-5α-androstan-3-one (XII)

A 5α-reductase inhibitor of somewhat different chemical structure was discovered by the Merck, Sharp and Dohme research group (Brooks et al., 1981). This 4-azasteroid (XII) proved to be a potent reversible inhibitor of the enzyme with a K_1 of 5×10^{-9} M. It had moderate affinity for the androgen receptor ($K_d = 3 \times 10^{-6}M$), thereby revealing an antiandrogenic component in its biological spectrum (Liang and Heiss, 1981). Its effect on the ventral prostate of mature male rats following 67 days' treatment with sc-administered steroid [in methanol–sesame oil (1:9)] is given in Table III (Brooks et al., 1981, 1982).

B. Active-Site-Directed Inhibitors (k_{cat} Inhibitors)

6-Methylene-4-pregnene-3,20-dione (XIII; R = H)

Because the driving force behind the catalytic activity of 5α-reductase appears to reside in polarization of the 3-oxo group of testosterone (Fig. 2), Petrow and Lack (1981) concluded that extension of conjugation beyond C-$_5$ and its proximal NADPH moiety might lead to a system able, on enzymatic activation, to bind covalently by a concerted mechanism to a proximal nucleophilic residue in the 5α-reductase active site. Their study of a series of αβ-unsaturated 3-oxo-4-dienic steroids led to the discovery that certain 6-methylenic 4-en-3-ones were in

TABLE III

Effect of 17β-*N,N*-Diethylcarbamoyl-4-methyl-4-aza-5α-androstan-3-one (XII) on the Ventral Prostate of Mature Rats following 67 Days' Treatment

Treatment (mg/rat/day)	Ventral prostate (mg)	Body weight gain (g)
Control	617 ± 25	139 ± 12
10 mg **XII**	396 ± 115	114 ± 12
50 mg **XII**	271 ± 14	111 ± 8

fact irreversible inhibitors of the k_{cat} type in the presence of NADPH. The mechanism given in Fig. 8 was proposed. No inhibition was shown in the absence of cofactor, thereby indicating the interesting possibility that the latter plays a determinant role in specificity. Kinetic studies showed that 17α-acetoxy-6-methylene-4-pregnene-3,20-dione (**XIII**; R = OAc) has a K_i of 1.25×10^{-6} *M* and k_{cat} of 4.8×10^{-3} sec^{-1} (Petrow *et al.*, 1981). Unfortunately it proved to be only slightly active *in vivo*. The simpler 6-methylene-4-pregnenen-3,20-dione (**XIII**; R = H), previously synthesized by the first author some 20 years ago (Burn *et al.*, 1964), and found at that time to be of no particular value, proved to be of outstanding biological interest on *in vivo* study (Petrow *et al.*, 1982). Thus on daily sc administration to 3-week-old Harlan–Sprague–Dawley rats for 35 days, a major antiprostatic effect was observed as shown in Table IV.

In assessing these data it should be noted that the developing immature rat

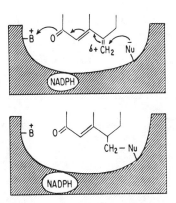

Fig. 8. Proposed interaction of Δ^4-unsaturated 3-ketosteroids bearing a 6-methylene substituent with the enzyme yielding an irreversibly inactivated enzyme. Nu is a hypothetical nucleophilic element in this area of the enzyme. (From Petrow *et al.*, 1981, by permission of the publishers.)

TABLE IV

Effect of 6-Methylene-4-pregnene-3,20-dione (XIII; R = H) on the Body Weight and Growth of Ventral Prostate, Seminal Vesicles, Testes, Kidneys, and Adrenals of Immature Rats[a]

	Effect		
Parameter	Treated (N = 10)	Control (N = 10)	p
Initial body weight (g)	39 ± 3.3	36 ± 4.2	NS[b]
Final body weight (g)	229 ± 3.3	261 ± 5.3	<.001
Ventral prostate (mg)	41 ± 4	205 ± 19	<.001
Seminal vesicles (mg)	84 ± 10	399 ± 26	<.001
Testes (g)	2.07 ± 0.13	2.96 ± 0.07	<.001
Kidneys (g)	1.74 ± 0.05	2.15 ± 0.07	<.001
Adrenals (mg)	50 ± 4	71 ± 7	<.03

[a]From Petrow et al. (1982). Reproduced by permission of the publishers.
[b]NS, not significant.

prostate is particularly responsive to changes in trophic support. The prostate of the mature rat, in contrast, has already passed through its period of growth and maturation and has reached a steady state. Aging, moreover, has been accompanied by a gradual reduction in R_{DHT} content (Shain et al., 1975). The effect of 6-methylene-4-pregnene-3,20-dione (**XIII;** R = H) on the ventral prostate of the intact mature rat is given in Table V. Under the conditions of this experiment, a significant effect on the prostate required 12 days' treatment, in contrast to the 7

TABLE V

Effect of 6-Methylene-4-pregnene-3,20-dione (XIII; R = H) on the Weight of Seminal Vesicles and Ventral Prostate of Mature Rats[a]

	Effect on weight		
Organ weight	Treated	Vehicle only	p
7-Day study			
Seminal vesicles (mg)	424 ± 64	770 ± 45	<.01
Ventral prostate (mg)	194 ± 23	248 ± 22	NS[b]
12-Day study			
Seminal vesicles (mg)	361 ± 35	916 ± 41	<.001
Ventral prostate (mg)	190 ± 18	339 ± 21	<.001
Initial body weight (g)	234 ± 7.7	227 ± 9.6	NS
Final body weight (g)	286 ± 6.6	290 ± 6.5	NS

[a]From Petrow et al. (1982). Reproduced by permission of the publishers.
[b]NS, not significant.

TABLE VI

Effect of 6-Methyleneprogesterone (XIII) on the 5α-Reductase Content of the Prostate in Castrated Adult Male Rats

Treatment	Number of rats	T reduced/mg protein (pmol)	Reduction of 5α-Reductase in Prostate (%)
TP (1 mg/kg)	5	5.29	34
TP (1 mg/kg) + **XIII** (100 mg/kg)	5	3.50	
Untreated	4	5.10	61
XIII (100 mg/kg)	5	1.96	

days necessary for prostatic involution following castration. This is to be expected, because castration leads to total elimination of trophic support and other changes (see Table I; cf. also Bruchovsky and Craven, 1975; Shimazaki *et al.*, 1969; Moore and Wilson, 1973), whereas treatment with the 5α-reductase inhibitor leads only to partial elimination of DHT from the prostate. This is illustrated by an initial study in which we treated adult rats 24 hr after castration with TP, either alone or in admixture with **XIII** (sc in oil), followed by sacrifice 24 hr later and determination of the 5α-reductase content of the prostate. The results shown in Table VI were obtained.

That a 5α-reductase inhibitor can totally eliminate trophic support from the prostate has still to be established. If the arguments presented here are valid, however, such total elimination of DHT will not be required for the palliative treatment of prostatic cancer. Only time within the crucible of experiment can provide the answer.

XI. SUMMARY

Both presumptive and experimental evidence points to the following conclusions:

1. The aim of palliative therapy of prostatic cancer should be directed toward attenuation or inhibition of neoplastic growth by partial elimination of DHT from the prostate.
2. Partial elimination of trophic support can be achieved by administration of a 5α-reductase inhibitor.
3. Treatment with such a 5α-reductase inhibitor may be expected (*a*) to show a prophylactic effect in genetically susceptible individuals, and (*b*) to prolong patient life during the endocrine-responsive phases of the disease.

Acknowledgments

We thank Mrs. Rachel Hougom for her excellent secretarial assistance.

Addendum

We now find that growth of the Dunning R-3327H prostatic adenocarcinoma in the intact male Copenhagen × Fisher rat is markedly supressed by the 5α-reductase inhibitor 6-methylene progesterone (XIII; R = H) (Petrow *et al.*, 1984).

REFERENCES

Ablin, R. J., Bush, I. M., Bruns, G. R., and Guinan, P. D. (1979a). Modulatory effects of oestrogen therapy on immunological responsiveness. *Cancer Detect. Prev.* **2**, 453–470.

Ablin, R. J., Bhatti, R. A., Guinan, P. D., and Khin, W. (1979b). Modulatory effects of oestrogen on immunological responsiveness. II. Suppression of tumour-associated immunity in patients with prostatic cancer. *Clin. Exp. Immunol.* **38**, 83–91.

Abul-Hajj, Y. J. (1972). Stereospecificity of hydrogen transfer from NADPH by steroid Δ^4-5α- and Δ^4-5β-reductase. *Steroids* **20**, 215–222.

Anderson, K. M., and Liao, S. (1968). Selective retention of dihydrotestosterone by prostatic nuclei. *Nature (London)* **219**, 277–279.

Asselin, J., Labrie, F., Gourdeau, Y., Bonne, C., and Raynaud, J.-P. (1976). Binding of [^{3}H]methyltrienolone (R 1881) in rat prostate and human benign prostatic hypertrophy. *Steroids* **28**, 449–459.

Azadian-Boulanger, G., Bucourt, R., Nedelec, L., and Nomine, G. (1975). Steroides trieniques androgenes et anabolisants. *Eur. J. Med. Chem.* **10**, 353–359.

Bailar, J. C., III, and Byar, D. P. (1970). Estrogen treatment for cancer of the prostate. Early results with 3 doses of diethylstilbestrol and placebo. *Cancer* **26**, 257–261.

Bard, D. R., and Lasnitzki, I. (1977). The influence of oestradiol on the metabolism of androgens by human prostatic tissue. *J. Endocrinol.* **74**, 1–9.

Baulieu, E.-E., and Jung, I. (1970). A prostatic cytosol receptor. *Biochem. Biophys. Res. Commun.* **38**, 599–606.

Baulieu, E. E., Lasnitzki, I., and Robel, P. (1968). Metabolism of testosterone and action of metabolites on prostate glands grown in organ culture. *Nature (London)* **219**, 1155–1156.

Beecham Group Ltd. (1976). Belg. P. 839, 751 (Sept. 20).

Blackard, C. E. (1975). The Veterans' Administration cooperative urological research group studies of carcinoma of the prostate. A review. *Cancer Chemother. Rep., Part 1* **59**, 225–227.

Blackard, C. E., Doe, R. P., Mellinger, G. T., and Byar, D. P. (1970). Incidence of cardiovascular disease and death in patients receiving diethylstilbestrol for carcinoma of the prostate. *Cancer* **26**, 249–256.

Bouton, M. M., Pornin, C., and Grandadam, J. A. (1981). Estrogen regulation of rat prostate androgen receptor. *J. Steroid Biochem.* **15**, 403–408.

Boyns, A. R., Cole, E. N., Golder, M. P., Danutra, V., Harper, M. E., Brownsey, B., Cowley, T., Jones, G. E., and Griffiths, K. (1972). *Proc. Tenovus Workshop* **4**, 207.

Brooks, J. R., Baptista, E. M., Berman, C., Haw, E. A., Hichens, M., Johnston, D. B. R., Primka, R. L., Rasmusson, G. H., Reynolds, G. F., Schmitt, S. M., and Arth, G. E. (1981). Response of rat ventral prostate to a new and novel 5α-reductase inhibitor. *Endocrinology (Baltimore)* **109**, 830–836.

Brooks, J. R., Berman, C., Hichens, M., Primka, R. L., Reynolds, G. F., and Rasmusson, G. H. (1982). Biological activities of a new steroidal inhibitor of Δ^4-5α-reductase. *Proc. Soc. Exp. Biol. Med.* **169,** 67–73.

Bruchovsky, N., and Craven, S. (1975). Prostatic involution: Effect on androgen receptors and intracellular androgen transport. *Biochem. Biophys. Res. Commun.* **62,** 837–843.

Bruchovsky, N., and Rennie, P. S. (1979). New considerations in the hormonal induction and regulation of animal tumours. *U.I.C.C. Tech. Rep. Ser.* **48,** 220–232.

Bruchovsky, N., and Wilson, J. D. (1968a). The conversion of testosterone to 5α-androstan-17β-ol-3-one by rat prostate *in vivo* and *in vitro*. *J. Biol. Chem.* **243,** 2012–2021.

Bruchovsky, N., and Wilson, J. D. (1968b). The intranuclear binding of testosterone and 5α-androstan-17β-ol-3-one by rat prostate. *J. Biol. Chem.* **243,** 5953–5960.

Buller, H. R., Boon, T. A., Henry, C. P., Dabhoiwala, N. F., and ten Cate, J. W. (1982). Estrogen-induced deficiency and decrease in antithrombin III activity in patients with prostatic cancer. *J. Urol.* **128,** 72–74.

Burn, D., Cooley, G., Davies, M. T., Ducker, M. W., Ellis, B., Feather, P., Hiscock, A. K., Kirk, D. N., Leftwick, A. P., Petrow, V., and Williamson, D. M. (1964). Modified steroid hormones. XXXIII. Steroidal 6-formyl-3-alkoxy-3,5-dienes and some of their transformations. *Tetrahedron* **20,** 597–609.

Butenandt, A., Tscherning, K., and Hanish, G. (1935). Über einige neue Vertreter der Androsteron-Gruppe (1935). *Ber. Dtsch. Chem. Ges.* **68,** 2097–2102.

Butler, W. S. S., III, and Schade, A. L. (1958). The effect of castration and androgen replacement on the nucleic acid composition, metabolism and enzymatic capacity of the rat ventral prostate. *Endocrinology (Baltimore)* **63,** 271–279.

Callow, R. K., and Deansley, R. (1935). CLXXIV. Effect of androsterone and of male hormone concentrates on the accessory reproductive organs of castrated rats, mice and guinea pigs. *Biochem. J.* **29,** 1424–1445.

Chopra, D. P., and Wilkoff, L. J. (1976). Inhibition and reversal by β-retinoic acid of hyperplasia induced in a cultured mouse prostate tissue by 3-methylcholanthrene or *N*-methyl-*N'*-nitro-*N*-nitrosoguanidine. *JNCI, J. Natl. Cancer, Inst.* **56,** 583–587.

Cowan, R. A., Cowan, S. K., Giles, C. A., and Grant, J. F. (1976). Prostatic distribution of sex hormone-binding globulin and cortisol-binding globulin in benign hyperplasia. *J. Endocrinol.* **71,** 121–131.

David, K., Dingemanse, E., Freud, J., and Laquer, E. (1935). Über Krystallinsches mannliches Hormon aus Hoden (Testosteron), wirksamen als aus Harn oder aus Cholesterin bereitetes Androsteron. *Z. Physiol. Chem.* **233,** 281–282.

Davidson, S. J., and Talalay, P. (1966). Purification and mechanism of action of a steroid Δ^4-5β-dehydrogenase. *J. Biol. Chem.* **241,** 906–915.

Davidson, J. M., Camargo, C. A., and Smith, E. R. (1979). Effect of androgen on sexual behaviour in hypogonadal men. *J. Clin. Endocrinol. Metab.* **48,** 955–958.

Dorfman, R. I. (1969). Androgens and anabolic agents. *In* "Methods in Hormone Research" (Dorfman, R. I., ed.), Vol. IIA, pp. 151–220. Academic Press, New York.

Dorfman, R. I., and Kincl, F. A. (1963). Relative potency of various steroids in an anabolic-androgenic assay using the castrated rat. *Endocrinology (Baltimore)* **72,** 259–266.

Dorfman, R. I., and Ungar, F. (1965). "Metabolism of Steroid Hormones." Academic Press, New York.

Drago, J. R., Goldman, L. B., Maurer, R. E., Eckels, D. D., and Gershwin, M. E. (1980). Histology, histochemistry, and acid phosphatase of noble (Nb) rat prostate adenocarcinomas and treatment of an androgen-dependent Nb rat prostate adenocarcinoma. *JNCI, J. Natl. Cancer Inst.* **64,** 931–937.

Eisenberg, E., and Gordon, G. S. (1950). The levator ani muscle of the rat as an index of myotrophic activity of steroidal hormones. *J. Pharmacol. Exp. Ther.* **99,** 38–44.

Fang, S., and Liao, S. (1969). Antagonistic action of antiandrogens on the formation of a specific dihydrotestosterone-receptor protein complex in rat ventral prostate. *Mol. Pharmacol.* **5,** 428–431.

Fang, S., Anderson, K. M., and Liao, S. (1969). Receptor proteins for androgens. On the role of specific proteins in selective retention of 17β-hydroxy-5α-androstan-3-one by rat ventral prostate *in vivo* and *in vitro. J. Biol. Chem.* **244,** 6584–6595.

Farnsworth, W. E. (1966). Metabolism of 19-nortestosterone by human prostate. *Steroids* **8,** 825–843.

Farnsworth, W. E. (1975). Human prostatic dehydroepiandrosterone sulfate sulfatase. *In* "Normal and Abnormal Growth of the Prostate" (M. Goland, ed.), pp. 160–170. Thomas, Springfield, Illinois.

Farnsworth, W. E., and Brown, J. R. (1963). Testosterone metabolism in the prostate. *Natl. Cancer Inst. Monogr.* **12,** 323–325.

Farnsworth, W. E., and Brown, J. R. (1976). Androgen of the human prostate. *Endoc. Res. Commun.* **3,** 105–117.

Fisher, L. K., Kogut, M. D., Moore, R. J., Goebelsmann, J. E., Weitzman, J. J., Isaacs, H., Jr., Griffin, J. E., and Wilson, J. D. (1978). Clinical, endocrinological, and enzymatic characterization of two patients with 5α-reductase deficiency: Evidence that a single enzyme is responsible for the 5α-reduction of cortisol and testosterone. *J. Clin. Endocrinol. Metab.* **47,** 653–664.

Forchielli, E., and Dorfman, R. I. (1956). Separation of Δ⁴-5α- and Δ⁴-5β-hydrogenases from rat liver homogenate. *J. Biol. Chem.* **223,** 443–448.

Forchielli, E., Brown-Grant, K., and Dorfman, R. I. (1958). Steroid Δ⁴-hydrogenases of rat liver. *Proc. Soc. Exp. Biol. Med.* **99,** 594–596.

Foulds, L. (1969). "Neoplastic Development," Vol. 1, p. 73. Academic Press, New York.

Frederiksen, D. W., and Wilson, J. D. (1971). Partial characterization of the nuclear reduced nicotinamide adenine dinucleotide phosphate: Δ⁴-3-ketosteroid 5α-oxidoreductase of rat prostate. *J. Biol. Chem.* **246,** 2584–2953.

Geller, J., Cantor, T., and Albert, J. (1975). Evidence for a specific dihydrotestosterone-binding cytosol receptor in the human prostate. *J. Clin. Endocrinol. Metab.* **41,** 854–862.

Gloyna, R. E., and Wilson, J. D. (1969a). A comparative study of the conversion of testosterone to 17β-hydroxy-5α-androstan-3-one (dihydrotestosterone) by prostate and epididymis. *Endocrinology (Baltimore)* **29,** 970–977.

Gloyna, R. E., and Wilson, J. D. (1969b). Evidence that dihydrotestosterone may be involved in prostatic growth. *Clin. Res.* **17,** 284.

Goldzieher, J. W., and Acevedo, H. F. (1962). Metabolism of androstenedione by hypertrophic and carcinomatous prostate glands. *44th Meet. Endoc. Soc., Chicago,* p. 7.

Graef, V., Golf, S. W., and Tuschen, M. (1981). NADPH:4-ene-3-oxosteroid-5α-reductase and NADH:4-ene-3-oxosteroid-5α-reductase in liver microsomes of different species of animals. *J. Steroid Biochem.* **14,** 883–887.

Habib, F. K., Lee, I. R., Stitch, S. R., and Smith, P. H. (1976). Androgen levels in the plasma and prostatic tissues of patients with benign hypertrophy and carcinoma of the prostate. *J. Endocrinol.* **71,** 99–107.

Hammond, G. L. (1978). Endogenous steroid levels in the human prostate from birth to old age: A comparison of normal and diseased tissues. *J. Endocrinol.* **78,** 7–19.

Hartiala, V., Uotila, P., and Nienstedt, W. (1976). Metabolism of testosterone in the isolated perfused rat lungs. *J. Steroid Biochem.* **7,** 527–533.

Hawkins, E. F., Nijs, M., and Brassinne, C. (1976). Enzymatic binding of corticosterone to protein in cytosols of human benign prostatic hypertrophy tissue. *J. Endocrinol.* **69,** 17P.

Hemsell, D. L., Grodin, J. M., Brenner, P. F., Siiteri, P. K., and Macdonald, P. C. (1974). Plasma precursors of estrogen. II. Correlation of the extent of conversion of plasma androstenedione to estrone with age. *J. Clin. Endocrinol. Metab.* **38**, 476–479.

Henderson, B. E., Ross, R. K., Pike, M. C., and Casagrande, J. T. (1982). Endogenous hormones as a major factor in human cancer. *Cancer Res.* **42**, 3232–3239.

Hermann, W. M., and Beach, R. C. (1976). Psychotropic effects of androgens: A review of clinical observations and new human experimental findings. *Pharmakopsychiatr. Neuropsychophar-makol.* **9**, 205–219.

Huggins, C., and Hodges, C. V. (1944). Studies on prostatic cancer. I. The effects of castration, of estrogen, and of androgen injection on serum phosphatases in metastatic carcinoma of the prostate. *Cancer Res.* **1**, 293–297.

Huggins, C., Stevens, R. E., Jr., and Hodges, C. V. (1941). Studies on prostatic cancer. II. The effects of castration on advanced carcinoma of the prostate gland. *Arch. Surg.* **43**, 209–223.

Hutchison, G. B. (1981). Incidence and etiology of prostate cancer. *Urology, Suppl.* **17**, 4–10.

Imperato-McGinley, J., Guerro, L., Gautier, T., and Peterson, R. E. (1974). Steroid 5α-reductase deficiency in man. An inherited form of male pseudohermaphroditism. *Science* **186**, 1213–1215.

Johansson, S., and Ljunggren, E. (1981). Prostatic carcinoma cured with hormonal therapy. *Scand. J. Urol. Nephrol.* **15**, 331–332.

Josso, N. (1973). *In vitro* synthesis of Müllerian-inhibiting hormone by seminiferous tubules from the calf fetal testis. *Endocrinology (Baltimore)* **93**, 829–834.

Kao, L. W. L., and Weisz, J. (1979). Inhibition of steroid 5α-reductase *in vivo:* Effect on suppression of luteinizing hormone and stimulation of accessory sex organs by testosterone in the orchidectomized rat. *J. Endocrinol.* **81**, 209–220.

King, R. J. B., and Mainwaring, W. I. P. (1974). "Steroid Cell Interactions." Butterworths, London.

Kliman, B., Prout, G. R. Jr., McLaughlin, R. A., and Griffin, P. P. (1978). Altered androgen metabolism in metastatic prostate cancer. *J. Urol.* **119**, 623–626.

Kliman, R. A., McLaughlin, R. A., and Prout, G. R., Jr. (1980). Effect of diethylstilbestrol on androgen receptors in human benign prostatic hyperplasia. *62nd Annu. Meet., Endocrinol. Soc., Abstr.* 829, p. 282.

Kochakian, C. D. (1937). Testosterone and testosterone acetate and the protein and energy metabolism of castrate dogs. *Endocrinology (Baltimore)* **21**, 750–755.

Kochakian, C. D. (1950). Comparison of the protein anabolic property of various androgens in the castrated rat. *Am. J. Physiol.* **160**, 53–61.

Kochakian, C. D. (1976). "Anabolic–Androgenic Steroids." Springer-Verlag, Berlin and New York.

Lemm, U., and Wenzel, M. (1977). Enzymatische Synthese von [5α-T-]-Dihydrotestosterone. *J. Labelled Compd. Radiopharm.* **13**, 67–73.

Lemon, H. M., Wotiz, H. H., and Robitscher, T. (1953). Metabolism of testosterone by neoplastic human prostate. *J. Clin. Endocrinol.* **13**, 948–956.

Lepor, H., Ross, A., and Walsh, P. C. (1982). The influence of hormonal therapy on survival of men with advanced prostatic cancer. *J. Urol.* **128**, 335–340.

Leshin, M., and Wilson, J. D. (1982). Inhibition of steroid 5α-reductase in human skin fibroblasts by 17β-*N,N*-diethylcarbamoyl-4-methyl-4-aza-5α-androstan-3-one. *J. Steroid Biochem.* **17**, 245–250.

Liang, T., and Heiss, C. E. (1981). Inhibition of 5α-reductase, receptor binding, and nuclear uptake of androgens in the prostate by a 4-methyl-4-aza-steroid. *J. Biol. Chem.* **256**, 7998–8005.

Lotz, W. (1980). Importance of 5α-reduction for the trophic effects of androgens on rat accessory sex organs and LH control. *J. Steroid Biochem.* **13**, 1261–1264.

McGuire, J. S., and Tomkins, G. M. (1959). The multiplicity and specificity of Δ⁴-3-ketosteroid hydrogenases (5α). *Arch. Biochem. Biophys.* **82,** 476–477.

McGuire, J. S., Jr., and Tomkins, G. M. (1960). The heterogeneity of Δ⁴-3-ketosteroid reductases (5α). *J. Biol. Chem.* **235,** 1634–1638.

McGuire, J. S., Jr., Holls, V. W., Jr., and Tomkins, G. M. (1960). Some characteristics of the microsomal steroid reductases (5α) of rat liver. *J. Biol. Chem.* **235,** 3112–3117.

McNeal, J. E. (1979). New morphologic findings relevant to the origin and evolution of carcinoma of the prostate and BPH. *U.I.C.C. Tech. Rep. Ser.* **48,** 24–37.

Mainwaring, W. I. P. (1969). A soluble androgen receptor in the cytoplasm of rat prostate. *J. Endocrinol.* **45,** 531–541.

Mainwaring, W. I. P. (1970). The separation of androgen receptor and 5α-reductase activities in subcellular fractions of rat prostate. *Biochem. Biophys. Res. Commun.* **40,** 192–198.

Mainwaring, W. I. P. (1975). A review of the formation and binding of 5α-dihydrotestosterone in the mechanism of action of androgens in the prostate of the rat and other species. *J. Reprod. Fertil.* **44,** 377–393.

Mainwaring, W. I. P. (1977). "The Mechanism of Action of Androgens." Springer-Verlag, Berlin and New York.

Mainwaring, W. I. P., and Peterken, B. M. (1971). A reconstituted cell-free system for the specific transfer of steroid-receptor complexes into nuclear chromatin isolated from rat ventral prostate gland. *Biochem. J.* **125,** 285–295.

Mainwaring, W. I. P., and Milroy, E. V. G. (1973). Characterization of the specific androgen receptors in the human prostate gland. *J. Endocrinol.* **57,** 371–384.

Marks, T., and Petrow, V. (1983). Effect of the pre-estrogen 4-androstene-3,17-dion-19-al on the Dunning R3327 prostatic adenocarcinoma. *Cancer Res.* **43,** 3687–3690.

Menon, M., Tananis, C. E., Hicks, L. L., Hawkins, E. F., McLaughlin, M. G., and Walsh, P. C. (1978). Characterization of the binding of a potent synthetic androgen, methyltrienolone, to human tissues. *J. Clin. Invest.* **61,** 150–163.

Milewich, L., Parker, P. S., and MacDonald, P. C. (1978). Testosterone metabolism by human lung tissue. *J. Steroid Biochem.* **9,** 29–32.

Miller, B. E., Miller, F. R., and Heppner, G. H. (1981). Interactions between tumor subpopulations affecting their sensitivity to the antineoplastic agents cyclophosphamide and methotrexate. *Cancer Res.* **41,** 4378–4381.

Moore, R. A. (1944). Benign hypertrophy and carcinoma of the prostate. *Surgery (St. Louis)* **16,** 152–157.

Moore, R. J., and Wilson, J. D. (1972). Localization of the reduced nicotinamde adenine dinucleotide phosphate: Δ⁴-3-ketosteroid 5α-oxidoreductase in the nuclear membrane of the rat ventral prostate. *J. Biol. Chem.* **247,** 958–967.

Moore, R. J., and Wilson, J. D. (1973). The effect of androgenic hormones on the reduced nicotinamde adenine dinucleotide phosphate: Δ⁴-3-ketosteroid 5α-oxidoreductase of rat ventral prostate. *Endocrinology (Baltimore)* **93,** 581–582.

Moore, R. J., and Wilson, J. D. (1974). Extraction of the reduced adenine dinucleotide phosphate: Δ⁴-3-ketosteroid 5α-oxidoreductase of rat prostate with digitonin and potassium chloride. *Biochemistry* **13,** 450–456.

Moore, R. J., and Wilson, J. D. (1975). Reduced nicotinamide adenine dinucleotide phosphate: Δ⁴-3-Ketosteroid 5α-reductase of rat ventral prostate. *In* "Methods in Enzymology" (B. O'Malley and J. G. Hardman, eds.), Vol. 36, pp. 466–474. Academic Press, New York.

Murota, S., Shikita, M., and Tamaoki, B. (1965). Androgen formation in the testicular tissue of patients with prostatic carcinoma. *Biochim. Biophys. Acta* **117,** 241–246.

Murphy, G. P., Saroff, J., Joiner, J., and Gaeta, J. (1975). Prostatic carcinoma treated at Categorical Center, 1960–69. *N.Y. State J. Med.* **75,** 1663–1669.

Nayfeh, S. N., and Baggett, B. (1969). Metabolism of progesterone by rat testicular homogenates. III. Inhibitory effects of intermediates and other steroids. *Steroids* **14**, 269–283.

Nicol, T., Helmy, I. D., and Abou-Zikry, A. (1952). A histological explanation for the beneficial action of endocrine therapy in carcinoma of the prostate. *Br. J. Surg.* **40**, 166–172.

Noble, R. L. (1977a). Hormonal control of growth and progression in tumours of Nb rats and a theory of action. *Cancer Res.* **37**, 82–94.

Noble, R. L. (1977b). Sex steroids as a cause of adenocarcinoma of the dorsal prostate in Nb rats, and their influence on the growth of transplants. *Oncology* **34**, 138–141.

Noble, R. L. (1977c). The development of prostatic adenocarcinoma in Nb rats following prolonged sex hormone administration. *Cancer Res.* **37**, 1929–1933.

Noble, R. L. (1979). Carcinoma of the prostate may be caused by the sequential action of antagonistic sex hormones—Transplants in Nb rats show unique hormone responses. *AACR Abst.* p. 26.

Nuti, K. M., and Karavolas, H. J. (1977). Effect of progesterone and its 5α-reduced metabolites on gonadotrophin levels in estrogen-primed ovariectomized rats. *Endocrinology (Baltimore)* **100**, 777–781.

Pearlman, W. H. (1963). Metabolism of Δ^4-androstene-3,17-dione-7-^{3}H and its localization in the rat. *Natl. Cancer Inst. Monogr.* **12**, 309–315.

Peterson, R. E., Imperato-McGinley, J., Gautier, T., and Sturla, E. (1977). Male pseudohermaphroditism due to steroid 5α-reductase deficiency. *Am. J. Med.* **62**, 170–191.

Petrow, V., and Lack, L. (1981). Studies on a 5α-reductase inhibitor and their therapeutic implications. *In* "The Prostatic Cell: Structure and Function" (G. P. Murphy, A. A. Sandberg, and J. P. Karr, eds.), Part B, pp. 283–297. Alan R. Liss, New York.

Petrow, V., Wang, Y., Lack, L., and Sandberg, A. (1981). Prostatic cancer. I. 6-Methylene-4-pregnen-3-ones as irreversible inhibitors of rat prostatic Δ^4-3-ketosteroid 5α-reductase. *Steroids* **38**, 121–140.

Petrow, V., Padilla, G. M., Kendle, K., and Tantawi, A. (1982). Inhibition of prostatic growth in rats by 6-methylene-4-pregnene-3,20-dione. *J. Endocrinol.* **95**, 311–313.

Petrow, V., Wang, C., Lack, L., Sandberg, A., Kadohama, N., and Kendle, K. (1983). Prostatic cancer. II. Inhibitors of rat prostatic Δ^4-3-ketosteroid 5α-reductase derived from 6-methylene-4-androsten-3-ones. *J. Steroid Biochem.* **19**, 1491–1502.

Petrow, V., Padilla, G. M., Mukherji, S., and Marts, S. (1984). Endocrine dependence of prostatic cancer upon dihydrotestosterone and not upon testosterone. *J. Pharm. Pharmacol.* **36**, 352–353.

Pollard, M., Luckert, P. H., and Schmidt, M. A. (1982). Induction of prostate adenocarcinoma in Lobund Wistar rats by testosterone. *Prostate* **3**, 563–568.

Pontes, J. E., Karr, J. P., Kirdani, R. Y., Murphy, G. P., and Sandberg, A. A. (1982). Estrogen receptors and clinical correlations with human prostatic disease. *Urology* **19**, 399–403.

Poste, G., Doll, J., and Fidler, I. J. (1981). Interactions among clonal subpopulations affect stability of the metastatic phenotype in polyclonal populations of B16 melanoma cells. *Proc. Natl. Acad. Sci. U.S.A.* **78**, 6226–6230.

Rotkin, I. D. (1979). Epidemologic factors associated with prostatic cancer. *U.I.C.C. Tech. Rep. Ser.* **48**, 56–80.

Ruberg, I., Senge, T., and Neumann, F. (1982). Microautoradiographic studies on distribution of 5α-dihydrotestosterone, cyproterone acetate and oestradiol-17β in human prostatic hyperplasia tissue transplated in juvenile rats. *Acta Endocrinol.* **101**, 144–153.

Ruzicka, L., and Goldberg, M. W. (1935). Sexual hormone. XI. Partielle Verseifung von Di-estern des Androstan-3-cis, 17-transdiols sowie dessen partielle Veresterung, Beiträge zur Spezifität der Sexualhormonwirkung. *Helv. Chim. Chim. Acta* **19**, 99–156.

Saenger, P., Goldman, A. S., Levine, L. S., Korthschutz, S., Muecke, E. C., Katsumata, M.,

Doberne, Y., and New, M. I. (1978). Prepubertal diagnosis of steroid 5α-reductase deficiency. *J. Clin. Endocrinol. Metab.* **46,** 627–634.

Sar, M., Liao, S., and Stumpf, W. E. (1970). Nuclear concentration of androgens in rat seminal vesicles and prostate demonstrated by dry-mount autoradiography. *Endocrinology (Baltimore)* **86,** 1008–1011.

Saunders, F. J. (1963). Some aspects of relation of structure of steroids to their prostate-stimulating effects. *Natl. Cancer. Inst. Monogr.* **12,** 139–159.

Schneider, J. J. (1952). Conversion of desoxycorticosterone to four allopregnane metabolites by rat liver *in vitro. J. Biol. Chem.* **199,** 235–244.

Schoonees, R., Schalch, D. S., Reynoso, G., and Murphy, G. P. (1972). Bilateral adrenalectomy for advanced prostatic carcinoma. *J. Urol.* **108,** 123–125.

Shain, S. A., Boesel, R. W., and Axelrod, L. R. (1975). Aging in the rat prostate. Reduction in detectable ventral prostate androgen receptor content. *Arch. Biochem. Biophys.* **167,** 247–263.

Shain, S. A., McCullough, B., Nitchuk, N., and Boesel, R. W. (1977a). Prostate carcinogenesis in the A × C rat. *Oncology* **34,** 114–122.

Shain, S. A., Nitchuk, W. M., and McCullough, B. (1977b). Steroid Metabolism by spontaneous adenocarcinoma of the A × C rat ventral prostate. *JNCI, J. Natl. Cancer. Inst.* **58,** 747–751.

Shain, S. A., Boesel, R. W., Radwin, H. M., and Lamm, D. B. (1979). Cytoplasmic and nuclear androgen receptors of human prostate. *In* "Prostate Cancer and Hormone Receptors" (G. P. Murphy and A. Sandberg, eds.), pp. 33–49. Alan R. Liss, New York.

Shaw, E. (1980). Design of irreversible inhibitors. *In* "Enzyme Inhibitions and Drugs" (M. Sandler, ed.), pp. 25–42. Unwin Bros., Ltd., Surrey, United Kingdom.

Shimazaki, J., Kurihara, H., Ito, Y., and Shida, K. (1965). Metabolism of testosterone in prostate. (1st Report and 2nd Report). Separation of prostatic 17β-ol-dehydrogenase and 5α-reductase *Gunma J. Med. Sci.* **14,** 313–325 and 326–333.

Shimazaki, J., Matsushita, I., Furuya, N., Yamanaka, H., and Shida, K. (1969). Reduction of 5α-position of testosterone in the rat ventral prostate. *Endocrinol. Jpn.* **16,** 453–458.

Siiteri, P. K. (1982). Review of studies on estrogen biosynthesis in the human. *Cancer. Res., Suppl.* **42,** 3269s–3273s.

Siiteri, P. K., and Wilson, J. D. (1970). Dihydrotestosterone in prostatic hypertrophy. The formation and control of dihydrotestosterone in the hypertrophic prostate of man. *J. Clin. Invest.* **49,** 1737–1745.

Siiteri, P., and Wilson, J. D. (1974). Testosterone formation and metabolism during male sexual differentiation in the human embryo. *J. Clin. Endocrinol. Metab.* **38,** 113–125.

Smith, P. H., Robinson, M. R. G., and Cooper, E. H. (1976). Carcinoma of the prostate: A focal point of divergent disciplines. *Eur. J. Cancer* **12,** 937–944.

Smith, T., Chisholm, G. D., and Habib, F. K. (1982). Failure of human benign prostatic hyperplasia to aromatise testosterone. *J. Steroid Biochem.* **17,** 119–120.

Thompson, E. A., Jr., and Siiteri, P. K. (1974). Utilization of oxygen and reduced nicotinamide adenine dinucleotide phosphate by human placental microsomes during aromatisation of androstenedione. *J. Biol. Chem.* **249,** 5364–5372.

Tomkins, G. (1957). The enzymatic reduction of Δ⁴-3-ketosteroids. *J. Biol. Chem.* **225,** 13–23.

Tomkins, G., and Isselbacher, K. J. (1954). Enzymatic reduction of cortisone. *J. Am. Chem. Soc.* **76,** 3100–3101.

Tschopp, E. (1935). Die physiologischen Wirkungen des kunstlichen mannlichen Sexualhormons (Androsteron). *Klin. Wochschr.* **14,** 1064–1068.

Tveter, K. J., and Attramadal, A. (1968). Selective uptake of radioactivity in ventral prostate following administration of testosterone-1,2-³H. *Acta Endocrinol.* **59,** 218–226.

Tymockzo, J. L., Liang, T., and Liao, S. (1978). Androgen receptor interactions in target cells:

Biochemical evaluation. *In* "Receptors and Hormone Action" (B. W. O'Malley and L. Birnbaumer, ed.), Vol. II, pp. 121–156. Academic Press, New York.

Van Doorn, E., and Bruchovsky, N. (1978). Mechanisms of replenishment of nuclear androgen receptors in rat ventral prostate. *Biochem. J.* **174,** 9–16.

Van Doorn, E., Craven, S., and Bruchovsky, N. (1976). The relationship between androgen receptors and the hormonally controlled responses of rat ventral prostate. *Biochem. J.* **160,** 11–21.

Verhoeven, G., Lamberigts, G., and De Moor, P. (1974). Nucleus-associated steroid 5α-reductase activity and androgen responsiveness. A study in various organs and brain regions of rats. *J. Steroid Biochem.* **5,** 93–100.

Vermulen, A., and Verdonck, L. (1976). Radioimmunoassay of 17β-hydroxy-5α-androstan-3-one, 4-androstene-3,17-dione, dehydroepiandrosterone, 17-hydroxyprogesterone and progesterone and its application to human male plasma. *J. Steroid Biochem.* **7,** 1–10.

Voigt, W., and Hsia, S. L. (1975). Novel methods of inhibiting the activity of testosterone 5α-reductase. *U.S. Patent 3,917,829* (Nov. 4, 1975, to Research Corporation, N.Y.).

Voigt, W., Fernandez, E. P., and Hsia, S. L. (1970). Transformation of testosterone into 17β-hydroxy-5α-androstan-3-one by microsomal preparations of human skin. *J. Biol. Chem.* **245,** 5594–5599.

Wagner, R., Shulze, K. H., and Jungblut, P. W. (1975). Estrogen and androgen receptor in human prostate and prostatic tumour tissue. *Acta Endocrinol., Suppl.* **193,** 52.

Walsh, P. C., and Wilson, J. D. (1976). The induction of prostatic hypertrophy in the dog with androstanediol. *J. Clin. Invest.* **57,** 1093–1097.

Walsh, P. C., Madden, J. D., Harrod, M. J., Goldstein, J. L., MacDonald, P. C., and Wilson, J. D. (1974). Familial incomplete male pseudohermaphroditism, type 2. Decreased dihydrotestosterone formation in pseudovaginal perineoscrotal hypospadias. *N. Engl. J. Med.* **291,** 944–949.

Westphal, U. (1969). *Abstr., 4th Meet. Int. Study Group Steroid Horm., Rome* p. 9.

Wiebert, D. M., Griffin, J. E., and Wilson, J. D. (1983). Characterization of the cytosol androgen receptor of the human prostate. *J. Clin. Endocrinol. Metab.* **56,** 113–120.

Yates, J., and Deshpande, N. (1975). Evidence for the existence of a single 3β-hydroxysteroid dehydrogenase/$\Delta^{5,4}$-oxosteroid isomerase complex in the human andrenal gland. *J. Endocrinol.* **64,** 195–196.

9

Aromatase: A Target Enzyme in Breast Cancer

J. O'NEAL JOHNSTON AND BRIAN W.
METCALF*

*Merrell Dow Research Institute
Cincinnati, Ohio*

I. Introduction 307
II. Aromatase System 309
    A. Mechanism of Aromatization 309
    B. Inhibition of Aromatase 310
    C. Suicide Inhibition 312
III. Biological Evaluations 317
    A. *In Vitro* Aromatase Inhibition 317
    B. *In Vivo* Aromatase Inhibition 320
    C. Hormone Activity of Aromatase Inhibitors 322
    D. Effect of Aromatase Inhibitors on Endocrine-Dependent Rodent
       Mammary Tumors 323
IV. Summary 324
    References 324

I. INTRODUCTION

Hormones are often implicated in various aspects of genesis and growth of cancer. Malignant cells tend to lose their ability to differentiate, but some malignant tumors retain their responsiveness to the specific hormones that were neces-

*Present address: Smith Kline & French Laboratories, 1500 Spring Garden Street, Philadelphia, Pennsylvania 19101.

Novel Approaches to Cancer Chemotherapy
Copyright © 1984 by Academic Press, Inc.
All rights of reproduction in any form reserved.
ISBN 0-12-676980-X

sary for growth and maintenance of function in the normal tissue from which the tumor originated. Hormonal dependence was suggested in 1896 by the clinical experiments of Sir George Beatson, who achieved regression of metastatic breast carcinoma by oophorectomy. Endocrine ablative therapy for breast cancer was significantly advanced with the introduction of bilateral adrenalectomy and accompanying cortisone replacement (Huggins and Bergenstal, 1952) and hypophysectomy (Pearson and Ray, 1960). The rationale of endocrine therapy in treatment of breast cancer has progressed empirically from surgical removal of hormone-secretory organs to the paradoxical response to administration of pharmacological doses of estrogens or androgens. These conventional forms of endocrine therapy have similar objective response rates (26–36%) among large groups of patients whose selection is based only on menopausal status (Henderson and Canellos, 1980). In patients who responsd to endocrine manipulations, the fraction of cells synthesizing DNA declines and histological cell necrosis is associated with tumor mass shrinkage. This is not observed in patients who fail to respond (Nordenskjöld *et al.,* 1976; Kennedy, 1974).

Approximately one-third of the 110,000 annual new breast carcinoma cases in the United States will be classified as hormone dependent. This subgroup is characterized by the presence of estrogen and progesterone receptors in tumor tissues. In patients with hormone-responsive neoplasms, the withdrawal of estrogen following surgical ablation or treatment with antiestrogens, which alters estrogen action, results in tumor regression (McGuire, 1975). Subsequent investigations have focused on inhibitors of estrogen biosynthesis, since aromatase (estrogen synthetase) is the rate-limiting enzyme in the conversion of androgens to estrogens. This enzyme could have regulatory roles in both the pathogenesis and the treatment of hormone-dependent breast cancer, thus making aromatase a target enzyme in the treatment of breast cancer. This concept has been substantiated by clinical experience with two compounds, aminoglutethimide and Δ^1–testololactone, used for the treatment of breast cancer (Santen and Wells, 1980; Segaloff *et al.,* 1962), which also inhibit aromatase (Santen *et al.,* 1978; Barone *et al.,* 1979). Improvement in the aromatase-inhibitory activity may be possible by development of mechanism-activated inhibitors of aromatase. Such compounds should have a higher affinity for the enzyme and consequently greater specificity than the current clinically available agents. Longer duration of pharmacological action would be expected when the enzyme is inactivated by covalent binding of the inhibitor in the enzyme-active site. Suicide enzyme inactivation may prove to be a successful approach for development of drugs that achieve their therapeutic effect by inhibiting enzyme systems (Sjoerdsma, 1981; Walsh, 1982).

The sites of estrogen production differ according to the reproductive status of the patient. In premenopausal women the primary site of estrogen production is the ovary, where androstenedione and testosterone are converted to estrone and estradiol, respectively. In postmenopausal women, extraglandular aromatization of androstenedione to estrone accounts for nearly all endogenous estrogen synthesis (MacDonald *et al.*, 1967; Grodin *et al.*, 1973; Longcope, 1971). Peripheral estrogen biosynthesis has been shown to occur in tissues such as adipose tissue (Schindler *et al.*, 1972; Nimrod and Ryan, 1975), muscle (Longcope *et al.*, 1978), liver (Smuk and Schwers, 1977), hair follicles (Schweiket *et al.*, 1975), brain (Naftolin *et al.*, 1971), and breast tumors. (Abul-Hajj *et al.*, 1979; Adams and Li, 1975; Miller and Forrest, 1976; Perel *et al.*, 1980). Postmenopausal women can produce physiological amounts of estrogen to activate target tissues. Conditions such as obesity, hepatic disease, or hyperthyroidism are associated with increased risk for endometrial (Gordon *et al.*, 1975; MacDonald *et al.*, 1978) and breast cancer (Siiteri *et al.*, 1980). These disease states are also known to be associated with increased aromatization of androstenedione to estrogen (Forney *et al.*, 1981; Southren *et al.*, 1974). In women with endometrial (Davidson *et al.*, 1981) and breast cancer (Siiteri *et al.*, 1981) biological response to circulating estrogens in obese individuals is enhanced by the suppression of serum sex hormone-binding globulin (SHBG), which results in a higher level of circulating free estradiol (Gambone *et al.*, 1982). An increase in the unbound estradiol, the biologically active fraction in both breast and endometrial cancer patients, is highly suggestive that the free estrogen can promote cell proliferation in estrogen-dependent normal and malignant tissues. Estrogen stimulation may act in a permissive role by allowing or facilitating the primary action of other agents, such as viruses, other hormones, or carcinogens to initiate neoplastic change. There is very limited evidence that steroids have a primary or direct carcinogenic effect in human breast cancer.

II. AROMATASE SYSTEM

A. Mechanism of Aromatization

The aromatase system is an enzyme complex involving a flavoprotein, cytochrome P-450 reductase, that transfers electrons from NADPH to the terminal enzyme, cytochrome P-450 aromatase (Salhanick, 1982). By analogy with the better-studied cholesterol side-chain cleavage enzyme, cytochrome P-450$_{scc}$, the substrate androst-4-ene-3,17-dione probably binds to the cytochrome P-450 in the oxidized state. The heme, after reduction, interacts with molecular oxygen, and hydroxylation occurs. Two sequential hydroxylations take place at the androgen C-19 position, followed by a third at 2β. The products of these hydroxylations are 19-hydroxyandrost-4-ene-3,17-dione, 19-oxoandrost-4-ene-3,17-dione, and estrone (Scheme 1). Estrone results from the spontaneous collapse of the intermediate 2β-hydroxy-19-oxoandrost-4-ene-3,17-dione with liberation of formic acid

(Fishman and Goto, 1981). This is in accordance with the known stoichiometry, which demands the consumption of three molecules of O_2 and NADPH for each molecule of estrogen formed (Thompson and Siiteri, 1974b).

In apparent contradiction to Fishman's finding that the third hydroxylation occurs at 2β (Goto and Fishman, 1977) is the demonstration by Akhtar et al. (1982) that the enzymatic aromatization of 19-oxoandrost-4-ene-3,17-dione in the presence of $^{18}O_2$ yields formic acid containing one atom of ^{18}O. Akhtar has invoked the cyclic hemiacetal intermediate shown in Scheme 1 to rationalize the two results.

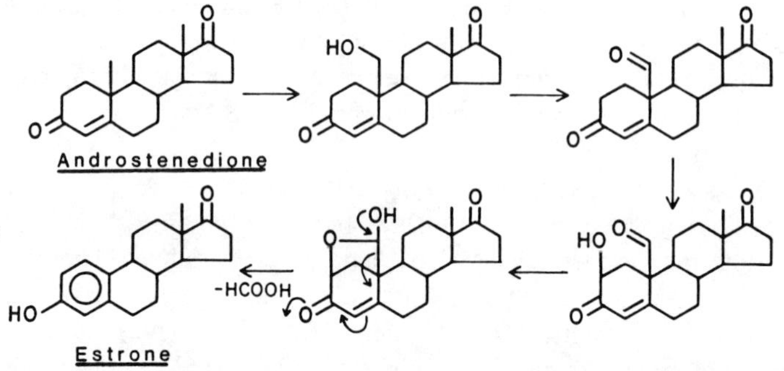

SCHEME 1

Hydroxylation at C-2 occurring after hydroxylations at C-19 is difficult to accommodate in a single active-site hypothesis. Fishman and Goto (1981) have proposed multiple active sites based on the differential inhibition by 19-hydroxyandrost-4-ene-3,17-dione and 19-oxoandrost-4-ene-3,17-dione on the conversion of androst-4-ene-3,17-dione and 19-hydroxylated products and to estrone. The 19-oxoandrost-4-ene-3,17-dione inhibited the two 19-hydroxylations to a lesser extent than it did the 2β hydroxylation, while 19-hydroxy-androst-4-ene-3,17-dione inhibited all three hydroxylations to a similar degree.

B. Inhibition of Aromatase

Aminoglutethimide (**1**), initially studied as an anticonvulsant, has since been found to be a general inhibitor of steroid biosynthesis by virtue of its binding to cytochrome *P*-450 complexes. Clinical observations of adrenal insufficiency led to the finding that **1** blocks the conversion of cholesterol to pregnenolone (Dexter *et al.*, 1967). Somewhat later Thompson and Siiteri (1973) observed its inhibitory effects on aromatase. While steroidal substrates and inhibitors exhibit type I high-spin spectra on binding either to cholesterol scc enzyme [cholesterol monooxygenase (side chain cleaving); EC 1.14.15.6] or to aromatase (Thompson and Siiteri, 1974a), aminoglutethimide binding results in type II low-spin spectra (Uzgiris *et al.*, 1977, Salhanick, 1982). The cholesterol scc enzyme, which has been purified, has been thoroughly studied. It has been suggested that aminoglutethimide binds in such a manner as to prevent the reduction of substrate-bound cytochrome P-450 by the electron transport system (Salhanick, 1982). Presumably the mechanism of inhibition of aromatase by aminoglutethimide is similar. Aminoglutethimide is a competitive inhibitor of human placental aromatase with a K_i of 1 μM (Thompson and Siiteri, 1973), while it inhibits cholesterol scc with a K_i of 30 μM (Salhanick, 1982). Santen and Misbin (1981) have estimated inhibitory concentrations of aminoglutethimide for a number of cytochrome P-450-dependent hydroxylations: aromatase (0.3 μM), 18-hydroxylase (0.2 μM), cholesterol scc (3.5 μM), and 11-hydroxylase (120 μM).

A number of steroids bind to placental aromatase in a reversible manner (Schwarzel *et al.*, 1973). Among the most potent of the competitive inhibitors is 5α-androstane-3,17-dione, which binds to the enzyme with an affinity similar to that of testosterone. Indeed, 5α reduction has been suggested to be a mechanism of physiological control of estrogen biosynthesis (Siiteri and Thompson, 1975). Other competitive inhibitors have been designed to take advantage of an apparent lipophilic binding site that can accommodate substituents at C-7. Thus, 7α-(4'-amino)phenylthio-androst-4-ene-3,17-dione (**3**) binds with a K_i of 18 nM. The apparent K_m for androstene-dione is 63 nM (Brueggemeier *et al.*, 1978).

Δ^1-Testololactone (**2**), which is used clinically in the treatment of breast cancer (Segaloff *et al.*, 1962), has also been described as a competitive inhibitor of aromatase (Siiteri and Thompson, 1975). The decrease in circulating estrone with Δ^1-testololactone administration presumably explains its antitumor properties (Barone *et al.*, 1979).

4-Hydroxy- (**4**) and 4-acetoxyandrost-4-ene-3,17-dione (**5**) have also been described as potent competitive inhibitors of placental aromatase (Brodie *et al.*, 1977, 1979). Recent findings with **2, 4,** and **5,** however, have shown that the inhibition process is more complex than simple competitive inhibition. The compounds are in fact members of a class of compounds commonly called "suicide inhibitors," which will be described in the next section.

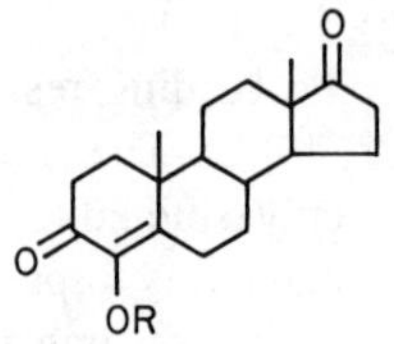

4, R = H
5, R = COCH$_3$

C. Suicide Inhibition

An attractive approach to the irreversible inactivation of enzymes is the use of inhibitors possessing latent reactive functionalities that are unmasked at the enzyme's active site. Since the enzyme becomes inactivated as a consequence of its own mechanism of action, such inhibitors have been referred to as "suicide inhibitors." An inhibitor acting by such a mechanism would be expected to be extremely specific, because it should inactivate only those enzymes for which it is a substrate. It could also be expected to exhibit long-lasting biochemical and pharmacological effects *in vivo*, as the enzyme should remain inactivated even after free inhibitor is no longer present. Resumption of enzymatic activity would depend on new enzyme synthesis. The reader is referred to a review by Walsh (1982), which offers the most comprehensive mechanistic summary of this area, whereas Sjoerdsma (1981) has reviewed the status of several suicide inhibitors under clinical development.

Definitive mechanistic studies have been announced by Ortiz de Montellano and co-workers on the inactivation of the inducible hepatic cytochrome *P*-450's by olefinic and acetylenic substrates (Ortiz de Montellano *et al.*, 1982). As these enzymes presumably operate by a mechanism similar to that of the cytochrome *P*-450-dependent aromatase, conclusions drawn from inactivation studies on the hepatic enzymes may be pertinent to aromatase inhibition. Acetylene inactivates hepatic cytochrome *P*-450 *in vitro*, and a green pigment has been isolated from the livers of acetylene-treated rats and shown to be *N*-(2-oxoethyl) heme. Since vinyl fluoride treatment gives rise to the same pigment, Ortiz de Montellano has proposed the mechanism of inactivation by acetylene shown in Scheme 2. Simi-

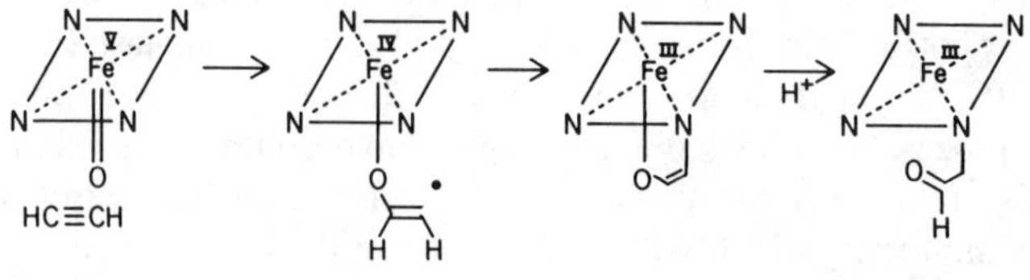

SCHEME 2

larly ethylene, which is also an inactivator, gives rise to a N-(2-hydroxyethyl) heme (Ortiz de Montellano *et al.*, 1981). Allenes also inactivate cytochrome *P*-450, although heme adducts have not been isolated (Ortiz de Montellano and Kunze, 1980). Presumably the mechanism by which allenes inactivate is related to that of acetylenes and olefins.

Based on similar considerations we synthesized the 10-allenyl steroid **6** with the hope that oxygen atom insertion by aromatase would lead to an allene oxide intermediate that would alkylate either prosthetic heme or surrounding protein as shown in Scheme 3. In addition we prepared the 10-propargyl steroid **7** (Metcalf *et al.*, 1981). Compound **7** (Scheme 4a) was postulated to inactivate aromatase via an oxygen insertion mechanism. The proposed oxirene may be a discrete intermediate, or inactivation may occur from a radical intermediate as proposed by Ortiz de Montellano *et al.* (1982) for acetylene itself. Alternately, **7** could undergo sequential hydroxylations at C-19 to afford the conjugated acetylene (Scheme 4b). Such an acetylene would be expected to be an active Michael acceptor that could alkylate some enzyme nucleophile.

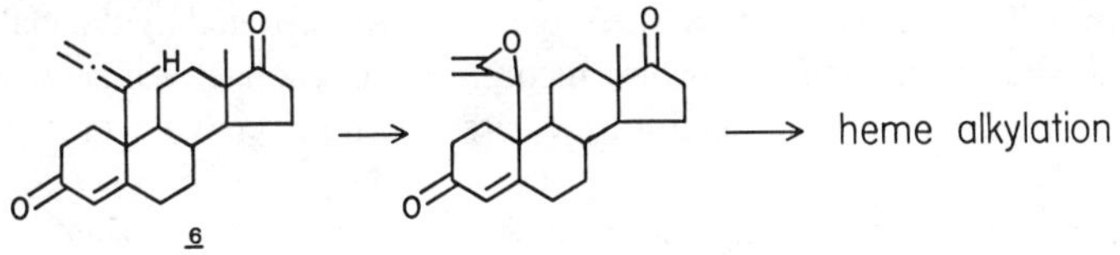

SCHEME 3

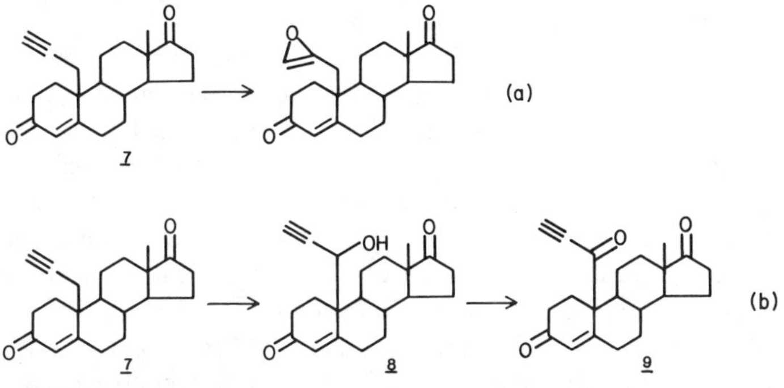

SCHEME 4

Incubation of the aromatase preparation (Reed and Ohno, 1976) to which an NADPH-generating system had been added for varying time periods with different concentrations of **6** and **7** resulted in a time-dependent loss of enzyme activity that followed pseudo-first-order kinetics for more than two half-lives. When the enzyme half-life at these different inhibitor concentrations is plotted against the reciprocal of the inhibitor concentration as described by Kitz and Wilson (1962), the K_i values for **6** and **7** are found to be 14 nM and 5 nM (K_m for testosterone is 45 nM), and the calculated enzyme half-lives at infinite inhibitor concentration are 26 and 11 min, respectively (Fig. 1A). These observed saturation kinetics indicate that a step subsequent to reversible formation of the Michaelis–Menten complex is rate limiting. The inhibition process is active-site directed, as demonstrated by protection against inactivation by the substrate testosterone; at a concentration of **7** at 5 nM, the enzyme half-life increases from 45 to 215 min when the testosterone concentration during preincubation is increased from 45 to 450 nM. There is no time-dependent loss of enzyme activity in the absence of the NADPH-generating system (Fig. 1B). The latter result is evidence that both inhibitors require activation by a functioning aromatase before inactivation can occur. The presence of dithiothreitol (10 mM) in the preincubation medium and the absence of lag time before the onset of inhibition rule out the possibility of inhibition via an affinity-labeling mode by a diffusible alkylating species. The inhibition observed at zero time presumably represents a competitive component of inhibition. The irreversibility of the process is demonstrated by the inability of dialysis at 4°C against the incubation medium to regenerate aromatase activity over a 24-hr period, under conditions where a control enzyme preparation is stable.

Although compounds bearing allenic or acetylenic functions are inactivators of the broadly specific cytochrome P-450 of rat hepatic microsome (Ortiz de Montellano *et al.*, 1981, 1982), neither **6** nor **7** has any inhibitory activity (1 μM, 1 hr incubation) toward the cytochrome P-450-dependent dealkylation of ethyl morphine. In addition, no significant inhibition of the steroid 11β-hydroxylase system was observed on incubation of **6** or **7** at 1 μM for 30 min before monitoring the conversion of deoxy[1,2-^{3}H]corticosterone to corticosterone. Evidently, in the case of **6** and **7** the positioning of the allene or propargylic function at the 10β position confers specificity toward aromatase. While the inactivation of aromatase by **6** most likely involves the intermediacy of an allene oxide, two distinct possibilities exist for inactivation by **7**. If **7** induced inactivation according to Scheme 4b, the proposed intermediate **9** could be expected to be an affinity label for aromatase of activity comparable to **7**. In addition, a kinetic isotope effect on the rate of inactivation induced by 19,19-dideuterio-**7** may be observable if the mechanism of Scheme 4b, but not that of Scheme 4a, is operative and binding of substrate is not rate determining. We find that **9** does not significantly inactivate aromatase at a concentration of 1 μM (during a 20-min incubation in presence of the NADPH-generating system and absence of dithiothreitol and ethylenediaminetetraacetic acid), nor is the rate of inactivation induced by 19,19-dideuterio-**7** significantly different from that induced by **7**. Thus, we favor the mechanism involving oxene attack on the triple bond for the inactivation of

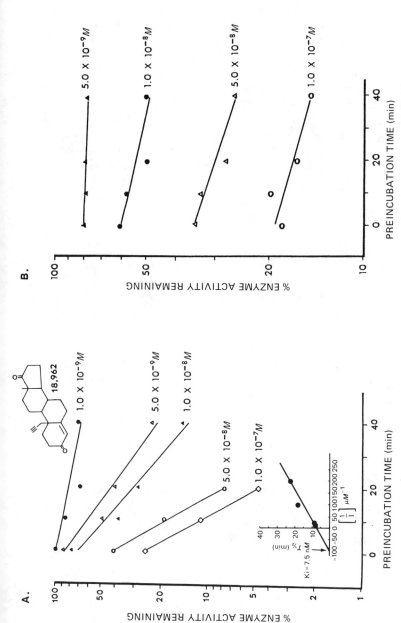

Fig. 1. Aromatase inhibition by inhibitor **7**. (A) Time-dependent enzyme inactivation was obtained after preincubation of **7** with placental aromatase, 450 μg microsomal protein, and NADPH-generating system. Aromatase activity was determined after the addition of [1β,2β-^{3}H]testosterone (450 nM, 0.9 μCi) for a 10-min assay at 25°C. Product formation based on accumulation of ^{3}H$_2$O from the stereospecific elimination of tritium. Insert shows the analysis of the inactivation rates. (B) Incubation conditions same as (A), except the NADPH-generating system was absent from the preincubation medium (Johnston *et al.*, 1984b).

aromatase by **7.** The 10-propargyl steroid **7** has also been synthesized independently by others (Covey *et al.,* 1981; Marcotte and Robinson, 1982a).

Covey *et al.* (1981) have also prepared the propargyl alcohol **8** and have demonstrated that it too is a suicide inactivator of aromatase. Once again several possible mechanisms exist. Compound **8** may be hydroxylated to the ketone **9** as suggested by Covey *et al.,* or it may undergo oxygen atom insertion into the triple bond as in the Ortiz de Montellano type of mechanism. The apparent K_i of **9** is approximately 1000 times higher than that of **7,** which may argue against **8** being an intermediate in the inactivation process induced by **7.**

19,19-Difluoroandrost-4-ene-3,17-dione (**10,** Scheme 5) has been found by Marcotte and Robinson (1982b) to inactivate aromatase in a suicidal manner with a K_i of 1 μM. The proposed mechanism of inactivation involves oxidative conversion of the difluoro group to an acyl fluoride that acylates the enzyme (Scheme 5).

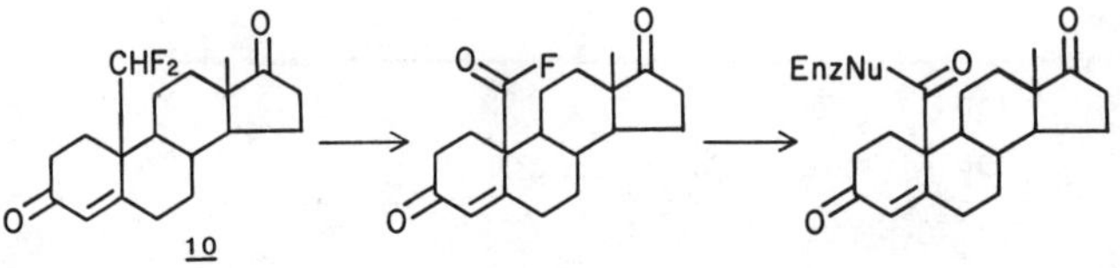

SCHEME 5

This recent flurry of interest in the design of suicide inactivators for aromatase has led to a reexamination of the kinetics of inhibition of previously known competitive inhibitors. Thus, it now appears that the presence of a Δ^1 double bond leads to suicide inactivators. Δ^1-Testololactone (**2**) inactivates aromatase in a NADPH-dependent process with an apparent K_i of 35 μM. On the other hand, testololactone itself, which lacks the Δ^1 double bond, is a simple competitive inhibitor. Similarly androsta-1,4-diene-3,17-dione (**11**) is an irreversible inhibitor with a K_i of 0.32 μM (Covey and Hood, 1982a), while androsta-1,4,6-triene-3,17-dione (**12**) is also a time-dependent inactivator with a K_i of 0.18 μM (Covey and Hood, 1981). It is possible that the irreversibility of inhibition associated with the inclusion of a Δ^1 double bond is a result of an Ortiz de Montellano type of mechanism acting at the normal 2β-hydroxylation step. More difficult to explain are the recent findings that 4-hydroxy-(**4**) and 4-acetoxyandrost-4-ene-3,17-dione (**5**), long known as competitive inhibitors (Brodie *et*

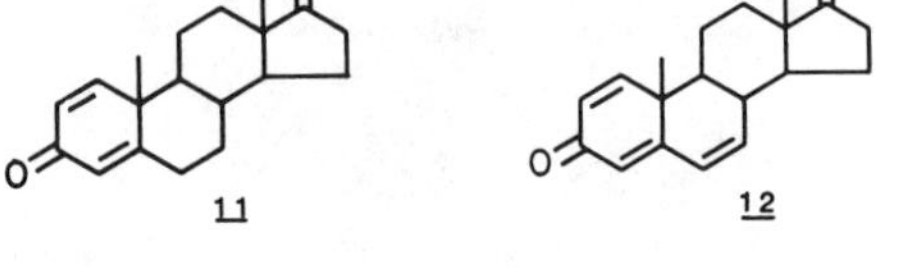

al., 1977, 1979), are also suicide inactivators (Brodie *et al.*, 1981a; Covey and Hood, 1982b). A highly speculative mechanism has been offered (Covey and Hood, 1982a).

While a number of competitive and suicide inactivators are now available, the 10-propargyl steroid 7 and 4-hydroxyandrost-4-ene-3,17-dione (4) are clearly the most potent. Future studies will undoubtedly concentrate on these two substances.

III. BIOLOGICAL EVALUATIONS

A. *In Vitro* Aromatase Inhibition

Compounds that inhibit peripheral aromatization should lower endogenous estrogens and would be of clinical interest in the treatment of metastatic breast cancer. As previously described, aminoglutethimide (1) and Δ^1-testololactone (2) inhibited placental aromatization *in vitro* and lowered estrogen in postmenopausal women with breast cancer. Therefore, we evaluated these clinical agents and the new suicide inhibitors for their ability to inhibit aromatization using assay conditions for first-order inhibition kinetics (Metcalf *et al.*, 1981). These inhibitors were also evaluated using *in vitro* cell cultures of human choriocarcinoma trophoblast (JAr) cells that have maintained their capacity to synthesize estrogens (Bellino *et al.*, 1978). In the trophoblast assay, approximately 10^6 JAr cells were cultured for 24 hr. The inhibitor was then added to the culture at varying intervals up to 1 hr before addition of [1-^{3}H]androstene-dione (40 nM). The product formed was determined during a 30-min assay (Johnston *et al.*, 1984a). Pseudo-first-order inhibition kinetics were obtained for suicide-type inhibitors (Fig. 2). The clinically proven compounds, 1 and 2, had lower affinities for aromatase, since their apparent inhibition constants (K_i) were approximately 75 times greater than those observed for the suicide inhibitors (Table I). Δ^1-Testololactone (2) showed time-dependent kinetics in placental microsomes as previously reported by Covey and Hood (1982a). The suicide-type inhibition was also present in trophoblast cells treated with 2. The inactivation of aromatase occurs at approximately the same rate as the newer suicide inhibitor 6 and 10. This rate of inactivation presumably accounts for the inhibition of peripheral aromatization observed in breast cancer patients following treatment with Δ^1-testololactone (2) (Barone *et al.*, 1979; Judd *et al.*, 1982).

The 4-hydroxyandrostenedione (4) inhibits aromatase about four times faster than the 10-propargyl analog of androstenedione (7) in both microsomal preparations and trophoblast cells. The latter compound (7) has two to three times greater affinity for the enzyme active site than 4-hydroxyandrostenedione (4), which contributes to the greater competitive inhibition observed at 0 min of

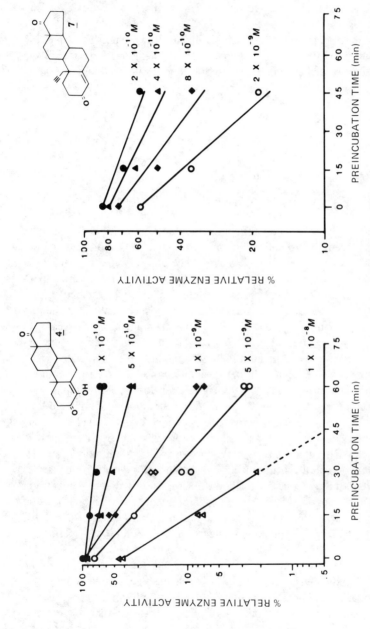

Fig. 2. Time-dependent kinetics of suicide aromatase inhibitors of estrogen synthesis of trophoblast cells. Trophoblast cells were cultured for 24 hr before medium replacement with 1.8 ml of fresh medium. At time intervals from 0 to 60 min, inhibitor **4** or **7** was added in 0.1 ml of medium. Following these preincubation periods, the aromatase was started with the addition of 0.1 ml of medium containing 40 n*M* of [1-³H]androstenedione followed by 30 min of incubation.

TABLE I

Comparative Aromatase Inhibition Kinetics[a]

| Aromatase inhibitor | | Inhibitor properties[b] | | | | | |
| Common or chemical name | Structure number | Human placental microsomes | | | Human trophoblast cell cultures | | |
		K_i (nM)	$t_{1/2}$ (min)	k_{cat} (sec^{-1})	K_i (nM)	$t_{1/2}$ (min)	k_{cat} (sec^{-1})
Aminoglutethimide	1	750	NTD[c]	—	830	NTD[c]	—
Δ1-Testololactone	2	770	21.0	5.5×10^{-4}	844	69.1	1.7×10^{-4}
4-Hydroxyandrost-4-ene-3,17-dione	4	10.2	2.9	4.1×10^{-3}	2.1	6.1	1.9×10^{-3}
10-(1,2-Propadienyl)estr-4-ene-3,17-dione	6	13.6	25.9	4.5×10^{-4}	74.8	69.6	1.7×10^{-4}
10-(2-Propynyl)estr-4-ene-3,17-dione	7	4.5 ± 1.3	11.2 ± 0.7	1.0×10^{-3}	0.6	26.0	4.4×10^{-4}
10β-Difluoromethylestr-4-ene-3,17-dione[d]	10	1066	23.7	4.9×10^{-4}	104	55.5	2.1×10^{-4}
Androsta-1,4,6-triene-3,17-dione	12	110	29.8	3.9×10^{-4}	17.1	23.0	5.0×10^{-4}

[a]Time-dependent assays for placental and cell cultures (Metcalf et al., 1981; Johnston et al., 1984a,b).

[b]Apparent K_i, k_{cat} values and $t_{1/2}$, enzyme half-life at infinite inhibitor concentration, were determined by method of Kitz and Wilson (1962). NTD, Not time dependent; apparent K_i estimated from V_0/V_i vs [I] at 0 min of preincubation. K_i(app) $= K_i$(observed)/$[(K_m + S)/K_m]$.

[c]NTD, Not time dependent.

[d]Compound 10 was a gift from C. H. Robinson, Johns Hopkins University School of Medicine, Baltimore, Maryland.

319

preincubation (Fig. 2). Calculation of an apparent K_i using data from the 0 min of preincubation provided K_i (app) values of 3.5 nM for **4** and 2.1 nM for **7**. In human hormone-responsive mammary cancer cells these latter compounds exhibited potent half-maximum inhibition (IC_{50}) values for estradiol biosynthesis during 6 hr incubation of MCF-7 cells (MacIndoe *et al.*, 1982). In these tumor cells, **4** and **7** were 4000 and 8000 times more potent inhibitors than aminoglutethimide (**1**), with IC_{50} values of 100 and 50 pM, respectively. No cytotoxicity was detected in these cell cultures when the aromatase inhibitors were present at 5 μM. In breast carcinoma tissue, both **4** and **7** maximally inhibited the formation of estrone and estradiol from androstenedione at 85 to 350 nM (Perel *et al.*, 1981).

B. *In Vivo* Aromatase Inhibition

Pregnant mare's serum gonadotrophin (PMSG) stimulated ovarian aromatase and maintained a steady state of ovarian estrogen secretion in rats (Brodie *et al.*, 1976). Injection of PMSG-treated rats with 50 mg/kg of **4** or **12** caused a marked reduction in both ovarian aromatase activity and ovarian vein estrogen levels by 4 hr posttreatment. At 48 hr posttreatment both ovarian aromatase activity and estrogen concentrations had returned to control values for rats treated with **12** (Brodie *et al.*, 1982a). Ovarian aromatase activity in rats receiving **4** was approximately 85% inhibited at 48 hr, while the plasma estrogen levels were about 50% of control values (Brodie *et al.*, 1981a, 1982b). Ovarian vein estrogen concentrations were decreased by 73% in proestrous rats at 4 hr after a single sc injection of 50 mg/kg of **4**. A differential effect was evident on estrogen synthesis and interconversion, since estradiol levels were inhibited by 82% while estrone was reduced by only 16% (Brodie *et al.*, 1977).

Ovarian aromatase activity was stimulated with PMSG in immature mice implanted with silastic tubes containing about 5 or 15 mg of **7** with an estimated delivery rate of about 0.3 and 1 mg/kg/day (Fig. 3). In nonstimulated mice, **7** inhibited ovarian aromatase by 58%. In PMSG-stimulated animals, the gonadotrophin treatment increased ovarian aromatase activity along with an increase in uterine weight due to the greater estrogen biosynthesis. A dose-related decrease in ovarian aromatase was associated with a 30% decrease in uterine weight occurring in PMSG-treated mice. This suggested that **7** can decrease estrogen biosynthesis with a subsequent inhibition of the physiological response to estrogen in its target tissue (Johnston *et al.*, 1984b).

Peripheral aromatization was inhibited by 90% of control values in four monkeys treated with 50 mg/kg of **4**. The metabolic clearance rate of androstenedione and estrone was not altered, nor was the interconversion of androgens, estrogens, or 5α-reduced androgens (Brodie and Longcope, 1980). However, the clearance rate of **4** was about twice as rapid as that observed for androstenedione

OVARIAN WEIGHT   AROMATASE ACTIVITY   UTERINE WEIGHT

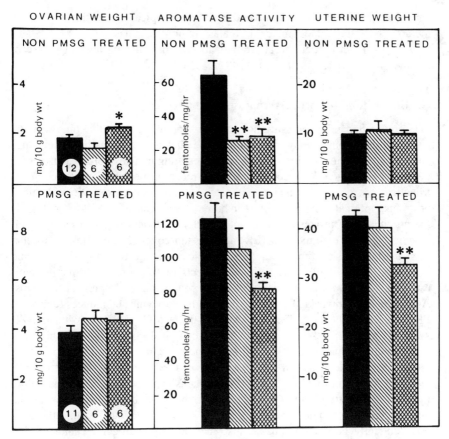

Fig. 3.   Ovarian aromatase activity and target organ response. Immature mice received either a control blank silastic implant (solid), or implants containing 3 mm (hatched) or 10 mm (cross-hatched) of inhibitor **7.** The following day, half of the mice received 20 IU sc of PMSG or vehicle. Three days later ovarian and uterine weights and ovarian aromatase activity were determined. Data expressed as mean ± SE. Treatments that are statistically different from blank implant controls are indicated as * for $p \leq .05$ and ** for $p \leq .01$ (Johnston *et al.*, 1984b).

in monkeys. This rapid clearance of **4** would require that large doses be administered via sustained-release methods to achieve pharmacological effects (Brodie *et al.*, 1981b). The major metabolite of **4** in rats was 3β-hydroxy-5α-androstane-4,17-dione (20–50%). This metabolite retained only 10% of the *in vitro* aromatase-inhibitory activity of the parent inhibitor (Marsh *et al.*, 1982). The contribution of this metabolite to the rapid clearance of **4** in the monkey has not been established. The 4-hydroxytestosterone, which is about 65% as active as **4,** was the only unconjugated metabolite (<2%) reported for the rhesus monkey (Brodie *et al.*, 1981b). These pharmacokinetic and metabolic profiles of **4** will have a major influence on its potential pharmacological application for cancer therapy. The other major suicide aromatase inhibitor (7) has not yet been evaluated for its effect on peripheral aromatization in primates because of its recent discovery in 1981 (Metcalf *et al.*, 1981).

C. Hormone Activity of Aromatase Inhibitors

Hormone-dependent breast tumors contain steroid receptors that bind with the hormone. This complex is translocated in the nucleus to chromatin-binding sites and initiates a series of biochemical events resulting in a physiological effect. In the case of estrogen-dependent tumors, the receptor-mediated events may contribute to the growth or maintenance of the tumor. An example of induced posttranscriptional protein synthesis in human breast cancer cells (MCF-7 line) is the production of progesterone receptors (PR). This is a result of estrogen interacting with its own receptor (ER) and the subsequent nuclear processing that occurs after translocation of the ER complexes in the nucleus (Horwitz and McGuire, 1978, 1979). The antitumor effects of the clinically effective antiestrogen, tamoxifen, are probably mediated via estrogen receptor mechanisms. At low concentrations (<0.1 μM) tamoxifen is estrogenic and induces functional PR synthesis, whereas at higher levels (1 μM) MCF-7 cell growth and PR synthesis are suppressed. At these pharmacological concentrations, this antiestrogen also depletes cytosol ER and blocks its nuclear processing, which contributes to the reduction in cell growth and PR synthesis (Horwitz *et al.*, 1978; Horwitz and McGuire, 1978). Androgens can also antagonize the induction of PR by estrogen in MCF-7 cells, which can be blocked by nonsteroidal antiandrogens (MacIndoe and Etre, 1981). These results suggest that the antiestrogenic effects of androgens are also mediated by androgen receptor mechanisms. Similar antagonistic responses are apparent in therapeutic use of androgens in breast cancer.

The hormonal responsiveness of these MCF-7 cells in culture provided a unique opportunity for evaluation of effects of both receptor-mediated events and steroidal metabolism of androgens and estrogen (MacIndoe, 1979; MacIndoe and Woods, 1981). Therefore, several aromatase inhibitors were investigated for their effects on estrogenic activity as assessed by depletion of cytosol ER, induction of PR, and binding to PR of MCF-7 mammary cancer cells (MacIndoe *et al.*, 1982). In these studies competitive aromatase inhibitors, aminoglutethimide (1), 5α-dihydrotestosterone, and "suicide-type" inhibitors, Δ^1-testololactone (2), 4-hydroxyandrostenedione (4), and 10-(2-propynyl)estr-4-ene-3,17-dione (7), were incubated in subconfluent MCF-7 cultures for 5 days before determination of the effect of these inhibitors on ER and PR concentrations. Only 4 interacted with ER and induced synthesis of PR in a dose-related response similar to the results observed from incubating equimolar concentrations of estradiol in these cell cultures. However, in overnight incubation **4** weakly bound to ER of MCF-7 cytosol, suggesting that the prolonged exposure of **4** to intact MCF-7 cells for 5 days resulted in stimulation of PR synthesis, which was mediated via estrogen receptor mechanism. This apparent dichotomy can be explained by the intracellular conversion of **4** to a more potent estrogenic metabolite (MacIndoe *et al.*, 1982). An alternate explanation is that the metabolite is an androgen-like steroid, since androgens can also induce estrogen receptor translocation and subsequent synthesis of PR in MCF-7 cells (Zava and McGuire, 1978). Rodent uterotrophic bioassays of **4** did not demonstrate marked estrogenic activity *in vivo* (Brodie *et al.*, 1977). However, the rat may have a high rate of first-pass hepatic metabolism of 4-hydroxyandrostenedione (**4**), as has been demonstrated in the monkey (Brodie *et al.*, 1981b). Since only 1.4% of the original compound (**4**) remained at 1 hr following iv injection in rats (Marsh *et al.*, 1982), the ability of these metabolites to induce translocation of ER and synthesis of PR has not been established.

The allene (**6**) and acetylene (**7**) analogs of androstenedione did not exhibit significant binding to androgen, estrogen, or progestin receptors. These compounds induced minimal uterotrophic activity when administered to immature mice for 3 days at doses up to 100 mg/kg/day (Johnston *et al.*, 1981a,b; 1984b). These data suggest that these suicide inhibitors have minimal intrinsic hormonal activity.

D. Effect of Aromatase Inhibitors on Endocrine-Dependent Rodent Mammary Tumors

Administration of the carcinogen 7,12-dimethylbenz[a]anthracene (DMBA) to rats induces mammary tumors of which approximately 80% are hormone dependent (Huggins *et al.*, 1959). This rodent model has been used to evaluate the effect of aromatase inhibitors on mammary tumor growth. The androstenedione analogs (**4, 5, 12**) all caused significant tumor regression, in that the tumor was reduced to less than half of its original size in about 80 to 90% of the tumors after 4 weeks of treatment. These compounds were injected subcutaneously and/or a silastic implant was used, so that the total daily dose was usually 50 mg/kg/day (Brodie *et al.*, 1977, 1979, 1982a,b). In experiments with **5**, estrogen secretion rates were decreased without alteration of gonadotrophin concentrations in peripheral plasma. Tumor regression following treatment of tumor-bearing rats with **5** for 2 weeks could be reversed by the addition of estrogen. Treatment of DMBA-induced tumors with 50 mg/kg/day testosterone also caused tumor regression, but the aromatase suicide inhibitors were two to three times more effective (Brodie *et al.*, 1979). These studies indicate that the hormone-responsive DMBA-induced mammary tumors will regress upon treatment with aromatase inhibitors. The specificity of this response is somewhat ambiguous, since prolactin plays a predominant role in the growth of these rodent neoplasms (Manni *et al.*, 1977). Estrogen may act indirectly to influence tumor growth by stimulating prolactin secretion (Meites, 1972) and by maintaining both prolactin (Arafah *et al.*, 1980) and insulin receptors (Shafie and Hilf, 1978). No definite role for prolactin has yet been found in human breast cancer, where estrogens appear to be of much greater importance than prolactin.

IV. SUMMARY

Aromatase, the rate-limiting enzyme in the conversion of androgens to estrogens, represents a unique target enzyme for the regulation of estrogen-dependent mammary tumors. The ongoing development of a new class of mechanism-based "suicide-type" inhibitors may provide potential therapeutic agents that exhibit a high degree of specificity and selectivity in the regulation of hormone biosynthesis. These new inhibitors are expected to provide long-lasting biochemical and pharmacological effects *in vivo*, since enzyme activity, and consequently estrogen biosynthesis, is irreversibly blocked. Recovery of hormone levels will then be dependent on new enzyme synthesis. The increased effectiveness of enzyme suicide inhibitors in comparison to the inhibitory activity of the agents currently in clinical use may lead to an improvement in the treatment of endocrine-dependent breast cancer.

REFERENCES

Abul-Hajj, Y. J., Iverson, R., and Kiang, D. T. (1979). Aromatization of androgens by human breast cancer. *Steroids* **33,** 205–222.

Adams, J. B., and Li, K. (1975). Biosynthesis of 17β-oestradiol in human breast carcinoma tissues and a novel method for its characterization. *Br. J. Cancer* **31,** 429–433.

Akhtar, M., Calder, M. R., Corina, D. L., and Wright, J. N. (1982). Mechanistic studies on C-19 demethylation in oestrogen biosynthesis. *Biochem. J.* **201,** 569–580.

Arafah, B. M., Manni, A., and Pearson, O. H. (1980). Effect of hypophysectomy and hormone replacement on hormone receptor levels and the growth of 7,12-dimethylbenz(a)anthracene-induced mammary tumors in the rat. *Endocrinology (Baltimore)* **107,** 1364–1368.

Barone, R. M., Shamonki, I. M., Siiteri, P. K., and Judd, H. L. (1979). Inhibition of peripheral aromatization of androstenedione to estrone in postmenopausal women with breast cancer using Δ^1-testololactone. *J. Clin. Endocrinol. Metab.* **49,** 672–676.

Beatson, G. T. (1896). On the treatment of inoperable cases of carcinoma of the mamma: Suggestion for a new method of treatment with illustrative cases. *Lancet* **2,** 104–107, 162–165.

Bellino, F. L., Hussa, R. O., and Osawa, Y. (1978). Estrogen synthetase in choriocarcinoma cell culture. Stimulation by dibutyryl cyclic adenosine monophosphate and theophylline. *Steroids* **32,** 37–44.

Brodie, A. M. H., and Longcope, C. (1980). Inhibition of peripheral aromatization by aromatase inhibitors, 4-hydroxy- and 4-acetoxy-androstenedione. *Endocrinology (Baltimore)* **106**, 19–21.

Brodie, A. M. H., Schwarzel, W. C., and Brodie, H. J. (1976). Studies on the mechanism of estrogen biosynthesis in the ovary—I. *J. Steroid Biochem.* **7**, 787–793.

Brodie, A. M. H., Schwarzel, W. C., Shaikh, A. A., and Brodie, H. J. (1977). The effect of an aromatase inhibitor, 4-hydroxy-4-androstene-3,17-dione, on estrogen-dependent processes in reproduction and breast cancer. *Endocrinology (Baltimore)* **100**, 1684–1695.

Brodie, A. M. H., Marsh, D. A., and Brodie, H. J. (1979). Aromatase inhibitors. IV. Regression of hormone-dependent, mammary tumors in the rat with 4-acetoxyandrostene-3,17-dione. *J. Steroid Biochem.* **10**, 423–429.

Brodie, A. M. H., Garrett, W. M., Hendrickson, J. R., Tsai-Morris, C., Marcotte, P. A., and Robinson, C. H. (1981a). Inactivation of aromatase *in vitro* by 4-hydroxy-4-androstene-3,17-dione and 4-acetoxy-4-androstene-3,17-dione and sustained effects *in vivo*. *Steroids* **38**, 693–702.

Brodie, A. M. H., Romanoff, L. P., and Williams, K. I. H. (1981b). Metabolism of the aromatase inhibitor 4-hydroxy-4-androstene-3,17-dione by male rhesus monkeys. *J. Steroid Biochem.* **14**, 693–696.

Brodie, A. M. H., Brodie, H. J., Garrett, W. M., Hendrickson, J. R., Marsh, D. H., and Tsai-Morris, C. H. (1982a). The effects of aromatase inhibitor: 1,4,6-Androstatrienedione (ATD) on DMBA-induced mammary tumors in the rat and its mechanism of action *in vivo*. *Biochem. Pharm.* **31**, 2017–2023.

Brodie, A. M. H., Garrett, W. M., Hendrickson, J. R., and Tsai-Morris, C. H. (1982b). Effects of aromatase inhibitor 4-hydroxyandrostenedione and other compounds in the 7,12-dimethyl-benz(a) anthracene-induced breast carcinoma model. *Cancer Res., Suppl.* **42**, 3360–3364.

Brueggemeier, R. W., Floyd, E. E., and Counsell, R. E. (1978). Synthesis and biochemical evaluation of inhibitors of estrogen biosynthesis. *J. Med. Chem.* **21**, 1007–1011.

Covey, D. F., and Hood, W. F. (1981). Enzyme-generated intermediates derived from 4-androstene-3,6-17-trione and 1,4,6-androstatriene-3,17-dione cause a time-dependent decrease in human placental aromatase activity. *Endocrinology (Baltimore)* **108**, 1597–1598.

Covey, D. F., and Hood, W. F. (1982a). A new hypothesis based on suicide substrate inhibitor studies for the mechanism of aromatase. *Cancer Res., Suppl.* **42**, 3327–3333.

Covey, D. F., and Hood, W. F. (1982b). Aromatase enzyme catalysis is involved in the potent inhibition of estrogen biosynthesis caused by 4-acetoxy- and 4-hydroxy-4-androstene-3,17-dione. *Mol. Pharmacol.* **21**, 173–180.

Covey, D. F., Hood, W. F., and Parikh, V. D. (1981). 10β-Propynyl-substituted steroids. Mechanism-based enzyme activated irreversible inhibitors of estrogen biosynthesis. *J. Biol. Chem.* **256**, 1076–1079.

Davidson, B. J., Gambone, J. C., Lagasse, L. D., Castaldo, T. W., Hammond, G. L., Siiteri, P. K., and Judd, H. L. (1981). Free estradiol in postmenopausal women with and without endometrial cancer. *J. Clin. Endocrinol. Metab.* **52**, 404–408.

Dexter, R. N., Fishman, L. M., Ney, R. L., and Liddle, G. W. (1967). Inhibition of adrenal corticoid synthesis by aminoglutethimide: Studies of the mechanism of action. *J. Clin. Endocrinol. Metab.* **27**, 473–480.

Fishman, J., and Goto, J. (1981). Mechanism of estrogen biosynthesis. Participation of multiple enzyme sites in placental aromatase hydroxylations. *J. Biol. Chem.* **256**, 4466–4471.

Forney, J. P., Milewich, L., Chen, G. T., Garlock, J. L., Schwarz, B. E., Edman, C. D., and MacDonald, P. C. (1981). Aromatization of androstenedione to estrone by human adipose tissue *in vitro*. Correlation with adipose tissue mass, age, and endometrial neoplasia. *J. Clin. Endocrinol. Metab.* **53**, 192–199.

Gambone, J. C., Pardridge, W. M., Lagasse, L. D., and Judd, H. L. (1982). *In vivo* availability of circulating estradiol in postmenopausal women with and without endometrial cancer. *Obstet. Gynecol.* **59,** 416–421.

Gordon, G. G., Olivo, J., Rafii, R., and Southren, A. L. (1975). Conversion of androgens to estrogens in cirrhosis of the liver. *J. Clin. Endocrinol. Metab.* **40,** 1018–1026.

Goto, J., and Fishman, J. (1977). Participation of a nonenzymatic transformation in the biosynthesis of estrogens from androgens. *Science* **195,** 80–81.

Grodin, J. M., Siiteri, P. K., and MacDonald, P. C. (1973). Source of estrogen production in postmenopausal women. *J. Clin. Endocrinol. Metab.* **36,** 207–214.

Henderson, I. C., and Canellos, G. P. (1980). Cancer of the breast. The past decade. *N. Eng. J. Med.* **302,** 17–30, 78–90.

Horwitz, K. B., and McGuire, W. L. (1978). Estrogen control of progesterone receptor in human breast cancer: Correlation with nuclear processing of estrogen receptor. *J. Biol. Chem.* **253,** 2223–2228.

Horwitz, K. B., and McGuire, W. L. (1979). Estrogen control of progesterone receptor induction in human breast cancer. Role of nuclear estrogen receptor. *Adv. Exp. Med. Biol.* **117,** 95–110.

Horwitz, K. B., Koseki, Y., and McGuire, W. L. (1978). Estrogen control of progesterone receptor in human breast cancer: Role of estradiol and antiestrogen. *Endocrinology (Baltimore)* **103,** 1742–1751.

Huggins, C., and Bergenstal, D. M. (1952). Inhibition of human mammary and prostatic cancers by adrenalectomy. *Cancer Res.* **12,** 134–141.

Huggins, C., Briziarelli, G., and Sutton, H. (1959). Rapid induction of mammary carcinoma in the rat and the influence of hormones on tumors. *J. Exp. Med.* **109,** 25–42.

Johnston, J. O., Wright, C. L., and Metcalf, B. W. (1981a). Irreversible inhibition of aromatase by 10-(2-propynyl)estr-4-ene-3,17-dione (RMI 18,962). Proceedings 63rd Annual Endocrine Society Meeting. *Endocrinology (Baltimore)* **109,** 651. (Abstr.)

Johnston, J. O., Wright, C. L., and Metcalf, B. W. (1981b). Inhibition of estrogen biosynthesis via substrate-induced inactivation with 10-allenyl-estr-4-en-3,17-dione (RMI 18,882). *Physiologist* **24,** 71. (Abstr.)

Johnston, J. O., Wright, C. L., and Metcalf, B. W. (1984a). Time-dependent inhibition of aromatase in trophoblastic tumor cells in tissue cultures. *J. Steroid Biochem.* **20,** 1221–1226.

Johnston, J. O., Wright, C. L., and Metcalf, B. W. (1984b). Biochemical and endocrine properties of a mechanism-based inhibitor of aromatase. *Endocrinology (Baltimore)* **115,** 776–785.

Judd, H. L., Barone, R. M., Laufer, L. R., Gambone, J. C., Monfort, S. L., and Lasley, B. L. (1982). *In vivo* effects of Δ^1-testololactone on peripheral aromatization. *Cancer Res., Suppl.* **42,** 3345–3348.

Kennedy, B. J. (1974). Hormonal therapies in breast cancer. *Semin. Oncol.* **5,** 119–130.

Kitz, R., and Wilson, I. B. (1962). Esters of methanesulfonic acid as irreversible inhibitors of acetylcholinesterase. *J. Biol. Chem.* **237,** 3245–3249.

Longcope, C. (1971). Metabolic clearance and blood production rates of estrogen in postmenopausal women. *Am. J. Obstet. Gynecol.* **111,** 778–781.

Longcope, C., Pratt, J. H., Schneider, S. H., and Fineberg, S. E. (1978). Aromatization of androgens by muscle and adipose tissue *in vivo*. *J. Clin. Endocrinol. Metab.* **46,** 146–152.

MacDonald, P. C., Rombaut, R. P., and Siiteri, P. K. (1967). Plasma precursors of estrogen. I. Extent of conversion of plasma androstenedione to estrone in normal males and non-pregnant, normal, castrate and adrenalectomized females. *J. Clin. Endocrinol. Metab.* **27,** 1103–1111.

MacDonald, P. C., Edman, C. D., Hemsell, D. L., Porter, J. C., and Siiteri, P. K. (1978). Effect of obesity on conversion of plasma androstenedione to estrone in postmenopausal women with and without endometrial cancer. *Am. J. Gynecol.* **130,** 448–455.

McGuire, W. L. (1975). Endocrine therapy in breast cancer. *Sel. Top. Clin. Sci. Annu. Rev. Med.* **26,** 353–363.

MacIndoe, J. H. (1979). Estradiol formation from testosterone by continuously cultured human breast cancer cells. *J. Clin. Endocrinol. Metab.* **49,** 272–277.

MacIndoe, J. H., and Etre, L. A. (1981). An antiestrogenic action of androgens in human breast cancer cells. *J. Clin. Endocrinol. Metab.* **53,** 836–842.

MacIndoe, J. H., and Woods, G. R. (1981). Steroid metabolizing enzymes in human breast cancer cells. II. 5α-Reductase, 3α-hydroxysteroid oxidoreductase, and 17β-oxidoreductase. *Endocrinology (Baltimore)* **108,** 1407–1413.

MacIndoe, J. H., Woods, G. R., Etre, L. A., and Covey, D. F. (1982). Comparative studies of aromatase inhibitors in cultured human breast cancer cells. *Cancer Res., Suppl.* **42,** 3378–3381.

Manni, A., Trujillo, J. E., and Pearson, O. H. (1977). Predominant role of prolactin in stimulating the growth of 7,12-dimethylbenz(a)anthracene-induced rat mammary tumor. *Cancer Res.* **37,** 1216–1219.

Marcotte, P. A., and Robinson, C. H. (1982a). Synthesis and evaluation of 10β-substituted 4-estrene-3,17-diones as inhibitors of human placental microsomal aromatase. *Steroids* **39,** 325–344.

Marcotte, P. A., and Robinson, C. H. (1982b). Inhibition and inactivation of estrogen synthetase (aromatase) by fluorinated substrate analogues. *Biochemistry* **21,** 2773–2778.

Marsh, D. A., Romanoff, L., Williams, K. I. H., Brodie, H. J., and Brodie, A. M. H. (1982). Synthesis of deuterium- and tritium-labeled 4-hydroxyandrostene-3,17-dione, an aromatase inhibitor, and its metabolism *in vitro* and *in vivo* in the rat. *Biochem. Pharmacol.* **31,** 701–705.

Meites, J. (1972). Relation of prolactin and estrogen to mammary tumorigenesis in the rat. *JNCI, J. Natl. Cancer Inst.* **48,** 1217–1224.

Metcalf, B. W., Wright, C. L., Burkhart, J. P., and Johnston, J. O. (1981). Substrate-induced inactivation of aromatase by allenic and acetylenic steroids. *J. Am. Chem. Soc.* **103,** 3221–3222.

Miller, W. R., and Forrest, A. P. M. (1976). Oestradiol synthesis from C_{19} steroids by human breast cancers. *Br. J. Cancer* **33,** 116–118.

Naftolin, F., Ryan, K. J., and Petro, Z. (1971). Aromatization of androstenedione by the diencephalon. *J. Clin. Endocrinol. Metab.* **33,** 368–370.

Nimrod, A., and Ryan, K. J. (1975). Aromatization of androgens by human abdominal and breast fat tissue. *J. Clin. Endocrinol. Metab.* **40,** 367–372.

Nordenskjöld, B., Löwhagen, T., Westerberg, H., and Zajicek, J. (1976). ^{3}H-Thymidine incorporation into mammary carcinoma cells obtained by needle aspiration before and during endocrine therapy. *Acta Cytol.* **20,** 136–143.

Ortiz de Montellano, P. R., and Kunze, K. L. (1980). Inactivation of hepatic cytochrome P-450 by allenic substrates. *Biochem. Biophys. Res. Commun.* **94,** 443–449.

Ortiz de Montellano, P. R., Beilan, H. S., Kunze, K. L., and Mico, B. A. (1981). Destruction of cytochrome P-450 by ethylene. Structure of the resulting heme adduct. *J. Biol. Chem.* **256,** 4395–4399.

Ortiz de Montellano, P. R., Kunze, K. L., Beilan, H. S., and Wheeler, C. (1982). Destruction of cytochrome P-450 by vinyl fluoride, fluroxene, and acetylene. Evidence for a radical intermediate in olefin oxidation. *Biochemistry* **21,** 1331–1339.

Pearson, O. H., and Ray, B. S. (1960). Hypophysectomy in the treatment of metastatic mammary cancer. *Am. J. Surg.* **99,** 544–552.

Perel, E., Wilkins, D., and Killinger, D. W. (1980). The conversion of androstenedione to estrone, estradiol, and testosterone in breast tissue. *J. Steroid Biochem.* **13,** 89–94.

Perel, E., Davis, S. P., Covey, D. F., and Killinger, D. W. (1981). Effects of 4-hydroxy-4-androstene-3,17-dione and 10-propargylestr-4-ene-3,17-dione on the metabolism of androstenedione in human breast carcinoma and breast adipose tissues. *Steroids* **38,** 397–405.

Reed, K. C., and Ohno, S. (1976). Kinetic properties of human placental aromatase. Applications of an assay measuring ^3H_2O release from $1\beta,2\beta$-^{3}H-androgens. J. Biol. Chem. 251, 1625–1631.

Salhanick, H. A. (1982). Basic studies on aminoglutethimide. Cancer Res., Suppl. 42, 3315–3321.

Santen, R. J., and Misbin, R. I. (1981). Aminoglutethimide: Review of pharmacology and clinical use. Pharmacotherapy 1, 95–120.

Santen, R. J., and Wells, S. A., Jr. (1980). The use of aminoglutethimide in the treatment of patients with metastatic carcinoma of the breast. Cancer 46, 1066–1074.

Santen, R. J., Santner, S., Davis, B., Veldhuis, J., Samojlik, E., and Ruby, E. (1978). Aminoglutethimide inhibits extraglandular estrogen production in postmenopausal women with breast carcinoma. J. Clin. Endocrinol. Metab. 47, 1257–1265.

Schindler, A. E., Ebert, A., and Friedrich, E. F. (1972). Conversion of androstenedione to estrone by human fat tissue. J. Clin. Endocrinol. Metab. 35, 627–630.

Schwarzel, W. C., Kruggel, W. G., and Brodie, H. J. (1973). Studies on the mechanism of estrogen biosynthesis. VIII. The development of inhibitors of the enzyme system in human placenta. Endocrinology (Baltimore) 92, 866–880.

Schweikert, H. U., Milewich, L., and Wilson, J. D. (1975). Aromatization of androstenedione by isolated hairs. J. Clin. Endocrinol. Metab. 40, 413–417.

Segaloff, A., Weeth, J. B., Meyer, K. K., Rongone, E. L., and Cunningham, M. E. G. (1962). Hormonal therapy in cancer of the breast. XIX. Effect of oral administration of Δ^1-testololactone on clinical course and hormonal excretion. Cancer 15, 633–635.

Shafie, S. M., and Hilf, R. (1978). Relationship between insulin and estrogen binding to growth response in 7,12-dimethylbenz(a)anthracene-induced rat mammary tumors, Cancer Res. 38, 759–764.

Siiteri, P. K., and Thompson, E. A. (1975). Studies of human placental aromatase. J. Steroid Biochem. 6, 317–322.

Siiteri, P. K., Nisker, J. A., and Hammond, G. L. (1980). Hormonal basis of risk factors for breast and endometrial cancer. Prog. Cancer Res. Ther. 14, 499–505.

Siiteri, P. K., Hammond, G. L., and Nisker, J. A. (1981). Increased availability of serum estrogens in breast cancer: A new hypothesis. Banbury Rep. 8, 87–101.

Sjoerdsma, A. (1981). Suicide inhibitors as potential drugs. Clin. Pharm. Exp. Ther. 30, 3–22.

Smuk, M., and Schwers, J. (1977). Aromatization of androstenedione by human hair. J. Clin. Endocrinol. Metab. 45, 1009–1012.

Southren, A. L., Olivo, J., Gordon, G. G., Vittek, J., Brener, J., and Rafii, F. (1974). The conversion of androgens to estrogens in hyperthyroidism. J. Clin. Endocrinol. Metab. 38, 207–214.

Thompson, E. A., and Siiteri, P. K. (1973). Studies on the aromatization of C-19 androgens. Ann. N.Y. Acad. Sci. 212, 378–391.

Thompson, E. A., and Siiteri, P. K. (1974a). Utilization of oxygen and reduced nicotinamide adenine dinucleotide phosphate by human placental microsomes during aromatization of androstenedione. J. Biol. Chem. 249, 5364–5372.

Thompson, E. A., and Siiteri, P. K. (1974b). The involvement of human placental microsomal cytochrome P-450 in aromatization. J. Biol. Chem. 249, 5373–5378.

Uzgiris, V. I., Graves, P. E., and Salhanick, H. A. (1977). Ligand modification of corpus luteum mitochondrial cytochrome P-450 spectra and cholesterol mono-oxygenation. An assay of enzyme specific inhibitors. Biochemistry 16, 593–600.

Walsh, C. (1982). Suicide substrates: Mechanism-based enzyme inactivators. Tetrahedron 38, 871–909.

Zava, D. T., and McGuire, W. L. (1978). Androgen action through estrogen receptors in human breast cancer cell line. Endocrinology (Baltimore) 103, 624–631.

10

Cell Membranes: Targets for Selective Antitumor Chemotherapy

SUSAN J. FRIEDMAN AND PHILIP SKEHAN

Department of Pharmacology, and Oncology Research Group
Faculty of Medicine
University of Calgary
Calgary, Alberta, Canada

I.	Is Cancer a Disease of Abnormal Growth or of Cell Recognition? . . .	329
II.	Membrane Targets and Strategies for Selective Antitumor Therapy . .	333
	A. Selectively Toxic Amino Sugars	334
	B. Host Cell Protection from Cytotoxicity	341
	C. Surface Galactosyltransferase Acceptors	342
	D. Targeted Drug Delivery	343
	E. Macrophage-Mediated Tumor Cell Killing	344
III.	Summary	345
	References	346

I. IS CANCER A DISEASE OF ABNORMAL GROWTH OR OF CELL RECOGNITION?

The concept of cancer as a disease of abnormal cell growth is a hypothesis, not an established fact. Surprisingly, there does not appear to be a single literature report that presents a formal comparison of normal and tumor growth kinetics, and detailed growth kinetics have not been established for either. All that is presently known with certainty is that deceleratory growth—a process in which the specific growth rate slows gradually but progressively with time—is the kinetic pattern for both normal and malignant tissues (reviewed in Skehan and Friedman, 1982).

329

Novel Approaches to Cancer Chemotherapy
Copyright © 1984 by Academic Press, Inc.
All rights of reproduction in any form reserved.
ISBN 0-12-676980-X

As a test of the hypothesis that cancer is a disease of abnormal growth, we performed a computer analysis of 46 literature data bases of *in vivo* normal and malignant growth processes in higher vertebrates (P. Skehan and S. J. Friedman, manuscript in preparation). From measurements of tissue size as a function of time we calculated specific growth rate values for each successive pair of data points and examined the ability of 18 different growth equations to model these data bases. What we found was that for both normal and malignant tissues, growth was predominantly or exclusively deceleratory, that growth inhibition progressed much more rapidly at small tissue size than at large, and that inverse *N*th-root equations provided the best overall fits to both normal and tumor data. Thus, for the present data bases, the predominant kinetic growth pattern of mammalian tissues *in vivo* is qualitatively identical to that of normal tissues. Although it is of course possible that the two differ quantitatively (e.g., tumor cells might proliferate more rapidly), we were not able to compare growth rate coefficients and minimum doubling times of tumors with corresponding normal tissues from the same host species, since this information was not available in the literature. However, a comparison of tumor and normal tissue doubling times obtained from [^{3}H]thymidine cell cycle analysis and presented in Steel's comprehensive tabulation (1977) fails to support the generality of the hypothesis that tumor cells proliferate more rapidly than normal cells. Certain kinds of tumors tend to have shorter doubling times, others longer doubling times, and still others the same doubling time as their normal counterparts. On balance, there is no sensible pattern of difference in doubling time between tumors as a group and normal tissues as a group.

A second conclusion that can be drawn from our analysis is that tumor growth is highly regulated, and the underlying mechanism—mass inhibition—is probably the same one that governs the growth of normal tissues. Mass inhibition results when cells within a population exert a negative-feedback control over one another's growth by means of inhibitory signals whose overall intensity increases with tissue size (mass or volume). The central feature of mass inhibition is a specific growth rate that decreases monotonically as a function of momentary tissue size but is independent of tissue age and inoculum size. There was a strong suggestion in the normal tissue data bases that the deceleratory growth phase was produced by mass inhibition of growth. Mass inhibition could be positively identified in a number of the tumor data bases, because host animals received multiple inoculum sizes in several experiments.

In summary, our analysis of *in vivo* growth kinetics leads to the following generalizations (to which some individual exceptions clearly exist):

1. Tumor growth is highly regulated.
2. This regulation results from mass inhibition.
3. There is no sensible difference either qualitatively or quantitatively be-

tween the kinetic growth-regulatory patterns of tumors and normal tissues.

4. Cancer is not (in most cases) a disease of growth abnormality.

Thus, a critical question arises. If cell growth is not the central lesion in cancer, what is? The phenomenon of mass inhibition offers a possible answer. Mass inhibition results from a growth-inhibitory negative-feedback communication between member cells within a multicellular community. These signals appear to be tissue specific in most cases, in that heterotypic interactions are usually ineffective or less effective than homotypic ones. Mass inhibition can be mediated by at least three intercellular communication mechanisms: soluble growth inhibitors (chalones), the extracellular matrix, and direct surface contact interactions. All appear to act at the cell surface. Each exhibits a target tissue specificity that effectively constitutes a cellular recognition mechanism. Thus, deceleratory growth caused by mass inhibition involves two separate steps. The first is a cellular recognition that acts as a switch to turn on mass inhibition, while the second is the actual operation of the mass inhibition machinery per se. Mass inhibition can only occur if an appropriate recognition has already been established.

This suggests that neoplastic transformation may arise from an alteration in the surface recognition process that mediates the mass inhibition of growth. Tumors behave as if they were new types of tissues with unique surface-recognitive determinants but normal growth-regulatory machinery. Thus, neoplastic transformation may be a process of tissue neogenesis.

With mass inhibition, growth is fastest at infinitesimal size. An initiated cell undergoing preneoplastic phenotypic progression within a mature adult tissue will possess the same recognitive determinant(s) as a normal cell and will therefore respond normally to the tissue's mass inhibition signals. When that same cell undergoes a phenotypic change in its surface-recognitive determinants, it will no longer respond to the normal tissue's mass inhibition signals. Because the transformed cell is unique and has no access to other cells with the same recognitive determinants, neither will it be able to mass inhibit itself. As a result, neoplastic transformation will trigger an explosive acceleratory increase in the growth rate of the transformed cell. As growth enlarges the tumor population, mass inhibition will gradually develop and the tumor's growth rate will progressively slow, giving rise to deceleratory kinetics. Eventually growth will stop altogether when the tumor reaches its equivalent of a mature adult tissue size, provided of course that it does not first kill the host. What causes the tumor to temporarily grow faster than its normal tissue counterpart is not a change in either its growth or growth-regulatory machinery but rather the sudden loss of access to cells with identical recognitive determinants. The ostensibly faster growth of tumors, so widely asserted in the literature yet contradicted by available cell cycle data (Steel, 1977), is in actuality an artifact of analysis. There is no evidence that the kinetic parameters of normal tissue and tumor growth show any consistent differences when sizes are comparable. Tumors wrongly appear to grow faster than normal tissues only when relatively small tumors are compared with large and fully mature tissues. This is not a valid comparison. While a tumor may sometimes experience a change in its growth machinery so that it will grow either faster or slower than its normal counterpart *at a specific size,* this change is incidental to neoplastic transformation and is not required for progressive neoplastic growth.

1. Implications for Tumor Therapy

Antiproliferative chemotherapy is only effective against rapidly growing tumors, and tumors grow most rapidly when they are very small. The downward convexity of most tumor-specific growth rate versus size curves predicates that the antiproliferatives will only be effective at small tumor burden when growth rate is high. This situation generally occurs only during the earliest stages of neoplastic disease before tumors reach clinically detectable size, or following the elimination of most tumor burden by surgery or other therapeutic modalities. The latter consideration provides a powerful theoretical argument for adjuvant antiproliferative chemotherapy. The former suggests that because of their considerable toxicity toward rapidly proliferating host tissues and their relative ineffectuality against all but very small tumors, the antiproliferatives are likely to be counterproductive in the treatment of many tumors by the time they reach clinically detectable size.

Where mass inhibition is mediated by soluble inhibitors that can act over large distances, any reduction of tumor mass—whether by resection, radiation, or chemotherapy—is likely to actually shorten patient life span. Mass inhibition by soluble inhibitors allows multiple tumors within a single host to be growth controlled not by their individual sizes but by the entire tumor burden within the host (DeWys, 1972; Gorelik *et al.,* 1981; Ketcham *et al.,* 1961; Schatten, 1958; Simpson-Herren *et al.,* 1977). Thus, when a large primary tumor is removed from a patient who also has disseminated disease, the result will be an almost complete release from mass inhibition and a corresponding explosive growth acceleration of the micrometastases. Where metastatic foci are situated in potentially more life-threatening localities than the primary focus, reduction of the primary mass may actually reduce patient life span by promoting the explosive growth of the more dangerously located metastases (Simpson-Herren *et al.,* 1977).

The involvement of mass inhibition in tumor growth regulation and the strong possibility that surface recognition processes may play an important role in neoplastic disease indicate the need to develop new strategies of chemotherapy to complement the existing but limited arsenal of antiproliferatives. In particular, cellular recognitive determinants together with the plasma membrane and cell surface region in which they are situated are new and potentially important targets for chemotherapeutic attack.

II. MEMBRANE TARGETS AND STRATEGIES FOR SELECTIVE ANTITUMOR THERAPY

Neoplastic transformation is accompanied by a wide variety of plasma membrane and cell surface changes (Friedman and Skehan, 1981; Hynes, 1979; Nicolson, 1976b; Poste, 1977; Wallach, 1975; Table I). There does not appear to be any order, pattern, or sequence to these changes, and individually none reliably correlates with or is diagnostic of the neoplastic state (Skehan and Friedman, 1981). Instead, the changes appear to be part of the gradual accumulation of random, independent, and unpredictable phenotypic alterations that accompanies preneoplastic and neoplastic progression (Farber and Cameron, 1980; Foulds, 1969; Prehn, 1976). Although none of these alterations is essential to the neoplastic process, their acquisition can confer important biological capabilities to a cell that intensify its malignancy. As new phenotypic variants arise, the host environment selects for those most efficient at exploiting available resources (Kreider and Bartlett, 1981). This selection leads to an improved environmental fitness and a progressive speciation of the tumor cell population. The improved

TABLE I

Membrane and Membrane-Mediated Cell Behavioral Changes in Transformed Cells and Malignant Tissues

Property	References
Nutrient transport rates	Hatanaka, 1974; Pardee, 1975
Ionic fluxes	Boynton et al., 1982
Activity of membrane enzymes	Lamont, 1982; Nicolson, 1976b, 1982
Cholesterol	Chen et al., 1978; Coleman and Lavietes, 1981
Glycosphingolipids	Hakomori, 1981; Yogeeswaran, 1983
Glycoproteins	Friedman and Skehan, 1981; Hynes, 1976; Nicolson, 1982; Warren et al., 1978; Yogeeswaran, 1983
Tumor antigens	Herberman, 1977; Klein and Klein, 1977; Levine, 1982
Extracellular matrix	Alitalo and Vahari, 1982
Cell separation and locomotion	Sträuli and Weiss, 1977; Weiss, 1976a
Cell deformability	Lichtman and Weed, 1976; Sato et al., 1977; Weiss, 1976b
Cytoskeletal–membrane interactions	Carraway et al., 1983; Nicolson, 1976a,b
Cell interactions	Ruoslahti, 1981; Tarin, 1976

fitness tends to increase tumor aggressiveness, while the speciation produces tumor heterogeneity. The heterogeneity in turn tends to create new subpopulations of tumor cells some of which possess an increased metastatic capacity or therapeutic resistance. This cellular evolution is frequently mediated by changes in the cell surface and plasma membrane, suggesting that these structures may be obligatory targets of chemotherapeutic attack for the control of many neoplastic diseases. Several novel and potentially selective antitumor therapies directed at cellular membrane targets are reviewed in the following paragraphs, as well as in other chapters in this volume (Chapters 2, 5, 9, 11).

A. Selectively Toxic Amino Sugars

1. D-Glucosamine

D-Glucosamine is a naturally occurring sugar and a major carbohydrate component of glycoproteins, glycolipids, and glycosaminoglycans. The antitumor activity of D-glucosamine was first demonstrated in 1953 by Quastel and Cantero for the mouse sarcoma 37 tumor. Subsequent work in a number of laboratories established that glucosamine was cytotoxic toward a variety of other animal tumors as well (Ball *et al.*, 1957; Bekesi *et al.*, 1969a,b; Bekesi and Winzler, 1970; Friedman and Skehan, 1981; Lindner *et al.*, 1960; Molnar and Bekesi, 1972). Cytotoxicity by glucosamine has also been demonstrated for human tumor xenographs grown in athymic nude mice (Friedman and Skehan, 1981; Helson *et al.*, 1979). The most significant finding throughout all of these studies is the apparently complete lack of glucosamine toxicity toward normal host tissues at *in vivo* concentrations that are strongly tumoricidal. This unusual lack of host toxicity makes glucosamine a potentially attractive chemotherapeutic agent in its own right and raises the possibility that it might be used in combination to reduce the clinical dosage of other antitumor drugs with greater host toxicity side effects.

Cells accumulate extracellular glucosamine by facilitated transport (Plagemann and Erbe, 1973). Intracellularly glucosamine is rapidly phosphorylated to glucosamine 6-phosphate, which serves as the starting point for its entry into intermediary metabolism (Fig. 1). Glucosamine exerts two separate effects on cell culture systems. In the concentration range 1–10 mM, it produces a reversible, dose-dependent inhibition of cell growth (Friedman and Skehan, 1980, 1981; Krug *et al.*, 1983). The effect is independent of cell cycle phase, and glucosamine-inhibited cells have microspectrophotometric DNA distributions identical to control distributions (P. Skehan, J. Thomas, and S. Friedman, unpublished observations). Growth inhibition is accompanied by a marked increase in the glycerolipid content of malignant human epithelial cell lines (Krug *et al.*, 1983) and a lipid vesicle accumulation in rat C_6 gliomas (Friedman and Skehan,

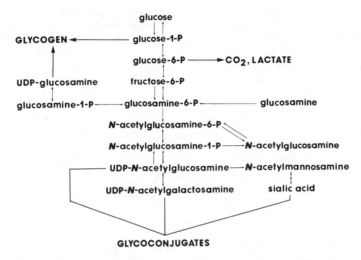

Fig. 1. Metabolism of D-Glucosamine. (Adapted from Warren, 1972.)

1980). At concentrations above 10 mM, glucosamine is cytotoxic and produces cell lysis in 24 to 48 hr (Friedman and Skehan, 1980, 1983).

A variety of drugs with local anesthetic activity potentiate glucosamine's tumoricidal effect. These potentiators include several different classes of membrane-active drugs that are not usually considered to be local anesthetics but that possess some degree of local anesthetic activity (Table II). Glucosamine and anesthetic concentrations that are individually cytostatic interact synergistically in combination to produce growth inhibition and cell lysis (Table III).

Studies with rat C_6 glioma cells suggested that cellular membranes are primary targets of glucosamine's tumoricidal activity. Cytostatic concentrations of glucosamine produced rapid ultrastructural changes in gliomas, particularly in cell

TABLE II

Membrane-Active Drugs That Potentiate Cell Lysis by Glucosamine

Drug	Clinical/experimental use	Structure
Lidocaine	Local anesthetic	Aromatic amine
Adiphenine	Smooth-muscle relaxant	Aromatic amine
Chlorprothixene	Antipsychotic tranquilizer	Thioxanthine
Thioridazine	Antipsychotic tranquilizer	Phenothiazine
Papaverine	Smooth-muscle relaxant	Benzylisoquinoline
Haloperidol	CNS depressant, tranquilizer	Butyrophenone
Ketamine	Anesthetic	Cyclohexanone

TABLE III

Cytotoxicity of Glucosamine in Combination with Membrane-Active Drugs[a]

Cell line	Drug	Inhibition (%)	Cell lysis
RL ♂ mouse leukemia	Glucosamine (1.8 mM)	31	−
	Lidocaine (0.7 mM)	54	−
	Combination	82	+
P-388 mouse leukemia	Glucosamine (7.3 mM)	46.7	−
	Lidocaine (1.7 mM)	28.8	−
	Combination	71.6	+
P-815 mouse mastocytoma	Glucosamine (3.6 mM)	57.6	−
	Lidocaine (0.8 mM)	35	−
	Combination	83.5	+
C_6 rat glioma	Glucosamine (10 mM)	45	−
	Lidocaine (2.5 mM)	40	−
	Combination	97	+
C_6 rat glioma	Glucosamine (3 mM)	26	−
	Papaverine (0.1 mM)	48	−
	Combination	70	+
C_6 rat glioma	Glucosamine (3 mM)	26	−
	Chlorprothixene (2.5 μM)	12	−
	Combination	44	+
C_6 rat glioma	Glucosamine (3 mM)	26	−
	Thioridazine (3 μM)	24	−
	Combination	62	+
C_6 rat glioma	Glucosamine (3 mM)	26	−
	Adiphenine (0.35 mM)	30	−
	Combination	55	+
C_6 rat glioma	Glucosamine (10 mM)	45	−
	Haloperidol (50 μM)	42	−
	Combination	92	+
C_6 rat glioma	Glucosamine (10 mM)	45	−
	Ketamine (1 mM)	12	−
	Combination	68	+

[a]Results are shown for several separate experiments. Duplicate cultures were collected 48 hr after drug treatment was begun. Protein contents or cell numbers of duplicate cultures differed from the average ±5% or less. Cell lysis was assessed by phase-contrast microscopy. For each cell line, the percentage inhibition for the drug combination was significantly greater than that expected for summation of mutually exclusive inhibitors (Friedman and Skehan, 1980). Percentage inhibition or cell number per flask was measured as 100 (1 − test/control) (data taken from Friedman and Skehan, 1980, 1983).

TABLE IV

Changes in Ultrastructure of Rat C_6 Glioma Cells following Treatment with Glucosamine, Lidocaine, and Glucosamine plus Lidocaine[a]

Drug treatment	Ultrastructural changes
Glucosamine (10 mM)	Condensed nucleoli and mitochondria; accumulation of lipoid bodies, Golgi complexes, and vacuoles; autophagosomes; dilated fragmented rough endoplasmic reticulum
Lidocaine (2.5 mM)	Accumulation of small membrane vesicles, electron-opaque Golgi complexes, lipoid bodies; membranous sheetlike structures originating from lipoid bodies
Glucosamine (10 mM) + lidocaine (2.5 mM)	Greatly increased accumulation of membranous vacuoles, lipoid bodies, electron-opaque Golgi complexes, dilated rough endoplasmic reticulum, membranous sheets;; autophagosomes; evaginated mitochondrial membranes; membranous whorls

[a]Adapted from Friedman and Skehan, 1983.

membranes (Table IV). These changes were detected within the first 3 hr of treatment and became increasingly severe until cell lysis occurred between 24 and 48 hr. Lidocaine produced comparable membrane ultrastructural changes with a similar time course, and the use of glucosamine in combination with lidocaine accelerated and intensified these changes.

These results raised the possibility that glucosamine alone or in combination with a local anesthetic might produce membrane damage by interfering with a fundamental membrane-synthetic process such as glycosylation or lipid synthesis. Glucosamine and the glucosamine-containing antibiotic tunicamycin both are glycosylation inhibitors in a number of mammalian cells including C_6 gliomas (Friedman and Skehan, 1981; Schwarz and Datema, 1982). These drugs are known to interfere with viral glycoprotein synthesis and replication (Scholtissek, 1975; Scholtissek et al., 1975; Schwarz et al., 1979; Schwarz and Datema, 1982), and tunicamycin is reported to be selectively toxic to virally infected mammalian cells (Duksin and Bornstein, 1977; Olden et al., 1979). The use of isotopic precursors of carbohydrates and lipids to screen for biochemical synergism of glucosamine–lidocaine combinations failed to reveal inhibitory effects on the synthesis of glycoproteins, glycolipids, or lipids other than sterols that could not be explained by the actions of D-glucosamine alone. However, within the same period of time required for ultrastructural changes in cellular membranes, glucosamine inhibited the incorporation of [2-^{14}C]acetate into sterols and into an unidentified 400-dalton lipid that migrated close to sterols on thin-layer chromatograms. This inhibition was potentiated by lidocaine and increased over the same range of D-glucosamine concentrations that led to increased cell toxicity after a 48-hr treatment (Friedman and Skehan, 1980). Glucosamine alone produced a dose-dependent inhibition of sterol synthesis (Friedman and Skehan, 1978b), and all of the potentiating local anesthetic-type drugs inhibited sterol synthesis and the uptake of exogenous cholesterol (Friedman and Skehan, 1978a, 1979). These findings suggested that the critical lesion responsible for glucosamine's tumoricidal activity was damage to the endomembrane system produced by an inhibition of cholesterol biosynthesis.

How might the inhibition of cholesterol synthesis contribute to the selective tumoricidal activity of glucosamine? It is not yet known why D-glucosamine is selectively toxic to *in vivo* tumors. Normal and tumor cells may differ in their ability to take up or metabolize glucosamine, or to repair sublethal damage produced by the drug. Alternatively, they may differ either in their requirements for sterols and other metabolites generated from the cholesterol biosynthesis pathway, or in their ability to regulate these biosynthetic processes.

Cholesterol is an important structural and functional regulator of biological membranes. Through its effects on membrane fluidity and cooperativity (Oldfield and Chapman, 1972; Quinn, 1981; Shattil and Cooper, 1976; Shinitzky and Inbar, 1976; Sinensky, 1978; Wallach, 1975), cholesterol can influence a wide range of membrane, organelle, and cellular functions including transmembrane fluxes of inorganic ions, membrane electrical properties, permeability to water and small molecules, transport processes, activities of membrane-bound enzymes and receptors, endocytosis, mitochondrial respiration, cell adhesion, and cell proliferation (Alderson and Green, 1975; Alivisatos *et al.*, 1977; Baldassare *et al.*, 1979; Benz and Cross, 1978; Cavenee *et al.*, 1981; Coleman and Lavietes, 1981; Demel *et al.*, 1972; Graham and Green, 1969; Heiniger *et al.*, 1976; Jain, 1975; Kandutsch and Chen, 1977; Kutchai *et al.*, 1980; Papahadjopoulos, 1976; Sabine, 1977; Szabo, 1974; Wiley and Cooper, 1975). The multiple aberrations of membrane structure and function in tumors might arise in part from defects in the regulation of cholesterol metabolism and the interrelated pathway of dolichol-mediated glycoprotein assembly (Brown and Goldstein, 1980; Gough and Hemming, 1970; James and Kandutsch, 1979; Mills and Adamany, 1978, 1981). The absence of dietary feedback control of cholesterol biosynthesis is characteristic of a number of experimental tumors (Chen *et al.*, 1978; Coleman and Lavietes, 1981; Philippot *et al.*, 1977; Sabine, 1976; Siperstein, 1970; Wallach, 1975; Wiley and Siperstein, 1976). Cholesterol biosynthesis rates are frequently elevated in tumors, as are the levels of cholesterol and the cholesterol:phospholipid ratio in their cell and organelle membranes (Coleman and Lavietes, 1981; Fumagalli *et al.*, 1964; Wallach, 1975). These alterations might well provoke a cascade of compensatory changes in cellular respiratory metabolism and membrane function that permit the tumors to survive their cholesterol imbalance (Coleman and Lavietes, 1981).

In certain circumstances the inhibition of cholesterol biosynthesis might itself be sufficient to cause a loss of cell viability. Cellular cholesterol is derived partly

from dietary sources and partly by de novo synthesis from acetyl-CoA. If cells
are deprived of an exogenous source of cholesterol such as low-density lipopro-
tein (LDL), or are prevented from using it, the mevalonate generated at the 3-
hydroxy-3-methylglutaryl (HMG)-CoA reductase step in the biosynthetic pathway is shunted almost entirely into cholesterol biosynthesis (Brown and Goldstein, 1980) (Fig. 2). A pronounced inhibition of the pathway depletes cells both
of cholesterol and of several nonsterol metabolites such as ubiquinone and dolichol, which are produced from mevalonate and required for growth and viability
(Brown and Goldstein, 1980; Habenicht *et al.,* 1980; Kaneko *et al.,* 1978;
Quesney-Huneeus *et al.,* 1979). A reduction in membrane cholesterol can be
expected to cause pronounced changes in plasma membrane mechanical stability, surface potential, transmembrane ion fluxes, and permeability to water
(Benz and Cross, 1978; Demel *et al.,* 1972; Jain, 1975; Kutchai *et al.,* 1980;
Szabo, 1974; Wiley and Cooper, 1975). Cell death could easily result from the
attendant changes in cellular ion concentrations and/or osmotic pressure.

The inhibition of cholesterol production per se would not be important in cells
whose cholesterol requirements were satisfied by exogenously provided cholesterol. Under these conditions, de novo cholesterol biosynthesis is suppressed to
low levels and most of the mevalonate produced is preferentially shunted into
collateral nonsterol pathways for which farnesyl pyrophosphate is a direct pre-

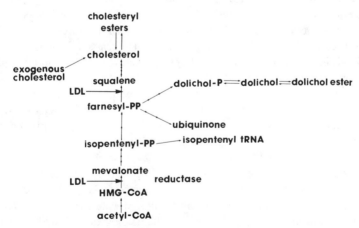

Fig. 2.   Cholesterol metabolism and interrelated pathways. HMG-CoA reductase, the major rate-
limiting enzyme of mevalonate synthesis, is regulated by a multifeedback mechanism involving
LDL-derived cholesterol [or an oxygenated metabolite (Kandutsch *et al.,* 1978)] and one or more
nonsterol products of mevalonate metabolism (Brown and Goldstein, 1980). The synthesis of cholesterol, dolichol, isopentenyl-tRNA, and ubiquinone is coordinately regulated (Brown and Goldstein,
1980; Faust *et al.,* 1979; Mills and Adamany, 1981). The heavy arrows indicate sites of feedback
inhibition by LDL.

cursor (Brown and Goldstein, 1980; Gough and Hemming, 1970). With such cells, a severe inhibition of farnesyl pyrophosphate synthesis (or of rate-limiting enzymes distal to farnesyl pyrophosphate that are involved in the synthesis of essential nonsterol metabolites) might suffice to initiate irreversible damage leading to cell death. It has been demonstrated that a pronounced impairment of dolichol synthesis and protein glycosylation occurs in cells grown in normal serum-containing medium and treated with the HMG-CoA reductase inhibitor 25-hydroxycholesterol (Mills and Adamany, 1978). Defective protein glycosylation can alter secondary and higher-order protein structures, modify their susceptibility to proteolytic cleavage, and interfere with intracellular transport and secretion of glycoproteins (Olden *et al.,* 1982; Schwarz and Datema, 1982). Studies with tunicamycin point to possible differences between normal and transformed cell responses to an inhibition of glycoprotein synthesis (Olden *et al.,* 1979). Cultured cells transformed by oncogenic viruses are selectively killed by tunicamycin while normal embryo cells or nontransformed established cell lines remain viable. The selective toxicity of the drug is proposed to result from a difference in sensitivity of normal and transformed cells to an inhibition of glucose metabolism and nutrient transport caused by tunicamycin treatment. These findings may be relevant to the observation that tunicamycin-treated B_{16} melanoma cells are unable to metastasize following iv inoculation into animal hosts (Irimura *et al.,* 1981).

In addition to its direct effects on tumor cells, glucosamine may also act *in vivo* to enhance host immune responses. Bekesi and Winzler observed that animals whose tumors regressed after high-dose glucosamine infusion were able to reject subsequent transplants of the same tumor (Bekesi and Winzler, 1970). In human cancer patients infused with doses of glucosamine that produce plasma levels equal to or greater than 4 m*M,* natural killer (NK) cell activity is significantly augmented (Matheson *et al.,* 1983). Glucosamine, at concentrations several orders of magnitude lower than required for tumoricidal activity, directly activates natural killer function of nonadherent normal peripheral blood mononuclear cells *in vitro* by a mechanism that appears to involve thymidine metabolism (Matheson *et al.,* 1984).

The effectivensss of D-glucosamine and glucosamine–anesthetic drug combinations in the therapy of human cancers remains to be established. Phase 1 clinical trials of glucosamine are currently in progress at our institution. Thus far, glucosamine has not been found to produce hematological or blood biochemical changes in any of the 13 patients tested. Preliminary clinical pharmacological studies indicate that the drug-distributional and elimination phases can be fitted to a two-compartment open-system pharmacokinetic model. The distributional phase (α) has a half-life of 12 min or less and is followed by a slower elimination phase (β) with a half-life of 1 to 2 hr (Table V). Glucosamine may be of potential benefit for the treatment of central nervous system (CNS) tumors and pleural

TABLE V

Pharmacokinetic Data from Pretrial Bolus Infusions of D-Glucosamine[a]

Patient	α[b]	$t_{1/2}\alpha$ (hr)	β	$t_{1/2}\beta$ (hr)	V1 (liters/kg)	k_{el} (hr^{-1})	Plasma clearance (k_{el} V1) (liters/kg/hr)
1	9.33	0.07	0.52	1.35	0.08	2.06	0.158
2	6.48	0.11	0.45	1.55	0.05	1.66	0.078
3	3.36	0.21	0.36	1.92	0.07	2.86	0.194
4	2.26	0.31	0.32	2.17	0.27	0.58	0.156

[a]Glucosamine was administered by infusion over a 10-min interval at a dose of 9 g/m^2. Plasma glucosamine levels were analyzed at 5, 8, 12, 16, 20, 25, 30, 60, 180, and 360 min from the start of the infusion. Pharmacokinetic data were obtained from semilog plots of plasma concentration versus time curves according to the procedure of Mitenko and Ogilvie (1972).

[b]Explanation of symbols: α, hybrid disposition rate constant for the rapid phase; $t_{1/2}\alpha$, α-phase half-life; β, hybrid disposition rate constant for the slow phase; $t_{1/2}\beta$, β-phase half-life; V1, volume of the central compartment; k_{el}, elimination rate constant.

effusions, in that intravenously infused drug appears to distribute effectively into cerebrospinal fluid (CSF) and pleural effusion fluid.

2. D-Mannosamine

Another naturally occurring amino sugar, D-mannosamine, is cytotoxic to T-cell leukemia lines but not to phytohemagglutinin (PHA)-stimulated normal T lymphocytes (Onoda et al., 1982). Its cytotoxicity is potentiated by sodium oleate. The amino sugar itself rapidly induces cell fusion in T-cell leukemia cultures, suggesting that it may act to perturb either lipid bilayer structure or ion fluxes. The effects of mannosamine and glucosamine on macromolecular synthesis are similar (Bekesi et al., 1969a; Onoda et al., 1982), although mannosamine appears to have a different membrane mode of action. In the C_6 glioma system, mannosamine toxicity was not potentiated by lidocaine, while glucosamine was devoid of fusogenic activity (S. J. Friedman and P. Skehan, unpublished observations).

B. Host Cell Protection from Cytotoxicity

Several studies in the literature suggest the possibility of using membrane-reactive natural and synthetic products to enhance the therapeutic index of conventional antitumor drugs. Kinders et al. have isolated growth-inhibitory glycopeptides from mouse cerebral cortex that are potent reversible inhibitors of protein synthesis and cell growth in normal but not transformed or tumorigenic cell lines (Kinders et al., 1980, 1982; Kinders and Johnson, 1981; McGhee et *al.*, 1983). The glycopeptides are bound by normal and transformed cells, but the latter avoid growth inhibition either by degrading the inhibitor(s) (Kinders and Johnson, 1981) or by reducing their membrane content of the ganglioside GM_1, which is required for the inhibitory effect (Kinders *et al.*, 1982). *In vitro* experiments have demonstrated the selective protection of nonmalignant cells from the cytotoxic effects of 5-bromodeoxyuridine (BUdR) (McGhee *et al.*, 1983). Using a different approach, Paterson, Cass, and co-workers have demonstrated that nitrobenzylthioinosine (NBMPR), a potent but reversible inhibitor of nucleoside transport, protects cultured cells against the antiproliferative effects of cytotoxic nucleoside analogs (reviewed in Paterson *et al.*, 1981a). The inhibitor binds tightly and reversibly to plasma membrane nucleoside transporters and blocks the entry of structurally diverse nucleosides and their synthetic analogs into cultured cells. When administered to tumor-bearing animals in the form of NBMPR-phosphate, which is converted by cellular ecto-5'-nucleotidase into NBMPR, the inhibitor protects normal tissues from the cytotoxic effects of potentially lethal doses of adenosine analogs, nebularine, toyocamycin, tubericidin, and deazauridine-Ara-C combinations (Kolassa *et al.*, 1982; Lynch *et al.*, 1981; Paterson *et al.*, 1979, 1981b). Significant antineoplastic effects were observed in animals with Ehrlich ascites tumors, colon carcinomas, and L1210 [HGPRTase⁻ (hypoxanthine-guanine phosphoribosyltransferase)] tumors when NBMPR-phosphate was used in combination with high doses of nebularine. Interestingly, the transport inhibitor not only protected normal tissues but also contributed to the observed therapeutic effects, possibly by becoming converted to a 6-thiopurine metabolite (Paterson *et al.*, 1981b). For reasons not yet understood, neoplastic cells are less sensitive to the inhibitor than normal tissues. The protective effect of NBMPR-phosphate on normal tissues correlated with their decreased ability to accumulate cytotoxic drugs (Kolassa *et al.*, 1982). The mechanism by which the inhibitor alters the tissue distribution of nucleoside drugs causing some tissues to increase and others to decrease their uptake may be due to tissue differences in the conversion of NBMPR-phosphate to its active form, in the kinetic characteristics of nucleoside transport, or in the rates of NBMPR-insensitive nucleoside transport (Kolassa *et al.*, 1982).

C. Surface Galactosyltransferase Acceptors

Podolsky *et al.* have reported the presence of a low molecular weight galactosyltransferase acceptor in human malignant effusions that selectively inhibits the growth of *in vitro*-transformed cells and virally induced solid tumor in hamsters (Podolsky and Isselbacher, 1982; Podolsky *et al.*, 1983). The cancer-associated galactosyltransferase acceptor (CAGA) preferentially inhibits the incorporation of sugars into acid-precipitable cellular material in CAGA-sensitive cells, and to a much lesser extent produces a delayed inhibition of protein and nucleic acid synthesis. CAGA requires both carbohydrate and peptide portions of the molecule and possibly cellular internalization for its activity. Both transformed and nontransformed cells bind CAGA, but there are quantitative differences in binding capacity. This and events subsequent to binding may be important for its tumoricidal effects.

D. Targeted Drug Delivery

The cell surface can bind a wide array of extracellular molecules and can form adhesive associations with a variety of multimolecular surfaces. Some of these associations possess a high degree of target specificity. Antibodies bind to specific antigens, lectins to a narrow spectrum of carbohydrate mono- or oligosaccharides, and hormones to specific binding sites.

These differential affinities constitute a recognition mechanism and provide a theoretical basis for selective chemotherapy by targeted drug delivery (Edwards and Thorpe, 1981; Widder et al., 1979). Cytotoxic drugs incorporated into antibody, lectin, hormone, liposome, or microsphere carriers can in principle be preferentially delivered to an in vivo target cell population such as a tumor for which the carrier has a particularly high affinity. During neoplastic progression, transformed cells gradually accumulate extensive alterations in their surface composition. Both quantitative and qualitative changes are common in the surface concentrations of proteins, glycoproteins, glycosaminoglycans, phospholipids, glycolipids, sphingolipids, and sterols (Wallach, 1975; Table I). In addition, there frequently occur changes in the degree of glycosylation, phosphorylation, and sulfation of particular surface molecular species. To the extent that one of these changes increases a tumor cell's affinity for a carrier vehicle significantly above that of normal host tissues, it becomes a potential attack point for targeted drug delivery.

In practice, drug targeting has encountered a number of obstacles. Among the most important of these is the very neoplastic progression process that creates tumor cell surface alterations in the first place. Neoplastic progression operates independently in each cell within a tumor population (Foulds, 1969; Prehn, 1976). Thus, as time passes different cells experience different phenotypic alterations and speciate into microevolutionarily distinct lineages. By the time they reach clinically detectable size, most tumors contain multiple subpopulations that differ from one another—often qualitatively—in their surface composition and therefore binding affinities for drug-targeting vehicles (Dalianis et al., 1979; Kerbel, 1979; Miller and Heppner, 1979; Olsson and Ebbesen, 1979; Prehn, 1970). Successful destruction of subpopulations with a high affinity for a carrier vehicle will temporarily reduce tumor burden. But it will also stimulate the rapid growth of surviving low-affinity subpopulations by reducing tumor burden and therefore mass inhibition of growth (DeWys, 1972; Gorelik et al., 1981; Ketcham et al., 1961; Miller et al., 1980; Schatten, 1958; Simpson-Herren et al., 1977). The surviving subpopulations will tend to be refractory to the original treatment (Goldin and Johnson, 1977; Kerbel, 1979; Olssen and Ebbeson, 1979). The use of highly target-specific vehicles—such as monoclonal antibodies directed against a single antigenic determinant—is therefore unlikely to be capable of eradicating entire tumor populations in the absence of other therapeutic measures.

Several additional obstacles to successful target drug delivery have been encountered. The reticuloendothelial system sequesters and degrades macromolecular carriers, thereby reducing the cytotoxin available for reaction with tumors (Souhami et al., 1981; Widder et al., 1979). Efforts to overcome this nonspecific blockade have not yet been successful (Souhami et al., 1981). Carriers are subject to degradation by plasma enzymes, can have difficulty crossing endothelial barriers to gain access to tumor tissue, and are not always sufficiently selective to distinguish effectively between normal and neoplastic target cells (Widder et al., 1979).

Targeted drug delivery may prove particularly useful in the management of metastasis. With many tumors, general metastases are not formed by cells that have migrated directly from a primary mass, but instead are seeded by cells that have colonized a small handful of special tissues, particularly reticuloendothelial tissues that serve as generalizing sites for metastatic dispersal (Bross and Blumenson, 1976; De Baetselier et al., 1981). Thus, the propensity for reticuloendothelial tissues to sequester carriers may be therapeutically advantageous.

E. Macrophage-Mediated Tumor Cell Killing

When treated with macrophage-activating factor (MAF), bacterial endotoxin, or certain serum factors, macrophages acquire the ability to kill tumor cells selectively in vitro (Cameron and Churchill, 1979; Chapman and Hibbs, 1977; Fidler, 1978; Hibbs et al., 1972, 1977, 1978; Hibbs, 1973). Activated macrophages are tumoricidal toward a broad spectrum of transformed cells, and the effect operates across the species barrier (reviewed in Hibbs et al., 1978). Tumor cell killing requires close contact between target and effector cells and is nonphagocytic. The mechanism by which macrophages recognize tumor cells is not known, but presumably involves a membrane phenotypic change that occurs with high frequency in many types of cells undergoing neoplastic progression.

The acquisition of tumoricidal activity is the result of a complex differentiative process (Hibbs et al., 1977). It is regulated by microenvironmental chemical signals, and is thought to involve progressive changes in the physical properties of the macrophage plasma membrane (Chapman and Hibbs, 1977, 1978; Hibbs et al., 1978). The final stage in the maturation process is the transformation of nontumoricidal activated macrophages into killer cells. This step can be reversibly blocked by exposing the macrophages to plasma lipoproteins or by elevating their membrane cholesterol content with cholesterol-rich liposomes (Chapman and Hibbs, 1977). These treatments cause tumoricidal macrophages to lose their antitumor activity, as does protease exposure (Chapman and Hibbs, 1977).

Macrophages appear to be recruited to sites of neoplastic growth, and in some (but not all) experimental tumors their presence in large numbers within the tumor is associated with decreased metastatic activity (Alexander, 1976; Birbeck and Carter, 1972; Eccles and Alexander, 1974a,b; Gershon et al., 1967). Tumors that are depleted of macrophages prior to host transplantation tend to exhibit metastatic enhancement (Wood and Gillespie, 1975). Conversely, poorly metastatic tumors show increased metastatic activity when transplanted into macrophage-defective hosts (Nicholson et al., 1982). The presence of large numbers of activated macrophage within a tumor does not ensure its destruction, however (Eccles and Alexander, 1974a; Evans, 1972), since tumors appear to be able to condition their environment with factors that suppress the tumoricidal activation step (Hibbs et al., 1978; Spitalny and North, 1977) and may also be able to inhibit directly the expression of tumoricidal activity by transferring cholesterol into membranes of macrophages with which they come into contact (Chapman and Hibbs, 1977). Macrophages isolated from experimental tumor tissue have been found to be reversibly inactivated, but can be triggered to become tumoricidal in vitro in the presence of suitable activators (Russell et al., 1977). The intravenous injection of liposomes containing macrophage activators such as MAF or muramyl dipeptide into tumor-bearing mice inhibits tumor growth and metastatic spread and prolongs the life span of the treated animals (Fidler, 1980; Fidler et al., 1981; Schroit and Fidler, 1982), suggesting the potential usefulness of liposome-encapsulated macrophage activators for antimetastatic therapy in humans.

All tumors are not equally sensitive to macrophage-mediated killing (Roder et al., 1979; Wiltrout et al., 1982), and even variants within a single tumor population may exhibit vastly different sensitivities (Miner et al., 1982; Miner and Nicholson, 1983). From studies on tumor cell susceptibility to humoral and cell-mediated killing (Schlager et al., 1978; Schlager and Ohanian, 1979, 1980; Schlager, 1982), it appears that tumors can modify their membrane lipid composition to prevent triggering of the lytic process or to repair sublethal damage produced by interaction with immune effectors.

III. SUMMARY

Available evidence suggests that most cancers arise not from primary lesions in cell growth-regulatory machinery, but from an alteration in the surface recognition process that mediates the mass inhibition of growth. Tumors behave as if they were new types of tissues with unique surface-recognitive determinants that enable them to function independently of surrounding normal tissues. Thus, in many cases cancer may be a disease of tissue neogenesis. Within these new tissue growths, clonal diversification proceeds at a rapid rate and creates subpopulations that are antigenically heterogeneous, drug resistant, and metastatic. Therapeutic intervention in this process requires knowledge of the cellular mechanisms that give rise to tumor cell heterogeneity and promote metastatic dissemination of cells from the primary tumor. Targeted drug delivery systems, which are preferentially taken up by some tissues reported to serve as generalizing sites, may prove to be useful for eradicating tumor cells lodged in these tissues either directly or through tumoricidally activated macrophages.

Selective toxicity, which has been so successfully achieved in antimicrobial therapy, continues to present a challenge for cancer therapists. Tumor cell membranes are potentially important targets for selective chemotherapeutic attack. These are abnormal both structurally and functionally and must be considered to play a fundamental role as mediators of the abnormal cell interactions that characterize malignant behavior. The existence of membrane-active drugs and tumoricidal macrophages that are selectively toxic to tumors suggests that membrane defects common to a broad spectrum of tumors exist and can be therapeutically exploited. The development of therapies that are capable of selectively perturbing tumor cell membranes is still in its infancy. Further research is needed to elucidate the functional consequences of structural and conformational changes in cell membrane molecules to permit the development of new classes of selectively toxic antitumor drugs.

REFERENCES

Alderson, J. C. E., and Green, C. (1975). Enrichment of lymphocytes with cholesterol and its effect on lymphocyte activation. *FEBS Lett.* **52**, 208–211.

Alexander, P. (1976). Dormant metastases which manifest on immunosuppression and the role of macrophages in tumours. *In* "Fundamental Aspects of Metastasis" (L. Weiss, ed.), pp. 227–239. North-Holland Publ., Amsterdam.

Alitalo, K., and Vahari, A. (1982). Pericellular matrix in malignant transformation. *Adv. Cancer Res.* **37**, 111–158.

Alivisatos, S., Papastavrou, C., Drouka-Liapati, E., Molyvdas, A., and Nikitopoulou, G. (1977). Enzymatic and electrophysiological changes of the function of membrane proteins by cholesterol. *Biochem. Biophys. Res. Commun.* **79**, 677–683.

Baldassare, J. J., Saito, Y., and Silbert, D. F. (1979). Effect of sterol depletion on LM cell sterol mutants. *J. Biol. Chem.* **254**, 1108–1113.

Ball, J. A., Wick, A. N., and Sanders, C. (1957). Influence of glucose antimetabolites on the Walker Tumor. *Cancer Res.* **17**, 235–239.

Bekesi, J. G., and Winzler, R. J. (1970). Inhibitory effects of D-glucosamine on the growth of Walker 256 carcinosarcoma and protein, RNA, and DNA synthesis. *Cancer Res.* **30**, 2905–2912.

Bekesi, J. G., Bekesi, E., and Winzler, R. J. (1969a). Inhibitory effect of D-glucosamine and other sugars on the biosynthesis of protein, ribonucleic acid, and deoxyribonucleic acid in normal and neoplastic tissues. *J. Biol. Chem.* **244**, 3766–3772.

Bekesi, J. G., Molnar, Z., and Winzler, R. J. (1969b). Inhibitory effect of D-glucosamine and other sugar analogs on the viability and transplantibility of ascites tumor cells. *Cancer Res.* **29**, 353–359.

Benz, R., and Cross, D. (1978). Influence of sterols on ion transport through lipid bilayer membranes. *Biochim. Biophys. Acta* **506**, 265–280.

Birbeck, M. S. C., and Carter, R. L. (1972). Observations on the ultrastructure of two hamster lymphomas with particular reference to infiltrating macrophages. *Int. J. Cancer* **9**, 249–257.

Boynton, A. L., McKeehan, W. L., and Whitfield, J. F., eds. (1982). "Ions, Cell Proliferation, and Cancer." Academic Press, New York.

Bross, I. D. J., and Blumenson, L. E. (1976). Metastatic sites that produce generalized cancer: Identification and kinetics of the generalizing sites. In "Fundamental Aspects of Metastasis" (L. Weiss, ed.), pp. 359–375. North-Holland Publ., Amsterdam.

Brown, M. S., and Goldstein, J. L. (1980). Multivalent feedback regulation of HMG Co A reductase, a control mechanism coordinating isoprenoid synthesis and cell growth. *J. Lipid Res.* **21**, 505–517.

Cameron, D. J., and Churchill, W. H. (1979). Cytotoxicity of human macrophages for tumor cells. *J. Clin. Invest.* **63**, 977–984.

Carraway, C. A. C., Jung, G., and Carraway, K. L. (1983). Isolation of actin-containing transmembrane complexes from ascites adenocarcinoma sublines having mobile and immobile receptors. *Proc. Natl. Acad. Sci. U.S.A.* **80**, 430–434.

Cavenee, W. K., Chen, H. W., and Kandutsch, A. A. (1981). Cell-substratum and cell-monolayer adhesion are dependent upon cellular cholesterol biosynthesis. *Exp. Cell Res.* **131**, 31–40.

Chapman, H. A., and Hibbs, J. B. (1977). Modulation of macrophage tumoricidal capability by components of normal serum: A central role for lipid. *Science* **197**, 282–285.

Chapman, H. A., and Hibbs, J. B. (1978). Modulation of macrophage tumoricidal capability by polyene antibiotics: Support for membrane lipid as a regulatory determinant of macrophage function. *Proc. Natl. Acad. Sci. U.S.A.* **75**, 4349–4353.

Chen, H. W., Kandutsch, A. A., and Heiniger, H. J. (1978). The role of cholesterol in malignancy. *Prog. Exp. Tumor Res.* **22**, 275–316.

Coleman, P. S., and Lavietes, B. B. (1981). Membrane cholesterol, tumorigenesis, and the biochemical phenotype of neoplasia. *CRC Crit. Rev. Biochem.* **11**, 341–393.

Dalianis, T., Klein, G., and Andersson, B. (1979). Selection of a low antigenic variant subline from the TA3St ascites carcinoma by repeated passage of antibody-coated cells through anti-immunoglobulin columns. *JNCI, J. Natl. Cancer Inst.* **63**, 383–388.

De Baetselier, P., Gorelik, E., Eshhar, Z., Ron, Y., Katzav, S., Feldman, M., and Segal, S. (1981). Metastatic properties conferred on non-metastatic tumors by hybridization of spleen B-lymphocytes with plasmacytoma cells. *JNCI, J. Natl. Cancer Inst.* **67**, 1079–1086.

Demel, R. A., Bruckdorfer, K. R., and Van Deenen, L. L. M. (1972). The effect of sterol structure on the permeability of liposomes to glucose, glycerol and Rb+. *Biochim. Biophys. Acta* **255**, 321–330.

DeWys, W. D. (1972). Studies correlating the growth rate of a tumor and its metastases and providing evidence for tumor-related systemic growth-retarding factors. *Cancer Res.* **32**, 374–379.

Duksin, D., and Bornstein, P. (1977). Changes in surface properties of normal and transformed cells caused by tunicamycin, an inhibitor of protein glycosylation. *Proc. Natl. Acad. Sci. U.S.A.* **74,** 3433–3437.

Eccles, S. A., and Alexander, P. (1974a). Macrophage content of tumours in relation to metastatic spread and host immune reaction. *Nature (London)* **250,** 667–669.

Eccles, S. A., and Alexander, P. (1974b). Sequestration of macrophages in growing tumors and its effect on the immunological capacity of the host. *Br. J. Cancer* **30,** 42–49.

Edwards, D. C., and Thorpe, P. E. (1981). Targeting toxins—the retiarian approach to chemotherapy. *Trends Biochem. Sci.* **6,** 313–316.

Evans, R. (1972). Macrophages in syngeneic animal tumours. *Transplantation* **14,** 468–473.

Farber, E., and Cameron R. (1980). The sequential analysis of cancer development. *Adv. Cancer Res.* **31,** 125–226.

Faust, J. R., Goldstein, J. L., and Brown, M. S. (1979). Synthesis of ubiquinone and cholesterol in human fibroblasts: Regulation of a branched pathway. *Arch. Biochem. Biophys.* **192,** 86–99.

Fidler, I. J. (1978). Recognition and destruction of target cells by tumoricidal macrophages. *Isr. J. Med. Sci.* **14,** 177–191.

Fidler, I. J. (1980). Therapy of spontaneous metastases by intravenous injection of liposomes containing lymphokines. *Science* **208,** 1469–1471.

Fidler, I. J., Sone, S., Fogler, W. E., and Barnes, Z. L. (1981). Eradication of spontaneous metastases and activation of alveolar macrophages by intravenous injection of liposomes containing muramyl dipeptide. *Proc. Natl. Acad. Sci. U.S.A.* **78,** 1680–1684.

Foulds, L. (1969). "Neoplastic Development." Academic Press, New York.

Friedman, S. J., and Skehan, P. (1978a). Anesthetics inhibit sterol metabolism in glioma cells. *J. Cell Biol.* **79,** 240a.

Friedman, S. J., and Skehan, P. (1978b). Membrane effects of D-glucosamine. *In Vitro* **14,** 336.

Friedman, S. J., and Skehan, P. (1979). The inhibition of sterol synthesis by anesthetics. *FEBS Lett.* **102,** 235–240.

Friedman, S. J., and Skehan, P. (1980). Membrane-active drugs potentiate the killing of tumor cells by D-glucosamine. *Proc. Natl. Acad. Sci. U.S.A.* **77,** 1172–1176.

Friedman, S. J., and Skehan, P. (1981). Malignancy and the cell surface. *In* "The Transformed Cell" (I. L. Cameron and T. B. Pool, eds.), pp. 67–133. Academic Press, New York.

Friedman, S. J., and Skehan, P. (1983). Membrane-active drugs in cancer chemotherapy: Cellular mechanisms. *Proc. 13th Int. Cong. Chemother., Vienna* Pt. 284, 44–47.

Fumagalli, R., Grossi, E., Paoletti, P., and Paoletti, R. (1964). Studies on lipids in brain tumours. I. Occurrence and significance of sterol precursors of cholesterol in human brain tumours. *J. Neurochem.* **11,** 561–565.

Gershon, R. K., Carter, R. L., and Lane, N. J. (1967). Studies on homotransplantable lymphomas in hamsters. IV. Observations on macrophages in the expression of tumor immunity. *Am. J. Pathol.* **51,** 1111–1133.

Goldin, A., and Johnson, R. K. (1977). Resistance to antitumor agents. *In* "Recent Advances in Cancer Treatment" (H. J. Tagnon and M. J. Staquet, eds.), pp. 155–169. Raven, New York.

Gorelik, E., Segal, S., and Feldman, M. (1981). On the mechanism of tumor "concomitant immunity." *Int. J. Cancer* **27,** 847–856.

Gough, D. P., and Hemming, F. W. (1970). The characterization and stereochemistry of biosynthesis of dolichols in rat liver. *Biochem. J.* **118,** 163–166.

Graham, J. M., and Green, C. (1969). The binding of hormones and related compounds by normal and cholesterol-depleted plasma membranes of rat liver. *Biochem. Pharmacol.* **18,** 493–502.

Habenicht, A. J. R., Glomset, J. A., and Ross, R. (1980). Relation of cholesterol and mevalonic acid to the cell cycle in smooth muscle and Swiss 3T3 cells stimulated to divide by platelet-derived growth factor. *J. Biol. Chem.* **255**, 5134–5140.

Hakomori, S. I. (1981). Glycosphingolipids in cellular interactions, differentiation and oncogenesis. *Annu. Rev. Biochem.* **50**, 733–764.

Hatanaka, M. (1974). Transport of sugars in tumor cell membranes. *Biochim. Biophys. Acta* **355**, 77–104.

Heiniger, H. J., Kandutsch, A. A., and Chen, H. W. (1976). Depletion of L-cell sterol depresses endocytosis. *Nature (London)* **263**, 515–517.

Helson, L., Helson, C., Sordillo, P., and Skehan, P. (1979). Inhibition of human neuroblastoma cells by D-glucosamine and papaverine. *Proc. Am. Assoc. Cancer Res.* **20**, 248.

Herberman, R. B. (1977). Immunogenicity of tumor antigens. *Biochim. Biophys. Acta* **473**, 93–119.

Hibbs, J. B. (1973). Macrophage nonimmunologic recognition: Target cell factors related to contact inhibition. *Science* **180**, 868–870.

Hibbs, J. B., Lambert, L. H., and Remington, J. S. (1972). Possible role of macrophage mediated nonspecific cytotoxicity in tumour resistance. *Nature (London), New Biol.* **235**, 48–50.

Hibbs, J. B., Taintor, R. R., Chapman, H. A., and Weinberg, J. B. (1977). Macrophage tumor killing: Influence of the local environment. *Science* **197**, 279–282.

Hibbs, J. B., Chapman, H. A., and Weinberg, J. B. (1978). The macrophage as an antineoplastic surveillance cell: Biological perspectives. *J. Reticuloendothel. Soc.* **24**, 549–570.

Hynes, R. O. (1976). Cell surface proteins and malignant transformation. *Biochim. Biophys. Acta* **458**, 73–107.

Hynes, R. O., ed. (1979). "Surface of Normal and Malignant Cells." Wiley, New York.

Irimura, T., Gonzalez, R., and Nicolson, G. L. (1981). Effects of tunicamycin on B16 metastatic melanoma cell surface glycoproteins and blood-borne arrest and survival properties. *Cancer Res.* **41**, 3411–3418.

Jain, M. K. (1975). Role of cholesterol in biomembranes and related systems. *Curr. Top. Membr. Transp.* **6**, 1–57.

James, M. J., and Kandutsch, A. A. (1979). Interrelationships between dolichol and sterol synthesis in mammalian cell cultures. *J. Biol. Chem.* **254**, 8442–8446.

Kandutsch, A. A., and Chen, H. W. (1977). Consequences of blocked sterol synthesis in cultured cells: DNA synthesis and membrane composition. *J. Biol. Chem.* **252**, 409–415.

Kandutsch, A. A., Chen, H. W., and Heiniger, H. J. (1978). Biological activity of some oxygenated sterols. *Science* **201**, 498–501.

Kaneko, I., Hazama-Shimada, Y., and Endo, A. (1978). Inhibitory effects on lipid metabolism in cultured cells of ML-236B, a potent inhibitor of 3-hydroxy-3-methyl-glutaryl-coenzyme A reductase. *Eur. J. Biochem.* **87**, 313–321.

Kerbel, R. S. (1979). Implications of immunological heterogeneity of tumours. *Nature (London)* **280**, 358–360.

Ketcham, A. S., Kinsey, D. L., Wexler, H., and Mantel, N. (1961). The development of spontaneous metastases after the removal of a primary tumor. *Cancer* **14**, 875–881.

Kinders, R. J., and Johnson, T. C. (1981). Glycopeptides prepared from mouse cerebrum inhibit protein synthesis and cell division in baby hamster kidney cells, but not in their polyoma virus-transformed analogs. *Exp. Cell Res.* **136**, 31–41.

Kinders, R. J., Milenkovic, A. G., Nordin, P., and Johnson, T. C. (1980). Characterization of cell-surface glycopeptides from mouse cerebral cortex that inhibit cell growth and protein synthesis. *Biochim. J.* **190**, 605–614.

Kinders, R. J., Rintoul, D. A., and Johnson, T. C. (1982). Ganglioside GM1 sensitizes tumor cells to growth inhibitory glycopeptides. *Biochem. Biophys. Res. Commun.* **107**, 663–669.

Klein, G., and Klein, E. (1977). Immune surveillance against virus-induced tumors and nonrejectability of spontaneous tumors: Contrasting consequences of host versus tumor evolution. *Proc. Natl. Acad. Sci. U.S.A.* **74,** 2121–2125.

Kolassa, N., Jakobs, E. S., Buzzell, G. R., and Paterson, A. R. P. (1982). Manipulation of toxicity and tissue distribution of tubericidin in mice by nitrobenzylthioinosine-5'-monophosphate. *Biochem. Pharmacol.* **31,** 1863–1874.

Kreider, J. W., and Bartlett, G. L. (1981). The Shope papilloma–carcinoma complex of rabbits: A model system of neoplastic progression and spontaneous regression. *Adv. Cancer Res.* **35,** 81–110.

Krug, E., Dussaulx, E., Roxen, R., Griglio, S., de Gasquet, P., and Zweibaum, A. (1983). D-Glucosamine-induced increase of the glycerol-containing lipids in growing cultures of human malignant epithelial cells. *JNCI, J. Natl. Cancer Inst.* **70,** 57–61.

Kutchai, H., Cooper, R. A., and Forster, R. E. (1980). The effects of anesthetic alcohols and alterations in the level of membrane cholesterol. *Biochim. Biophys. Acta* **600,** 542–552.

Lamont, J. T. (1982). Glycosyltransferases in fetal, neonatal, and adult colon: Relationship to differentiation. *In* "The Glycoconjugates" (M. I. Horwitz, ed.), Vol. III, pp. 187–195. Academic Press, New York.

Levine, A. J. (1982). Transformation-associated tumor antigens. *Adv. Cancer Res.* **37,** 75–109.

Lichtman, M. A., and Weed, R. I. (1976). Cellular deformability of normal and leukemic hematopoietic cells: A determinant of marrow and vascular egress. *In* "Fundamental Aspects of Metastasis" (L. Weiss, ed.), pp. 319–325. North-Holland Publ., Amsterdam.

Lindner, J., Schweinitz, H. A., and Becker, K. (1960). Über die geschwulsthemmende Wirkung von Grundsubstanzbestandteilen. II. Mitteilung Stoffwechseluntersuchugen. *Klin. Wochenschr.* **38,** 763–768.

Lynch, T. P., Paran, J. H., and Paterson, A. R. P. (1981). Therapy of mouse leukemia L1210 with combinations of nebularine and nitrobenzylthioinosine-5'-monophosphate. *Cancer Res.* **41,** 560–565.

McGhee, J. E., Johnson, B., Kinders, R., and Johnson, T. C. (1983). Selective protection of nonmalignant cells by a novel cell surface glycopeptide. *Cancer Res.* **43,** 2015–2017.

Matheson, D. S., Green, B. J., and Friedman, S. J. (1984). The effects of D-glucosamine on human natural killer activity *in vitro. J. Biol. Resp. Modif.* **3,** 345–453.

Matheson, D. S., Wong, E., Green, B. J., Van Olm, M., and Friedman, S. J. (1983). Effect of D-glucosamine on human natural killer cell activity. *Proc. 13th Int. Cong. Chemother., Vienna* Pt. 265, 32–35.

Miller, F. R., and Heppner, G. H. (1979). Immunologic heterogeneity of tumor cell subpopulations from a single mouse mammary tumor. *JNCI, J. Natl. Cancer Inst.* **63,** 1457–1463.

Miller, B. E., Miller, F. R., Leith, J., and Heppner, G. H. (1980). Growth interaction in vivo between tumor subpopulations derived from a single mouse mammary tumor. *Cancer Res.* **40,** 3977–3981.

Mills, J. T., and Adamany, A. M. (1978). Impairment of dolichyl saccharide synthesis and dolichol-mediated glycoprotein assembly in the aortic smooth muscle cell in culture by inhibitors of cholesterol biosynthesis. *J. Biol. Chem.* **253,** 5270–5273.

Mills, J. T., and Adamany, A. M. (1981). The role of phosphorylated dolichols in membrane glycoprotein biosynthesis: Relation to cholesterol biosynthesis. *Int. Rev. Cytol.* **73,** 104–147.

Miner, K. M, and Nicolson, G. L. (1983). Differences in the sensitivities of murine metastatic lymphoma/lymphosarcoma variants to macrophage-mediated cytolysis and/or cytostasis. *Cancer Res.* **43,** 2063–2067.

Miner, K. M., Klostergaard, J., Granger, G. A., and Nicolson, G. L. (1982). Differences in cytotoxic effects of activated murine peritoneal macrophages and J774 monocytic cells on metastatic variants of B16 melanoma. *JNCI, J. Natl. Cancer Inst.* **70,** 717–724.

Mitenko, P. A., and Ogilvie, R. I. (1972). Rapidly achieved plasma concentration plateaus, with observations on theophylline kinetics. *Clin. Pharmacol. Ther.* **13,** 329–335.

Molnar, Z., and Bekesi, J. G. (1972). Cytotoxic effects of D-glucosamine on the ultrastructure of normal and neoplastic tissues *in vivo. Cancer Res.* **32,** 756–765.

Nicolson, G. L. (1976a). Transmembrane control of the receptors on normal and tumor cells. I. Cytoplasmic influence over cell surface components. *Biochim. Biophys. Acta* **457,** 57–108.

Nicolson, G. L. (1976b). Transmembrane control of the receptors on normal and tumor cells. II. Surface changes associated with transformation and malignancy. *Biochim. Biophys. Acta* **458,** 1–72.

Nicolson, G. L. (1982). Cancer metastasis. Organ colonization and the cell surface properties of malignant cells. *Biochim. Biophys. Acta* **695,** 114–176.

Nicolson, G. L., Mascali, J. J., and McGuire, E. J. (1982). Metastatic RAW 117 lymphosarcoma as a model for malignant-normal cell interactions. *Oncodev. Biol. Med.* **4,** 149–159.

Olden, K., Pratt, R. M., and Yamada, K. M. (1979). Selective cytotoxicity of tunicamycin for transformed cells. *Int. J. Cancer* **24,** 60–66.

Olden, K., Parent, J. B., and White, S. L. (1982). Carbohydrate moieties of glycoproteins. A reevaluation of their function. *Biochim. Biophys. Acta* **650,** 209–232.

Oldfield, E., and Chapman D. (1972). Dynamics of lipids in membranes. Heterogeneity and the role of cholesterol. *FEBS Lett.* **23,** 285–297.

Olsson, L., and Ebbesen, P. (1979). Natural polyclonality of spontaneous AKR leukemia and its consequences for so-called specific immunotherapy. *JNCI, J. Natl. Cancer Inst.* **62,** 623–627.

Onoda, T., Morikawa, S., Harada, T., Suzuki, Y., Inoue, K., and Nishigami, K. (1982). Antitumor acticity of D-mannosamine in vitro: Different sensitivities among human leukemia cell lines possessing T-cell properties. *Cancer Res.* **42,** 2867–2871.

Papahadjopoulos, D. (1976). The role of cholesterol as a membrane component: Effects on lipid-protein interactions. *Lipids* **1,** 187–196.

Pardee, A. B. (1975). The cell surface and fibroblast proliferation. Some current research trends. *Biochim. Biophys. Acta* **417,** 153–172.

Paterson, A. R. P., Jakobs, E. S., Lauzon, G. J., and Weinstein, W. M. (1979). Drug sequence-dependent toxicity and small bowel mucosal injury in mice treated with low doses of 3-deazauridine and 1-β-D-arabinofuranosylcytosine. *Cancer Res.* **39,** 2216–2219.

Paterson, A. R. P., Kolassa, N., and Cass, C. E. (1981a). Transport of nucleoside drugs in animal cells. *Pharmacol. Ther.* **12,** 515–536.

Paterson, A. R. P., Kolassa, N., Lynch, T. P., Jakobs, E. S., and Cass, C. E. (1981b). In vitro studies with an inhibitor of nucleoside treatment, nitrobenzylthioinosine-5′-monophosphate. *In* "Nucleosides in Cancer Treatment" (M. H. N. Tattersall and R. M. Fox, eds.), pp. 84–95. Academic Press, New York.

Philippot, J. R., Cooper, A. G., and Wallach, D. F. H. (1977). Regulation of cholesterol biosynthesis by normal and leukemic (L2C) guinea pig lymphocytes. *Proc. Natl. Acad. Sci. U.S.A.* **74,** 956–960.

Plagemann, P. G. W., and Erbe, J. (1973). Transport and metabolism of D-glucosamine by cultured Novikoff rat hepatoma cells and effects on nucleotide pools. *Cancer Res.* **33,** 482–492.

Podolsky, D. K., and Isselbacher, K. J. (1982). Transformation-specific cell killing by a cancer-associated galactosyltransferase acceptor and cellular binding. *Biochem. J.* **208,** 249–259.

Podolsky, D. K., Fournier, D., and Isselbacher, K. J. (1983). Inhibition of carbohydrate incorporation in transformed cells by a cancer-associated galactosyltransferase acceptor (CAGA). *J. Cell Physiol.* **115,** 23–30.

Poste, G. (1977). The cell surface and metastasis. *In* "Cancer Invasion and Metastasis: Biologic

Mechanisms and Therapy'' (S. B. Day, W. P. Laird Myers, M. G. Lewis, P. Stansly, and S. Garattini, eds.), pp. 19–47. Raven, New York.

Prehn, R. T. (1970). Analysis of antigenic heterogeneity within individual 3-methylcholanthrene-induced mouse sarcomas. *JNCI, J. Natl. Cancer Inst.* **45,** 1039–1045.

Prehn, R. T. (1976). Tumor progression and homeostasis. *Adv. Cancer Res.* **23,** 203–236.

Quastel, J. H., and Cantero, A. (1953). Inhibition of tumor growth by D-glucosamine. *Nature (London)* **171,** 252–254.

Quesney-Huneeus, V., Wiley, M. H., and Siperstein, M. D. (1979). Essential role of mevalonate synthesis in DNA replication. *Proc. Natl. Acad. Sci. U.S.A.* **76,** 5056–5060.

Quinn, P. J. (1981). The fluidity of cell membranes and its regulation. *Prog. Biophys. Mol. Biol.* **38,** 1–104.

Roder, J. C., Lohmann-Matthes, M. L., Domzig, W., Kiessling, R., and Haller, O. (1979). A functional comparison of tumor killing by activated macrophages and natural killer cells. *Eur. J. Immunol.* **9,** 283–288.

Ruoslahti, E. (1981). Cell-matrix tissue interactions in development and neoplasia. *Oncodevel. Biol. Med.* **2,** 295–303.

Russell, S. W., Doe, W. F., and McIntosh, A. T. (1977). Functional characterization of a stable, noncytolytic stage of macrophage activation in tumors. *J. Exp. Med.* **146,** 1511–1520.

Sabine, J. R. (1976). Progressive loss of cellular metabolic controls during hepatic carcinogenesis. *In* ''Control Mechanisms in Cancer'' (W. E. Criss, T. Ono, and J. R. Sabine, eds.), pp. 351–361. Raven, New York.

Sabine, J. R. (1977). ''Cholesterol.'' Dekker, New York.

Sato, H., Khato, J., Sato, T., and Suzuki, M. (1977). Deformability and filtrability of tumor cells through nucleopore filter with reference to viability and metastatic spread. *Gann. Monogr. Cancer Res.* **20,** 3–13.

Schatten, W. E. (1958). An experimental study of postoperative tumor metastases. *Cancer* **11,** 455–459.

Schlager, S. I. (1982). Ability of tumor cells to resist humoral versus cell-mediated immune attack is controlled by different membrane physical properties. *Biochim. Biophys. Res. Commun.* **106,** 58–64.

Schlager, S. I., and Ohanian, S. H. (1979). Physico-chemical properties of tumor cells that influence their susceptibility to humoral immune killing. *Biochem. Biophys. Res. Commun.* **91,** 1512–1520.

Schlager, S. I., and Ohanian, S. H. (1980). Modulation of tumor cell susceptibility to humoral immune killing through chemical and physical manipulation of cellular lipid and fatty acid composition. *J. Immunol.* **125,** 1196–1200.

Schlager, S. I., Ohanian, S. H., and Borsos, T. (1978). Identification of lipids associated with the ability of tumor cells to resist humoral immune attack. *J. Immunol.* **120,** 472–480.

Scholtissek, C. (1975). Inhibition of the multiplication of enveloped viruses by glucose derivatives. *Curr. Top. Microbiol. Immunol.* **70,** 101–119.

Scholtissek, C., Rott, R., and Klenk, H. D. (1975). Two different mechanisms of the inhibition of the multiplication of enveloped viruses by D-glucosamine. *Virology* **63,** 191–200.

Schroit, A. J., and Fidler, I. J. (1982). Stimulation of macrophage-mediated destruction of tumor cells by liposomes containing a lipophilic derivative of muramyl dipeptide. *In* ''Current Concepts in Human Immunology and Cancer Immunomodulation'' (B. Serrou, C. Rosenfeld, J. C. Daniels, and J. P. Saunders, eds.), pp. 631–637. Elsevier, Amsterdam.

Schwarz, R. T., and Datema, R. (1982). Inhibition of lipid-dependent glycosylation. *In* ''The Glycoconjugates'' (M. I. Horowitz, ed.), Vol. III, Part A, pp. 47–79. Academic Press, New York.

Schwarz, R. T., Schmidt, M. F. G., and Datema, R. (1979). Inhibition of glycosylation of viral glycoproteins. *Trans. Biochem. Soc.* **7**, 322–325.

Shattil, S. J., and Cooper, R. A. (1976). Membrane microviscosity and human platelet function. *Biochemistry* **15**, 4832–4837.

Shinitzky, M., and Inbar, M. (1976). Microviscosity parameters and protein mobility in biological membranes. *Biochim. Biophys. Acta* **433**, 133–149.

Simpson-Herren, L., Springer, T. A., Sanford, A. H., and Holmquist, J. P. (1977). Kinetics of metastases in experimental tumors. *Progr. Cancer Res. Ther.* **5**, 117–133.

Sinensky, M. (1978). Defective regulation of cholesterol biosynthesis and plasma membrane fluidity in a Chinese hamster ovary cell mutant. *Proc. Natl. Acad. Sci. U.S.A.* **75**, 1247–1249.

Siperstein, M. D. (1970). Regulation of cholesterol biosynthesis in normal and malignant tissues. *Curr. Top. Cell Regul.* **2**, 65–100.

Skehan, P., and Friedman, S. J. (1981). Malignant transformation: In vivo methods and in vitro correlates. *In* "The Transformed Cell" (I. L. Cameron and T. B. Pool, eds.), pp. 8–65. Academic Press, New York.

Skehan, P., and Friedman, S. J. (1982). Deceleratory growth by a rat glial tumor line in culture. *Cancer Res.* **42**, 1636–1640.

Souhami, R. L., Patel, H. M., and Ryman, B. E. (1981). The effect of reticuloendothelial blockade on the blood clearance and tissue distribution of liposomes. *Biochim. Biophys. Acta* **674**, 354–371.

Spitalny, G. L., and North, R. J. (1977). Subversion of host defense mechanisms by malignant tumors: An established tumor as a privileged site for bacterial growth. *J. Exp. Med.* **145**, 1264–1277.

Steel, G. G. (1977). "Growth Kinetics of Tumors." Oxford Univ. Press (Clarendon), London and New York.

Sträuli, P., and Weiss, L. (1977). Cell locomotion and tumor penetration. *Eur. J. Cancer* **13**, 1–12.

Szabo, G. (1974). Dual mechanism for the action of cholesterol on membrane permeability. *Nature (London)* **252**, 47–49.

Tarin, D. (1976). Cellular interactions in neoplasia. *In* "Fundamental Aspects of Metastasis" (L. Weiss, ed.), pp. 151–289. North-Holland Publ., Amsterdam.

Wallach, D. F. H. (1975). "Membrane Molecular Biology of Neoplastic Cells." Elsevier, Amsterdam.

Warren, L. (1972). The biosynthesis and metabolism of amino sugars and amino sugar-containing heterosaccharides. *In* "Glycoproteins, their Composition, Structure and Function" (A. Gottschalk, ed.), Part B, pp. 1097–1126. Elsevier, Amsterdam.

Warren, L., Buck, C. A., and Tuszynski, G. P. (1978). Glycopeptide changes and malignant transformation. A possible role for carbohydrate in malignant behavior. *Biochim. Biophys. Acta* **516**, 97–127.

Weiss, L. (1976a). Biophysical aspects of the metastatic cascade. *In* "Fundamental Aspects of Metastasis" (L. Weiss, ed.), pp. 51–70. North-Holland Publ., Amsterdam.

Weiss, L. (1976b). Cell deformability: Some general considerations. *In* Fundamental Aspects of Metastasis" (L. Weiss, ed.), pp. 305–310. North-Holland Publ., Amsterdam.

Widder, K. J., Senyei, A. E., and Ranney, D. F. (1979). Goals and problems of targeted cancer chemotherapy. *In* "Advances in Pharmacology and Chemotherapy" (R. J. Schnitzer, ed.), pp. 213–271. Academic Press, New York.

Wiley, J. S., and Cooper, R. A. (1975). Inhibition of cation cotransport by cholesterol enrichment of human red cell membranes. *Biochim. Biophys. Acta.* **413**, 425–431.

Wiley, M. H., and Siperstein, M. D. (1976). Control of cholesterol synthesis in normal and malignant cells. *In* "Control Mechanisms in Cancer" (W. E. Criss, T. Ono, and J. R. Sabine, eds.), pp. 343–350. Raven, New York.

Wiltrout, R. H., Brunda, M. J., and Holden, H. T. (1982). Variation in selectivity of tumor cell cytolysis by murine macrophages, macrophage-like cell lines and NK cells. *Int. J. Cancer* **30**, 335–342.

Wood, G. W., and Gillespie, G. Y. (1975). Studies on the role of macrophages in regulation of growth and metastasis of murine chemically induced fibrosarcomas. *Int. J. Cancer* **16**, 1022–1029.

Yageeswaran, G. (1983). Cell surface glycolipids and glycoproteins in malignant transformation. *Adv. Cancer Res.* **38**, 289–350.

11

Intervention of Sodium Flux as a Target for Cancer Chemotherapy

IVAN L. CAMERON

Department of Cellular and Structural Biology
The University of Texas Health Science Center at San Antonio
San Antonio, Texas

I. Introduction	355
II. Ionic Differences between Normal and Tumor Cells	356
III. Common Ionic Events Associated with the Stimulation of Quiescent Cells to Divide	360
IV. Properties and Mode of Action of Amiloride	362
V. Effect of Amiloride on Inhibition of Normal and Tumor Cell Proliferation	363
VI. Search for Other Blockers of Electrolyte Flux as Potential Inhibitors of Cell Proliferation	364
References	372

I. INTRODUCTION

A fundamental premise for rational cancer chemotherapy is that, if a real difference exists between normal and cancer cells, then this difference can be exploited therapeutically to inhibit or kill the cancer cells selectively. Our research has led us to conclude that the intracellular concentration of sodium (Na) is significantly elevated in all of the cancer cells from solid tumors that we have tested. Having established this as a difference between tumor cells and their normal counterpart cells, we are beginning to test approaches to lowering intracellular Na in an attempt to inhibit tumor cell growth selectively. This report

355

constitutes a summary and a progress report of our efforts to establish this new basis and this new approach to cancer chemotherapy.

II. IONIC DIFFERENCES BETWEEN NORMAL AND TUMOR CELLS

As long ago as 1905, Beebe recognized that the ratio of potassium concentration over sodium concentration was less than one in rapidly dividing embryonic and cancer tissue cell populations, but was greater than one in slowly or nondividing normal tissue cell populations of mature animals. This suggests that ion concentrations might mediate mitogenic or oncogenic processes.

In 1971, Cone formalized a unified theory on the basic mechanism of normal mitotic control and oncogenesis. Specifically, he stated that high intracellular concentrations of Na^+ directly influenced the stimulation of mitogenic events. That a high intracellular concentration of Na^+ might be associated with oncogenesis was supported by his later observation of elevated Na^+ level in a mitotically active sarcoma compared to adjacent mitotically inactive normal tissue (Cone, 1974).

The advent of energy-dispersive X-ray microanalysis (EDS) in association with appropriate cell and tissue preparative procedures has allowed several laboratories to test Cone's prediction that the intracellular levels of Na^+ and K^+ are changed in rapidly dividing and neoplastically transformed cells as compared to slowly dividing or nondividing normal cells. This advantage of EDS is that quantitative data are obtained on several elements in a single analysis. Thus, this morphoanalytical technique allows us to determine the subcellular level of Na, Mg, P, S, Cl, K, and sometimes Ca on a millimole per kilogram dry-weight basis. It should be mentioned that EDS, like many other techniques does not tell us about the free or bound state of the elements measured. A summary of our EDS findings from normal and tumor cell types is provided here.

Table I compares cellular data from several tumor versus normal counterparts (Cameron *et al.,* 1980). Table II summarizes our data on the concentrations of Na, Cl, and K in (1) normal, (2) preneoplastic, and (3) overt tumor cells during the course of cell transformation. Since Cone and his co-workers have presented evidence to suggest that elevated intracellular concentrations of Na may be mitogenic, we decided to compare the mean values of elemental concentrations from a variety of cells grouped according to their proliferative capacity. We asked, are elevations in the intracellular concentrations of Na and Cl, as well as changes in other elements, characteristic of tumor cells or of dividing cells in general? Thus, we grouped the elemental concentrations that we have determined from a variety of cell types by EDS into four categories as follows: group I, nontumor cell types—the normal counterparts of tumor cells we have analyzed; group II, tumor cell types; group III, rapidly proliferating cells—normal cells,

TABLE I

Element Concentration Differences between Tumor and Nontumor Cell Types and between Rapidly and Slowly Dividing Cell Types[a,b]

Group number and cell population classification	N	Na	Mg	P	S	Cl	K
Group I, nontumor cell types	11	138	44	495	173	142	339
Group II, tumor cell types	8	451	44	527	215	329	348
p value of difference between groups I and II		<.001	NS[d]	NS	NS	<.001	NS
Group III, rapidly proliferating[c]	9	196	63	626	242	206	549
Group IV, slowly proliferating	21	140	50	515	213	159	389
p value of difference between groups III and IV		<.001	<.005	<.10	NS	<.001	<.001
p value of difference between groups II and III		<.005	<.005	<.10	NS	<.001	<.001

[a]Adapted from Cameron et al., 1980.
[b]Mean concentration (millimoles per kilogram dry weight).
[c]Rapidly dividing cell populations are defined as cell populations with a turnover time of 7 days or less, or with a mitotic index of 1.5% or greater.
[d]NS, not significant.

classified as rapidly dividing because each has a turnover time of 7 days or less (Cameron, 1971) or has a mitotic index of 1.5% or greater; group IV, slowly proliferating—normal cells that fall short of the criteria established for group III. Cell types included in group III were duodenal interphase crypt cells, 2-day-old cardiac myocytes, and 4-day-old cardiac myocytes from the mouse and colonic epithelium and thymus cortex from the rat. Cell types included in group IV were lactating mammary epithelium, thymus medulla, duodenal smooth muscle, pancreatic acinar cells, and normal hepatocytes from tumor-bearing host rats and lactating mammary epithelium, 16-day-old cardiac myocytes, 32-day-old cardiac myocytes, pancreatic acinar cells, bladder transitional epithelium, and hepatocytes from both normal and mice and from those bearing a transplantable hepatoma. A statistical comparison of the mean elemental concentrations from these four groups is given in Table I. In each class of cell populations, the nuclear cytoplasmic ratio of element concentration was determined and was subjected to a statistical analysis of variance (Cameron et al., 1980). No significant pattern of elemental concentration in either the nuclear or cytoplasmic location could be attributed to any of the four classes of cell populations. In the comparisons between tumor cell types and their nontumorous counterparts (group II versus group I in Table I), the Na and Cl concentrations showed large and significant increases for the tumor cell types. No other elements showed concentration differences between these two cell types. When groups III and IV were compared, the rapidly proliferating cell populations showed significant increases in the concentration of Na, Cl, Mg, P, and K compared to the slowly dividing cell types. Although Na and Cl concentrations were seen to be increased in the rapidly dividing populations, the magnitude of the increase was not as great as between the tumor cell types and their nontumorous counterpart cells. When tumor cell types were compared to rapidly dividing normal cell types (group II vs group III), Na and Cl were both in higher concentration in the tumor cell types, while P, Mg, and K were in higher concentration in the rapidly dividing cell types. Thus, an increased intracellular concentration of Na appears to be related to mitogenesis; however, the much higher concentration of Na in cancer cells suggests that an increased Na concentration is more dramatically related to oncogenesis than to mitogenesis. This conclusion could apply equally for the concentration of Cl, but Cl is known to follow the electrochemical gradient established by Na under a variety of conditions, which therefore implicated Na as a causal factor in mitogenesis and/or oncogenesis.

Although the role of the high intracellular levels of Na in transformed cells is not known, it has been speculated that the high level of Na is mitogenic and/or oncogenic. These observations coupled with our findings that 8 weeks of treatment with dimethyl hydrazine (DMH), a carcinogen known to induce colon cancer, induces an irreversible hyperplasia in the colonic epithelium of rats (Heitman et al., 1983), caused us to ask if the intracellular concentration of Na might be used as an indicator or marker of the progression of carcinogenesis in the colon of DMH-treated rats. A study was designed to answer this question. Briefly, it was found that the intracellular concentration of Na does give an accurate indication of neoplastic progression in the DMH-treated rats.

The experiment involved use of male Sprague–Dawley rats, 6 weeks old, which were randomly divided into three groups. One group of rats was given 16 weekly subcutaneous (sc) injections of DMH at a dosage of 9.5 mg/kg body weight, the second group was given 16 weekly injections of the vehicle solution, and the third group was given eight weekly injections of DMH starting 8 weeks after injections in the first two groups were started. Four weeks after the last injection, all rats were killed by decapitation and a portion of their descending colon 1 cm above the rectum was cryofixed for X-ray microanalysis while an adjacent portion of colon was fixed for light microscopy.

Nuclei within the proliferative zone of the colon crypts of adenocarcinoma in the submucosa were analyzed for element content. X-ray pulse–height distribution was measured in the energy range of 0 to 10.22 keV with a resolution of 20 eV/channel. The Tracor Nothern Super M1 (multiple least squares) program was used to deconvolute the spectra and to calculate elemental peak:continuum ratios for each element in each spectrum. Continuum was arbitrarily designated as 4.50 to 5.00 keV, an energy interval in which no characteristic peaks were generated from the samples. For each of the detectable elements of biological relevance,

TABLE II

Effect of DMH Treatment on the Intracellular Element Content of Colonic Columnar
Epithelial Cells and of Colonic Adenocarcinoma Cells[a]

Conditions	N	Content (mmol/kg dry weight)		
		Sodium	Chlorine	Potassium
A, No DMH, vehicle control	7[b]	244±17[c]	182±15	506±25
B, 8 weeks of DMH treatment	5[b]	271±15	173±16	488±16
C, 16 weeks of DMH treatment	5[b]	323±18	204±11	458±33
ANOVA[d]				
F value		4.80	1.46	0.63
p value		<.05	NS	NS
D, adenocarcinoma, 16 weeks of DMH treatment	50[e]	364±14	213±8	344±10

[a]Only cells in the proliferative zone of the crypts were subjected to electron probe X-ray microanalysis. Goblet cells were not analyzed. Only adenocarcinoma cells that had invaded the submucosa
were analyzed. The rats were killed 4 weeks after the last injection of DMH or of the vehicle (control)
to allow recovery from the acute toxic effects of the drug.

[b]N = number of rats analyzed. At least 10 cells were measured to obtain the mean value for each
rat. The rats in condition C showed no evidence of overt adenocarcinomas.

[c]Mean ± SEM.

[d]ANOVA = analysis of variance; NS = not significant.

[e]The mean ± SE in this case was derived from analysis of 50 neoplastic cells from one of two rats
with overt adenocarcinomas.

the two groups of data were subjected to the analysis-of-variance statistical test.
Quantification of data was performed with a series of standards.

The results from the electron probe X-ray microanalysis are given in Table II.
For conditions A–C a one-way analysis of variance (ANOVA) was run for each
of the three elements listed in Table II. The concentrations of Cl and K were not
found to be significantly different among conditions A–C. The concentration of
Na is significantly different as determined by the one-way ANOVA, and a
Student-Newman-Keul's multiple-range test revealed that the values in condition
A (controls) were significantly lower than the values in condition C (16 weeks of
DMH treatment) at $p < .01$. Condition A was not significantly different from
condition B. There is a pattern of increase in intracellular Na from the normal
state to the invasive adenocarcinoma cell state; however, a larger number of

cancerous rats still need to be analyzed before the adenocarcinoma study is complete.

Our earlier studies showed that eight injections of DMH at the same dosage and schedule were sufficient to induce a significant and irreversible hyperplasia in the colon crypts. The data in Table II do not show a significant increase in Na content until the rats were treated with DMH for 16 weeks.

Thus, a significant increase in cell proliferation was found after 8 weeks of carcinogen treatment. A significant increase in intracellular Na was detected after 16 weeks of DMH treatment. The data have more than one interpretation. One interpretation is that the cell proliferation increase occurs before an increase in intracellular Na. This would indicate that this colon carcinogenesis model has at least three sequential steps: (1) increase in cell proliferation, (2) increase in intracellular Na, and (3) overt neoplastic transformation. Another interpretation is that the detection of changes in cell proliferation is a more sensitive marker of the progression of carcinogenesis than is the detection of intracellular Na concentration changes. Improvements in the X-ray microanalysis that we have instituted, along with an increase in the number of rats used in the study, should aid in deciding if the cell proliferation change precedes the change in intracellular Na. Nevertheless, the present data are adequate to conlcude that a significant increase in intracellular Na occurs before overt neoplastic transformation in the DMH colon carcinogenesis model we have used. Thus, information on the intracellular concentration of Na provides a new and useful indicator of the progression of carcinogenesis in the colon of DMH-treated rats. These findings indicate that an elevation in intracellular Na concentration is indeed linked to carcinogenic progression to the neoplastic state.

III. COMMON IONIC EVENTS ASSOCIATED WITH THE STIMULATION OF QUIESCENT CELLS TO DIVIDE

The stimulation of quiescent mammalian cells, the fertilization of sea urchin eggs, and the hormonal stimulation of oocyte maturation division in amphibians appear to have in common (1) an increased flux of Na^+ and K^+, (2) a surge in the intracellular concentration of free Ca^{2+}, and (3) an increase (alkaline surge) in intracellular pH (Leffert and Koch, 1980; Rosengurt and Mendoza, 1980; Epel, 1980; Johnson et al., 1976; LaBadie and Cameron, 1981; Cameron et al., 1983; Lee and Steinhardt, 1981; Moreau et al., 1980; Wasserman et al., 1980). A compendium of much of the research on this topic has been published by Boynton et al. (1982). Thus, there appear to be common ionic events associated with the stimulation of many types of quiescent cells.

Cone's theory of mitogenesis and oncogenesis predicted that the stimulation of cell proliferation would be accompanied by an increase in the ionic activity of Na^+. We have tested this prediction in the fully grown amphibian oocytes that are arrested in first meiotic metaphase. Such arrested oocytes can be removed from the ovaries and can be induced by the hormone progesterone to undergo maturation, which consists of ger .inal vesicle (nuclear envelope) breakdown (GVBD), completion of the meiotic division, and the extrusion of the first polar body. We wanted to determine the normal sequence of ionic events and to define more adequately the involvement of Na^+ and other ions in the resumption of amphibian oocyte meiosis.

Oocytes from the toad *Xenopus laevis* were therefore stimulated by progesterone to complete their first maturation division (GVBD) in 4 to 7 hr. To determine the role of ionic events in this process, we and others have measured the time course of changes in oocyte volume, water content, concentration of Na^+, K^+, Cl, Ca^{2+}, Mg^{2+}, and H^+ and the nuclear magnetic resonance (NMR) spin-lattice relaxation time of oocyte water protons (Cameron *et al.*, 1983). Figure 1 summarizes many of the findings. Initially the oocyte has a relatively low intracellular free Na^+ and free K^+ concentration. The experimental findings are interpreted to indicate that progesterone causes an increase in the

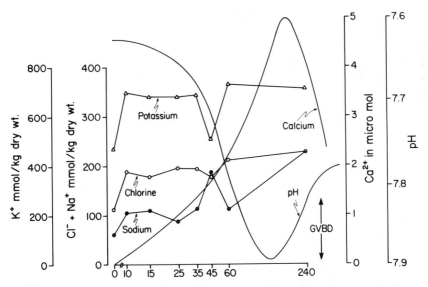

Fig. 1. Summary of changes in the concentration of ions during maturation of *Xenopus* oocytes. Time is plotted on a logarithmic scale. The sodium (●), potassium (△), and cholorine (○) data are taken from an electron probe X-ray microanalysis study (Cameron *et al.*, 1983); the hydrogen ion data are taken from a pH microelectrode study (Lee and Steinhardt, 1981); and the calcium data are taken from a calcium-ion-selective microelectrode study (Moreau *et al.*, 1980). GVBD, first maturation division.

motional freedom of water molecules and increases the permeability of the oocyte membrane to Na^+ and K^+ influx, but also promotes their release from bound intracellular stores. Some of these stores are closely associated with macromolecules. An increasing intracellular free Na^+ may enhance a Na^+ – Ca^{2+} exchange at available Ca^{2+} storage sites, such as mitochondria, cytoplasmic vesicles, calcium-binding macromolecules, pigment granules, or cortical granules. Which of these sites will be tuilized depends on which of the sites contain sufficient Ca^{2+} and on the presence of external Ca^{2+}. Once the free-Ca^{2+} surge reaches a threshold point, maturation events proceed and the free-Ca^{2+} surge by itself is sufficient to allow GVBD. The early Na^+ and/or K^+ surge may stimulate a Na^+,K^+-ATPase pump in the oocyte. It also appears that the surge of free Na^+ at 45 min is temporally coupled to a Na^+–H^+ exchange allowing an alkaline shift. The surge of Na^+ at 45 min in the stimulated oocyte is blocked by amiloride (LaBadie and Cameron, 1981), which may in turn block the Na^+–H^+ exchange. That oocyte maturation can occur in isosmotic sucrose (I. L. Cameron, unpublished observation) indicates that intracellular ionic stores are adequate to permit necessary ionic surges and that ionic influx is not essential for meiotic maturation in this species.

It seems reasonable to assume that pharmacological interference with essential ion flux events might inhibit the stimulation of cell proliferation. Support for this assumption is provided by several recent drug studies. For example, amiloride, a drug that blocks the passive influx of Na^+ into the stimulated cells, interferes with (1) cell proliferation via the stimulation of quiescent mammalian cells (Leffert and Koch, 1980, 1982; Rosengurt and Mendoza, 1980; Pool et al., 1981; Sparks et al., 1982, 1983), (2) the fertilization and activation of development of sea urchin eggs (Johnson et al., 1976; Epel, 1980), and (3) the hormonal stimulation of amphibian oocyte maturation division cycle (LaBadie and Cameron, 1981). Amiloride has also been shown to inhibit the proliferation of tumor cells accompanied by the lowering of the intracellular sodium ion concentration (Sparks et al., 1983).

Before proceeding to a more complete discussion of the effects of amiloride on inhibition of cell proliferation in normal and tumor cells, it seems important to review its properties and its mode of action as an inhibitor of facilitated Na^+ entry and Na^+–H^+ exchange.

IV. PROPERTIES AND MODE OF ACTION OF AMILORIDE

Amiloride was synthesized by Cragoe and his colleagues at the Merck, Sharp and Dohme Research Laboratories in their search for a nonsteroidal diuretic that had modest natriuretic activity along with antikaluretic (potassium-sparing) activity. Amiloride is dealt with in two detailed works (Cuthbert *et al.*, 1978; Benos, 1982). Only a brief review about amiloride is given here. The chemical structure of amiloride is shown in Table III. The chemical name of amiloride is 3,5-diamino-6-chloropyrazinecarboxamide, and its trade name is Midamor (amiloride hydrochloride).

Amiloride has proved to be a clinically important drug for the management of edema, congestive heart failure, and hypertension in humans. Studies in humans have indicated that the minimum dose that will effectively cause potassium retention with increased excretion of water and sodium is 5 mg/day. The drug can be taken orally and has a half-life of about 10 hr in humans. Amiloride is not metabolized in mammals and is eliminated in urine.

Amilordie has also proved to be especially useful as a pharmacological agent for elucidating the molecular mechanisms of Na entry into electrically highly resistant "tight" epithelia and in Na^+-H^+ electroneutral exchange systems such as in the "leaky" epithelium of the renal proximal tubule. It appears to inhibit Na influx in the cells and tissues of a wide variety of animal species. This drug acts rapidly and in a completely reversible fashion when the drug is removed.

As mentioned earlier, amiloride-sensitive Na transport systems are divided into two types. The tight epithelial sodium transport system often shows a 50% inhibition of Na-dependent short-circuit current at a concentration of less than $1 \mu M$. The concentration of amiloride needed to give 50% inhibition in the Na^+-H^+ electroneutral exchange system is higher, about 1 mM.

Amiloride is highly fluorescent and can be excited by ultraviolet light at 215, 288, and 360 nm, and emits at 420 nm. It can be dissolved in water up to 16 mM. Although the primary site of action is thought to be at the plasma membrane, it has also been found within the cell when used in higher concentrations. It is therefore conceivable that amiloride blocks cell proliferation, not by blocking Na^+ flux, but by direct inhibition of protein translation within the cell. Leffert and Koch (1982) have explored this possibility and have found that at a concentration of 4 μM initiation of cellular DNA synthesis is inhibited, but it does not inhibit cell-free protein synthesis at this concentration. Thus, amiloride remains useful as a probe of Na^+ flux independent of its effects on protein synthesis. However, caution is advised in the use of amiloride in attempts to establish a direct causal relationship between Na^+ flux and cell proliferation.

V. EFFECT OF AMILORIDE ON INHIBITION OF NORMAL AND TUMOR CELL PROLIFERATION

Because of amiloride's known ability to block passive influx of Na^+ into cells that are stimulated to divide, we initiated a series of experiments to see if amiloride would inhibit proliferation of normal and transformed cells *in vivo* and *in vitro*. We also wanted to see if a relationship could be established between the intracellular content of Na or other ions and the rate of cell proliferation. Much of this work is reviewed in detail elsewhere (Cameron *et al.*, 1983; Sparks *et al.*, 1982, 1983), and only a brief summary will be given here.

Amiloride, when given in a series of injections, inhibited both DMA/J mammary adenocarcinoma and H6 hepatoma growth *in vivo* in a dose-dependent fashion (Sparks *et al.*, 1983). Amiloride caused no changes in the mean profile diameters of metaphase or interphase H6 hepatoma or DMA/J mammary adenocarcinoma cells, suggesting that the action of amiloride on tumor growth was not due to cell volume changes. It was also found that three injections of amiloride, spaced 8 hr apart and given at a dose of 1.0 μg/g body weight into mice bearing H6 hepatomas, resulted in a significant decrease in the intranuclear content of Na but not the content of Mg, Cl, or K as measured by electron probe X-ray microanalysis in the H6 hepatoma cells. Likewise, the intracellular level of Na, but not the level of Mg, Cl, or K, was decreased in the rapidly dividing duodenal crypt cells in the same amiloride-treated animals. This decrease in Na level in the H6 tumor cells and in rapidly dividing normal duodenal crypt cells was correlated to a significant decrease in the proliferation of both cell types as measured by the tritiated thymidine autoradiography labeling index (Sparks *et al.*, 1983; Cameron and Hunter, 1983). These data show that amiloride both inhibited tumor growth and decreased the proliferation of the tumor cells in the H6 hepatomas and in rapidly dividing duodenal crypt cells, which was correlated with a decreased intranuclear Na content.

It appears from our *in vitro* studies using H6 hepatoma cells that colonies of rapidly proliferating primary liver cells in culture are inhibited from proliferation by concentrations of amiloride (0.1 mM) that have no inhibitory effect on colonies of slowly proliferating primary liver cells in the same culture dish (Sparks *et al.*, 1982). Clearly the rapidly dividing cells are more sensitive to amiloride than are the slowly dividing cells *in vitro*. However, it is yet to be established if rapidly dividing tumor cells are more sensitive to the inhibitory effects of amiloride than are rapidly dividing normal cells. If tumor cells are more sensitive to amiloride, it could establish a basis for selective inhibition of cancer cells.

VI. SEARCH FOR OTHER BLOCKERS OF ELECTROLYTE FLUX AS POTENTIAL INHIBITORS OF CELL PROLIFERATION

Based on the common ionic events associated with stimulation of cells to proliferate, we decided that the progesterone-stimulated amphibian oocyte maturation system might be a good system to screen for drugs that might be expected to interfere with ionic events and therefore with cell proliferation. Drugs that interfere with stimulation of cell proliferation in one cell system presumably will interfere with stimulation of cell proliferation in other cell systems. The drugs tested in our first screening test include amiloride and seven of its analogs, as well as seven substances of other structural types, all of which control electrolyte transport.

The amphibian oocyte assay is designed to give information on (1) the toxicity of each drug, (2) the effective inhibitory dose of each drug, and (3) the ability of the oocytes to recover from the drug's inhibitory effect. It is to be hoped that such findings can be used to predict inhibitory properties of each drug and the drug dosage that might be expected to inhibit cell proliferation when tested on rapidly dividing normal and tumor cell populations in mammals. The code number, chemical structure, molecular weight (MW), and method of dissolution of each drug tested are listed in Table III.

Using the least-squares linear regression slope analysis, the millimolar concentration of each compound required to cause a 50% inhibition of GVBD was calculated. To measure the oocyte's ability to recover from the inhibitory effects of each compound, the oocytes were removed from the compound following 24 hr exposure. The oocytes were then kept for another 24 hr in drug-free Ringer's solution. The percentage GVBD for each concentration of each test compound was again scored, and a least-squares linear regression analysis slope for each compound was again calculated. The ratio of the slope value for the first 24 hr exposure to the compound divided by the slope value after the second 24 hr gives an index of the ability of the oocytes to recover. Table IV summarizes the experimental findings. In the concentration range studied, compounds **1, 6, 9,** and **12** showed no reversibility of inhibition while compounds **7, 8,** and **14** showed high reversibility.

All oocytes were exposed to a solution of 0.3% trypan blue after the end of the reversibility test. The toxicity data at the 1 mM concentration of each test compound showed less than 70% survival for compounds **3, 4, 5, 11, 12,** and **13.** The other compounds showed greater than 80% survival.

That a drug does not demonstrate reversibility may be due either to irreversible cellular alterations not involving cytotoxicity, or to cytotoxic damage. The ability to exclude trypan blue, tested at the end of the drug reversibility test, gives some information on these two possibilities. As an example, compounds **4** and **5** were highly potent inhibitors of GVBD but showed low reversibility and low survival values. Thus, at the specified concentrations these two drugs are cytotoxic, but we cannot be sure whether the irreversibility is due to cytotoxicity or to an irreversible cellular alteration. This is not true for drug **1** where survival is high, but inhibition is highly irreversible. We can therefore say that this drug caused an irreversible cellular alteration with little or no cytotoxicity. The value of such screening data can be evaluated by comparisons to data on other cell

TABLE III

Structure of Some Compounds That Block Electrolyte Flux[a]

Compound number	Structure	References	MW	Method of dissolution[b]	Comments	Reference
1		a	333.785	A	Analog of amiloride	Cragoe et al., 1967
2		a	401.835	B	Analog of amiloride	Cragoe et al., 1967
3		a	409.28	A	Analog of amiloride	Cragoe et al., 1967
4		a	369.815	A	Analog of amiloride	Cragoe et al., 1967

No.	Structure		MW	Category	Description	Reference
5	$CH_3(CH_2)_3$, H_3C, Cl–N=C–CON, NH_2, C–NH_2, N, NH_2	a	299.773	A	Analog of amiloride	Cragoe ett al., 1967
6	(cyclopentyl indanone structure) CH_3, Cl, Cl, $HOOCH_2C$–O	b	357.2	D	Loop diuretic in rats, dogs, and humans	Woltersdorf et al., 1977
7	CH=$C(COCH_3)_2$, Cl, Cl, $HOOCH_2C$–O	c	331.15	C	Loop diuretic in dogs	Bicking et al., 1976
8	$CH_2NH_2 \cdot HCl$, OH, I, $C(CH_3)_3$	d	341.632	B	Loop diuretic in rats, dogs, chimpanzees, and humans	Stokker et al., 1980
9	$COCC_2H_5$, CH_2, Cl, Cl, $HOOC(CH_2)_3$–O	e	331.206	C	Not a diuretic but inhibits electrolyte transport in some other tissues; homolog of ethacrynic acid	Woltersdorf et al., 1978

(continued)

TABLE III (*Continued*)

Compound number	Structure	References	MW	Method of dissolution[b]	Comments	Reference
10	 NaO$_2$C(CH$_2$)$_3$O$_2$ ¼ H$_2$O	f	411.8	E	Not a diuretic but is an inhibitor of Cl$^-$ transport in the brain; homolog of compound **6**	Cragoe et al., 1982
11	 HOOCH$_2$C—O	b	355.22	C	Not a diuretic but an inhibitor of Cl$^-$ transport in some other tissues	Woltersdorf et al., 1977
12	 CH$_3$(CH$_2$)$_2$—N CH$_3$(CH$_2$)$_3$	a	327.825	A	Analog of amiloride	Cragoe et al., 1967

13		g	303.153	C	Loop diuretic; also blocks edema in the brain (ethacrynic acid)	Schultz et al., 1962
14		h	302.147	F	Amiloride	Bicking et al., 1965
15		a	383.244	F	Analog of amiloride called benzamil	Cragoe et al., 1967

[a] Reproduced from Cameron et al., 1984, with permission of Blackwell Scientific Publications Ltd., Oxford.

[b] Method of dissolution: (A) A soluble isethionate salt is formed by suspending a weighed quantity of the solid in water and adding a slight excess of one molecular equivalent of isethionic acid based on the molar quantity of amiloride analog. The mixture is stirred and heated briefly to effect solution, after which it may be diluted to the final volume. If difficulty is encountered in achieving solution, some dimethyl sulfoxide (DMSO) is added. (B) This compound is already in the form of one of its salts, so the procedure outlined in A is followed except that no isethionic acid is added. (C) A soluble sodium salt is formed by suspending a weighed quantity of the compound in water and adding a slight excess of a molecular equivalent of sodium bicarbonate, warming, and stirring. The solution is then diluted to the appropriate volume. Limited heating and storage are required to prevent degradation of this compound. (D) Same as C except that solutions are stable to heating and storage. (E) Same as D except that the compound is already in the form of its sodium salt, and therefore, no sodium bicarbonate is added. (F) Soluble in water.

369

TABLE IV

Screening of Test Compounds for Their Ability to Cause Inhibition of Germinal Vesicle Breakdown (GVBD), Reversibility of the Inhibitory Effect, and Survival of Progesterone-Stimulated Oocytes[a,b]

Test compound number	GVBD during first 24 hr in test compound concentration response Slope 1 (% per mM)	r[c]	Inhibitory concentration (50% mM)	GVBD in second 24 hr after removal of test compound Slope 2 (% per mM)	Reversibility of inhibition ratio[d] slope 1/slope 2	Survival (%) at 1 mM dose[e]
1	−29.82	0.78	1.68	−29.82	1.00	83
2	−30.47	0.87	1.64	−25.46	1.20	84
3	−26.57	0.51	1.88	−29.22	0.91	67
4	−61.38	0.72	0.82	−64.35	0.95	52
5	−38.63	0.47	1.29	−54.23	0.71	43
6	− 3.47	0.99	14.41	− 3.47	1.00	80
7	−12.06	0.91	4.15	− 0.05	262.00	81
8	−18.27	0.96	2.74	− 1.80	10.15	83
9	−21.55	0.95	2.32	−21.55	1.00	86
10	−14.63	0.97	3.42	− 7.85	1.86	81
11	−17.52	0.97	2.85	− 4.81	3.64	67
12	−44.90	0.77	1.11	−44.90	1.00	61
13	−19.31	0.92	2.59	−16.55	1.17	59
14	−14.99	0.90	3.34	− 1.93	7.77	100
15	−19.16	0.87	2.61	− 7.86	2.44	97

[a]Reproduced from Cameron et al., 1984, with permission of Blackwell Scientific Publications Ltd., Oxford.

[b]From 25 to 50 progesterone-stimulated Xenopus oocytes were scored for each of five different concentrations for each test compound. A linear dose–response slope was fitted to the data.

[c]Correlation coefficient.

[d]The higher the ratio value the more reversible the inhibition.

[e]At the end of the 48 hr of treatment, the oocytes were exposed to 0.3% trypan blue; those oocytes that stain were judged to be dead. The progesterone-stimulated or non-progesterone-stimulated controls had 91% or higher survival. The vehicle controls, when diluted to the concentrations used in the analysis, had 85–100% survival.

proliferation systems. Considerable comparative data already exist in the case of amiloride. The comparative data on the effects of amiloride on different cell proliferation systems are summarized in Table V.

Some of the variation in the inhibitory dosage 50% on cell proliferation as shown in Table V is due to differential sensitivity in the different cell systems. This is best illustrated in the case of the primary liver cultures reported by Sparks et al. (1982). Primary liver cultures showed the cell colonies of rapidly proliferating hepatocytes to be far more sensitive to amiloride than were the cell

TABLE V

Effect of Amiloride on Inhibition of Cell Proliferation in Different Cell Systems[a]

System studied	Proliferative parameter measured	Inhibitory concentration (50% ED_{50})	Reference
1. Maturation division cycle of *Xenopus* oocytes stimulated with progesterone	Germinal vesicle	3.34 mM	Cameron *et al.,* 1984
2. Fertilized sea urchin eggs	Activation of development	0.2–0.5 mM	Johnson *et al.,* 1976
3. Serum-stimulated 3T3 cells in culture	%[^{3}H]TdR-Labeled nuclei	0.23 mM	Rozengurt and Mendoza, 1980
4. Fresh peptide-containing media on cultured hepatocytes from rats	% Labeled nuclei	~0.1 mM	Leffert and Koch, 1980
5. 70% hepatectomy in rats *in vivo*	% Labeled nuclei	~0.5 mg/100 g body weight	Leffert and Koch, 1980
6. Primary liver cell cultures from mouse			
a. Loosely aggregated rapidly dividing cells	% Labeled nuclei	~0.1 mM	Sparks *et al.,* 1982
b. Tightly aggregated slowly dividing cells	% Labeled nuclei	>1.0 mM	
7. Cultured H6 hepatoma cells from mouse	% Labeled nuclei and cell number	~0.1 mM	Sparks *et al.,* 1982
8. H6 hepatoma growth *in vivo*[b]	Tumor size and % labeled nuclei	~1 mg/100 g body weight	Sparks *et al.,* 1983

[a]Reproduced from Cameron *et al.,* 1984, with permission of Blackwell Scientific Publications Ltd., Oxford.

[b]Injections were every 6 or 8 hr and ranged from 3 to 17 injections.

colonies of slowly proliferating hepatocytes grown in the same culture dish. Such differential drug sensitivity will allow the selective inhibition of one cell population over another cell population. It will indeed be important to establish if tumor cells are more sensitive to the inhibitory effects of such drugs as compared to nontumor cell types.

We have already begun to test compounds **7** and **8** in our H6 hepatoma mouse system *in vivo* as potentially cytostatic inhibitors of cell proliferation in the dose range that was found to give inhibition of tumor growth in the case of amiloride. Our preliminary data show that compounds **7** and **8** when injected into tumorous mice at 5 mg/100 g body weight every 6 hr for 24 hr also caused tumor regression and inhibition of cell proliferation in host tissues. Unfortunately the 5 mg/100 g body weight dosage caused such marked and significant diuresis that it is not known if the tumor regression was due to a distrubance in the normal equilibrium between cell birth rate and cell death rate in the tumors and/or if the water content of the tumor decreased under the influence of diuretic treatment.

We are encouraged to continue our studies with amiloride as well as other diuretics and blockers of electrolyte flux as drugs that may be useful in the treatment of solid tumors. Further study is now needed to help establish the concentration and the optimal drug usage schedules that will be the safest and the most effective for cancer chemotherapy. Basic studies are also needed to help clarify the mechanism(s) of action of these drugs on cells both *in vitro* and *in vivo*.

The use of such diuretics are inhibitors of tumor growth appears to represent an excitingly new but rational approach to the cancer chemotherapy field.

Acknowledgments

This work was supported by the U.S. National Science Foundation Research Grant PCM 80484. I wish to acknowledge Dr. E. J. Cragoe, Jr., of The Merck, Sharp and Dohme Research Laboratories for the gift of the compounds listed in Table III and for helpful discussion and comments on this project.

REFERENCES

Beebe, S. P. (1905). The chemistry of malignant growths. II. The inorganic constituents of tumors. *Am. J. Physiol.* **12,** 167–172.

Benos, D. J. (1982). Amiloride: A molecular probe of sodium transport in tissues and cells. *Am. J. Physiol.* **242,** 131–145.

Bicking, J. B., Mason, J. W., Woltersdorf, O. W. Jr., Jones, J. H., Kwong, S. F., Robb, C. M. and Cragoe, E. J. Jr. (1965). Pyrazine diuretics. I. *N*-amidino-3-amino-6-halo-pyrazinecarbox-amides. *J. Med. Chem.* **8,** 638.

Bicking, J. B., Robb, C. M., Watson, L. S., and Cragoe, E. J. Jr. (1976). (Vinylaryloxy) acetic acids. A new class of diuretic agents, 1. (Diacylvinylaryloxy)acetic acids. *J. Med. Chem.* **19,** 530.

Boynton, A. L., McKeehan, W. L., and Whitfield, J. F. (1982). "Ions, Cell Proliferation, and Cancer." Academic Press, New York.

Cameron, I. L. (1971). Cell proliferation and renewal in the mammalian body. *In* "Cellular and Molecular Renewal in the Mammalian Body" (I. L. Cameron and J. D. Thrasher, eds.), pp. 45–85. Academic Press, New York.

Cameron, I. L., and Hunter, K. E. (1983). Effect of cancer cachexia and amiloride treatment on the intracellular sodium content in tissue cells. *Cancer Res.* **43,** 1074–1078.

Cameron, I. L., Smith, N. K. R., Pool, T. B., and Sparks, R. L. (1980). Intracellular concentration of sodium and other elements as related to mitogenesis and oncogenesis *in vivo. Cancer Res.* **40,** 1493–1500.

Cameron, I. L., LaBadie, D. R. L., Hunter, K. E., and Hazelwood, C. F. (1983). Changes in water proton relaxation times and in nuclear to cytoplasmic element gradients during meiotic matura-tion of *Xenopus* oocytes. *J. Cell. Physiol.* **116,** 87–92.

Cameron, I. L., Lum, J. B., and Cragoe, E. J., Jr. (1984). Amiloride, and other blockers of electrolytic flux as inhibitors of progesterone stimulated meiotic maturation in *Xenopus* oocytes. *Cell Tissue Kinet.* **17,** 161–169.

Cone, C. D., Jr. (1971). Unified theory on the basic mechanism of normal meiotic control and oncogenesis. *J. Theor. Biol.* **30,** 151–181.

Cone, C. D., Jr. (1974). The role of the surface electrical transmembrane potential in normal and malignant mitogenesis. *Ann. N. Y. Acad. Sci.* **238,** 420–435.

Cragoe, E. J. Jr., Woltersdoft, O. W., Jr., Bicking, J. B., Kwong, S. K., and Jones, J. H. (1967). Pyrazine diuretics. II. *N*-Amidino-3-amino-5-substituted-6-halopyrazinecarboxamides. *J. Med. Chem.* **10,** 66.

Cragoe, E. J., Jr., Gould, N. P., Woltersdorf, O. W., Jr., Bourke, R. S., Nelson, L. R., Simelberg, H. K., Waldman, J. B., Popp, A. J., and Sedransk, N. (1982). Agents for the treatment of brain injury, 1. (Aryloxy)alkanoic acids. *J. Med. Chem.* **25,** 567.

Cuthbert, A. W., Fanelli, G. M., Jr., and Scriabine, A. (1978). "Amiloride and Epithelial Sodium Transport." Urban & Schwarzenberg, Baltimore and Munich.

Epel, D. (1980). Ionic triggers in the fertilization of sea urchin eggs. *Ann. N. Y. Acad. Sci.* **339,** 74–85.

Heitman, D. W., Grubbs, B. G., Heitman, T. O., and Cameron, I. L. (1983). Effects of 1,2-dimethylhydrazine treatment and feeding regimen on rat colonic epithelial cell proliferation. *Cancer Res.* **43,** 1153–1162.

Johnson, J. D., Epel, D., and Paul, M. (1976). Intracellular pH and activation of sea urchin eggs after fertilization. *Nature (London)* **262,** 661–664.

LaBadie, D. R. L., and Cameron, I. L. (1981). Nuclear and cytoplasmic changes in sodium content during progesterone induced maturation of *Xenopus* oocytes: Involvement of net sodium influx. *J. Cell. Biol.* **91,** 2a.

Lee, S. C., and Steinhardt, R. A. (1981). pH changes associated with meiotic maturation in oocytes of *Xenopus laevis. Dev. Biol.* **85,** 358–369.

Leffert, H. L., and Koch, K. S. (1980). Ionic events at the membrane initiate rat liver regeneration. *Ann. N. Y. Acad. Sci.* **339,** 201–215.

Leffert, H. L., and Koch, K. S. (1982). Monovalent cations and the control of hepatocyte proliferation in chemically defined medium. *In* "Ions, Cell Proliferation, and Cancer (A. L. Boynton, W. L. McKeehan, and J. F. Whitfield, eds.), pp. 103–130. Academic Press, New York.

Moreau, M., Villain, J. P., and Guerrier, P. (1980). Free calcium changes associated with hormone action in amphibian oocytes. *Dev. Biol.* **78,** 201–214.

Pool, T. B., Cameron, I. L., Smith, N. K. R., and Sparks, R. L. (1981). Intracellular sodium and growth control: A comparison of normal and transformed cells. *In* "The Transformed Cell" (I. L. Cameron and T. B. Pool, eds.), pp. 398–420. Academic Press, New York.

Rozengurt, E., and Mendoza, S. (1980). Monovalent ion fluxes and the control of cell proliferation in cultured fibroblasts. *Ann. N. Y. Acad. Sci.* **339,** 175–190.

Schultz, E. M., Cragoe, E. J., Jr., Bicking, J. B., Bolhofer, W. A. and Sprague, J. M. (1982). α,β-Unsaturated ketone derivatives of aryloxyacetic acids. A new class of diuretics. *J. Med. Pharm. Chem.* **5,** 660.

Sparks, R. L., Pool, T. B., Smith, N. K. R., and Cameron, I. L. (1982). The role of ions, ion fluxes, and Na^+, K^+-ATPase activity in the control of proliferation, differentiation, and transformation. *In* "Genetic Expression in the Cell Cycle (G. M. Padilla and K. S. McCarty, Sr., eds.), pp. 363–392. Academic Press, New York.

Sparks, R. L., Pool, T. B., Smith, N. K. R., and Cameron, I. L. (1983). Effects of amiloride on tumor growth and intracellular element content of tumor cells *in vivo. Cancer Res.* **43,** 73–77.

Stokker, G. E., Deana, A. A., deSolms, S. J., Schultz, E. M., Smith, R. L., and Cragoe, E. J., Jr.

(1980). 2-(Aminomethyl)phenols, a new class of saluretic agents. 1. Effects of nuclear substitution. *J. Med. Chem.* **23**, 144.

Wasserman, W. J., Pinto, L. H., O'Conner, C. M., and Smith, I. D. (1980). Progesterone induces a rapid increase in Ca of *Xenopus laevis*. *Proc. Natl. Acad. Sci. U.S.A.* **77**, 1534–1536.

Woltersdorf, O. W., Jr., deSolms, S. J., Schultz, E. M., and Cragoe, E. J., Jr. (1977). (Acularyloxy)acetic acid diuretics. I. (2-Alkyl and 2,2-dialkyl-1-oxo-5-indanyl-oxy)acetic acids. *J. Med. Chem.* **20**, 1400.

Woltersdorf, O. W., Jr., deSolms, S. J., and Cragoe, E. J. (1978). Evolution of the (aryloxy)acetic acid diuretics: Diuretic agents. *ACS Symp. Ser.* No. 83, pp. 190–203.

Index

A

4-Acetoxyandrost-4-ene-3,17-dione, 311, 316–317
17α-Acetoxy-6-methylene-4-pregnen-3,20-dione, 295
17α-Acetoxy-6-methylene-4-pregnene-3,20-dione, 293–297
Acetylene, 312
α-Acetylenic ornithine, 104
α-Acetylenic putrescine, 105
N^1-Acetyltransferase, 96–97
Actinomycin D, 175–176
ADCC, see Antibody-dependent cellular cytotoxicity
Adenocarcinoma, 233, see also specific organ, adenocarcinoma of
Adenosine analogs, 342
S-Adenosylmethionine decarboxylase (SAMDC), 95, 98, 100–101, 105, 114
S-Adenosyl-2-methylornithine, 105
S-Adenosyl-3-thio-1,8-diaminooctane, 105
Adiphenine, 335–336
Adrenalectomy, 281–282
Adriamycin, see Doxorubicin
Aflatoxin, 135
AFP, see α-Fetoprotein
10-Allenyl steriod, 313–314
Amiloride, 362–372
γ-Aminobutyraldehyde, 97
Aminoglutethimide, 308, 310–311, 317, 319, 322–323
7α-(4'-Amino)phenylthio-androst-4-ene-3,17-dione, 311
Amino sugars, 334–341
Amphotericin B, 207
Androgens, 270–271, see also 5α-Dihydrotestosterone
action within prostatic cell, 276–278
receptor for, 273–274, 276–277, 283, 287, 322
5α-Androstane-3,17-dione, 311
Androsta-1,4-diene-3,17-dione, 316
Androsta-1,4,6-triene-3,17-dione, 316, 319–320, 323

Anesthetic, local, 335–337
Angiogenic response, 178–179
Antibody, multivalent, 38
Antibody-dependent cellular cytotoxicity (ADCC), 15, 252, 261
Antigen, see specific antigens
Antimetastatic agents
   inhibitors
      of arachidonic acid metabolism, 127–153
      of polyamine biosynthesis, 93–117
   tuftsin, 260
Antimicrobial agents, 207–208, 262–263
Antiproliferative agents, 332
Antisera, 25–27
Antitumor agents
   at cell membrane, 333–345
   conjugated to monoclonal antibodies, 53
   inhibitors
      of arachidonic acid metabolism, 127–153
      of polyamine biosynthesis, 93–117
   liposome-encapsulated, 53
   toxicity of, 214–215
   resistance to, 198–199
   targeting of, 62–63, 199–202, 343–344
   tuftsin, 258–262
   variation in tumor cell response to, 198–199
1-β-D-Arabinofuranosylcytosine (ara-C), 108, 112, 174–176, 185, 342
Ara-C, see 1-β-D-Arabinofuranosylcytosine
Arachidonic acid
   metabolites of, 128–133
      in initiation, 133–135
      in promotion, 135–138
      in tumor cell metastasis, 141–153
   release from cellular stores, 132
Arginase, 95
Aromatase, 285–286, 307–324
   inhibitors of, 308, 310–311
      effect on endocrine-dependent mammary tumors, 323–324
      hormone activity of, 322–323
      suicide, 312–317
      in vitro evaluation of, 317–320
      in vivo evaluation of, 320–322
   mechanism of aromatization by, 309–310

Aromatic amines, 134
Aspirin, 133, 135–137
Astrocytoma, 45
8-Azaguanine, 175

B

BCNU, see 1,3-Bis(2-chloroethyl)-1-
nitrosourea
Benzidine, 135
Benzo[a]pyrene (BP), 134
Biological response modifier, 204
1, 3-Bis(2-chloroethyl)-1-nitrosourea (BCNU),
8–9, 11–12, 109, 112, 174
Bladder
carcinoma of, 56
papilloma of, 5
Bleomycin, 214–215
Blood cells, 202–203
Blood group antigens, 50
Blood vessel, 152, see also Capillaries
Bone marrow, 184, 202–203
transplantation of, 54–57
Bone tumor, 145
BP, see Benzo[a]pyrene
Brain tumor, 102–103, 112
Breast
adenocarcinoma of, 142, 177, 364
carcinoma of, 5, 34, 40–41, 52–53, 56,
109–110, 138, 233, 307–324
tumor-associated antigens, 42
5-Bromodeoxyuridine (BUdR), 342
p-Bromophenacyl bromide, 134–135
BUdR, see 5-Bromodeoxyuridine

C

Calcium
channel blockers, 150–152
intracellular, 361–362
Cancer, see specific organ, cancer of
Capillaries
interaction with liposomes, 186–198
structural classes of, 187–189, 194
in tumors, 193–198
Carboquinone, 177
17β-Carboxy-4-androstene-3-one, 292–294
Carcinoembryonic antigen (CEA), 39, 48
Carcinogen, metabolic activation of,
134–135
Carcinogenesis, 101–102, 109–110
Carcinoma, see specific organ, carcinoma of

Carcinosarcoma, Walker, 142–144
Carrageenan, 260
Castration, 270, 281–282, 289–292
CEA, see Carcinoembryonic antigen
Cell adhesion, 143–144
Cell cycle, 97, 100, 107–108
Cell growth, 97–98, 106–107, 329–333
Cell membrane, 329–346
target for antitumor therapy, 333–345
Cell proliferation, 360–364
inhibitors of, 362–372
Cell recognition, 329–333, 346
Central nervous system tumor, 340–341
Chemotaxis, 256
Chemotherapeutic drugs, see Antitumor agents
Chemotherapy, 165–221
interferon treatment and, 8–9
multiagent, 198–199
Chloride, intracellular, 357–362
Chlorprothixene, 335–336
Cholesterol, 338–340
Choriocarcinoma, 43
Choriocarcinoma trophoblast cells, 317
Colon
adenocarcinoma of, 41
carcinoma of, 5, 40, 110, 233, 241–243,
342, 358–360
Colony-stimulating factor, 16
Colorectal carcinoma, 34, 39–40, 42, 52–53,
61–62
Cyclooxygenase pathway, 128–131
Cyclophosphamide, 111–112
Cytochrome P-450, 309–312, 314

D

Daunoblastin, 175
Daunomycin, 62
Deazauridine, 342
Dehydroacetylenic putrescine, 105
Dehydro-α-difluoromethylornithine, 104
Dehydro-α-difluoromethylputrescine, 105
Dehydro-α-monofluoromethylornithine, 104
Dehydro-α-monofluoromethylputrescine,
105
trans-3-Dehydroornithine, 104
Development, 97–98
DFMO, see α-Difluoromethylornithine
DHT, see 5α-Dihydrotestosterone
α, ω-Diamine, 105
Diamine oxidase, 96–97
Diaminoazobenzene, 101

1, 4-Diaminobutanone, 104
trans-1,4-Diamino-α-butene, 104
1,3-Diamino-2-propanol, 105
Dicyclohexylamine, 105
17β-*N,N*-Diethylcarbamoyl-4-methyl-4-aza-5α-androstan-3-one, 293–294
Diethylnitrosamine, 101–102
Differentiation, 98–100, 257, 279
19,19-Difluoroandrost-4-ene-3,17-dione, 316
10β-Difluoromethylestr-4-ene-3,17-dione, 319
α-Difluoromethylornithine (DFMO), 94, 98–100, 103–104, 108–109
  activity of
    antiproliferative, 106–107
    antitumor, 109–110
    inhibition of metastases, 113–116
  and clinical cancer, 116–117
  in combination chemotherapy, 111–113
  with tuftsin, 260
  monotherapy of experimental tumors with, 110–111
α-Difluoromethylputrescine, 105
5α-Dihydrotestosterone (DHT), 271–297, 322–323
  biosynthesis of, 271–273
  in human prostate, 277–279
  and prostatic cancer
    human studies, 281
    rat studies, 280–281
  receptor for, 273–277
7,12-Dimethylbenz[*a*]anthracene (DMBA), 109–110, 137–138, 323
Dimethyl hydantoin (DMH), 358–360
Dimethylhydrazine, 110, 137
16,16-Dimethyl-17β-hydroxy-4-androsten-3-one, 293
Dimethylnitrosamine acetate, 137
Diphtheria toxin, 56–57, 63
Dipryidamole, 141
Diuretics, 364–372
DMBA, *see* 7,12-Dimethylbenz[*a*]anthracene
DMH, *see* Dimethyl hydantoin
Doxorubicin, 112, 172, 174–177
Drug, *see* Antimicrobial agents; Antitumor agents

E

Eicosatetraynoic acid, 134, 137
Embryogenesis, 98
Endocrine therapy, 308
Endometrial cancer, 309

Epstein–Barr virus, 37–38, 66
Ehrlich ascites tumor cells, 174–177
Estrogens, 282, 285–286
  biosynthesis of, 308–309
  receptor for, 283, 308
Estrogen synthetase, *see* Aromatase
Estrogen therapy, 281–282, 287–292
Estrone, 280
Ethylene, 313

F

Fat emulsions, intravenous, 213
α-Fetoprotein (AFP), 39
Fibroblast, 241–243
Fibronectin, 139–140
Fibrosarcoma, 235, 260–261
Flufenamic acid, 136–137
5-Fluorouracil, 109, 176

G

Galactosyltransferase acceptor, 342–343
Ganglioside GM_1, 342
Gastrointestinal tract
  carcimona of, 41, 50, 53, 58, 61
  tumor-associated antigens, 42
Genitourinary tract, tumor-associated antigens, 43
Germ cell carcinoma, 43
Glioblastoma, 241–243
Glioma, 45, 51–52, 58, 61, 102, 334–337, 341
Glucocorticoid receptor, 283
D-Glucosamine, 334–341
Glycopeptides, growth-inhibitory, 341–342
Glycosyltransferase, 4
Graft-versus-host disease, 54–55, 58
Granulocytopenia, 15–16

H

Haloperidol, 335–336
Hematopoiesis, and interferon, 15–16
Hematoprophyrin, 62–63
Hemostatic mechanism, of metastasis, 140–141
Heparin, 141
Hepatocyte, 184, 370–371
Hepatoma, 39, 102, 112, 175–177, 364, 371–372
trans-Hex-2-en-5-yne-1,4-diamine, 104
5-Hexyne-1,4-diamine, 104

High-fat diet, 138
Hystiocytoma, 47
Hodgkin's disease, 208, 262
Hormone-dependent tumor, 307–309
Host resistance, 203–208
Human
    hybridoma, 37
    monoclonal antibodies, 36–38
Hybridoma, 25, 27
    human cell lines for, 31, 37
    production of, 29–32, 37
    screening of clones of, 32–35
    subcloning of, 35–36
α-Hydrazino-α-methylornithine, 104
α-Hydrazinoornithine, 104
Hydroperoxy fatty acids, 137, 145
4-Hydroxyandrost-4-ene-3,17-dione, 311,
    316–323
3β-Hydroxy-5-ene steroid oxidoreductase/5 →
    4-ene,3-ketosteroid isomerase, 284–285
3α-/3β-Hydroxyoxidoreductase, 285
17β-Hydroxyoxidoreductase, 285
15-Hydroxyprostaglandin dehydrogenase,
    129–131
Hydroxyurea, 108
Hyperthermia, 208–209

I

IFN, see Interferon
Illudin S, 174
Imaging, of tumor, 51–53
9,11-Iminoepoxyprosta-5,13-dienoic acid,
    148–150
Immune system
    activation by interferon, 3
    manipulation with monoclonal antibodies,
        63–64
Immunohistology, 40–51
Immunomodulator, 204–206, 251–263
Immunotoxin, 56–57, 62
Indomethacin, 133–138
Infection, 207–208, 233–234, 253, 262–263
Inflammation, 192–193, 210–211
Initiation, 101, 110, 133–135
Interferon (IFN), 1–16, 109
    activation of natural killer cells, 14–15
    activity of
        anticellular, 8–9
        antitumor, 3
        antiviral, 1–3

administration prior to surgery, 9–10
    cellular changes associated with, 4
    and chemotherapy, 8–9
    clinical trials of, 5–6
    combination interferon treatment, 6–9
    in combination with
        α-difluoromethylornithine, 113–114
    cytolysis of tumor cells by, 12–13
    and hematopoiesis, 15–16
    induction of, 2
    production of, 2–3
    refractory state toward, 5–6
    treatment of lymph node metastases with,
        10–12
    tumors sensitive to, 5
Interferon-α, 2, 6–8, 15–16
Interferon-β, 2, 6, 8, 15–16
Interferon-γ, 2, 5–8, 12–14, 16, 238–239
Interleukin 2, 14–15
Ion fluxes
    blockers of, 362–372
    and cell division, 360–362
    in normal versus tumor cells, 356–360
Ischemia, 192–193

K

Ketamine, 335–336
Kidney
    adenocarcinoma of, 176
    carcinogens in, 135

L

Laminin, 140
Laryngeal papilloma, juvenile, 5
Leiomyosarcoma, 47
Leukemia, 12, 54–57, 102, 110, 200, 203, 336
    acute, 5
    acute lymphocytic, 49
    acute myelocytic, 254
    acute myelogenous, 58
    chronic lymphocytic, 60
    chronic myelocytic, 263
    hairy cell, 208
    L1210, 112–113, 258–259, 261
    monocytic, 208
    myeloid, 34
    non-T-cell acute lymphoblastic, 59
    radiation-induced thymic, 14
    susceptibility to, 50

T-cell, 59, 341
  tumor-associated antigens, 44, 48
Leukocyte, 261–262
Leukokinase, 253
Leukotrienes, 127–153
Lidocaine, 335–337, 341
Lineage marker, reaction with monoclonal
    antibodies, 48–50
Liposome, 53, 63, 165–221, 343
  administered intravenously, 183–198
  and antimicrobial therapy, 207–208
  circulating
    localization on mononuclear phagocytes,
        182–184
    redistribution from mononuclear
        phagocytes, 184–186
  clearance from circulation, 183, 212
  as drug carriers
    clinical trials of, 215–219
    commercial development of, 215–219
    to lymph nodes, 210–212, 221
    therapy of experimental animal tumors,
        172–181
  interaction with capillaries
    in normal tissue, 186–192
    at sites of inflammation and ischemia,
        192–193
    in tumors, 193–198
  lymphokines in, 237–241
  preparation of, 168–172
  properties of, 168–172
  targeting of, 173, 178, 181–198, 219–221
    antibody-mediated, 199–202
    to mononuclear phagocytes, 203–208
    physiochemical, 208–210
    within vascular compartment, 202–203
  toxicity of, 212–215
Lipoxygenase pathway, 129–133, 137, 147
Liver
  cancer of, 101
  retention of liposomes by, 184
  tumor-associated antigens, 43
Lung
  adenocarcinoma of, 176
  carcinoma of, 41
    Lewis, 113–116, 142, 150, 176
    small cell, 34, 107, 111, 233
  tumor-associated antigens, 45
Lymph node, 182
  drug delivery to, 210–212, 221
  liposomes in, 210–212, 221

metastasis of cancer to, treatment with
    interferon, 10–12
Lymphocyte
  immortalization of, 36–38
  monoclonal antibodies to, 49
  transformation with Epstein-Barr virus,
      37–38
Lymphokines, 217
  activation
    of blood monocytes, 237–241
    of macrophages, 231–243
  liposome-encapsulated, 237–241
Lymphoma, 51, 56, 58, 102, 112, 177, 233,
    261
  B-cell, 60–61, 260
  cutaneous T-cell, 59, 62
  malignant, 49
  P-388, 12–13
  tumor-associated antigens, 45
Lymphosarcoma, 177
Lysosomal storage disease, 216

M

Macrophage, 3, 214, 220, 252, 255, 258–262,
    344–345
  activation of, 234, 236
    by lymphokines, 231–243
  infected, 207–208
  interaction with heterogeneous neoplasms,
      233–235
  in treatment of metastases, 235–237
Macrophage-activating factor, 344–345, *see
    also* Lymphokines
Magnesium, intracellular, 357–358, 361–362
Magnetic targeting, 57, 209–210
Major histocompatibility antigens, 50
Mammary epithelial antigens, 40
D-Mannosamine, 341
Mass inhibition, 330–332
Mastocytoma, 336
Meclofenamate, 135
Melanogenesis, 99, 111
Melanoma, 10–12, 40, 50–52, 58, 99, 107,
      111–114, 142, 233–243, 258–261, 340,
    see also Skin cancer
  tumor-associated antigens, 46–47
Melphalan, 177
Metabolic activation, of carcinogens, 134–135
Metastases, 220, 232–234, 345
  and arachidonic acid metabolites, 141–153

chemotherapy for, 178–181
growth of, 332
hemostatic mechanism of, 140–141
inhibition by α-difluoromethylornithine,
  113–116
to lymph nodes, 211–212
macrophages in, 205–206
treatment of, 240–243
  with interferon, 10
  with macrophages, 235–237
Metastatic cascade, 138–141
Methotrexate, 174–177, 201, 209
δ-Methylacetylinic putrescine, 105
Methylazoxymethanol acetate, 137
Methyl CCNU, 176
6-Methylene-4-pregnene-3,20-dione, 296–297
1,1'-[Methylethanediylidene(dinitrilo)]bis
  (3-aminoguanidine), 105
Methylglyoxal bis(guanylhydrazone) (MGBG),
  105, 107–109, 112–113
α-Methylornithine, 104–107
5'-Methylthioadenosine, 95–96
Methylthioadenosine phosphorylase, 95–96
Methyltrienolone, 283
MGBG, see Methylglyoxal
  bis(guanylhydrazone)
Microcapsule, 209–210
Microcirculation, interaction with liposomes,
  186–198
Micrometastases, see Metastases
Microorganisms, see also Infection
  host resistance to, 203–208
Microparticle, 218
Microsphere, 183, 209–210, 218–219
Monoamine oxidase, 96–97
Monoclonal antibody (MAb), 23–66, 217, 344
  binding to solubilized antigens, 34–35
  compared to conventional antisera, 25–27
  conjugated
    to drugs, 53, 62–63
    to magnetic compounds, 57
    to radionuclides, 62–63
    to toxins, 56–57, 62–63
  cross-reactivity of, 26–27
  definition of, 24–25
  diagnostic uses of, 39–53
  in drug targeting, 199–203
  human, 28
  immunohistochemical screening of, 34
  to lymphocyte subsets, 49
  manipulation of immune system with,
    63–64

mixtures of, 65
mouse, 36–37
panels of, 48, 50–51
production of, 27–38
  human, 36–38
  mass, 35–36
  mouse, 28–36
reaction with lineage markers, 48–50
serotherapy with, 57–62
therapeutic uses of, 53–66
  in bone marrow transplants, 54–57
  factors influencing efficiency of, 64–66
  in tumor imaging, 51–53
  viruses in preparations of, 66
  whole-cell binding assay for, 33–34
Monocyte, 254–257
  circulating blood, 183–184, 201–204, 214,
    237
    selective destruction of tumor cells by,
      241–243
α-Monofluoromethylornithine, 104
α-Monofluoromethylputrescine, 105
Mononuclear phagocyte, 182–186, 202–208,
  212–215, 220
Mouse, monoclonal antibodies, 28–37
Multiple myeloma, 5
Muramyl dipeptide, 207, 345
Mutagenicity, 134
Mycoses, 207–208
Myelofibrosis, 254
Myeloma cell, in hybridoma production,
  31–32

N

Nafazatrom, 147–148, 152
Nanoparticle, 104, 183, 218
Naproxen, 137
Nasopharyngeal carcinoma, 5, 263
Natural killer (NK) cell, 3, 14–15, 252, 255,
  261–262, 340
NBMPR, see Nitrobenzylthioinosine
Nebularine, 342
Neocarzinostatin, 175
Neuraminidase, 140
Neuroblastoma, 47, 49, 51, 57, 99
Neuroectodermal tumor, 45
Neurotensin, 255
Nifedipine, 150
Nimodipine, 150–151
Nitrobenzylthioinosine (NBMPR), 342
Nitrofuran, 134–135

Nitrosourea, 109
NK cell, *see* Natural killer cell
Nordihydroguaiaretic acid, 137
Nucleolar antigen, 41

O

ODC, *see* Ornithine decarboxylase
2′,5′-Oligoadenylate synthetase, 4
Oncogene, 167
Oocyte, amphibian, 361–362, 364–370
Ornithine, 95
Ornithine decarboxylase (ODC), 94–95,
 98–105, 110, 136
Osteogenic sarcoma, 47
Ovary
 carcinoma of, 5, 52–53, 233
 tumor-associated antigens, 44

P

Pancarcinoma, 42
Pancarcinoma antigen, 41
Pancreas
 carcinoma of, 39–40
 tumor-associated antigens, 43
Papaverine, 335–336
Papilloma, *see* specific organ, papilloma of
pH, of neoplastic tissue, 209
Phorbol myristate acetate, 143
Phosphodiesterase, 4, 144
Phospholipase, 132
Phosphorus, intracellular, 357–358
Platelet
 interaction with blood vessel walls, 152
 in metastasis, 140–153
cis-Platinum, 109, 112, 174, 176
PMN, *see* Polymorphonuclear leukocyte
 neutrophil
Polyamine oxidase, 96–97
Polyamines
 biosynthesis of, 94–96
  during chemical carcinogenesis, 101–102
  inhibitors of, 93–117
  during viral-induced transformation,
   100–101
 catabolism of, 96–97
 and cell cycle, 97, 100, 107–108
 in cell growth, 97–98, 106–107
 in clinical cancer, 102–103
 in development, 97–98
 and differentiation, 98–100

 in experimental animal tumors, 102
 interconversion of, 96
 structure of, 94
 urinary excretion of, 102
Polycyclic aromatic hydrocarbons, 134
Polyethylene glycol, 32
Polymorphonuclear leukocyte neutrophil
 (PMN), 252, 254–255, 258, 261–262
Potassium, intracellular, 357–362
Preneoplastic lesion, 41, 48
Progesterone, 283
 receptor, 308, 322
Promotion, 101, 110, 135–138
10-(1,2-Propadienyl)estr-4-ene-3,17-dione, 319
10-(2-Propynyl)estr-4-ene-3,17-dione, 313–323
Prostacylin
 agents that alter metabolism of, 147–148
 effect of
  on platelet-induced tumor cell adhesion,
   143–144
  on tumor-cell induced platelet
   aggregation, 142–143
 and tumor cell metastasis, 141–153
Prostacyclin synthase, 129–134, 137, 145
Prostaglandins, 127–153
Prostate
 carcinoma of, 5, 200, 269–297
  androgen-insensitive, 287
  androgen-responsive, 286–287
  hormone sensitivity of, 286–288
  latent lesion, 286
  palliative treatment of, 288–289
 hypertrophy of, 281
 steroid metabolism in, 282–286
 tumor-associated antigens, 44
Protein kinase, 4
Pseudohermaphrodite, human male, 279, 290
Putrescine, *see* Polyamines
Putrescine *N*-acetyltransferase, 96–97

Q

Quadroma, 38

R

Radionuclide, targeting of, 62–63
Receptor
 androgen, 273–277, 283, 287, 322
 androgen-progesterone, 283
 estrogen, 283, 308
 glucocorticoid, 283

progesterone, 308
  steroid, 282–283, 322
  tuftsin, 254–255, 257
5α-Reductase, 269–297
  characterization of, 275
  ˌˌficiency of, 279, 290
  inhibitors of, 285, 291–297
    active-site-directed, 294–297
    competitive reversible, 292–294
  mechanism of action of, 276
Renal cell carcinoma, 5
RES, *see* Reticuloendothelial system
Reticuloendothelial system (RES), 182–183,
    201–204, 212–215, 220–221, 344
  blockade of, 184–186, 197
Reticulosis, 208
Retrovirus, 66
Rheumatoid arthritis, 216
Ricin, 56–57, 63
RNase L, 4
Rous sarcoma virus, 101

S

SAMDC, *see* S-Adenosylmethionine
    decarboxylase
Sarcoma, 174–175, 259–260
  Kaposi's, 5
  tumor-associated antigens, 47–48
Scintigraphy, 51–53
Sendai virus, 32
Serological markers, 39–40
Serotherapy, with monoclonal antibodies,
    57–62
Skin cancer, 101, 234
Sodium flux, 355–372
Spermidine, *see* Polyamines
Spermidine synthase, 95, 105
Spermine, *see* Polyamines
Spermine synthase, 95, 105
Spleen, retention of liposomes by, 184
Splenectomy, 254, 262
Splenosis, 254
Steal hypothesis, 148–150, 152
Steroids
  anabolic, 271–274
  antiinflammatory, 136
  metabolism in prostatic cell, 282–286
  receptor for, 282–283, 322
Stomach, carcinoma of, 39–40, 233
Substance P, 255
Sulfatase, 284

Sulfur, intracellular, 357–358
Surgery, pretreatment with interferon, 9–10

T

Tamoxifen, 322
Targeting
  active, 182
  of drugs, 165–221
  of liposomes, 181–198
  passive, 182
  physical, 182
T cell, 3, 260–261
  removal from bone marrow for transplant,
    54–55
Terpenes, 136
Δ¹-Testololactone, 308, 316–317, 319,
    322–323
Testosterone, 271–297
  elimination from prostate, 281–282
Testosterone propionate, 280, 287
Tetradecanoyl phorbol acetate (TPA),
    135–138
Theophylline, 144–145
Thioridazine, 335–336
Thrombocytopenia, 140–141
Thromboxanes
  biosynthesis of, 127–153
  and tumor cell metastasis, 141–153
Thromboxane synthase, 129–132
  inhibitors of, 148–150
Thyroid cancer, 53
Toxin, targeting of, 62–63
Toyocamycin, 342
TPA, *see* Tetradecanoyl phorbol acetate
Transfer RNA, 4
Transformation, 100–103, 108, 331–334
Transplant of organs, 63–64
Trimethylamine carboxyborane, 174
Tubericidin, 342
Tuftsin, 113, 251–263
  abnormality of, 253–254
  activity of
    antimetastatic, 260
    antimicrobial, 262–263
    antitumor, 258–262
  biology of, 252–258
  chemical synthesis of, 257–258
  chemistry of, 252–258
  deficiency of, 253–254
  generation of, 252–253
  inhibitors of, 258

measurement of, 256
mechanism of action of, 257
purification of, 257–258
receptor for, 254–255, 257
toxicity of, 263
Tuftsin–endocarboxypeptidase, 253
Tumor
  growth kinetics of, 329–333
  imaging of, 51–53
Tumor-associated antigens, 25, 199–202
  detection with monoclonal antibodies, 39–51
Tumor cell
  destruction by activated monocytes,
    241–243
  drug-resistant, 233
  effect of interferon, 12–14
  heterogeneity of, 198–202, 232–233,
    333–334, 343–344, 346
  host resistance to, 203–208
  interaction of
    with blood vessel walls, 152
    with macrophages, 204–206, 233–235
  macrophage-mediated killing of, 344–345
  removal from bone marrow for transplant,
    55–57
Tunicamycin, 337, 340

U

Urinary bladder, carcinogens in, 135

V

Vascular system
  targeting of drugs within, 202–203
  tumor of, 193–198
Vindesine, 112
α-Vinylornithine, 104
α-Vinylputrescine, 105
Virus
  induction of transformation, 100–101
  in monoclonal antibody preparations, 66

W

Warfarin, 141
Wilms' tumor, 47

Y

Yolk sac carcinoma, 44

CELL BIOLOGY: A Series of Monographs

EDITORS

D. E. BUETOW

*Department of Physiology
and Biophysics
University of Illinois
Urbana, Illinois*

I. L. CAMERON

*Department of Anatomy
University of Texas
Health Science Center at San Antonio
San Antonio, Texas*

G. M. PADILLA

*Department of Physiology
Duke University Medical Center
Durham, North Carolina*

A. M. ZIMMERMAN

*Department of Zoology
University of Toronto
Toronto, Ontario, Canada*

G. M. Padilla, G. L. Whitson, and I. L. Cameron (editors). THE CELL CYCLE: Gene–Enzyme Interactions, 1969

A. M. Zimmerman (editor). HIGH PRESSURE EFFECTS ON CELLULAR PROCESSES, 1970

I. L. Cameron and J. D. Thrasher (editors). CELLULAR AND MOLECULAR RENEWAL IN THE MAMMALIAN BODY, 1971

I. L. Cameron, G. M. Padilla, and A. M. Zimmerman (editors). DEVELOPMENTAL ASPECTS OF THE CELL CYCLE, 1971

P. F. Smith. THE BIOLOGY OF MYCOPLASMAS, 1971

Gary L. Whitson (editor). CONCEPTS IN RADIATION CELL BIOLOGY, 1972

Donald L. Hill. THE BIOCHEMISTRY AND PHYSIOLOGY OF *TETRAHYMENA*, 1972

Kwang W. Jeon (editor). THE BIOLOGY OF AMOEBA, 1973

Dean F. Martin and George M. Padilla (editors). MARINE PHARMACOGNOSY: Action of Marine Biotoxins at the Cellular Level, 1973

Joseph A. Erwin (editor). LIPIDS AND BIOMEMBRANES OF EUKARYOTIC MICROORGANISMS, 1973

A. M. Zimmerman, G. M. Padilla, and I. L. Cameron (editors). DRUGS AND THE CELL CYCLE, 1973

Stuart Coward (editor). DEVELOPMENTAL REGULATION: Aspects of Cell Differentiation, 1973

I. L. Cameron and J. R. Jeter, Jr. (editors). ACIDIC PROTEINS OF THE NUCLEUS, 1974

Govindjee (editor). BIOENERGETICS OF PHOTOSYNTHESIS, 1975

James R. Jeter, Jr., Ivan L. Cameron, George M. Padilla, and Arthur M. Zimmerman (editors). CELL CYCLE REGULATION, 1978

Gary L. Whitson (editor). NUCLEAR–CYTOPLASMIC INTERACTIONS IN THE CELL CYCLE, 1980

Danton H. O'Day and Paul A. Horgen (editors). SEXUAL INTERACTIONS IN EUKARYOTIC MICROBES, 1981

Ivan L. Cameron and Thomas B. Pool (editors). THE TRANSFORMED CELL, 1981

Arthur M. Zimmerman and Arthur Forer (editors). MITOSIS/CYTOKINESIS, 1981

Ian R. Brown (editor). MOLECULAR APPROACHES TO NEUROBIOLOGY, 1982

Henry C. Aldrich and John W. Daniel (editors). CELL BIOLOGY OF *PHYSARUM* and *DIDYMIUM*, Volume I: Organisms, Nucleus, and Cell Cycle, 1982; Volume II: Differentiation, Metabolism, and Methodology, 1982

John A. Heddle (editor). MUTAGENICITY: New Horizons in Genetic Toxicology, 1982

Potu N. Rao, Robert T. Johnson, and Karl Sperling (editors). PREMATURE CHROMOSOME CONDENSATION: Application in Basic, Clinical, and Mutation Research, 1982

George M. Padilla and Kenneth S. McCarty, Sr. (editors). GENETIC EXPRESSION IN THE CELL CYCLE, 1982

David S. McDevitt (editor). CELL BIOLOGY OF THE EYE, 1982

P. Michael Conn (editor). CELLULAR REGULATION OF SECRETION AND RELEASE, 1982

Govindjee (editor). PHOTOSYNTHESIS, Volume I: Energy Conversion by Plants and Bacteria, 1982; Volume II: Development, Carbon Metabolism, and Plant Productivity, 1982

John Morrow. EUKARYOTIC CELL GENETICS, 1983

John F. Hartmann (editor). MECHANISM AND CONTROL OF ANIMAL FERTILIZATION, 1983

Gary S. Stein and Janet L. Stein (editors). RECOMBINANT DNA AND CELL PROLIFERATION, 1984

Prasad S. Sunkara (editor). NOVEL APPROACHES TO CANCER CHEMOTHERAPY, 1984

In preparation

B. G. Atkinson and D. B. Walden (editors). CHANGES IN EUKARYOTIC GENE EXPRESSION IN RESPONSE TO ENVIRONMENTAL STRESS, 1984